STEROIDS AND THE NERVOUS SYSTEM

ANNALS OF THE NEW YORK ACADEMY OF SCIENCES

Volume 1007

STEROIDS AND THE NERVOUS SYSTEM

Edited by GianCarlo Panzica and Roberto C. Melcangi

The New York Academy of Sciences
New York, New York
2003

Library of Congress Cataloging-in-Publication Data has been applied for.

International Meeting on Steroids and the Nervous System (2nd : 2003 : Turin, Italy)
Steroids and the nervous system / edited by GianCarlo Panzica and Roberto C. Melcangi.
p. ; cm. — (Annals of the New York Academy of Sciences ; v. 1007)
Proceedings of the 2nd International Meeting on Steroids and the Nervous System, Feb. 22–26, 2003, Turin, Italy. Includes bibliographical references and index.
ISBN 1-57331-486-2 (cloth : alk. paper) — ISBN 1-57331-487-0 (pbk. : alk. paper) 1. Neurohormones—Physiological effect—Congresses. 2. Steroid hormones—Physiological effect—Congresses. 3. Paracrine mechanisms—Congresses. 4. Autocrine mechanisms—Congresses.)
[DNLM: 1. Steroids—physiology—Congresses. 2. Nervous System Diseases—drug therapy—Congresses. 3. Nervous System Physiology—Congresses. 4. Receptors, Steroid—physiology—Congresses. 5. Steroids—therapeutic use—Congresses. WK 150 I62 2003] I. Panzica, GianCarlo. II. Melcangi, Roberto C. III. Title. IV. Series.
Q11.N5 vol. 1007
[QP356.4]
500 s—dc22
[612

2003027267

GYAT / PCP

Printed in the United States of America

ISBN 1-57331-486-2 (cloth)
ISBN 1-57331-487-0 (paper)
ISSN 0077-8923

ANNALS OF THE NEW YORK ACADEMY OF SCIENCES

Volume 1007
December 2003

STEROIDS AND THE NERVOUS SYSTEM

Editors
GIANCARLO PANZICA AND ROBERTO C. MELCANGI

International Scientific Committee
JACQUES BALTHAZART (*Liège, Belgium*)
LUIS MIGUEL GARCIA-SEGURA (*Madrid, Spain*)
ALLAN HERBISON (*Cambridge, UK*)
PHYLLIS WISE (*Davis, California, USA*)

This volume is the result of the **2nd International Meeting on Steroids and Nervous System**, sponsored by Fondazione Cavalieri Ottolenghi, Università degli Studi di Torino, Università degli Studi di Milano, National Science Foundation, International Brain Research Organization (IBRO), Regione Piemonte, Provincia di Torino, Comune di Torino, and held on February 22–26, 2003 in Turin, Italy.

CONTENTS

Part II. Pathological Correlations and New Tools in Therapeutical Approaches

Part III. Steroid Regulation of Reproduction

Part IV. Behavioral Effects

Part V. Glial Cells as a Target for Steroids

Part VI. Glucocorticoids and Mineralocorticoids: Synthesis, Mechanism of Action, and Effects

Financial assistance was received from:

- SERONO FOUNDATION

Introduction

Steroids and the Nervous System

ROBERTO C. MELCANGI[a] AND GIANCARLO PANZICA[b]

[a]*Department of Endocrinology and Center of Excellence on Neurodegenerative Diseases, 20133 Milan, Italy*

[b]*Department of Anatomy, Pharmacology, and Forensic Medicine, Laboratory of Neuroendocrinology, 10126 Torino, Italy*

The classical interpretation of the role of steroids in regulating the nervous system is based on their effects mediated through specific intracellular receptors. Moreover, steroids are generally considered as hormones produced by peripheral glands (e.g., adrenal, gonads) that have the central and peripheral nervous system as one of their multiple targets. This relatively simple view of the effects of steroids on neural circuits has been complicated by the discovery of membrane-bound receptors, by the synthesis and metabolism of steroids within the nervous system, and by the finding that glial cells are also important targets for steroids.

This increasing complexity in the relationships between steroids and the nervous system needs a forum in which current information is continually reviewed in light of ongoing new discoveries. This forum, the International Symposium on Steroids and the Nervous System, which both recapitulates information available thus far and identifies emerging topics, is held every two years in Torino, Italy.

The papers collected in this volume of the *Annals* comprise the invited lectures and selected oral communications presented during the 2nd International Symposium on Steroids and the Nervous System held in February 2003; the first meeting was published as a special issue of *Brain Research Reviews.*[1]

Several topics have been discussed during this meeting. For instance, the emerging importance of the **non-classical mechanisms of action of steroids** has been taken into consideration in a variety of experimental models. Estrogen rapidly alters the excitability of hypothalamic neurons that are involved in regulating numerous homeostatic functions including reproduction, stress responses, feeding, and motivated behaviors (Kelly *et al.*). Moreover, estrogens play an important role during midbrain development, promoting the differentiation and survival as well as physiological performance of midbrain dopaminergic cells (Beyer *et al.*). Non-genomic gonadal steroid feedback to neurosecretory hypothalamic neurons is mediated via neurosteroids acting as allosteric modulators of the postsynaptic $GABA_A$ receptors (Brussaard *et al.*). Neurosteroids in the ventral tegmental area (VTA) mediate lordo-

Address for correspondence: GianCarlo Panzica, Department of Anatomy, Pharmacology, and Forensic Medicine, Laboratory of Neuroendocrinology, corso M. D'Azeglio 52, 10126 Torino, Italy.

giancarlo.panzica@unito.it

Ann. N.Y. Acad. Sci. 1007: 1–5 (2003). © 2003 New York Academy of Sciences.
doi: 10.1196/annals.1286.040

sis of rodents (Frye *et al.*). The crucial role of neurosteroids as neurodegenerative and neuroprotective agents has been also upheld in a retinal excitotoxic paradigm (Guarneri *et al.*). In a murine cholinergic cell line from the basal forebrain, Marin *et al.* present evidence indicating that an estrogen receptor associated with the plasma membrane participates in estrogen-dependent reduction of induced neuronal death.

The importance of steroids is also highlighted by their **correlations with pathological status**. Menstrual cycle–linked disorders are caused by the action of endogenously produced GABA-acting steroids (Bäckström *et al.*). Estrogens are involved in the regulation of mood and cognitive functions and are probably implicated in the neuropathology of psychiatric disorders such as depression (Östlund *et al.*). Clinical investigations in humans produce evidence for an involvement of neuroactive steroids in conditions such as fatigue during pregnancy, premenstrual syndrome, postpartum depression, catamenial epilepsy and depressive disorders (Stoffel-Wagner).

Steroids have potential utilization as **therapeutic strategies** for neurodegenerative and neuropsychiatric disorders. Estrogen replacement therapy has shown potential both as a preventative measure and treatment for disorders such as Alzheimer's disease (Cutter *et al.*). Estrogen protects against ischemic injury in both the focal and global ischemia models by acting primarily via classical nuclear receptors (Merchenthaler *et al.*). Finally, estrogens could prove to be useful therapies in preventing brain damage from strokes (Yang *et al.*)

Steroids also exert a key role in the **neuroendocrine control of reproduction**. Discrepant effects of estrogens on gonadotropin-releasing hormone (GnRH) neurons were observed. GnRH biosynthesis is inhibited while GnRH secretion can be either stimulated, or unaffected or reduced, suggesting that the regulatory role of sex steroids (including estradiol) is very complex since it involves direct and indirect effects through genomic and/or non-genomic mechanisms (Matagne *et al.*). Etgen describes brain insulin-like growth factor-I (IGF-I) receptors as obligatory co-mediators of hormonal regulation of hypothalamic neuroendocrine function, as, for instance, the cooperation with estradiol in facilitating lordosis behavior. Glial cells are also important players in these regulations; in fact, steroid hormones and growth factors act in an integrated manner at the level of hypothalamic astrocytes to control GnRH neurons (Galbiati *et al.*). Estradiol targets multiple mechanisms (potassium currents, excitability) to alter GnRH neuron firing patterns, and the balance of stimulatory and inhibitory actions determines whether the integrated response is to increase or to decrease release (Moenter *et al.*). Outside the regulation of the GnRH system, the presence or absence of gonadal hormones during puberty is a major factor in the ability of steroids to activate reproductive behaviors in animal models (Sisk *et al.*). Finally, in the adult, steroid access to the brain could be modulated by photoperiodism, thus increasing the availability of steroids to the nervous structures during long days (Thiery and Malpaux).

Most **sex differences in brain functions** are attributed to sex differences in the effects of gonadal secretions. A variety of experimental models have been presented at the meeting. Arnold *et al.* review evidence that genetic sex of brain cells influences their sexual phenotype, and they critically discuss the relative advantages of mouse models in which the genetic sex of brain cells is independent of the gonadal type (testes vs. ovaries). Female ArKO mice, which cannot aromatize androgen to estrogen, showed reduced levels of lordosis behavior following adult treatment with estradiol and progesterone, suggesting therefore that estradiol is required for the development of neural mechanisms controlling this behavior in female mice. Thus, the classical view of sexual differentiation, that is, that the female brain develops in the absence of any hormonal secretion, needs to be re-examined (Bakker *et al.*). Androgens have dramatic influences on the development of the mammalian brain. As a consequence of these effects, levels of androgens during early life relate to sex-typical behavior across the lifespan (Hines). Lesion studies have identified a small group of large cells referred to as the magnocellular medial preoptic nucleus (MPN mag) whose integrity is required for normal mating behavior of rodents. The data, summarized by Swann *et al.*, indicate that the MPN mag is a sexually differentiated nucleus in a large steroid-responsive network that relays pheromonal signals from the sensory systems to the motor areas to affect behavior. Noradrenergic projections to the avian song system are involved in the latency to produce song and the ability to discriminate conspecific from heterospecific song. In addition, testosterone can regulate catecholamine steady-state levels and turnover in these regions. Thus the song control circuit may be modulated in significant ways via the androgen regulation of forebrain catecholamine systems (Ball *et al.*).

Steroid hormone receptors are the central component of the cellular machinery sensitive to steroid hormones. Blaustein reviews in his paper the effects of various neurotransmitters to upregulate or downregulate steroid hormone receptors in some neurons. This, in turn, presumably confers greater or decreased sensitivity to the particular factors that can activate the particular steroid receptor in those particular neurons. Therefore, steroid hormones are only one class of factors that can regulate and activate steroid hormone receptors.

Male gonadal hormones play a key role in inhibiting the **behavioral responses** to repeated nociceptive stimulation. Aromatase-immunoreactive neurons and aromatase activity are present in the dorsal horns of the spinal cord, suggesting that the control of pain thresholds may be mediated by estrogens produced at the spinal level and activating spinal nuclear estrogen receptors (Evrard and Balthazart). This suggests that the lower incidence of chronic pain syndromes in males could be due to the presence of these hormones (Aloisi *et al.*).

One important topic that has recently emerged in the study of the effects of steroids in the nervous system is that the effects are not directed only to neuronal compartments but that also **glial cells** exert a primary role in mediating such effects. The relationship between astrocytic and neuronal morphology during development is distinct for different brain regions and provides a fundamental basis for region-specific sexual differentiation. The functional significance of estradiol-induced differentiation of astrocytes and the cross-talk of these cells with neurons includes permanent changes in synaptic patterning and control of adult reproductive behaviors (McCarthy *et al.*). In the adult brain, reactive astrocytes, at injured sites, may express aromatase. This expression and the consecutive increase in the local production of estradiol in the brain is neuroprotective and may be an endogenous neural response to reduce the extent of neurodegenerative damage (Azcoitia *et al.*). Glia-originated neurotrophic factors and estradiol interact to control axogenic growth in hypothalamic neurons (Carrer *et al.*). Progesterone shows regenerative and myelinating properties following injury of the peripheral and central nervous system. These effects may be supportive of neuronal recuperation, as shown for several neuronal functional parameters that were normalized by progesterone treatment of spinal cord–injured animals (De Nicola *et al.*). Changes in gene expression caused by progesterone are being examined to identify additional factors that may control myelin formation in the peripheral nervous system (Rodriguez-Waitkus *et al.*). Neuroactive metabolites of progesterone, dihydroprogesterone and tetrahydroprogesterone, modify glial tube organization and decrease immunoreactivity for glia-associated proteins in the astrocytes of the subependymal layer (SEL). Moreover they reduce the proliferative activity within the SEL (Giachino *et al.*). The mRNA for Ndrg2, a member of the N-myc downregulated gene (NDRG) family with putative roles in neural differentiation, synapse formation, and axon survival, was localized to GFAP-positive astrocytes or radial glia in cerebral cortex and hippocampus. Its expression is under positive regulation by glucocorticoids *in vivo*. Since antidepressants may alleviate symptoms of depression by reversing the effects of glucocorticoids, these data suggest that further study of Ndrg2 regulation and function in glia could contribute to understanding of the pathogenesis and treatment of depression (Nichols). Multiple sclerosis (MS) occurs more commonly in females than males. However, the mechanisms resulting in gender differences in MS are unknown. Drew *et al.* review the role of sex steroids in modulating microglial cell function in relationship to MS.

Finally, several papers are dedicated to the **role of corticosteroids in regulating the nervous system**. Dysregulations and dysfunctions of corticosteroids and their receptors have been implicated in the pathogenesis of stress-related disorders, in particular in depression. Urani and Gass have analyzed several strains of mice with targeted mutations of corticosteroid receptors. Behavioral analyses have indicated that corticosteroid receptor mutant mice show alterations in their emotional behavior. The corticosteroid receptor–regulated target genes to be identified in these models may code for proteins that could represent new drug targets for the treatment of affective disorders. Compensating for the consequences of impaired corticosteroid receptor signaling is a novel strategy to discover better antidepressants (Holsboer). The amount of steroids available to activate receptors is not only dependent on the circulating levels, but also on pre-receptor metabolism of glucocorticoids occurring intracellularly. This metabolism is carried out by the enzymes 11β-hydroxysteroid dehydrogenases (11β-HSDs). There are two distinct isozymes: 11β-HSD type 2 inactivates glucocorticoids, while 11β-HSD type 1 elevates intracellular glucocorticoid levels. Holmes *et al.* highlight the important and very different roles that these two enzymes play in the brain, outlining recent results obtained from studying mice with a targeted gene deletion. Relationships among stress and serotonin are of particular interest. Activation of serotonin-1A receptors is attenuated in chronically stressed rats. Potentially, treatment with corticosteroid receptor antagonists can normalize the attenuated transmission after chronic stress (Joëls *et al.*).

The organization of this conference would have been impossible without the financial help of several granting agencies and local administrations. In particular, we would like to acknowledge the financial support of the University of Torino, University of Milano, and the Neuroscience Foundation Cavalieri-Ottolenghi (Torino). The Serono Foundation and IBRO generously supported travel grants and fellowships for young researchers attending the meeting. Finally, we have to thank the National Science Foundation (NSF) which, through a specific grant, allowed numerous U.S. students to participate in the meeting. With the help of the NSF we have also organized a special session dedicated to explaining to young researchers worldwide opportunities for funded research.

Moreover, we have to thank here the colleagues that helped us in reviewing the manuscripts collected for this volume of the *Annals:* A. Arnold (USA), T. Bäckström (Sweden), J. Bakker (Belgium), G.F. Ball (USA), J. Balthazart (Belgium), D. Belelli (UK), C. Beyer (Germany), W.J. Cutter (UK), A. Etgen (USA), C.F. Frye (USA), L.M. Garcia-Segura (Spain), A. Herbison (New Zealand), Y. Hurd (Sweden), M.J. Kelly (USA), M. McCarthy (USA), G. Mensah-Nyagan (France), F. Piva (Italy), M.A. Riva (Italy), J.M. Swann (USA), and P. Wise (USA).

Finally, we also would like to thank the editorial staff of the *Annals* of the New York Academy of Sciences for their professionalism and efficiency in seeing this volume through the press.

Information about this series of conferences is available at a dedicated website, <http://www.dafml.unito.it/anatomy/panzica/neurosteroids/index.html>, where the extended abstracts of the meeting,[2,3] as well as the program and list of participants are also available for downloading.

REFERENCES

1. Melcangi, R.C. & G.C. Panzica, Eds. 2001. Neuroactive Steroids for the Third Millennium. Brain Res. Rev. Vol. **37** (special issue).
2. Panzica, G.C. & S. Gotti, Eds. 2001. Trabajos del Instituto Cajal, Vol. LXXVIII, supplementum, pp. 1–186.
3. Panzica, G.C. & S. Gotti, Eds. 2003. Trabajos del Instituto Cajal, Vol. LXXIX, supplementum, pp. 1–287.

Estrogen Modulation of G-Protein–Coupled Receptor Activation of Potassium Channels in the Central Nervous System

MARTIN J. KELLY, JIAN QIU, AND OLINE K. RØNNEKLEIV

Department of Physiology & Pharmacology, Oregon Health & Science University, Portland, Oregon 97239, USA

ABSTRACT: Estrogen rapidly alters the excitability of hypothalamic neurons that are involved in regulating numerous homeostatic functions including reproduction, stress responses, feeding, and motivated behaviors. Neurosecretory neurons, such as gonadotropin-releasing hormone (GnRH) and dopamine neurons, and local circuitry neurons, such as pro-opiomelanocortin (POMC) and γ-aminobutyric acid (GABA) neurons, are among those involved. We have identified membrane-initiated, rapid-signaling pathways through which 17β-estradiol (E_2) alters synaptic responses in these neurons using whole-cell patch recording in hypothalamic slices from ovariectomized female guinea pigs. E_2 rapidly uncouples μ-opioid and $GABA_B$ receptors from G-protein–gated inwardly rectifying K^+ (GIRK) channels in POMC and dopamine neurons as manifested by a reduction in the potency of μ-opioid and $GABA_B$ receptor agonists to activate these channels. These effects are mimicked by the selective E_2 receptor modulators raloxifene and 4OH-tamoxifen, the membrane impermeable E_2-bovine serum albumin (BSA), but not by 17α-estradiol. Furthermore, the anti-estrogen ICI 182,780 antagonizes these rapid effects of E_2. Inhibitors of phospholipase C, protein kinase C, and protein kinase A block the actions of E_2, indicating that the E_2 receptor is G-protein–coupled to activation of this cascade. Conversely, estrogen enhances the efficacy of α_1-adrenergic receptor agonists to inhibit apamin-sensitive small-conductance, Ca^{2+}-activated K^+ (SK) currents in preoptic GABAergic neurons; it does so in both a rapid and sustained fashion. Finally, we observed a direct, steroid-induced hyperpolarization of GnRH neurons. These findings indicate that E_2 can modulate K^+ channels in hypothalamic (POMC, dopamine, GABA, GnRH) neurons that are involved in regulating numerous homeostatic functions through multiple intracellular signaling pathways.

KEYWORDS: dopamine; norepinephrine; POMC; GABA; K^+ channel; phospholipase C; protein kinase C; protein kinase A

Address for correspondence: Martin J. Kelly, Ph.D., Department of Physiology & Pharmacology, Oregon Health & Science University, Portland, Oregon 97239. Voice: 503-494-5833; fax: 503-494-4352.
kellym@ohsu.edu

Ann. N.Y. Acad. Sci. 1007: 6–16 (2003).
doi: 10.1196/annals.1286.001

INTRODUCTION

It is becoming increasingly evident that the gonadal steroid hormone estrogen (17β-estradiol, E_2) imparts a multifaceted influence over synaptic transmission in the mammalian central nervous system. Not only can E_2 alter synaptic responses via genomic mechanisms, but a wealth of information indicates that the steroid can also modulate cell-to-cell communication much more rapidly (for review see Ref. 1). These synaptic alterations are brought about via changes in the cellular responsiveness to the activation of various receptor systems (both G protein-coupled and ionotropic) to their respective first messengers. For example, E_2 can modulate the cellular responsiveness to ionotropic glutamate (both *N*-methyl-D-aspartate (NMDA) and non-NMDA) receptor activation.[2–4] In addition, it can alter the linkage of G protein-coupled receptor systems such as opioid (both μ and κ), γ-aminobutyric acid $(GABA)_B$ and dopamine D_2 receptors to their respective effector systems.[5-9] Furthermore, it now appears that the steroid can function as a first messenger by activating an estrogen receptor that couples directly to K^+ and Ca^{2+} channels by way of a pertussis toxin-sensitive G protein.[10,11] These fundamentally distinct signaling pathways give rise to a coordinated regulation by estrogen of complex physiological processes such as reproduction, stress responses, feeding and cognition. We will focus on the estrogenic modulation of K^+ channel activity in hypothalamic neurons involved in many of these physiological processes.

ESTROGEN MODULATION OF G-PROTEIN–COUPLED INWARDLY RECTIFYING K^+ (GIRK) CHANNELS

One of the principal actions of estrogen is to regulate the output of gonadotropin-releasing hormone (GnRH) from the mediobasal hypothalamus and hence the reproductive cycle. Although we demonstrated direct actions of estrogen to inhibit GnRH neuronal activity more than 15 years ago,[10,12] it has been only recently that estrogen receptors have been demonstrated in GnRH neurons.[13–15] In fact, estrogen responsiveness has been conferred to neurons closely juxtaposed to the GnRH cells.[16–21] Indeed, hypothalamic POMC and GABAergic neurons, both of which provide a prominent synaptic input onto GnRH neurons, express estrogen receptors and concentrate radiolabeled estradiol.[22–24] Opioid peptides and GABAergic ligands both serve to inhibit GnRH output[25–27] and thus luteinizing hormone (LH) release[25,28–30] from the anterior pituitary. While presynaptic interactions between opioid and GABAergic nerve terminals may help regulate this process,[31,32] it is clear that both μ-opioid and $GABA_B$ receptor agonists affect a direct, postsynaptic inhibition of GnRH neurons.[10]

Studies using *in vitro* slice preparation have revealed that μ-opioid receptor-mediated inhibition of GnRH neurons arises from the activation of a member of the G-protein–gated, inwardly rectifying K^+ channel subfamily known as GIRK1–4 (Kir3.1–3.4).[10,33,34] This elicits a robust hyperpolarization in current clamp, or outward current in voltage clamp. POMC and dopamine neurons are exquisitely responsive to μ-opioid receptor activation.[35,36] Acute E_2 exposure for no longer than 20 min results in a decreased potency of μ-opioid and $GABA_B$ receptor agonists to activate GIRKs in POMC and dopamine neurons.[37,38] The negative modulatory effect of estrogen (i.e., reduced potency of μ-opioid receptor and $GABA_B$ agonists in POMC and dopamine neurons) persists at least 24 h following systemic steroid administration.[6]

μ-Opioid and $GABA_B$ receptors serve as autoreceptors in their respective POMC and hypothalamic GABAergic neurons.[35,39,40] The fact that estrogen uncouples these autoreceptors from their GIRK channel implies that the steroid decreases the auto-inhibition of these cells, thereby increasing the release of these inhibitory neurotransmitters. Indeed, estrogen rapidly increases extracellular GABA concentrations in the preoptic area as measured by push/pull perfusion and microdialysis.[41,42] Coupled with the attenuated $GABA_B$ receptor-mediated autoinhibition of these GABAergic neurons, it stands to reason that estrogen would dramatically increase the firing rate of these neurons during negative feedback. Given that both POMC and hypothalamic GABAergic neurons synapse onto a number of neurosecretory neurons,[43–46] the collective modulation by estrogen of K^+ channel activity in these cells would greatly enhance the inhibitory tonus impinging on these neurons.

CELLULAR MECHANISMS OF ESTROGEN ACTIVATION OF PROTEIN KINASES

What is the underlying cause of this estrogen-induced decrease in the responsiveness of POMC and dopamine neurons to the μ-opioid and $GABA_B$ receptor-mediated activation of GIRK channels? One insight comes from studies that have examined μ-opioid receptor desensitization and opiate tolerance, both of which are associated with a refractoriness to μ-opioid receptor agonists, have implicated intracellular protein kinase pathways in these phenomena.[47–50] Indeed, we have shown that protein kinase A (PKA) inhibitors block the maintenance of cellular tolerance to μ-opioid receptor agonists after chronic morphine treatment that is observed in hypothalamic neurosecretory cells.[51] In addition, E_2 has been shown to rapidly stimulate PKA activity in peripheral (e.g., uterine) tissue, as well as to stimulate cyclic adenosine monophosphate responsive element binding protein (CREB) and c-fos expression.[52–56] Furthermore, PKA activators such as Sp-cAMP and forskolin mimic the effect of E_2 on the potency of the μ-opioid and $GABA_B$ receptor agonists.[38,57] In the presence of nonselective protein kinase inhibitors (e.g., staurosporine) or selective PKA inhibitors such as Rp-cAMP and KT5720, the effects of E_2 on the potency of the μ-opioid receptor agonist DAMGO or the $GABA_B$ receptor agonist baclofen are blocked. This demonstrates that the modulation by E_2 of the μ-opioid and $GABA_B$ receptor coupling to GIRK channels is due to increased PKA activity. In hippocampal CA1 pyramidal neurons, which are involved in learning and memory, estrogen activates a similar pathway to potentiate kainate currents.[3] Also, we know that multiple monoamine pathways activate PKA to inhibit small conductance, Ca^{2+}-activated K^+ (SK) channel activity in CA1 hippocampal pyramidal neurons,[58] and recently we have found that E_2 rapidly inhibits the SK current in the same neurons, probably via the same mechanism.[59]

There is considerable evidence for cross talk between various intracellular protein kinase pathways such as protein kinase C (PKC) and PKA in regulating effector systems.[60] PKA activators such as Sp-cAMP and forskolin and PKC activators such as phorbol esters mimic the effect of chronic morphine treatment in desensitizing the

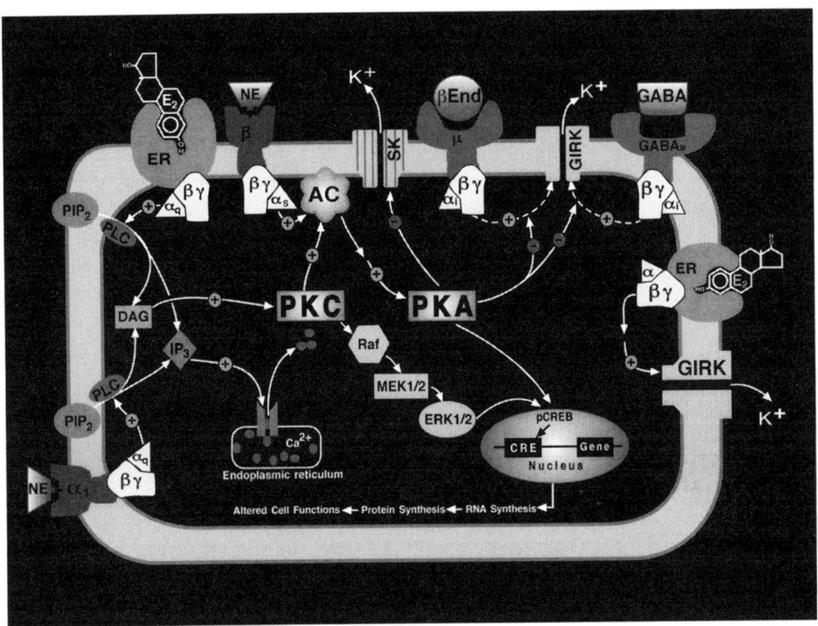

FIGURE 1. Schematic overview representing the short-term versus long-term estrogen-mediated modulation of G-protein–coupled receptors via a membrane-associated estrogen receptor in hypothalamic neurons. **Short term:** E_2 activates a membrane-associated ER that is $G\alpha_q$-coupled to activation of phospholipase C that catalyzes the hydrolysis of membrane-bound phosphatidylinositol 4,5-biphosphate (PIP_2) to inositol 1,4,5 triphosphate (IP_3) and diacylglycerol (DAG). Calcium is released from intracellular stores (endoplasmic reticulum) by IP_3, and DAG activates protein kinase C (PKC). Through phosphorylation, adenylyl cyclase (AC) activity is upregulated by PKC. The generation of cAMP activates PKA, which can rapidly uncouple μ-opioid (μ) and $GABA_B$ receptors from their effector system through phosphorylation of a downstream effector molecule (e.g., the inwardly rectifying K^+ channel, or GIRK). In addition, the β-adrenergic (β) receptor is $G\alpha_s$-coupled to activation of a adenylyl cyclase-PKA pathway that inhibits the small conductance, Ca^{2+}-dependent K^+ channel (SK), and this inhibition is potentiated by E_2 in hippocampal CA1 pyramidal neurons. On the other hand, the α_1-adrenergic receptor is $G\alpha_q$-coupled to the phosphatidylinositol pathway to activate PKC and PKA to phosphorylate the SK channel and inhibit its activity; this inhibition is potentiated by E_2 in hypothalamic neurons. ER-mediated modulation of kinase pathways either reduces the capacity of neuromodulators such as β-endorphin (β–End) and GABA to inhibit hypothalamic neuronal excitability, or augments the ability of neurotransmitters such as norepinephrine (NE) to increase neuronal excitability. Finally, in GnRH neurons, ER is $G\alpha_i$-coupled to activation of GIRK channels. **Long term**: Rapid ER-mediated activation of PKA can lead to phosphorylation of cAMP-responsive element binding protein (pCREB), which can then alter gene transcription through its interaction with the cAMP responsive element (CRE). Also, activation of PKC can stimulate the MAP kinase pathway (Raf-MEK1/2-ERK1/2) to cause further gene activation. Therefore, the "short-term" and "long-term" effects of E_2 are not mutually exclusive because the PKC-PKA pathway can also alter gene expression in an estrogen-response element-independent fashion.

μ-opioid receptor mediated responses.[47,51] In addition, PKC activators potentiate β-adrenergic receptor agonist stimulation of cyclic adenosine monophosphate (cAMP) accumulation in the preoptic area.[61] We have examined the involvement of PKC using selective inhibitors of PKC to block the effects of E_2 on the $GABA_B$ response.[62] First, treatment of neurons with bisindolymaleimide, which is an inhibitor of PKC that does not distinguish between conventional, atypical, and novel isoforms of PKC, eliminates all of the effects of E_2. Similar effects are seen with calphostin C, which is selective for the conventional and novel isoforms of PKC, on the E_2-induced decrease in DAMGO potency.[63] However, Gö6976, a selective inhibitor of conventional PKC isoforms is ineffective. In addition, when neurons are perfused internally with the rapid Ca^{2+} chelator BAPTA, the inhibition by E_2 is still observed. Since conventional isoforms of PKC are unlikely to be active with this level of calcium buffering, this result further supports a role for a Ca^{2+}-independent, PKC isoform (novel or atypical) in the estrogen-mediated effect. Finally, a selective PKC δ inhibitor, rottlerin, can fully block the effects of E_2 to inhibit the $GABA_B$ response, indicating that the novel PKC isoforms are involved in E_2 signaling.

Activation of PKC appears to be upstream from PKA based on the fact that forskolin can overcome the inhibition by the PKC inhibitor bisindolymaleimide. In addition, we believe that the E_2 receptor is Gq coupled because if we internally perfused neurons with a peptide that mimics the C terminal binding site of G_q,[64] the response to E_2 is significantly attenuated. If cells are dialyzed with the same concentration of a nonsense peptide of equal size, the response to E_2 is not affected.[38] Finally, G_q stimulates phospholipase C, and we have found that selective inhibitors of phopholipase C (i.e., U-73122) block the ability of E_2 to reduce the $GABA_B$ response in hypothalamic (dopamine, POMC) neurons.

Recent studies have shown that E_2 rapidly activates the MAP kinase pathway in primary cortical neuronal cultures and in cerebral cortical explant cultures.[65–67] However, inhibition of MAP kinase with inhibitors such as PD98059 does not prevent the E_2 modulation of the baclofen response. Therefore, the E_2-mediated inhibition of the $GABA_B$ (and μ–opioid) response appears to be mediated via a plasma membrane receptor that is $G\alpha_q$ coupled to activation of phospholipase C, protein kinase C, and protein kinase A (FIG. 1).

ESTROGEN MODULATION OF SMALL CONDUCTANCE, CA^{2+}-ACTIVATED K^+ (SK) CHANNELS

In addition to the inwardly rectifying K^+ channels, hypothalamic neurons also express small-conductance, Ca^{2+}-activated K^+ (SK) channels that are sensitive to antagonism by the peptidergic, honeybee toxin apamin.[68,69] These currents underlie the afterhyperpolarization (AHP) that is observed at the tail end of the action potential or a prolonged depolarizing stimulus.[69,70] In the preoptic area, we have found that the SK currents in GABAergic neurons are inhibited by β- and α_1-adrenergic receptor activation.[71] Of particular interest is that the α_1-adrenergic receptor-mediated inhibition of the SK current in these GABAergic neurons is markedly potentiated by a transient exposure to estrogen. This estrogen-induced enhancement of the coupling of α_1-adrenergic receptors to their effector SK channels lasts at least 24 h following systemic steroid administration, but most importantly these effects are manifested within 20 min following E_2, as measured in an *in vitro* slice preparation. The potentiation of the α_1-adrenergic receptor-mediated inhibition of the SK current in preoptic GABA neurons would facilitate the excitation caused by ascending noradrenergic input onto these cells.[24] In the hippocampus, E_2 rapidly augments the β-adrenergic inhibition of SK channel activity in CA1 neurons.[72] Although the mechanism(s) by which E_2 augments the α_1-adrenergic inhibition of the SK current in the hypothalamus, as well as the β-adrenergic inhibition of the SK current in the hippocampus, is probably via a similar cascade as described above (FIG. 1), the pathway needs to be elucidated.

ESTROGEN MODULATES DIRECTLY ION CHANNEL ACTIVITY THROUGH A G-PROTEIN LINKAGE

It has been known for some time that iontophoretically applied estrogen to preoptic area neurons alters their excitability primarily by inhibiting their firing rate.[73] This inhibition is associated with a membrane hyperpolarization due to the opening of a K^+ channel that has also been observed in the amygdala and arcuate nucleus.[10,74,75] This latter region contains GnRH neurons that are particularly responsive to this estrogenic inhibition.[10]

Estrogen also rapidly inhibits voltage-gated Ca^{2+} channels in medium spiny GABAergic neurons of the basal ganglia, an area that is involved in fine motor control. This effect of estrogen is mediated via a G protein.[11] Interestingly, the estrogen-induced augmentation of kainate currents in hippocampal CA1 pyramidal cells also involves an intervening G protein.[3] Thus, estrogen apparently is capable of relatively direct modulation of ion channel activity through a G protein, as well as more subtle modulation of G-protein–coupled receptor/K^+ channel coupling.

PHARMACOLOGICAL PROFILE OF THE RAPID ESTROGEN RESPONSE RECEPTOR

Earlier studies showed that the E_2 receptor mediating the rapid effects of E_2 in POMC neurons was highly selective.[57] The stereoisomer 17 α-estradiol could not mimic the actions of E_2 nor could the nonsteroidal agonist diethylstilbesterol. However, these actions of E_2 could be antagonized by the anti-estrogen ICI 164,384 with a K_i of 0.3 nM. Recently, we have further characterized the binding site for E_2 using a number of selective estrogen receptor modulators (SERMs).[38] As previously described, we have found that E_2 rapidly attenuates the outward K^+ current induced by the $GABA_B$ receptor agonist baclofen. The inhibitory effect of E_2 on the baclofen response are mimicked by the SERM raloxifene, but not by 17α-estradiol; and as expected from our earlier results, the response is antagonized by ICI 182,780. Furthermore, the membrane-impermeable conjugate E_2-BSA mimicked the actions of E_2. Therefore, collectively the results would indicate that E_2 binds to a G-protein– coupled (plasma membrane) receptor to activate a phospholipase C–protein kinase C–protein kinase A pathway to desensitize the μ-opioid and $GABA_B$ responses in POMC and dopamine neurons. Further evidence for a membrane receptor for E_2 has been provided by the recent studies of Toran-Allerand and colleagues,[76] who have shown both anatomical (electron microscopy) and biochemical (binding) evidence for plasma membrane estrogen receptor distinct from ERα and ERβ

SIGNIFICANCE

Estrogen modulates the excitability of a number of neurons that are involved in the control of homeostasis, including reproduction, stress responses, feeding, and motivated behaviors. Recently, we have gained some insight into the cellular mechanisms by which estrogen exerts its effects on these neurons. First, estrogen negatively modulates the coupling of the μ-opioid and/or $GABA_B$ receptors to their effector K^+ channel in β-endorphin, dopamine, and GABAergic neurons. This uncoupling requires the activation of a hierarchal, intracellular phosphorylation cascade involving phospholipase C, PKC, and PKA pathways (FIG. 1). These pathways also appear to be involved in the estrogen-induced augmentation of α_1-adrenergic inhibition of SK channel activity. It is known that PKA-dependent phosphorylation of the μ-opioid receptor hinders its association with $G_{i/o}$.[77,78] However, it remains to be seen whether the μ-opioid and $GABA_B$ receptors are the phosphorylation substrate that render them less prone to couple to its GIRK channel. More likely targets include $G_{i/o}$ subunits, GIRK channels, or protein regulators of G-protein–signaling that are common to both receptors. Future studies will endeavor to elucidate how the phosphorylation affects this uncoupling in POMC neurons.

Finally, estrogen itself can hyperpolarize and thereby inhibit some neurons like GnRH neurons by activating a K^+ channel. While it has long been thought that GnRH neurons do not contain estrogen receptors,[17–19] recent evidence indicates that these neurons express the β isoform of the estrogen receptor.[13–15,21] It is therefore conceivable that estrogen could interact with a membrane-associated receptor to effect a hyperpolarization of GnRH neurons by way of a G protein. Thus, there are multiple cellular mechanisms through which estrogen can exert rapid physiologic actions on hypothalamic neurons (FIG. 1).

ACKNOWLEDGMENTS

The experiments described in this review were supported by U.S. Public Health Service grants NS 35944, NS 38809, DA 05158, DA 00192 (Research Scientist Development Award to M.J.K.) and the National Institutes of Health Office of Research on Women's Health. The authors would like to recognize Martha A. Bosch, Rebecka D. Amodei and Barry R. Naylor for their expert technical contributions to these studies.

REFERENCES

1. KELLY, M.J. & E.J. WAGNER. 1999. Estrogen modulation of G-protein-coupled receptors. Trends Endocrinol. Metab. **10:** 369–374.
2. WAGNER, E.J., K.E. MOORE & K.J. LOOKINGLAND. 1993. Sexual differences in *N*-methyl-D-aspartate receptor-mediated regulation of tuberoinfundibular dopaminergic neurons in the rat. Brain Res. **611:** 139–146.

42. GRATTAN, D.R., M.S. ROCCA, K.I. STRAUSS, *et al.* 1996. GABAergic neuronal activity and mRNA levels for both forms of glutamic acid decarboxylase (GAD_{65} and GAD_{67}) are reduced in the diagonal band of Broca during the afternoon of proestrus. Brain Res. **733:** 46–55.
43. GOLDSMITH, P.C., J.E. BOGGAN & K.K. THIND. 1991. Opioid synapses on vasopressin neurons in the paraventricular and supraoptic nuclei of juvenile monkeys. Neuroscience **45:** 709–719.
44. LERANTH, C., N.J. MACLUSKY, H. SAKAMOTO, *et al.* 1985. Glutamic acid decarboxylase-containing axons synapse on LHRH neurons in the rat medial preoptic area. Neuroendocrinology **40:** 536–539.
45. LERANTH, C., N.J. MACLUSKY, M. SHANABROUGH & F. NAFTOLIN. 1988. Immunohistochemical evidence for synaptic connections between pro-opiomelanocortin-immunoreactive axons and LH-RH neurons in the preoptic area of the rat. Brain Res. **449:** 167–176.
46. HORVATH, T.L., F. NAFTOLIN & C. LERANTH. 1992. GABAergic and catecholaminergic innervation of mediobasal hypothalamic β–endorphin cells projecting to the medial preoptic area. Neuroscience **51:** 391–399.
47. CHEN, Y. & L. YU. 1994. Differential regulation by cAMP-dependent protein kinase and protein kinase C of the μ–opioid receptor coupling to a G protein-activated K^+ channel. J. Biol. Chem. **269:** 7839–7842.
48. NARITA, M., M. NARITA, H. MIZOGUCHI, & L.F. TSENG. 1995. Inhibition of protein kinase C, but not of protein kinase A, blocks the development of acute antinociceptive tolerance to an intrathecally administered μ-opioid receptor agonist in the mouse. Eur. J. Pharmacol. **280:** R1–R3.
49. MESTEK, A., J.H. HURLEY, L.S. BYE, *et al.* 1995. The human μ-opioid receptor: modulation of functional desensitization by calcium/calmodulin-dependent protein kinase and protein kinase C. J. Neurosci. **15:** 2396–2406.
50. WANG, L., V.M. MEDINA, M. RIVERA & A.R. GINTZLER. 1996. Relevance of phosphorylation state to opioid responsiveness in opiate naive and tolerant/dependent tissue. Brain Res. **723:** 61–69.
51. WAGNER, E.J., O.K. RØNNEKLEIV & M.J. KELLY. 1998. Protein kinase A maintains cellular tolerance to μ–opioid receptor agonists in hypothalamic neurosecretory cells with chronic morphine treatment: convergence upon a common pathway with estrogen in modulating μ-opioid receptor/effector coupling. J. Pharmacol. Exp. Ther. **285:** 1266–1273.
52. ARONICA, S.M. & B.S. KATZENELLENBOGEN. 1993. Stimulation of estrogen receptor mediated transcription and alteration in the phosphorylation state of the rat uterine estrogen receptor by estrogen, cyclic adenosine monophosphate, and insulin-like growth factor-I. Mol. Endocrinol. **7:** 743–752.
53. NAKHLA, A.M., M.S. KHAN, N.P. ROMAS & W. ROSNER. 1994. Estradiol causes the rapid accumulation of cAMP in human prostate. Proc. Natl. Acad. Sci. USA **91:** 5402 5405.
54. ZHOU, Y., J.J. WATTERS & D.M. DORSA. 1996. Estrogen rapidly induces the phosphorylation of the cAMP response element binding protein in rat brain. Endocrinology **137:** 2163–2166.
55. GU, G., A.A. ROJO, M.C. ZEE, *et al.* 1996. Hormonal regulation of CREB phosphorylation in the anteroventral periventricular nucleus. J. Neurosci. **16:** 3035–3044.
56. WATTERS, J.J., J.S. CAMPBELL, M.J. CUNNINGHAM, *et al.* 1997. Rapid membrane effects of steroids in neuroblastoma cells: effects of estrogen on mitogen activated protein kinase signalling cascade and c-fos immediate early gene transcription. Endocrinology **138:** 4030–4033.
57. LAGRANGE, A.H., O.K. RØNNEKLEIV & M.J. KELLY. 1997. Modulation of G protein-coupled receptors by an estrogen receptor that activates protein kinase A. Mol. Pharmacol. **51:** 605–612.
58. PEDARZANI, P. & J.F. STORM. 1993. PKA mediates the effects of monoamine transmitters on the K^+ current underlying the slow spike frequency adaptation in hippocampal neurons. Neuron **11:** 1023–1035.

59. KELLY, M.J. & O.K. RØNNEKLEIV. 2002. Rapid membrane effects of estrogen in the central nervous system. *In* Hormones, Brain and Behavior. D.W. Pfaff, Ed.: 361–380. Academic Press. San Diego, CA.
60. MONS, N., M. YOSHIMURA, H. IKEDA, *et al.* 1998. Immunological assessment of the distribution of type VII adenylyl cyclase in brain. Brain Res. **788:** 251–261.
61. ANSONOFF, M.A. & A.M. ETGEN. 1998. Estradiol elevates protein kinase C catalytic activity in the preoptic area of female rats. Endocrinology **139:** 3050–3056.
62. WAY, K.J., E. CHOU & G.L. KING. 2000. Identification of PKC-isoform-specific biological actions using pharmacological approaches. Trends Pharmacol. Sci. **21:** 181–187.
63. KELLY, M.J., A.H. LAGRANGE, E.J. WAGNER, & O.K. RØNNEKLEIV. 1999. Rapid effects of estrogen to modulate G protein-coupled receptors via activation of protein kinase A and protein kinase C pathways. Steroids **64:** 64–75.
64. AKHTER, S.A., L.M. LUTTRELL, H.A. ROCKMAN, *et al.* 1998. Targeting the receptor-Gq interface to inhibit in vivo pressure overload myocardial hypertrophy. Science **280:** 574–577.
65. SINGH, M., JR., G. SETALO, X. GUAN, *et al.* 1999. Estrogen-induced activation of mitogen-activated protein kinase in cerebral cortical explants: convergence of estrogen and neurotrophin signaling pathways. J. Neurosci. **19:** 1179–1188.
66. SINGER, C.A., X.A. FIGUEROA-MASOT, R.H. BATCHELOR & D.M. DORSA. 1999. The mitogen-activated protein kinase pathway mediates estrogen neuroprotection after glutamate toxicity in primary cortical neurons. J. Neurosci. **19:** 2455–2463.
67. SINGH, M., G.J. SETALO, X. GUAN, *et al.* 2000. Estrogen-induced activation of the mitogen-activated protein kinase cascade in the cerebral cortex of estrogen receptor-alpha knock-out mice. J. Neurosci. **20:** 1694–1700.
68. ERICKSON, K.R., O.K. RØNNEKLEIV & M.J. KELLY. 1993. Role of a T-type calcium current in supporting a depolarizing potential, damped oscillations, and phasic firing in vasopressinergic guinea pig supraoptic neurons. Neuroendocrinology **57:** 789–800.
69. KIRKPATRICK, K. & C.W. BOURQUE. 1996. Activity dependence and functional role of the apamin-sensitive K^+ current in rat supraoptic neurones in vitro. J. Physiol. (Lond.) **494:** 389–398.
70. WAGNER, E.J., C. REYES-VAZQUEZ, O.K. RØNNEKLEIV & M.J. KELLY. 2000. The role of intrinsic and agonist-activated conductances in determining the firing patterns of preoptic area neurons in the guinea pig. Brain Res. **879:** 29–41.
71. WAGNER, E.J., O.K. RØNNEKLEIV & M.J. KELLY. 2001. The noradrenergic inhibition of an apamine-sensitive small conductance Ca^{2+}-activated K^+ channel in hypothalamic γ-aminobutyric acid neurons: pharmacology, estrogen sensitivity and relevance to the control of the reproductive axis. J. Pharmacol. Exp. Ther. **299:** 21–30.
72. KELLY, M.J., H. HUA & J.F. STORM. 1999. 17β-estradiol rapidly potentiates β-adrenergic inhibition of the slow afterhyperpolarization current in hippocampal CA1 pyramidal neurons. APS conference: biology of potassium channels. Physiologist **42.** A22.
73. KELLY, M.J., R.L. MOSS & C.A. DUDLEY. 1976. Differential sensitivity of preoptic-septal neurons to microelectrophoresed estrogen during the estrous cycle. Brain Res. **114:** 152–157.
74. KELLY, M.J., U. KUHNT & W. WUTTKE. 1980. Hyperpolarization of hypothalamic parvocellular neurons by 17β–estradiol and their identification through intracellular staining with procion yellow. Exp. Brain Res. **40:** 440–447.
75. NABEKURA, J., Y. OOMURA, T. MINAMI, *et al.* 1986. Mechanism of the rapid effect of 17β-estradiol on medial amygdala neurons. Science **233:** 226–228.
76. TORAN-ALLERAND, C.D., X. GUAN, N.J. MACLUSKY, *et al.* 2002. ER-X: a novel, plasma membrane-associated, putative estrogen receptor that is regulated during development and after ischemic brain injury. J. Neurosci. **22:** 8391–8401.
77. HARADA, H., H. UEDA, Y. WADA, *et al.* 1989. Phosphorylation of μ-opioid receptors—a putative mechanism of selective uncoupling of receptor-G_i interaction, measured with low-K_m GTPase and nucleotide-sensitive agonist binding. Neurosci. Lett. **100:** 221–226.
78. HARADA, H., H. UEDA, T. KATADA, *et al.* 1990. Phosphorylated μ-opioid receptor purified from rat brains lacks functional coupling with G_i1, a GTP-binding protein in reconstituted lipid vesicles. Neurosci. Lett. **113:** 47–49.

Regulation of Gene Expression in the Developing Midbrain by Estrogen

Implication of Classical and Nonclassical Steroid Signaling

CORDIAN BEYER, JUSTYNA PAWLAK, VERONICA BRITO, MAGDALENA KAROLCZAK, TATIANA IVANOVA, AND EVA KÜPPERS

Abteilung Anatomie und Zellbiologie, Universität Ulm, D-89069 Ulm, Germany

ABSTRACT: Estrogen plays an important role during midbrain development. This is indicated by the presence of nuclear estrogen receptors and the transient expression of the estrogen-forming enzyme aromatase. A number of recent studies have shown that estrogen promotes the differentiation and survival, as well as physiological performance, of midbrain dopaminergic cells. In addition, we have reported that both ways of cellular estrogen signaling (classical and nonclassical) as well as interactions with nonneuronal target cells are involved in the transmission of intra- and intercellular estrogen effects in this brain region. This study provides additional evidence that (i) estrogen is capable of regulating gene expression in cultured embryonic neurons and astrocytes differently and (ii) both signaling mechanisms, i.e., classically through nuclear receptors and nonclassically through the stimulation of membrane–estrogen receptors, which are coupled to distinct intracellular signal transduction cascades, contribute diversely to gene regulation. These data reveal a high degree of complexity of estrogen action at the genomic level in the developing brain. Further studies are warranted to unravel the exact contribution of the differently regulated genes for developmental estrogen action.

KEYWORDS: estrogen; midbrain; astroglia; neuron; gene expression; dd RT-PCR

INTRODUCTION

It is generally accepted that estrogen influences the cellular differentiation and neural network formation of distinct neuronal phenotypes during central nervous system (CNS) development.[1,2] The premise also applies to the differentiating midbrain. During development, the estrogen-synthesizing enzyme aromatase is transiently expressed,[3] and both types of nuclear estrogen receptors (α/β) are permanently found within distinct mesencephalic nuclei, i.e., the substantia nigra and ventral tegmental area.[4,5] These observations indicate that locally produced estrogen in the midbrain can act in a paracrine or even autocrine way to mediate its developmental effects. Dopaminergic neurons appear to be the major targets of es-

Address for correspondence: Cordian Beyer, Ph.D., Abteilung Anatomie und Zellbiologie, Universität Ulm, D-89069 Ulm, Germany. Voice: 49-(0)731-50-23228; fax: 49-(0)731-50-23217. cordian.beyer@medizin.uni-ulm.de

Ann. N.Y. Acad. Sci. 1007: 17–28 (2003).
doi: 10.1196/annals.1286.002

trogen action in the developing midbrain. Estrogen promotes the morphological maturation and synaptic plasticity of this neuronal cell population by influencing neurite extension and dendritic arborization.[6] Furthermore, it regulates the activity of dopaminergic neurons by the control of transmitter synthesis, metabolism, and clearance from the extracellular space.[7–9] Besides morphogenetic effects, estrogen additionally affects the survival of dopamine neurons.[10,11] On the other hand, midbrain GABAergic cells also represent cellular targets for estrogen although to a lesser extent.[12] These *in vitro* data have recently been validated by a knockout approach that is based on the deactivation of estrogen receptor-β signaling. In this study, Beyer and Raab have provided clear evidence that the interruption of estrogen signaling causes a reduction in the number of surviving midbrain dopaminergic neurons and a significant change in their cellular morphology compared to the wild type.[13] At this stage, it is noteworthy that the effects of estrogen on dopaminergic neurons during perinatal development do not show any sex-specific characteristics.[14] This is in contrast to other brain regions where estrogen appears to be pivotal for the sexual differentiation of brain structures and functions.[1,2] Concerning intracellular estrogen action, we have demonstrated in a series of *in vitro* and *in vivo* studies that estrogen action in the midbrain is transmitted through nuclear estrogen receptors but also via nonclassical estrogen signaling.[15] This involves interactions with putative membrane-associated estrogen receptors that are coupled to distinct intracellular signal transduction cascades.[16] In particular, we found that estrogen can activate the phosphatidyl inositol (PI)-3 kinase and cAMP/protein kinase A pathways in mesencephalic neurons,[6,17] as well as the MAP-kinase pathway in astrocytes.[18] The latter observation suggests that midbrain astroglial cells are responsive, as are neurons, to estrogen and are implicated in the mediation of estrogen effects.

Originating from these observations, we attempted to tackle the influence of estrogen on the regulation of gene expression in developing midbrain cells in more detail. By the application of differential display RT-PCR (dd RT-PCR) techniques, we investigated the effects of estrogen at the molecular level in both neurons and astrocytes separately. Pharmacological approaches were employed to discriminate between classical and nonclassical estrogen signaling.

METHODS

Cell Culturing and Treatment

Adult Balb/c mice were kept in a 12 h dark/light cycle and mated during a 12 h period. Day 0 of pregnancy was defined as the day after insemination. At the indicated developmental stage, pregnant mice and postnatal animals were anesthetized with 25% chloralhydrate (1 mL/100 g body weight) and killed by decapitation. The preparation of neuronal cell cultures was performed as previously described.[7] Briefly, the midbrain was excised from E15 fetuses and dissociated enzymatically (0.1% trypsin) and mechanically. Cells were plated at a density of 2×10^5 cells/cm^2 on poly-DL-ornithine-coated culture dishes (9 cm^2). Cultures were raised with serum-free neurobasal medium (NBM supplemented with 100 mL/L B27, Gibco, Eggenstein, Germany) with a daily medium change. The medium did not contain phenol red. To establish astroglial cultures, the midbrain of newborns was dissected and incubated in a Ca^{2+}- and Mg^{2+}-free Dulbecco's PBS containing 0.1% trypsin and 0.02% EDTA. After 20 min, trypsin action was terminated by transferring tissue pieces to a Ca^{2+}- and Mg^{2+}-free Hank's balanced salt solution containing 20% fetal calf serum. Tissues were then dissociated as described above and resuspended in NBM. Cells were seeded at a density of 4 × 104 cells/cm^2. Upon reaching confluency, cells were trypsinized and replated at lower densities. Neuronal and astroglial cell cultures were finally used for treatment after six days *in vitro* or after the second plating, respectively. Cultures were treated for 24 h with 17β-estradiol (E, 10-8 M, Sigma, Germany), or a membrane-impermeable estrogen-BSA construct (E-BSA, 10-8 M, Sigma, Germany), or 17β-estradiol (E, 10-8 M) together with the estrogen receptor antagonist ICI (ICI 182,780, 1 mM, Tocris, UK).

RNA Preparation and Differential Display RT-PCR

Total RNA wasisolated from cultures using peqGOLD RNApure (Peqlab, Germany) according to the manufacturer's instructions. Cultured cells were harvested by lysis with TRI reagent. After phenol/chloroform extraction and centrifugation (13,000 rpm for 15 min, 4°C), the aqueous phase was transferred and precipitated in 50% isopropanol for 1 h at 20°C. The pellet was washed with 1 mL 75% ice-cold ethanol and centrifuged as above. Finally, the pellet was dried and stored at –80°C.

To divide total RNA into three subpopulations, RNA was reverse transcribed using 3′-one-base anchored oligo-dT primers provided in the ready-to-use RNAimage kit (Gibco; H-T_{11}G, H-T_{11}A, H-T_{11}C). Total RNA (0.2 μg) RNA was denatured for 5 min at 65°C in a total volume of 19 μL containing 1× reverse transcription buffer, 20 mL dNTP, and 4 mol anchored primer. The mixture was preincubated for 10 min at 37°C. Reverse transcription was initiated by adding 100 U M-MLF and performed for 60 min. PCR was done in a total volume of 20 mL containing 1× PCR buffer, 2 mL dNTP, 2 mL DNA, 4 pmol of one of the following 5′arbitrary primers (5′-AAGCTTGATTGCC-3′, 5′-AAGCTTCGACTGT-3′, 5′-AAGCTT-GGTTCAG-3′, 5′-AAGCTTCTCAACG-3′, 5′-AAGCTTAGTAGGC-3′, 5′-AAGCTT-GCACCAT-3′, 5′-AAGCTTAACGAGG-3′, 5′-AAGCTTTTACCGC-3′), 4 pmol of 3′one-base anchored primers used in the reversed transcription, 10 μCi α[S] dATP (1,000 mCi/mmol), and 1.2 U Taq polymerase (Gibco). PCR conditions were as follows: 1 min denaturation at 94°C, 2 min annealing at 40°C, 2 min elongation at 72°C, 32 cycles followed by one cycle at 72°C for 5 min.

PCR products were separated by PAGE (6%) containing 8 M urea and Tris-boric buffer (89 mM, pH 8.0, plus 1 mM EDTA). After electrophoresis, the dried gel was exposed to a X-ray film at room temperature (RT) for 24 h together with a fluorescent marker. Autoradiograms were dried and adjusted. Bands of interest were excised, transferred to a tube, and soaked with filter paper in 100 μL H_20. Samples were boiled for 15 min and centrifuged for 2 min at 13,000 rpm. The supernatant was transferred and DNA was precipitated with 75% ethanol containing 0.05 M sodium acetate and 5 μg glycogen for 1 h at –80°C, and then centrifuged as above. Pellets were vacuum-dried and dissolved in 10 μL H_20. Four microliters of the samples were used for reamplification (as described but without isotopes). Reamplified products were separated on 2% low-melting agarose gels, thereafter cut out, and purified using the QIAquick gel extraction kit (Quiagen, Karlsruhe, Germany). DNA was then used for cycle sequencing. Four microliters of DNA were mixed with 1 μL salt solution and 1 mL TOPO® vector (Quiagen) and incubated for 5 min at RT. Two miroliters of this reaction were incubated for 30 min on ice with a one-shot competent *E. coli* strain. After an incubation for 30 s at 42°C, medium (250 μL) containing 20 g Bacto-tryptone, 5 g Bacto-yeast extract, 0.5 g NaCl, 2.5 mL 1 M KCl, 10 mL 1 M $MgCl_2$, and 20 mL 1 M glucose was added. Cells were gently mixed and propagated overnight at 37°C. For further analysis, colonies were picked and plasmids were isolated and analyzed by restriction analysis followed by sequencing.

Sequencing and Capillary Electrophoresis

Plasmid DNA from overnight *E. coli* cultures (5 mL; selected by 50 mg/mL ampicilline) was purified using a QIAprep miniprep kit (Quiagen). Pelleted bacteria were resuspended in 250 mL buffer (P1) and transferred. Thereafter, 250 mDye ready reaction kit (ABI, Hamburg, Germany) with 0.2 mg purified plasmid, 10 pmol M13 forward and M13 reverse primers, and 4 mL reaction mix (dNTP, AmpliTaq, FS, rTth, DNA polymerase, pyrophosphatase, $MgCl_2$, and fluorescent-labeled ddNTP terminators) in a total volume of 10 mL. PCR conditions were: denaturation 10 s at 9 annealing 10 s at 50°C, and elongation 3 min at 55°C. Five microliters of the sequence reaction were added to 20 mL water and denatured at 90°C for 2 min. Sequencing was performed using the ABI Prism 310 Genetic Analyzer (ABI). Samples were loaded onto POP6 polymer containing 310 ga capillaries for 60 s at 2.0 kV. Electrophoretic separation was done for 35 minat 15 kV at 50°C. Data were further analyzed using the corresponding ABI Prism sequencing analysis software. Obtained sequences were then compared with GenBank libraries.

Competitive RT-PCR

For conforming ddPCR data, total RNA from treated/untreated neuronal and astroglial cultures were semiquantitatively assessed by applyingcompetitive RT-PCR techniques (for details see Refs. 6, 8, 19, 20). Total RNA was isolated as described above. PCRs were performed with 3 μL samples of RT-reaction, 0.2 μM of sense and antisense primers,[8,20] 0.2 mM dNTP, 2.5 mM $MgCl_2$, and 1.2 U Taq polymerase (all from Gibco). To ensure that no genomic DNA contamination was present and for use in competition experiments, RT-PCR for hypoxanthinephosphoribosyltraferase (HPRT) was performed for each sample. As expected, only the 249 bp control band, but not the 1,100 bp genomic, band was seen, proving the amplified RT-PCR products were only derived from the respective mRNA. The amplification protocol was as follows: 32 cycles with denaturation for 1 min at 95°C, annealing for 1 min at 65°C, and elongation for 2 min at 72°C. The specificity of the PCR products was tested by sequence analysis. The linearity of the amplification protocol was assessed by running 28, 32, 36, 40, and 44 cycles using midbrain tissue from newborn animals. Since linear relationships (not shown) were found for the amplified genes between until 36 cycles, 32 cycles were applied for all competitive analyses. After RT-PCR, the products were electrophoretically separated in a 1.5% agarose gel and visualized with ethidium bromide. Gels were examined with a fluorescent gel scanner (ImageMaster, Pharmacia, Hamburg, Germany) and densitometrically analyzed using the manufacturer's software (ImageMaster USD version 2.0, Pharmacia). The absolute optical density (OD) of PCR products was normalized to the OD of the corresponding HPRT band. In order to avoid interassay variations, RNA isolation, RT-PCR, and quantification of the samples from each developmental stage and from each independent culture experiment were performed at the same time.

RESULTS

Differential display RT-PCR analysis was used to investigate the influence of estrogen on gene expression in midbrain neuronal and astroglial cell cultures. Reverse transcription with anchoring primers directed against the polyA-tail of mRNA allowed for the division of total RNA into three subpopulations. The further amplification of the obtained cDNAs with anchoring and arbitrary primers under unspecified conditions resulted in approximately 50 differently expressed transcripts in neuronal and astroglial cell cultures. In total, the ddPCR method yielded about 3,500 RT-PCR products (per investigated cell population) with molecular siz-

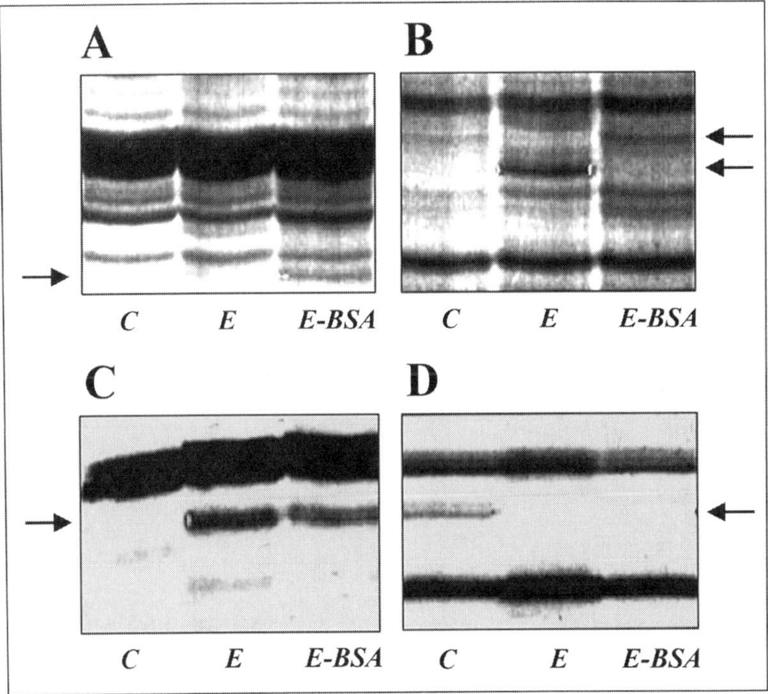

FIGURE 1. Autoradiogram of differential display RT-PCR analysis of gene expression in neuronal cell cultures of the embryonic mouse midbrain. Cultures were treated for 24 h with 17β-estradiol (E, 10^{-8} M), the membrane-impermeable estrogen construct 17β–estradiol-BSA hemisuccinate (E-BSA, 10^{-8} M), or left untreated (C). Note that only E-BSA (**A, B** *upper arrow*), or only E (**B**), or E and E-BSA to the same extent (**C**) are capable of inducing the expression of distinct transcripts. In contrast, both factors completely switch off the expression of another transcript (**D**).

es between 100 and 600 bp (a few examples are given in FIG. 1). After electrophoretic separation, sequencing, and competitive RT-PCR, only a few transcripts remained as candidate genes that were further characterized according to GenBank data. Generally, we observed different estrogen-dependent effects on gene regulation as presented in FIGURE 1 for neuronal cultures. Treatment with estrogen and/or E-BSA caused an increase as well as decrease in gene expression (FIG. 1C, D). Although both estrogen and E-BSA stimulated the expression of the same transcripts (FIG. 1C), they also targeted other genes separately (FIG. 1A, B). Because the ddRT-PCR method is not suitable to give reliable data on subtle differences in gene regulation, we have followed up only those transcripts that were characterized by a complete induction or reduction in expression or by increased or decreased expression levels compared to controls in the range of 50% and more (examples are given in FIG. 1). For the identification of regulated genes, usually up to 150 bp of the transcripts were sequenced. Homology levels were usually in the range of 70–100% as compared with data from the GenBank.

Regulation of Gene Expression in Neurons

Twenty-eight out of 48 estrogen-dependent and differentially regulated transcripts derived from neuronal cultures were identified by sequence analysis (data are

TABLE 1. List of genes in embryonic midbrain neuronal cell cultures that are differentially regulated by estrogen and estrogen-BSA

Gene	Regulation
Transmembrane GTPase	(–) estrogen
Translation factor IF2	
FUN12	
cas-S2 mitochondrial D-loop	
Cyclin D3	
Growth hormone	
Mammary-derived growth inhibitor	
tRNAs (Val, Leu, Phe)	(–) estrogen-BSA
12S and 16S ribosomal RNAs	
Regucalcin	(+) estrogen
Tyrosine hydrozylase	
JNKa	
Ryanodine receptor tyupe 2 (RyR2)	
Insulin receptor substrate-2	
Hexokinase II	
Serine/threonine kinase	
FGF-4	
Presenilin-1	
Tyrosine kinase receptor	(+) estrogen-BSA
IGIF precursor polypeptide	
Potassium channel KCNQ2	
Heat-shock protein dnaJ	
Glycine receptor-α1	
Brain-derived neurotrophic factor	

(+) Stimulated/inhibited; (–) downregulated/abolished.

summarized in TABLE 1). The other products revealed homologies of 30% and less compared to existing sequences in the mouse library and were therefore not further processed. Four genes appeared to be downregulated by estrogen and E-BSA exposure similarly, i.e., a putative transmembrane GTPase, the translation factor IF2, FUN12 protein, and cas-S2 mitochondrial D-loop, whereas E-BSA, but not estrogen, treatment abolished the expression of mitochondrial genes encoding for the tRNAs specific for Phe, Val, and Leu, and 12S and 16S ribosomal RNAs. Estrogen, but not E-BSA, inhibited the expression of cyclin D3, growth hormone, and mammary-derived growth inhibitor. Estrogen, but not E-BSA, stimulated the expression of tyrosine hydroxylase (TH), regucalcin, JNKa, ryanodine receptor type 2 (RyR2), insulin receptor substrate-2 (IRS2), hexokinase II, a serine/threonine kinase, FGF-4, and presenilin-1. Only E-BSA induced the expression of an unknown tyrosine kinase receptor, the IGIF precursor polypeptide, the potassium channel KCNQ2, LIM-kinase 1, heat-shock protein dnaJ, and glycine receptor α1 (GLRα1). Two examples are given for further competitive quantitative analysis of a classically and nonclassically regulated gene in midbrain neurons in FIGURE 2. The expression of the neurotrophin BDNF is increased after estrogen and E-BSA treatment. This effect is not

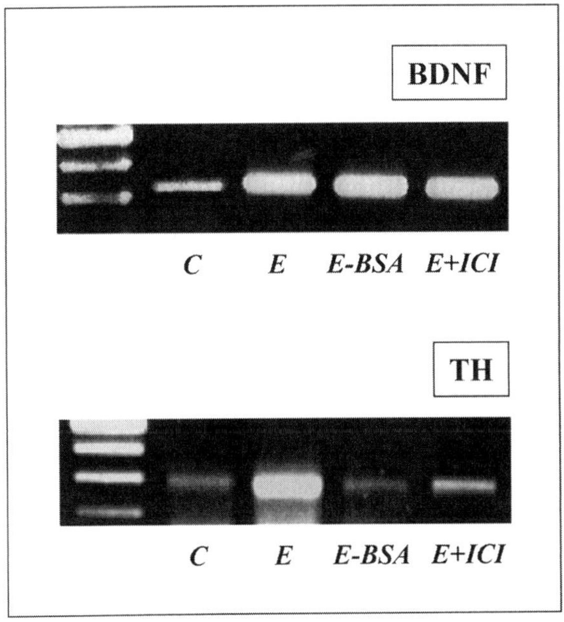

FIGURE 2. Effect of estrogen treatment (E, 10^{-8} M, 24 h) on brain-derived neurotrophic factor (BDNF) and tyrosine hydroxylase (TH) mRNA expression in neuronal midbrain cell cultures analyzed by competitive RT-PCR. Representative gels are shown. Note that the administration of E and E-BSA (a membrane-impermeable estrogen-BSA construct) stimulated similarly the expression of BDNF. This effect was not antagonized by ICI 182,780 (10^{-6} M, a potent inhibitor of nuclear estrogen receptors). In contrast, only E induced the expression of TH, whereas E-BSA was ineffective. This effect was completely blocked by ICI 182,780.

TABLE 2. List of genes in neonatal midbrain astroglial cell cultures that are differentially regulated by estrogen and estrogen-BSA

Gene	Regulation
ATP synthase 6 (mitochondrial) Histocompatibility antigen precursor (H47)	(–) estrogen
Casein kinase II β subunit (Csnk2β) Ribosomal protein S4	(–) estrogen-BSA
LIM-kinase TG integrating factor CD 80 antigen KIAA0916 protein	(+) estrogen
KIF14A protein Cytochrome c oxidase III (mitochondrial) Major histocompatibility complex region class II	(+) estrogen-BSA

(+) Stimulated/inhibited; (–) downregulated/abolished.

antagonized by ICI 182,780. In contrast, the expression of the dopamine synthesizing enzyme tyrosine hydroxylase is only induced after estrogen exposure but not by E-BSA. In addition, this effect is clearly abolished by ICI 182,780.

Regulation of Gene Expression in Astrocytes

In astroglial cultures, 12 out of 50 differentially regulated genes were identified after sequencing and comparison of the data with the GenBank Database. The other 38 had very low degrees of homology and were thus not further investigated. The list of identified genes is summarized in TABLE 2. Estrogen appears to induce the expression of KIAA0916 protein, cytochrome $P450_{arom}$, the CD 80 antigen, the TG-integrating factor, and the LIM-kinase. In contrast, E-BSA stimulated the expression of the major histocompatibility complex class II, mitochondrial cytochrome c oxidase III, and the KIF13A protein. Estrogen inhibited the expression of the histocompatible antigen precursor H47 and the mitochondrial ATP synthase 6, whereas E-BSA did so for the casein kinase II beta subunit (Csnk2β) and the ribosomal protein S4.

DISCUSSION

In the present study, we have attempted to analyze the role of estrogen in the developmental regulation of neuronal and astroglial gene expression in the mouse midbrain. In addition, we were interested in pinpointing the related intracellular signaling systems involved in this process. For that purpose, we used primary cell cultures that were treated either with 17β-estradiol or with a membrane-impermeable estrogen-BSA construct. For gene expression analysis, we employed ddPCR followed by gene sequencing and competitive semiquantitative RT-PCR. Our data reveal that depending on the investigated cell population the expression of different sets of transcripts is affected, ranging from growth factors to proteins implicated in intracellular signaling to membrane receptors. It is noteworthy that estrogen exposure caused down- as well as upregulation of subsets of genes. In addition, classical and nonclassical estrogen action regulated gene expression differently.

Estrogen has long been recognized as a modulator of developmental processes in the mammalian brain.[1,2] This also applies to the neostriatal complex and the developing midbrain. In both brain sites, nuclear estrogen receptors and the estrogen-synthesizing enzyme aromatase are found.[3,4,5,21,22,23] In the nigrostriatal system, dopaminergic cells appear to be estrogen sensitive. In addition, GABAergic neurons and nonneuronal cells such as astrocytes are also responsive to estrogen. One of the major estrogen effects iscritical involvement in the regulation of neurite extension, synapse plasticity, as well as neurotransmitter synthesis and catabolism in dopaminergic cells.[6–8] Another line of supportive evidence derives from studies that have demonstrated that (1) estrogen is essential for maintaining the cellular integrity of the nigrostriatal dopaminergic system in primates,[24] (2) estrogen exerts neuroprotective/antiapoptotic effects upon nigral dopamine neurons,[10] and (3) estrogen-mediated neuroprotection in the midbrain is likely to be mediated through the stimulation of the antiapoptotic PI3-kinase/Akt pathway.[17] These neuroprotective functions of estrogen either can be the consequence of a direct interaction with neurons, more precisely, with particular neuronal functions and survival cascades, or result from an interference of glial function. Our data and those of other groups ascribe the protective role of estrogen to both possibilities. Previously, we have shown that estrogen exhibits a sustained influence on the function of midbrain astrocytes through the stimulation of the MAP-kinase signaling pathway.[18] In this study, we can extend this predication because estrogen was found to regulate housekeeping genes in astroglial cells such as mitochondrial proteins/enzymes, but also cell surface antigens known to be important for the mediation of immune responses. This observation is in line with the well-established function of astroglia as a cellular mediator of estrogen-dependent neuroprotection in the CNS.[25–27] Concerning the cellular mechanisms involved in the regulation of astrocyte functionality in the midbrain by estradiol, our data clearly show that classical and nonclassical estrogen action is operating simultaneously in astrocytes. This is in accordance with the expression of nuclear estrogen receptors[25,28] and the presence of membrane-associated estrogen receptors as demonstrated by FACS analysis in our group (unpublished data) which are thought to be coupled to intracellular calcium- and MAP-kinase signaling.[12,18]

The duality of estrogen action in the midbrain is further underscored by the responsiveness of neurons. Again, our gene expression study reveals a considerable number of genes to be regulated differently by estrogen. Thus, early growth-regulating proteins, such as growth hormone and others, are downregulated; functional proteins ensuring neuronal performance and controlling cell activity, such as kinases and synthetic enzymes, as well as growth factors important for postnatal maturation such as BDNF and FGF-4, are upregulated. As described previously for astrocytes, estrogen and E-BSA appear to regulate different sets of genes in neurons and/or affect diverse neuronal populations differently. It is beyond the scope of this article to discuss in detail all genes differentially regulated. We rather focus on those associated with dopaminergic cell differentiation whereupon the observed estrogen-induced expression of BDNF and TH is of particular interest.[8,20] BDNF is a very important regulator not only of dopamine neuron development but also of dopamine neuron function.[29] Other studies in the past have also shown that estrogen is able to stimu late BDNF expression in the zebra finch forebrain[30] and in the rodent hippocampus.[31] Similarly, estradiol has been shown to increase TH expression in the rodent hypothalamus.[32] These two examples reveal the basic phenomenon that estrogen can directly interact with dopamine cells. It is also supported by the expression of estrogen receptors in this neuronal population,[5,23] which also controls neighboring cells providing differentiation-promoting signals to dopaminergic neurons. The regulation of TH expression in the midbrain (our study, in press[8]) and also in the locus coeruleus[33] occurs through the classical estrogen signaling mechanism that involves the activation of nuclear estrogen receptors. In contrast, estrogenic control of BDNF expression in the mouse midbrain as well as in the zebra finch forebrain[30] is due to nonclassical estrogen action and requires the activation of potential membrane estrogen receptors, which are coupled to distinct calcium-dependent, intracellular signaling pathways.[12,20] This clearly points out that nonclassical estrogen action is a more widespread phenomenon observed during brain development rather than an anomaly. A number of recent studies have analyzed estrogen-mediated control of gene expression in the developing CNS. They have revealed that estradiol controls the expression of several immediate early genes,such as *c-fos, c-jun,* and *jun-D* depending on the time intervals of steroid exposure.[34] In addition, nuclear RNA polymerase,[35] synapse-associated mRNAs,[36] growth hormone receptor mRNA,[37] and the proapoptotic protein Nip-2,[38] as well as the antiapoptotic proteins Bcl-2[39] and Bcl-xl,[40] represent further estrogen target genes in the developing brain. Our observations that estradiol is a pivotal regulator of growth factor supply, together with the data that estrogen positively interferes with intracellular death cascades, may form the basis for the observed neuroprotective function of this steroid hormone in the brain.[41]

In conclusion, we have presented evidence that estrogen triggers the expression of subsets of genes in developing mouse midbrain neurons and astrocytes. The high degree of complexity of estrogen action in the midbrain, however, involving different signaling systems and different target cells, makes it difficult at present to fully understand the developmental role of this steroid hormone. Nevertheless, it is safe to conclude that estrogen is crucial for the correct development and adult function of the nigrostriatal dopaminergic system.

ACKNOWLEDGMENTS

The authors acknowledge the technical assistance of G. Noack and N. Damm. This work was supported by the Deutsche Forschungsgemeinschaft (SFB 497).

REFERENCES

1. Beyer, C. 1999. Estrogen and the developing mammalian brain. Anat. Embryol. **199:** 379–390.
2. McEwen, B.S. 1992. Steroid hormones: effect on brain development and function. Horm. Res. **37:** 1–10.
3. Raab, H., C. Beyer, A. Wozniak, *et al.* 1995. Ontogeny of aromatase messenger ribonucleic acid and aromatase activity in the rat midbrain. Mol. Brain Res. **34:** 333–336.

4. RAAB, H., M. KAROLCZAK, I. REISERT & C. BEYER. 1999. Ontogenetic expression and splicing of estrogen receptor-α and -β mRNA in the rat midbrain. Neurosci. Lett. **275:** 21–24.
5. KRITZER, M.F. 1997. Selective colocalization of immunoreactivity for intracellular gonadal hormone receptors and tyrosine hydroxylase in the ventral tegmental area, substantia nigra and retrorubral fields in the rat. J. Comp. Neurol. **379:** 247–260
6. BEYER, C. & M. KAROLCZAK. 2000. Estrogenic stimulation of neurite growth in midbrain dopaminergic neurons depends on cAMP/protein kinase A signaling. J. Neurosci. Res. **59:** 107–116.
7. BEYER, C., C. PILGRIM & I. REISERT. 1991. Dopamine content and metabolism in mesencephalic and diencephalic cell cultures: sex differences and effects of sex steroids. J. Neurosci. **11:** 1325–1333.
8. IVANOVA, T. & C. BEYER. 2003. Estrogen regulates tyrosine hydroxylase expression in the neonate midbrain. J. Neurobiol. **54:** 638–647.
9. SIBUG, R., E. KÜPPERS, C. BEYER, *et al.* 1996. Genotype-dependent sex differentiation of dopaminergic neurons in primary cultures of embryonic mouse brain. Brain Res. **93:** 136–142.
10. SAWADA, H., M. IBI, T. KIHARA, *et al.* 2000. Mechanisms of antiapoptotic effects of estrogens in nigral dopaminergic neurons. FASEB J. **14:** 1202–1214.
11. CALLIER, S., M. LE SAUX, A.M. LHIAUBET, *et al.* 2002. Evaluation of the protective effect of oestradiol against toxicity induced by 6-hydroxydopamine and 1-methyl-4-phenylpyridinium ion (Mpp+) towards dopaminergic mesencephalic neurones in primary culture. J. Neurochem. **80:** 307–316.
12. BEYER, C. & H. RAAB. 1998. Nongenomic effects of estrogen: embryonic mouse midbrain neurons respond with a rapid release of calcium from intracellular stores. Eur. J. Neurosci. **10:** 255–262.
13. WANG, L., S. ANDERSSON, M. WARNER & J.-A. GUSTAFSSON. 2001. Morphological abnormalities in the brains of estrogen receptor β knockout mice. Proc. Natl. Acad. Sci. USA **98:** 2792–2796.
14. PILGRIM, C., C. BEYER & I. REISERT. 1999. The effects of sex and sex hormones on the development of dopaminergic neurons. *In* The Development of Dopaminergic Neurons. U. Di Porzio, R. Pernas-Alonso & C. Perrone-Capano, Eds.: 75–86. R.G. Landes. Austin, TX.
15. FALKENSTEIN, E., H.-C. TILLMANN, M. CHRIST, *et al.* 2000. Multiple actions of steroid hormones—a focus on rapid, nongenomic effects. Pharmacol. Rev. **52:** 513–555.
16. BEYER, C., T. IVANOVA, M. KAROLCZAK & E. KÜPPERS. 2002. Cell type-specificity of nonclassical estrogen signaling in the developing midbrain. J. Steroid Biochem. Mol. Biol. **81:** 319–325.
17. IVANOVA, T., P. MENDEZ, L.M. GARCIA-SEGURA & C. BEYER. 2002. Rapid stimulation of the PI3-kinase/Akt signaling pathway in developing midbrain neurones by oestrogen. J. Neuroendocrinol. **14:** 73–79.
18. IVANOVA, T., M. KAROLCZAK & C. BEYER. 2001. Estrogen stimulates the mitogen-activated protein kinase pathway in midbrain astroglia. Brain Res. **889:** 264–269.
19. IVANOVA, T., M. KAROLCZAK & C. BEYER. 2002. Estrogen stimulates GDNF expression in developing hypothalamic neurons. Endocrinology **143:** 3175–3178.
20. IVANOVA, T., M. KAROLCZAK, J. ENGELE & C. BEYER. 2001. Estrogen stimulates brain-derived neurotrophic factor expression in embryonic neurons through a membrane-mediated and calcium-dependent mechanism. J. Neurosci. Res. **66:** 221–230.
21. Küppers, E. & Beyer, C. 1999. Expression of estrogen receptor-a and –ß mRNA in the developing and adult mouse striatum. Neurosci. Lett. **276:** 95–98.
22. KÜPPERS, E. & C. BEYER. 1998. Expression of aromatase in the embryonic and postnatal mouse striatum. Mol. Brain. Res. **63:** 184–188.
23. CREUTZ, L.M. & M.F. KRITZER. 2002. Estrogen receptor-β immunoreactivity in the midbrain of adult rats: regional, subregional, and cellular localization in the A10, A9, and A8 dopamine cell groups. J. Comp. Neurol. **446:** 288–300.
24. LERANTH, C., R.H. ROTH, J.D. EISWORTH, *et al.* 2000. Estrogen is essential for maintaining nigrostriatal dopamine neurons in primates: implications for Parkinson's disease and memory. J. Neurosci. **20:** 8604–8609.

25. GARCIA-OVERJERO, D., S. VELGA, L.M. GARCIA-SEGURA & L.L. DONCARLOS. 2002. Glial expression of estrogen and androgen receptors after rat brain injury. J. Comp. Neurol. **450:** 256–271.
26. VIVIANI, B., E. CORSINI, M. BINAGLIA, *et al.* 2002. The anti-inflammatory activity of estrogen in glial cells is regulated by the PKC-anchoring protein RACK-1. J. Neurochem. **83:** 1180–1187.
27. DHANDAPANI, K.M. & D.W. BRANN. 2002. Estrogen-astrocyte interactions: implications for neuroprotection. BMC Neurosci. **3:** 6.
28. HÖSLI, E., K. JURASIN, W. RUHL, *et al.* 2001. Colocalization of estrogen and cholinergic receptors on cultured astrocytes of rat central nervous system. Int. J. Dev. Neurosci. **19:** 11–19.
29. HYMANN, C., M. HOFER, Y.A. BARDE, *et al.* 1991. BDNF is a neurotrophic factor for dopaminergic neurons of the substantia nigra. Nature **350:** 230–232.
30. DITTRICH, F., Y. FENG, R. METZDORF. & M. GAHR. 1999. Estrogen-inducible, sex-specific expression of brain-derived neurotrophic factor mRNA in a forebrain song control nucleus of juvenile zebra finch. Proc. Natl. Acad. Sci. USA **96:** 8241–8242.
31. SOLUM, D.T. & R.J. HANDA. 2002. Estrogen regulates the development of brain-derived neurotrophic factor mRNA and protein in the rat hippocampus. J. Neurosci. **22:** 2650–2659.
32. SIMERLY, R.B. 1989. Hormonal control of the development and regulation of tyrosine hydroxylase expression within a sexually dimorphic population of dopaminergic cells in the hypothalamus. Mol. Brain. Res. **6:** 297–310.
33. SEROVA, L., M. RIVKIN & E.L. SABBAN. 2002. Estradiol stimulates gene expression of norepinephrine biosynthetic enzymes in rat locus coeruleus. Neuroendocrinology **75:** 193–200.
34. SANTAGATI, S., Z.Q. MA, C. FERRARINI, *et al.* 1995. Expression of early genes in estrogen induced phenotypic conversion of neuroblastoma cells. J. Neuroendocrinol. **7:** 875–879.
35. PATNAIK, S.K. 1989. Evidence for estradiol-induced differential expression of genes for brain RNA polymerase during developmental stages of the rat. Biochem. Int. **18:** 721–729.
36. LUSTIG, R.H., P. HUA, M.C. WILSON & H.J. FEDEROFF. 1993. Ontogeny, sex dimorphism, and neonatal sex hormone determination of synapse-associated messenger RNAs in rat brain. Mol. Brain. Res. **20:** 101–110.
37. BENNETT, P.A., A. LEVY, D.F. CARMIGNAC, *et al.* 1996. Differential regulation of the growth hormone receptor gene: effects of dexamethasone and estradiol. Endocrinology **137:** 3891–3896.
38. GARNIER, M., D. DI LORENZO, A. ALBERTINI & A. MAGGI. 1997. Identification of estrogen-responsive genes in neuroblastoma SK-ER3 cells. J. Neurosci. **17:** 4591–4599.
39. ALKAYED, N.J., S. GOTO, N. SUGO, *et al.* 2001. Estrogen and bcl-2: gene induction and effect of transgene in experimental stroke. J. Neurosci. **21:** 7543–7550.
40. PIKE, C.J. 1999. Estrogen modulates neuronal Bcl-xl expression and beta-amyloid-induced apoptosis: relevance to Alzheimer's disease. J. Neurochem. **21:** 1552–1563.
41. KAJTA, M. & C. BEYER. 2003. Cellular strategies of estrogen-mediated neuroprotection during brain development. Endocrine **21:** 3–9.

Conditional Regulation of Neurosteroid Sensitivity of $GABA_A$ Receptors

ARJEN B. BRUSSAARD AND JAN-JURJEN KOKSMA

Department of Experimental Neurophysiology, Research Institute for Neurosciences, Faculty of Earth and Life Sciences, Vrije Universiteit Amsterdam, 1081 HV Amsterdam, the Netherlands

ABSTRACT: Nongenomic gonadal steroid feedback to oxytocin containing neurons in the supraoptic nucleus of the hypothalamus is mediated via the neurosteroid allopregnanolone (3α-OH-DHP) that acts as an allosteric modulator of the postsynaptic $GABA_A$ receptors. We found evidence to support the idea that neurosteroids not only potentiate $GABA_A$ receptor function but also prevent its suppression by PKC. In addition, we found that neurosteroid sensitivity of $GABA_A$ receptor itself is dependent on the balance between endogenous phosphatase and PKC activity and not, as previously suggested, on subunit composition changes of the $GABA_A$ receptor. These data imply that native $GABA_A$ receptors are only sensitive to 3α-OH-DHP if there is endogenous phosphatase activity. In contrast, when, due to endogenous release of oxytocin in the hypothalamus, the intracellular balance is shifted from high phosphatase activity toward a higher level of PKC-dependent phosphorylation, this leads to 3α-OH-DHP–insensitivity of the $GABA_A$ receptors. How the regulatory mechanisms of the $GABA_A$ receptor physiology for the hypothalamus may also account for alterations in GABA transmission observed in other brain areas is discussed.

KEYWORDS: $GABA_A$ receptor; lactation; parturition; synaptic plasticity; oxytocin; progesterone-metabolite; allopregnanolone; PKC; phosphatases

INTRODUCTION

The neurosteroid allopregnanolone (3α-OH-DHP) is a potent endogenous allosteric modulator of $GABA_A$ receptors[1–3] that acts via a specific binding-domain.[4,5] The neurosteroid allopregnanolone (3α-OH-DHP) is the most potent endogenous allosteric modulator of $GABA_A$ receptors and produces a benzodiazepine-like effect on the receptor's activity.[2] While desensitization of the postsynaptic GABA receptor channels can keep the receptor protein in an agonist-bound state, thereby slowing the rate of final ion-channel closure during the synaptic decay,[6] neurosteroids, by an effect on the recovery of the $GABA_A$ receptor from the desensitized state, may pro-

Address for correspondence: Prof. Dr. A.B. Brussaard, Department of Experimental Neurophysiology, Vrije Universiteit Amsterdam, de Boelelaan 1085,1081 HV Amsterdam, the Netherlands. Voice: +31 20 444 7098; fax: + 31 20 444 7112.
brssrd@cncr.vu.nl

Ann. N.Y. Acad. Sci. 1007: 29–36 (2003).
doi: 10.1196/annals.1286.003

long synaptic currents even further.[7] Variation in the efficacy of neurosteroids to modulate $GABA_A$ receptors, as observed in different types of neurons,[8–12] may arise from differences in subunit composition of the $GABA_A$ receptors. However, previous attempts to identify the specific $GABA_A$ receptor subunits that mediate neurosteroid effects did not give rise to an adequate explanation for the apparent correlation between diversity in receptor subtype and neurosteroid sensitivity.[9,10,13–18] Moreover, recent studies indicate that phosphorylation may affect neurosteroid modulation of recombinant[19] and native $GABA_A$ receptors.[20]

Using the oxytocin neurons in the supraoptic nucleus during the female reproduction cycle as a model, we aimed to explain the endogenous shift between different modes of neurosteroid sensitivity of $GABA_A$ receptor activity.[1,10–11] As argued, the shift in neurosteroid sensitivity is nongenomic and conditionally regulated by the cells expressing the $GABA_A$ receptors.[2]

GABA Regulates Oxytocin Neuron Activity

$GABA_A$ receptor signaling exerts powerful, reproductive state–specific effects on the functioning of oxytocin neurons. Approximately one-half of all axosomatic and axodendritic synapses on oxytocin neurons are GABAergic in nature, and essentially all spontaneous inhibitory postsynaptic currents (sIPSCs) in these cells arise through activation of the $GABA_A$ receptor. The $GABA_A$ receptors are composed of pentameric combinations of α1 and/or α2, β2 and/or β3, and γ2 subunits of the $GABA_A$ receptor. In late pregnancy, GABA input appears to prevent massive increases in oxytocin firing *in vitro*, and oxytocin secretion *in vivo*.[10] Further studies undertaken *in vivo* have highlighted the importance of $GABA_A$ receptor activation in enabling oxytocin neurons to exhibit intermittent high-frequency-bursting behaviours during lactation.[21]

$GABA_A$ Receptor Subunit Switching Affects Synaptic Current Decay

Long-term plasticity of postsynaptic $GABA_A$ receptors results from alterations in the subunit composition of these receptors expressed by oxytocin neurons.[21] In particular, it was found that the gene expression of the α1 subunit was elevated during the course of pregnancy, such that peak levels were obtained on day 19 of pregnancy and that cellular mRNA levels then declined precipitously over the final two days of pregnancy, before the onset of parturition. Electrophysiological analysis over the last two days of pregnancy revealed that this change in α1 subunit expression correlated with the presence of $GABA_A$ receptors displaying distinct pharmacological properties. In late pregnancy, the α1 subunit–dominant $GABA_A$ receptor subtype is characterized by a relatively short duration of the synaptic current that is prolonged by 3α-OH-DHP. In contrast, two days later at the time of parturition, the $GABA_A$ receptor subtype changes to one with a somewhat slower synaptic current duration,[10] and this isoform persists throughout subsequent lactation.[11] More importantly, however, correlated to this subunit switch, a change occurs in neurosteroid sensitivity of the $GABA_A$ receptors found in these cells; upon parturition the $GABA_A$ receptors were found to be markedly less sensitive to 3α-OH-DHP compared to during pregnancy.[10]

Unresolved Issues in $GABA_A$ Receptor Regulation

However, at that point, it was left unanswered what the causal relationship was between $GABA_A$ receptor subunit switching and alterations in short-term modulation of this receptor type by allosteric or metabotropic modulators.[21] We found previously that allosteric interaction between the extracellular 3α-OH-DHP molecules and the $GABA_A$ receptor clearly affects the intracellular signal transduction routes of receptor regulation.[1] However, it was unclear whether the reverse was true—that is, whether changes in intracellular signal transduction cascades might also affect neurosteroid sensitivity of $GABA_A$ receptors.

Neurosteroid sensitivity of $GABA_A$ receptors may differ in different brain areas,[22–24] suggesting a relation with receptor subunit composition. Indeed, *in vitro* expression studies indicated that $GABA_A$ receptor subunit composition determines neurosteroid sensitivity.[4,15,25] However, most subunit combinations of this receptor are sensitive to the allosteric effect of neurosteroids,[4] and conflicting data remain on the few subunits that have been implicated in reducing neurosteroid sensitivity of $GABA_A$ receptors.[9,16,17,26] In our laboratory, we found that $GABA_A$ receptors in the oxytocin neurons of WT mice and α1 –/– mice are equally sensitive to potentiation by 3α-OH-DHP.[2] Thus, in mouse oxytocin neurons, the α1 subunit was not required for allosteric modulation of $GABA_A$ receptors in oxytocin neurons by 3α-OH-DHP.

Hence, we hypothesized that an alternative mechanism must regulate neurosteroid sensitivity of $GABA_A$ receptors in oxytocin neurons, i.e., posttranslational modification of $GABA_A$ receptor. The causal relationships between neurosteroid regulation of $GABA_A$ receptors and putative endogenous, and oxytocin neuron-specific shifts in the balance of protein kinase and phosphatase activity, were investigated in detail to find support for this idea.

Conditional Expression of Neurosteroid-Insensitive $GABA_A$ Receptors

The postsynaptic $GABA_A$ receptors in oxytocin neurons are susceptible to allosteric modulation by 3α-OH-DHP during some stages of the female reproductive cycle, in particular during pregnancy.[11] In late pregnancy in mammals, the endogenous levels of progesterone, and consequently those of 3α-OH-DHP, are very high. These high concentrations of progesterone are maintained until term, when progesterone levels show an abrupt fall.[27] The concentration of progesterone increases again during lactation. The levels of 3α-OH-DHP in the brain follow the changes in progesterone.

As reported and reviewed previously, the increasing levels of circulating 3α-OH-DHP with advancing pregnancy[27] strongly potentiate the overall synaptic efficacy of the GABA input (by around 40%), in particular by directly increasing the sIPSC decay time constant.[21] This implies that neurosteroid potentiation of postsynaptic receptor activity is a predominant factor in the alteration of the impact of the GABA input observed during pregnancy. This marked increase in synaptic inhibition underlies the potent tonic restraining influence of the GABAergic input upon oxytocin neuron firing in late pregnancy and provides oxytocin neurons with a powerful safety switch to prevent premature release of oxytocin.

It was also shown that around the time of parturition $GABA_A$ receptors in oxytocin neurons become insensitive to modulation by 3α-OH-DHP.[10] The issue at hand then was how does such change comes about. In other words, what was the mechanism underlying the change in functional expression toward 3α-OH-DHP-insensitive $GABA_A$ receptors by oxytocin neurons around that time?

What Regulates Neurosteroid Sensitivity of $GABA_A$ Receptors?

We found that the endogenous $GABA_A$ receptor sensitivity to 3α-OH-DHP in oxytocin neurons during late pregnancy is brought about by an endogenously regulated constitutively high level of phosphatase activity, and can be suppressed temporarily by inducing a shift toward a relatively higher level of activity of PKC.[2] And, *vice versa*, after parturition, when $GABA_A$ receptors are insensitive to neurosteroids in these cells, both inhibition of PKC and stimulation of Ca^{2+}-dependent phosphatase 2A restored the 3α-OH-DHP sensitivity. We therefore propose that phosphatases and PKC have a converging effect, possibly acting on the same serine/threonine residue of one of the non-α $GABA_A$ receptor subunits.[28] Alternatively, PKC and phosphatases could also act on different phosphorylation sites or on other proteins of the postsynaptic density of the GABA synapse, including receptor-interacting and receptor-clustering proteins like gephyrin[29] and/or phosphatase-targeting proteins like spinophilin.[30]

This phosphorylation-dependent regulation of the effect of an allosteric modulator is distinct from direct effects of phosphorylation of residues of β and γ subunit on $GABA_A$ receptor channel desensitization properties.[31] We did not observe in oxytocin neurons any direct effect on sIPSC decay time constants of alteration in protein kinase or phosphatase activity, such as that reported for hippocampal neurons.[6,32]

The most conclusive evidence of the physiological significance of our thesis is that the shift toward higher levels of PKC activity may be explained by endogenous activation of oxytocin autoreceptors upon parturition,[2] i.e., in lactating females that normally display 3α-OH-DHP resistance of their $GABA_A$ receptors, we were able to restore receptor-sensitivity to this neurosteroid by pretreating the oxytocin neurons with an oxytocin antagonist.

Neurosteroid Modulation of $GABA_A$ Receptor Function

In summary, PKC and 3α-OH-DHP have distinct effects on the $GABA_A$ receptor, and these effects are mutually exclusive. Our current working model of how this bidirectional interaction between allosteric and metabotropic receptor modulation could be brought about at the level of the transmembrane receptor protein is shown in FIGURE 1. For simplicity, we have excluded receptor interaction (postsynaptic density) proteins that may also be phosphorylated and/or dephosphorylated to mediate the alterations in receptor function.

We propose that neurosteroid sensitivity of $GABA_A$ receptors in oxytocin neurons can be manipulated both by alterations in phosphatase and PKC activity.[2] Phosphatases and PKC converge onto the same site of action, possibly a phosphorylation site of the γ2 or the β2 subunit receptor subunits that are expressed in oxytocin neurons. In such a scenario, neurosteroid binding to the receptor prevents the intracellular action of PKC,[1] whereas the neurosteroid binding site of the $GABA_A$ receptor is only exposed if the receptor is dephosphorylated by phosphatases.

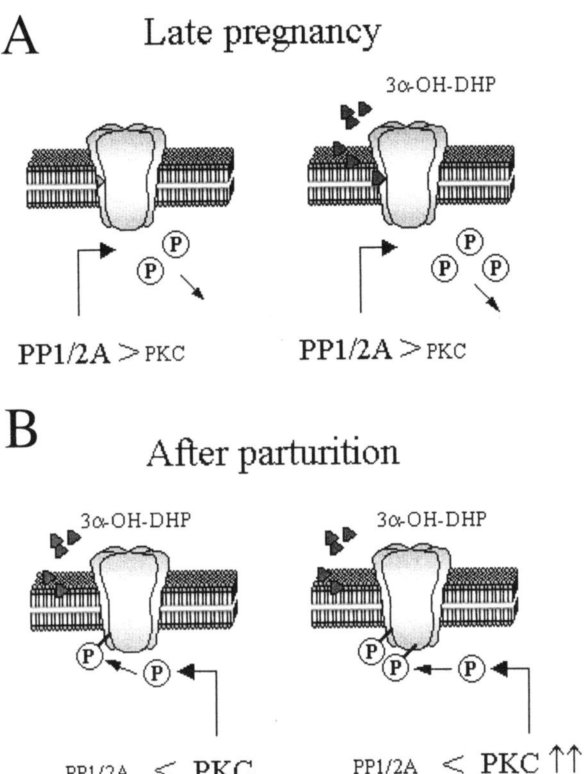

FIGURE 1. Receptor model for bidirectional interaction between PKC and 3α-OH-DHP. (**A**) When the balance between phosphatase and PKC activity is in the direction of dephosphorylation, $GABA_A$ receptors are susceptible to 3α-OH-DHP modulation. When 3α-OH-DHP is bound to the receptor, PKC can no longer affect the $GABA_A$ receptor activity. (**B**) When the balance is shifted toward higher levels of PKC activity, phosphorylation of the receptor affects the receptor in such a way that the binding site for 3α-OH-DHP is no longer exposed, or 3α-OH-DHP is no longer able to alter receptor properties.

Thus, neurosteroids not only prolong the synaptic current decay of $GABA_A$ receptor–mediated events, but also prevent subsequent metabotropic modulation by oxytocin autoreceptor activation within oxytocin neurons. However, the neurosteroid modulation of $GABA_A$ receptors itself in turn depends on the endogenous balance between Ca^{2+}-dependent phosphatase and protein kinase C activity. This type of nongenomic modulatory regulation may occur in a brain area–specific manner during particular periods of the behavioral physiology (e.g., pregnancy, stress, premenstrual syndrome). To elaborate further on this idea, it is noted that the type of conditional regulatory mechanism of $GABA_A$ receptor function described here is reminiscent of reports on $GABA_A$ receptors in transgenic mice lacking the PKC γ isomer in which alcohol sensitivity was affected[33] and in transgenic mice lacking

PKC ε isomer, being supersensitive to neurosteroids, as well as other allosteric modulators of the $GABA_A$ receptor, including alcohol.[34,35] It cannot be excluded that neurosteroids, in addition to their allosteric interaction with the $GABA_A$ recepors, play some role in translocation of particular PKC isomers toward the membrane, which in turn would affect the neurosteroid sensitivity of $GABA_A$ receptors being expressed. However, all available evidence argues in favor of a simple model as being the most parsimonious one (FIG. 1): neurosteroid sensitivity affects $GABA_A$ receptors in a bidirectional manner being dependent on but also affecting the metabotropic modulation of $GABA_A$ receptors. Because there appears to be no receptor-subunit specificity, we argue that this model presents a general concept that (a) also occurs in other brain areas and (b) one which neurosteroids and other allosteric modulators might have in common. If so, this implies that we have to look for novel routes of how to design mood-affecting agents. Indeed, since allopregnanolone is among the most potent neurosteroids currently known, its enhancing effects on $GABA_A$ receptor-mediated currents have already led to the development of related compounds for use as improved anxiolytic drugs with a reduced risk of tolerance as an alternative to benzodiazepines.[36] Modulation of the brain $GABA_A$ receptors by endogenous and, perhaps in the future, exogenous neurosteroids may affect a myriad of phenomena, such as memory, stress, anxiety, sleep, depression, seizures, and more.[37]

REFERENCES

1. BRUSSAARD, A.B., J. WOSSINK, J.C. LODDER & K.S. KITS. 2000. Progesterone-metabolite prevents protein kinase C-dependent modulation of gamma-aminobutyric acid type A receptors in oxytocin neurons. Proc. Natl. Acad. Sci. USA **97:** 3625–3630.
2. KOKSMA, J.-J., R.E. VAN KESTEREN, T.W. ROSAHL, *et al.* 2003. Oxytocin regulates neurosteroid modulation of $GABA_A$ receptors in supraoptic nucleus around parturition. J. Neurosci. **23:** 788–797.
3. TWYMAN, R.E. & R.L. MACDONALD. 1992. Neurosteroid regulation of $GABA_A$ receptor single-channel kinetic properties of mouse spinal cord neurons in culture. J. Physiol. **456:** 215–245.
4. TURNER, D.M., R.W. RANSOM, J.S. YANG & R.W. OLSEN. 1989. Steroid anesthetics and naturally occurring analogs modulate the γ-aminobutyric acid receptor complex at a site distinct from barbiturates. J. Pharmacol. Exp. Ther. **248:** 960–966.
5. LAMBERT, J.J., D. BELELLI, C. HILL-VENNING & J.A. PETERS. 1995. Neurosteroids and $GABA_A$ receptor function. Trends Pharmacol. Sci. **16:** 295–303.
6. JONES, M.V. & G.L. WESTBROOK. 1995. Desensitized states prolong $GABA_A$ channel responses to brief agonist pulses. Neuron **15:** 181–191.
7. ZHU, W.J. & S. VICINI. 1997. Neurosteroid prolongs $GABA_A$ channel deactivation by altering kinetics of desensitized states. J. Neurosci. **17:** 4022–4031.
8. HARRISON, N.L., S. VICINI & J.L. BARKER. 1987. A steroid anesthetic prolongs inhibitory postsynaptic currents in cultured rat hippocampal neurons. J. Neurosci. **7:** 604–609.
9. ZHU, W.J., J.F. WANG, K.E. KRUEGER & S. VICINI. 1996. δ subunit inhibits neurosteroid modulation of $GABA_A$ receptors. J. Neurosci. **16:** 6648–6656.
10. BRUSSAARD, A.B., K.S. KITS, R.E. BAKER, *et al.* 1997 Plasticity in fast synaptic inhibition of adult oxytocin neurons caused by switch in $GABA_A$ receptor subunit expression. Neuron **19:** 1103–1114.
11. BRUSSAARD, A.B., P. DEVAY, J.L. LEYTING-VERMEULEN & K.S. KITS. 1999. Changes in properties and neurosteroid regulation of GABAergic synapses in the supraoptic nucleus during the mammalian female reproductive cyle. J. Physiol. **516:** 513–524.

12. COOPER, E.J., G.A.R. JOHNSTON & F.A. EDWARDS. 1999. Effects of a naturally occurring neurosteroid on $GABA_A$ IPSCs during development in rat hippocampal or cerebellar slices. J. Physiol. **521:** 437–449.
13. THOMPSON, S.A., T.P. BONNERT, E. CAGETTI, *et al.* 2002. Overexpression of the $GABA_A$ receptor ε subunit results in insensitivity to anaesthetics. Neuropharmacology **43:** 662–668.
14. WOHLFARTH, K.M., M.T. BIANCHI & R.L. MACDONALD. 2002. Enhanced neurosteroid potentiation of ternary $GABA_A$ receptors containing the δ subunit. J. Neurosci. **22:** 1541–1549.
15. BELELLI, D., A. CASULA, A. LING & J.J. LAMBERT. 2002. The influence of subunit composition on the interaction of neurosteroids with $GABA_A$ receptors. Neuropharmacology **43:** 651–661.
16. DAVIES, P.A., M.C. HANNA, T.G. HALES & E.F. KIRKNESS. 1997. Insensitivity to anaesthetic agents conferred by a class of $GABA_A$ receptor subunit. Nature **385:** 820–823.
17. SMITH, S.S., Q.H. GONG, F.C. HSU, *et al.* 1998. $GABA_A$ receptor α4 subunit suppression prevents withdrawal properties of an endogenous steroid. Nature **392:** 926–930.
18. SMITH, S.S., Q.H. GONG, X. LI, *et al.* 1998. Withdrawal from 3α-OH-5α-pregnan-20-one using a pseudopregnancy model alters the kinetics of hippocampal $GABA_A$-gated current and increases the $GABA_A$ receptor α4 subunit in association with increased anxiety. J. Neurosci. **18:** 5275–5284.
19. LEIDENHEIMER, N.J., S.J. MCQUILKIN, L.D. HAHNER, *et al.* 1992. Activation of protein kinase C selectively inhibits the γ-aminobutyric acidA receptor: role of desensitization. Mol. Pharmacol. **41:** 1116–1123.
20. FANCSIK, A., D.M. LINN & J.G. TASKER. 2000. Neurosteroid modulation of GABA IPSCs is phosphorylation dependent. J. Neurosci. **20:** 3067–3075.
21. BRUSSAARD, A.B. & A.E. HERBISON. 2000. Long-term plasticity of postsynaptic $GABA_A$ receptor function in the adult brain: insights from the oxytocin neurone. Trends Neurosci. **23:** 190–195.
22. NGUYEN, Q., D.W. VAN SAPP, P.C. NESS & R.W. OLSEN. 1995. Modulation of $GABA_A$ receptor binding in human brain by neuroactive steroids: species and brain regional differences. Synapse **19:** 77–87.
23. POISBEAU, P., P. FELZ & R. SCHLICHTER. 1997. Modulation of $GABA_A$ receptor-mediated IPSCs by neuroactive steroids in a rat hypothalamo-hypophyseal coculture model. J. Physiol. **500:** 475–485.
24. COOPER, E.J., G.A.R. JOHNSTON & F.A. EDWARDS. 1999. Effects of a naturally occurring neurosteroid on $GABA_A$ IPSCs during development in rat hippocampal or cerebellar slices. J. Physiol. **521:** 437–449.
25. PUIA, G., M.R. SANTI, S. VICINI, *et al.* 1990. Neurosteroids act on recombinant human GABAA receptors. Neuron 4: 759–765.
26. WHITING, P.J., G. MCALLISTER, D. VASSILATIS, *et al.* 1997. Neuronally restricted RNA splicing regulates the expression of a novel $GABA_A$ receptor subunit conferring atypical functional properties. J. Neurosci. **17:** 5027–5037.
27. CONCAS, A., M.C. MOSTALLINO, P. PORCU, *et al.* 1998. Role of brain allopregnanolone in the plasticity of γ-aminobutyric acid type A receptor in rat brain during pregnancy and after delivery. Proc. Natl. Acad. Sci. U.S.A. **95:** 13284–13289.
28. MCDONALD, B.J. & S.J. MOSS. 1997. Conserved phosphorylation of the intracellular domains of $GABA_A$ receptor β2 and β3 subunits by cAMP-dependent protein kinase cGMP-dependent protein kinase protein kinase C and Ca^{2+}/calmodulin type II-dependent protein kinase. Neuropharmacology **36:** 1377–1385.
29. KNEUSSEL, M., J.H. BRANDSTATTER, B. GASNIER, *et al.* 2001. Gephyrin-independent clustering of postsynaptic $GABA_A$ receptor subtypes. Mol. Cell. Neurosci. **17:** 973–982.
30. HSIEH-WILSON, L.C., P.B. ALLEN, T. WATANABE, *et al.* 1999. Characterization of the neuronal targeting protein spinophilin and its interactions with protein phosphatase-1. Biochemistry **38:** 4365–4373.
31. KRISHEK, B.J., X. XIE, C. BLACKSTONE, *et al.* 1994. Regulation of $GABA_A$ receptor function by protein kinase C phosphorylation. Neuron **12:** 1081–1095.

32. Poisbeau, P., M.C. Cheney, M.D. Browning & I. Mody. 1999. Modulation of synaptic $GABA_A$ receptor function by PKA and PKC in adult hippocampal neurons. J. Neurosci. **19:** 674–683.
33. Harris, R.A., S.J. McQuilkin, R. Paylor, *et al.* 1995. Mutant mice lacking the γ isoform of protein kinase C show decreased behavioral actions of ethanol and altered function of γ-aminobutyrate type A receptors. Proc. Natl. Acad. Sci. USA **92:** 3658–3662.
34. Hodge, C.W., K.K. Mehmert, S.P. Kelley, *et al.* 1999. Supersensitivity to allosteric $GABA_A$ receptor modulators and alcohol in mice lacking PKCe. Nat. Neurosci. **2:** 997–1002.
35. Hodge, C.W., J. Raber, T. McMahon, *et al.* 2002. Decreased anxiety-like behavior, reduced stress hormones, and neurosteroid supersensitivity in mice lacking protein kinase C epsilon. J. Clin. Invest. **110:** 1003–1010.
36. Rupprecht, R. & F. Holsboer. 1999. Neuropsychopharmacological properties of neuroactive steroids. Steroids **64:** 83–91.
37. Majewska, M.D. 1992. Neurosteroids: endogenous bimodal modulators of the $GABA_A$ receptor. Mechanism of action and physiological significance. Prog. Neurobiol. **38:** 379–385.

Fluoxetine May Influence Lordosis of Rats through Effects on Midbrain 3α,5α-THP Concentrations

CHERYL A. FRYE,[a–c] SANDRA M. PETRALIA,[a] MADELINE E. RHODES,[a] AND BENJAMIN STEIN[a–c]

Departments of [a]Psychology, [b]Biological Sciences, and [c]The Center for Neuroscience Research, The University at Albany—State University of New York, 1400 Washington Avenue, Albany, New York 12222, USA

ABSTRACT: 5α-pregnan-3α-ol-20-one (3α,5α-THP) in the ventral tegmental area (VTA) mediates lordosis of rodents. If fluoxetine's effects on lordosis are mediated in part by midbrain 3α,5α-THP, then fluoxetine regimens that decrease and increase lordosis would be expected to respectively lower and elevate midbrain 3α,5α-THP levels. *Experiment 1:* Ovariectomized (ovx) rats received estradiol benzoate (EB; 5 μg, SC) at 0 and 24 h and fluoxetine (20 mg/kg, IP) or vehicle 30 min before sex testing and tissue collection. Other rats received fluoxetine (10 mg/kg, IP) or vehicle for 15 days followed by EB-priming and testing. Systemic acute or chronic fluoxetine significantly decreased lordosis and midbrain 3α,5α-THP levels compared to vehicle. *Experiment 2:* Ovx rats with unilateral cannula to the VTA were primed with EB (5 μg; 0, 24 h) and/or progesterone (0 or 100 μg; 44 h, SC). At 47.5 h, fluoxetine (3.6 μM) or vehicle was infused to the VTA. At 48 h, rats were tested. Administering fluoxetine to the VTA significantly increased lordosis and midbrain 3α,5α-THP levels compared to vehicle infusions. *Experiment 3:* Ovx EB-primed rats were tested prior to, and 30 min after, treatmemt with acute fluoxetine (20 mg/kg, IP). Rats were then infused with 3α,5α-THP (100 ng) or vehicle to the VTA and were retested. 3α,5α-THP, but not vehicle, to the VTA reversed acute fluoxetine's inhibitory effects on lordosis. Together, these data suggest fluoxetine may alter lordosis in part through actions of 3α-THP in the midbrain.

KEYWORDS: Nongenomic; neurosteroid; allopreganolone; 5α-pregnane-3α-ol-20-one; lordosis; progesterone; fluoxetine; depression; affect

INTRODUCTION

Progestins in the midbrain vental tegmental area (VTA) mediate lordosis, a behavior indicative of sexual receptivity of female rodents.[1] Administration of progesterone (P) to the VTA of ovariectomized (ovx), estradiol benzoate (EB)-primed rats, reliably facilitates lordosis.[1–2] Few intracellular progestin receptors (PRs) have been

Address for correspondence: Cheryl A. Frye, Ph.D., Department of Psychology, The University at Albany-SUNY, 1400 Washington Avenue, Albany, NY 12222. Voice: 518-442-4836; fax: 518-442-4867.
cafrye@cnsunix.albany.edu

Ann. N.Y. Acad. Sci. 1007: 37–41 (2003).
doi: 10.1196/annals.1286.004

localized to the VTA.[1,3] PR blockers infused to the VTA do not alter P-facilitated lordosis.[1] Further, progestins' affinity for PRs does not correspond to their facilitation of lordosis when applied to the VTA.[4] Thus, an important question that our laboratory has been investigating is how P has effects in the VTA for lordosis independent of actions at PRs.

Progesterone's actions in the VTA for facilitation of lordosis may involve its metabolite, 5α-pregnan-3α-ol-20-one (3α,5α-THP). Although circulating and midbrain P and 3α,5α-THP levels are significantly higher among receptive compared to nonreceptive rodents,[5–6] there is a stronger linear correlation between central 3α,5α-THP, rather than P, levels and lordosis.[7] Administration of 3α,5α-THP to the VTA is much more effective than is P itself at facilitating lordosis.[4]

Progesterone's actions in the VTA to facilitate lordosis may involve its metabolism to 3α,5α-THP. In the VTA, P is readily metabolized to dihydroprogesterone (DHP) through activity of the 5α-reductase enzyme, localized to this region.[1,8,9] DHP is then converted to 3α,5α-THP, and 3α,5α-THP can also be oxidized back to DHP through actions of the 3α-hydroxysteroid dehydrogenase (3α-HSD) enzyme in the midbrain VTA. [1,8,9] Inhibitors of 5α-reductase or 3α-HSD to the VTA of naturally receptive or hormone-primed rodents decrease sexual responses and midbrain 3α,5α-THP levels.[1] Thus, inhibiting P's metabolism to 3α,5α-THP in the VTA attenuates sexual receptivity.

Fluoxetine, a selective serotonin reuptake inhibitor (SSRI), can alter lordosis of rodents and may do so in part through effects on 3α,5α-THP levels. Acute (20 mg/kg, IP) or chronic (10 mg/kg, IP for 3 weeks) administration of fluoxetine decreases lordosis of naturally receptive rats or hamsters or hormone-primed rats.[10, 11] Fluoxetine can also alter synthesis of central 3α,5α-THP by shifting the enzymatic activity of 3α-HSD from the oxidative pathway that produces DHP toward the reductive pathway that produces 3α,5α-THP.[12] Because 3α,5α-THP levels in the VTA seem to have an important influence on lordosis of rodents, we investigated effects of fluoxetine on lordosis *and* midbrain 3α,5α-THP levels. We hypothesized that if fluoxetine's effects on lordosis are mediated by midbrain 3α,5α-THP levels, then fluoxetine dosing that decreases lordosis would reduce midbrain 3α,5α-THP levels, and fluoxetine regimen that enhances lordosis would elevate midbrain 3α,5α-THP levels.

METHODS

Adult, female Long-Evans rats were ovx and EB-primed (5 μg SC) at 0 and 24 h. All rats were tested for the incidence (LQ, % score) and intensity (LR on a four-point scale) of lordosis with a stimulus male. Immediately following testing, experimental female rats from experiments 1 and 2 were killed, and their midbrains rapidly dissected on ice. Tissues were stored at –70°C. 3α,5α-THP was measured according to previously published methods.[5–7]

Experiment 1. Rats were randomly assigned to one of three conditions. Some rats received acute systemic fluoxetine (20 mg/kg; IP) 30 min before testing. Other rats received chronic fluoxetine (10 mg/kg; IP for 15 days) and were tested 2 days later. The control condition involved acute or chronic injections of vehicle (saline; IP).

Experiment 2. Rats had unilateral guide cannula to the VTA and were EB-primed (5 μg SC) at 0 and 24 h. Half of the rats received systemic P (100 μg at 44 h). Within the EB-only and EB and P-primed groups, half of the rats received intra-VTA fluoxetine (3.6 μM) and the others received vehicle infusions 30 min prior to testing.

Experiment 3. Ovx rats with unilateral cannula to the VTA were EB-primed (5 μg SC) at 0 and 24 h and pretested for lordosis at 44 h. Rats were then administered fluoxetine (20 mg/kg; IP) and retested for sexual receptivity 30 min later. This was followed by an infusion to the VTA either of 3α,5α-THP (100 ng) or vehicle and retesting for sexual receptivity.

RESULTS

Experiment 1. Acute or chronic systemic fluoxetine significantly *reduced* LQs, LRs, and midbrain 3α,5α-THP levels, compared to vehicle administration to ovx, EB-primed rats. Control rats had mean LQs of 91 ± 2%, LRs of 2.1 ± 0.1, and midbrain 3α,5α-THP levels of 3.2 ± 0.6 ng/g. Acute fluoxetine significantly lowered LQs (48 ± 10%), LRs (0.7 ± 0.2), and midbrain 3α,5α-THP levels (1.2 ± 0.2 ng/g). Chronic fluoxetine also significantly decreased LQs (76 ± 12%), LRs (1.5 ± 0.8), and midbrain 3α,5α-THP levels (1.8 ± 0.3 ng/g), although not to the extent of acute fluoxetine.

Experiment 2. Intra-VTA infusions of fluoxetine to EB or EB and P-primed rats, significantly *increased* LQs, LRs, and midbrain 3α,5α-THP levels compared to vehicle infusions. EB-primed rats infused with vehicle had LQs of 38 ± 9%, LRs of 0.6 ± 0.2, and midbrain 3α,5α-THP levels of 2.4 ± 0.4 ng/g, which were increased to 54 ± 8%, 1.0 ± 0.2, and 3.8 ± 0.7 ng/g following infusions of fluoxetine. The same effect was observed in EB and P-primed rats, which had LQs of 43 ± 8%, LRs of 0.8 ± 0.2, and midbrain 3α,5α-THP levels of 5.7 ± 0.6 ng/g following infusions of vehicle. Fluoxetine infusions to EB and P-primed rats increased LQs to 76 ± 6%, LRs to 1.8 ± 0.2, and midbrain 3α,5α-THP levels to 6.8 ± 1.1 ng/g.

Experiment 3. Infusions of 3α,5α-THP to the VTA of rats reinstated lordosis that had been decreased by acute dosing with systemic fluoxetine. Pre-fluoxetine LQs and LRs of EB-primed rats were 62 ± 5% and 0.8 ± 0.3, respectively. Acute dosing with fluoxetine (20 mg/kg; IP) significantly reduced LQs (20 ± 7%) and LRs (0.3 ± 0.1) compared to their pretest levels. Infusions of 3α,5α-THP to the VTA reinstated LQs (84 ± 6%) and LRs (1.9 ± 0.2) to levels above that observed on the pretest, whereas infusions of vehicle did not (LQs: 28 ± 6%; LRs: 0.5 ± 0.1).

DISCUSSION

The hypothesis that fluoxetine's effects on sexual behavior were due in part to altering 3α,5α-THP levels in the midbrain VTA was supported by the data. Acute or chronic systemic administration of fluoxetine decreased the incidence and intensity of lordosis of female rats and decreased levels of 3α,5α-THP in the midbrain. Infusions of 3.6 μM fluoxetine to the VTA significantly increased the incidence and intensity of lordosis and elevated levels of midbrain 3α,5α-THP compared to rats that received vehicle. Notably, infusions of 3α,5α-THP to the VTA reinstated lordosis of rats that had decreased sexual receptivity due to acute, systemic fluoxetine dosing. These data suggest fluoxetine's effects on lordosis may be in part due to 3α,5α-THP's actions in the midbrain VTA.

These data confirm and extend previous reports of 3α,5α-THP and fluoxetine's effects on lordosis in three important ways. First, 3α,5α-THP levels in the midbrain VTA influence lordosis. Naturally receptive and mated rats have higher midbrain 3α,5α-THP levels than do nonreceptive rats.[5–6] 3α,5α-THP is the most effective progestin in facilitating lordosis when applied to the VTA of rodents.[4] Inhibiting or enhancing P's metabolism to 3α,5α-THP in the VTA respectively decreases and increases lordosis.[1] The present results extend these findings to demonstrate that a therapeutic drug, fluoxetine, can alter lordosis due to effects on midbrain 3α,5α-THP levels. Second, results of experiment 1 confirm findings of prior studies using systemic fluoxetine which found that lordosis was decreased among naturally receptive rats or hamsters or hormone-primed rats.[10–11] Results of experiments 2 and 3 extend these findings to show that central fluoxetine can have effects opposite to those of systemic fluoxetine. Third, prior *in vitro* studies demonstrated that fluoxetine can enhance synthesis of central 3α,5α-THP by shifting the enzymatic activity of 3α-HSD away from the oxidative pathway that produces DHP and toward the reductive pathway that produces 3α,5α-THP.[12] Our results, like those of previous *in vivo* studies, confirm that fluoxetine can either increase or decrease 3α,5α-THP production depending on the regimen used.[13–15]

There are several important implications of the findings that fluoxetine's effects on lordosis may be associated with midbrain 3α,5α-THP levels. First, administration of a phosphodiesterase inhibitor can counter fluoxetine's inhibitory effects on lordosis of rodents.[10] Investigations of 3α,5α-THP's actions in the VTA for lordosis have focused on mechanisms through ionotropic receptors. Perhaps future investigations of 3α,5α-THP's mechanisms in the VTA should consider actions involving phosphodiesterase. Second, fluoxetine's induction of 3α,5α-THP has effects on depressive behavior in animals.[16–17] The brain areas that underlie fluoxetine's effects on depression or its sexual side-effects are not known. The current findings indicate the VTA should be considered in addition to other brain regions. Third, fluoxetine increases 3α,5α-THP levels in the cerebral spinal fluid of clinically-depressed men concomitant with reducing depressive symptoms.[15] Women are more vulnerable to depression than are men, and women also have higher and more labile 3α,5α-THP levels than do men.[18] Some data suggest anti-depressants that stabilize 3α,5α-THP levels may be beneficial for some women.[19] Thus, fluoxetine may have different therapeutic effects (or side effects) in men and women that depend upon their endogenous variations and/or sensitivity to 3α,5α-THP.

In summary, the present results suggest fluoxetine has different effects on lordosis that depend in part upon fluoxetine's effects on midbrain 3α,5α-THP levels. There is a high incidence of sexual dysfunction among people taking SSRIs, such as fluoxetine, for the treatment of various clinical conditions.[20] It is important to understand further the mechanisms that may underlie the beneficial therapeutic effects of fluoxetine, as well as the potential deleterious side effects, because such effects may compromise compliance of this pharmacotherapy.

ACKNOWLEDGMENT

This research is supported by The National Science Foundation (grants IBN 98-96263 and IBN 03-16083).

REFERENCES

1. FRYE, C.A. 2001. The role of neurosteroids and non-genomic effects of progestins and androgens in the ventral tegmental area in mediating sexual receptivity of rodents. Brain Res. Brain Res. Rev. **37:** 201–222.
2. PLEIM, E.T. *et al.* 1991. A contributory role for midbrain progesterone in the facilitation of female sexual behavior in rats. Horm. Behav. **25:** 19–28.
3. MUNN, A.R. *et al.* 1983. Topographic distribution of progestin target cells in hamster brain and pituitary after injection of [^{3}H]R5020. Brain Res. **274:** 1–10.
4. FRYE, C.A. & J.M. VONGHER. 1999. Progestins' rapid facilitation of lordosis when applied to the ventral tegmentum corresponds to efficacy at enhancing $GABA_A$ receptor activation. J. Neuroendocrinol. **11:** 829–837.
5. FRYE, C.A. & L.E. BAYON. 1999. Mating stimuli influence endogenous variations in the neurosteroids 3α,5α-THP and 3α-Diol.J. Neuroendocrinol. **11:** 839–847.
6. FRYE, C.A. & J.M. VONGHER. 1999. 3α,5α-THP in the midbrain ventral tegmental area of rats and hamsters is increased in exogenous hormonal states associated with estrous cyclicity and sexual receptivity. J. Endocrinol. Invest. **22:** 455–464.
7. FRYE, C.A. & J.M. VONGHER. 2001. Progesterone and 3α,5α-THP enhance sexual receptivity in mice. Behav. Neurosci. **115:** 1118–1128.
8. MELLON, S.H. *et al.* 2001. Biosynthesis and action of neurosteroids. Brain Res. Brain Res. Rev. **37:** 3–12.
9. ZANISI, M. *et al.* 1984. Physiological role of the 5α-reduced metabolites of progesterone. *In* Metabolism of Hormonal Steroids in the Neuroendocrine Structures. F. Celotti, Ed.: 171–182. Raven Press. New York.
10. FRYE, C.A. & M.E. RHODES. 2003. Zaprinast, a phosphodiesterase 5 inhibitor, overcomes sexual dysfunction produced by fluoxetine, a selective serotonin reuptake inhibitor in hamsters. Neuropsychopharmacol. **28:** 310– 316.
11. MATUSZCZYK, J.V. *et al.* 1998. Subchronic administration of fluoxetine impairs estrous behavior in intact female rats. Neuropsychopharmacology **19:** 492–498.
12. GRIFFIN, L.D. & S.H. MELLON. 1996. Selective serotonin reuptake inhibitors directly alter activity of neurosteroidogenic enzymes. Proc. Natl. Acad. Sci. USA **96:** 13512–13517.
13. SERRA, M. *et al.* 2001. Opposite effects of short- versus long-term administration of fluoxetine on the concentrations of neuroactive steroids in rat plasma and brain. Psychopharmacology **158:** 48–54.
14. UZUNOV, D.P. *et al.* 1996. Fluoxetine-elicited changes in brain neurosteroid content measured by negative ion mass fragmentography. Proc. Natl. Acad. Sci. USA **93:** 12599–12604.
15. UZUNOVA, V. *et al.* 1998. Increase in the cerebrospinal fluid content of neurosteroids in patients with unipolar major depression who are receiving fluoxetine or fluvoxamine. Proc. Natl. Acad. Sci. USA **95:** 3239–3244.
16. GUIDOTTI, A. *et al.* 2001. The socially-isolated mouse: a model to study the putative role of allopregnanolone and 5α-dihydroprogesterone in psychiatric disorders. Brain Res. Brain Res. Rev. **37:** 110–115.
17. KHISTI, R.T. & C.T. CHOPDE. 2000. Serotonergic agents modulate anti-depressant-like effect of the neurosteroid 3α-hydroxy-5α-pregnan-20-one in mice. Brain Res. **865:** 291–300.
18. PEARSON MURPHY, B.E. & C.M. ALLISON. 2000. Determination of progesterone and some of its neuroactive ring A-reduced metabolites in human serum. J. Steroid Biochem. Mol. Biol. **74:** 137–142.
19. FREEMAN, E.W. *et al.* 2002. Allopregnanolone levels and symptom improvement in severe premenstrual syndrome. J. Clin. Psychopharmacol. **22:** 516–520.
20. BAYLON, R. 1995. Fluoxetine and sexual dysfunction. JAMA **273:** 1489.

Pathogenesis in Menstrual Cycle–Linked CNS Disorders

TORBJÖRN BÄCKSTRÖM, AGNETA ANDERSSON, LOTTA ANDREÉ, VITA BIRZNIECE, MARIE BIXO, INGER BJÖRN, DAVID HAAGE, MONICA ISAKSSON, INGA-MAJ JOHANSSON, CHARLOTT LINDBLAD, PER LUNDGREN, SIGRID NYBERG, INGA-STINA ÖDMARK, JESSICA STRÖMBERG, INGER SUNDSTRÖM-POROMAA, SAHRUH TURKMEN, GÖRAN WAHLSTRÖM, MINGDE WANG, ANNA-CARIN WIHLBÄCK, DI ZHU, AND ELISABETH ZINGMARK

Umeå Neurosteroid Research Center, Department of Clinical Sciences, Obstetrics and Gynecology, Norrlands University Hospital, SE-901 85 Umeå, Sweden

ABSTRACT: That 3alpha-hydroxy-5alpha/beta-pregnane steroids (GABA steroids) have modulatory effects on the GABA-A receptor is well known. In behavioral studies in animals high exogenous dosages give concentrations not usually reached in the brain under physiological conditions. Animal and human studies show that GABA-A receptor-positive modulators like barbiturates, benzodiazepines, alcohol, and allopregnanolone have a bimodal effect. In pharmacological concentrations they are CNS depressants, anesthetic, antiepileptic, and anxiolytic. In low dosages and concentrations, reached endogenously, they can induce adverse emotional reactions in up to 20% of individuals. GABA steroids can also induce tolerance to themselves and similar substances, and rebound occurs at withdrawal. Menstrual cycle–linked disorders can be understood by the concept that they are caused by the action of endogenously produced GABA-steroids through three mechanisms: (a) direct action, (b) tolerance induction, and (c) withdrawal effect. Examples of symptoms and disorders caused by the direct action of GABA steroids are sedation, memory and learning disturbance, clumsiness, increased appetite, worsening of petit mal epilepsy, negative mood as tension, irritability and depression during hormone treatments, and the premenstrual dysphoric disorder (PMDD). A continuous exposure to GABA steroids causes tolerance, and women with PMDD are less sensitive to GABA-A modulators. A malfunctioning GABA-A receptor system is related to stress sensitivity, concentration difficulties, loss of impulse control, irritability, anxiety, and depression. An example of withdrawal effect is "catamenial epilepsy," when seizures increase during menstruation after the withdrawal of GABA steroids. Similar phenomena occur at stress since the adrenals produce GABA steroids during stress.

KEYWORDS: menstrual cycle; premenstrual dysphoric disorder; epilepsy; GABA; neurosteroid; allopregnanolone; progesterone

Address for correspondence: Torbjörn Bäckström, M.D., Ph.D., Professor, Umeå Neurosteroid Research Center, Department of Clinical Sciences, Obstetrics and Gynecology, Norrlands University Hospital, SE-901 85 Umeå, Sweden. Voice: +46-90 785 2144; fax: +46-90 776006.
Torbjorn.Backstrom@Obgyn.umu.se

Ann. N.Y. Acad. Sci. 1007: 42–53 (2003).
doi: 10.1196/annals.1286.005

The effects of ovarian hormones on mood and CNS-related disorders is an issue of great interest today, especially since it was discovered that some of the ovarian steroids are potent modulators of neurotransmitter systems in the brain. Several conditions and symptoms show menstrual cycle–linked patterns. Examples of such conditions are the premenstrual dysphoric disorder (PMDD) or premenstrual syndrome (PMS), catamenial epilepsy, and menstrual migraine. Symptoms that change with the menstrual cycle are, for example, menstrual cycle–linked mood changes, memory and learning disturbances, menstrual cycle–linked insomnia, menstrual cycle–linked changes in eating behavior and alcohol usage, disturbance in concentration, increased stress sensitivity, loss of impulse control, and difficulty in controlling emotions. Many of these symptoms are part of the premenstrual dysphoric disorder, PMDD/PMS, a model condition of a menstrual cycle–linked CNS related condition, which we will discuss in more detail later in this paper.

SYMPTOM PATTERNS DURING THE OVULATORY MENSTRUAL CYCLE

Three different patterns of symptom distribution in relation to the ovulatory menstrual cycle are often seen. The first and most common pattern is an increase in symptom severity during the luteal phase, starting at the time of ovulation. The maximum severity occurs during the last 5 days of the menstrual cycle and the first two days of the next cycle. This pattern is seen in mood changes of the premenstrual dysphoric disorder (PMDD) or premenstrual syndrome (PMS).[1] This symptom pattern is also seen in women with petit mal absence epilepsy where the disease remains in adulthood.[2] The second pattern is an increase in symptoms at the time of menstruation. That is, the symptoms start at or just before full menstrual bleeding starts and end within the first 4 days of the next cycle. An example of a diseases having this pattern is in women with partial epilepsy, where there is an epileptic focus in cerebral cortex. There is a period with few seizures during the luteal phase and an increased seizure frequency during menstruation.[3] A similar pattern is seen among women with migraine, who also have an increased frequency of attacks during menstruation.[6] This pattern is called a "catamenial pattern." The third pattern is an increase in symptoms during the mid-cycle ovulatory phase. During this period there is an increase in energy, vigilance, and excitability. This pattern does not always represent a negative experience and is not then considered as a symptom. In premenstrual syndrome there is often a period of well-being during the periovulatory period.[1] However, in partial "focal" epilepsy, an increased seizure frequency can be noted during this part of the menstrual cycle in certain patients.[4,5]

MECHANISMS BEHIND MENSTRUAL CYCLE–LINKED SYMPTOM PATTERNS

We know that the ovarian hormones and their metabolites have fundamental effects in the brain. In anovulatory cycles no corpus luteum is formed and progesterone, allopregnanolone, and other luteal steroids are not synthesized. The classical hormonal nuclear receptors for estradiol and progesterone are present in neurons and uniquely distributed in certain regions.[7,8] The effects of the hormones via the classical receptors, called "genomic" effects, are mediated via transcription of specific genes, followed by protein synthesis, and take some time to achieve. Besides the "genomic" effects it is well known that certain 3alpha-hydroxy-5alpha/beta metabolites of progesterone (allopregnanolone and pregnanolone) and tetra-hydro-desoxycorticosterone (THDOC) are very potent positive modulators of the rapid GABA effect on the GABA-A receptor (GABA steroids).[9,10] This effect is called a direct "non-genomic" effect.[11] We know that many of progesterone's CNS effects are mediated via metabolism to 3alpha-hydroxy-5alpha/beta-pregnan-20-one.[12] This metabolism can occur within the brain. Estradiol is excitatory and seems to have modulatory effects via the excitatory glutamate system, increasing brain excitability and, in hippocampus, the synaptic spine density.[13–15] Since many symptom changes seen during the menstrual cycle can be interpreted as effects via non-genomic mechanisms, we will therefore concentrate in this review on the non-genomic mechanisms of allopregnanolone and estradiol. We are aware of the facts that the ovarian hormones also influence the function of several other transmitter systems, but a complete review of all effects is beyond the scope of this paper. Although some authors claim that central progesterone receptors are involved in PMS pathophysiology, treatment with mifepristone, a progesterone receptor antagonist that provides effective blockade of the progesterone receptors, did not alleviate premenstrual symptoms,[16] and therefore we concentrate on the non-genomic effects of allopregnanolone in this paper. However, more research is required to settle this controversy.

Changes in plasma concentration of estradiol, progesterone, and allopregnanolone are reflected in the brain.[17–19] In women, plasma levels of allopregnanolone increase from 1 nM in the follicular phase to approximately 4–12 nM in the luteal phase.[20] Allopregnanolone plasma levels are highly correlated with plasma levels of progesterone,[20,21] and it is conceivable that the corpus luteum is the major source for progesterone metabolites in fertile women.[22] Postmortem studies in fertile and postmenopausal women show the highest levels of allopregnanolone in the substantia nigra and basal hypothalamus, with concentrations ranging from 60–130 nmol/kg.[19] During the third trimester of pregnancy, plasma levels of allopregnanolone and pregnanolone are about 100 nM.[23] In non-pregnant women, plasma concentrations between 80–160 nM cause sedation[24] and 530–700 nM cause anesthesia.[25]

EFFECTS OF ALLOPREGNANOLONE VIA THE GABA-A RECEPTOR SYSTEM

The effect of allopregnanolone on the GABA-A receptor has several similarities to the effects of benzodiazepines, barbiturates, and alcohol. There are also differences in the effect, but we will here mainly discuss the similarities. These GABA-A receptor–active substances have some positive effects, but they also have a number of negative adverse side effects. Many of these negative effects become symptoms and diseases when occurring as a result of endogenous production of the GABA-A receptor–active steroids. These effects can be characterized as: (1) symptoms induced via direct effects on GABA-A receptor function; (2) effects via indirect changes in the function of the GABA-A system, and/or induction of tolerance; and (3) effects or symptoms caused by abstinence after withdrawal of allopregnanolone after a certain period of allopregnanolone exposure.

Direct Effects

Several GABA-A receptor agonists, such as benzodiazepines, barbiturates, alcohol, and allopregnanolone, show biphasic effects on mood and behavior. In high dosages or concentrations a general enhancement of many GABA-A receptors in several regions appears, and thereby more general effects are the result. In high dosages in both humans and animals, the progesterone metabolites pregnanolone and allopregnanolone are sedative, hypnotic, and even anesthetic.[25–27] In animal studies these steroids have also shown anxiolytic and antiepileptic effects.[28–30] However, GABA-A receptor agonists, including allopregnanolone, have, in addition, shown negative effects such as inhibition of learning and memory,[31] increase of appetite,[32] disturbances of motor function[30,33] and worsening of petit mal epilepsy,[34,35] and, in very high dosages, allopregnanolone has an abuse-potential effect.[36]

In low dosages or with low serum allopregnanolone concentrations, as seen during physiological situations, benzodiazepines, barbiturates, alcohol, and allopregnanolone induce loss of impulse control, negative mood, and aggression/irritability in certain individuals. This phenomenon, called disinhibition, seems to induce severe negative mood symptoms in 2–6% of individuals and mild symptoms in up to 20%.[37–39] The frequency of individuals (2–6%) having severe negative mood symptoms on GABA-A modulators is similar to the frequency of women in the general population having a severe form of menstrual cycle–linked condition, PMDD. The milder form, PMS, is found in 15–25% of the general population.[40] A number of hypotheses for the mechanism behind disinhibition have been presented, but the mechanism is not completely understood. In line with the above, allopregnanolone can induce anxiety in low physiological dosages or serum concentrations. In an animal model claiming to resemble PMS premenstrual syndrome, allopregnanolone induced increased anxiety and hippocampal expression of the alpha4 subunit of the GABA-A receptor.[41] The negative effect on mood of low dosages or serum concentrations has been shown both in humans and animals for allopregnanolone,[42,43] benzodiazepines,[37,44] barbiturates,[38,45,46] and ethanol.[39] A biphasic effect on negative mood has also been noted from different dosages of medroxyprogesterone and natural progesterone in postmenopausal women. Postmenopausal women taking sequential HRT feel worse on 10 mg MPA compared to 20 mg MPA[47] and worse on 400 mg/d vaginal progesterone compared to 800 mg/d[48] but both dosages were worse than placebo.[47,48]

Tolerance

Continuous and long exposure to benzodiazepines and GABAsteroids (3alpha-hydroxy-5alpha/beta-steroids) causes a malfunctioning of the GABA-A receptor system.[49–51] A tolerance develops and this tolerance leads to a lessening of the effect of allopregnanolone and similar steroids. A cross-tolerance occurs with lessening of the effect of benzodiazepines, alcohol, and other GABA-A receptor agonists. Several papers show changes in GABA-A receptor subunit composition, downregulation, and decreased GABA function after long-term exposure to GABA steroids.[49,51]

Similarly, reduced benzodiazepine, alcohol, and pregnanolone sensitivity during the luteal phase has been shown in women with PMS.[26,52,53] The action of GABA steroids has been found to be a factor which reinforces drug dependency. This has been the focus of extensive research and allopregnanolone shows a relation to dependence-induction. In addition there is a relation between premenstrual syndrome and increased alcohol consumption during the luteal phase as well as increased risk of alcohol abuse in women with PMS.[36,54,55–57]

Rebound Effect after Withdrawal

After continuous exposure to GABA-A receptor agonists, a withdrawal effect often occurs when the exposure is ended. This phenomenon occurs, for instance, during menstruation, when the production of GABA steroids by the corpus luteum of the ovary is interrupted. For GABA agonists, the withdrawal syndrome is characterized by sleep disturbance, irritability, increased tension and anxiety, panic attacks, hand tremor, clumsiness, sweating, difficulty in concentration, increased stress sensitivity, loss of impulse control, nausea, palpitations, headache, muscular pain and stiffness. Sometimes more serious symptoms appear like seizures, depression, and psychotic reactions.[58] Many of these symptoms are common in PMS and other CNS–linked conditions that are influenced by the menstrual cycle in a similar way as in PMS. In addition they are often linked to a simultaneous presence of PMS as in fibromyalgia.[59] Another example of a condition that is influenced by this withdrawal/ absence is partial epilepsy, where the patient has an epileptic focus in the cerebral cortex; a worsening occurs at the withdrawal period during menstruation. This phenomenon is called "catamenial epilepsy." Other examples are menstrual period–related migraine.[3–6,60] Also, during withdrawal of allopregnanolone, changes in GABA-A receptor subunits have been shown.[61]

ESTROGEN EFFECTS ON EXCITABILITY

Estradiol has been shown to decrease electroshock seizure threshold in a dose-dependent fashion.[13] In women with partial epilepsy, an increased frequency of epileptic discharges from an epileptic focus was noted in 11 of 14 women only 5 minutes after an i.v. injection of Premarin, an estrogen product. Grand mal seizures were provoked within 15 minutes after the injection in 4 of 14 patients.[62] It is also possible to induce an epileptic focus by applying estradiol directly to the cerebral cortex.[62] The result demonstrates an excitatory effect of estrogen on brain activity. As mentioned above estradiol is excitatory and seems to have its major effects via the excitatory glutamate system.[14,15]

PREMENSTRUAL SYNDROME (PMS) OR PREMENSTRUAL DYSPHORIC DISORDER (PMDD)

It has been debated for a long time whether PMS should be considered as a disease or a normal phenomenon not needing treatment. This is largely due to the failure to appreciate that the severity varies tremendously. Although most women experience mild mood and somatic symptoms premenstrually, a small but significant number (2–6% of fertile women) are severely disabled by the disorder and 15–20% of fertile women show disabling menstrual cycle–linked changes in several symptoms.[40,63] With the diagnostic criteria published by American Psychiatric Association's *Diagnostic and Statistical Manual of Mental Disorders* (4th edition),[64] a severe form of PMS with mood symptoms can be defined as premenstrual dysphoric disorder (PMDD). This has made the research more stringent, and now more knowledge of the background to menstrual cycle–linked mood changes is emerging.

The close link between the temporal symptom variations during the menstrual cycle and the luteal phase of the cycle indicates that a factor produced by the corpus luteum is involved in provoking premenstrual symptoms.[1] The symptoms start at ovulation and the intensity increases during the luteal phase in parallel with the rise in serum progesterone and allopregnanolone concentrations. The maximum symptom severity occurs 3–5 days after the progesterone and allopregnanolone peak in the luteal phase. The highest severity occurs during the last 5 premenstrual days or the first day of menstruation. The symptoms disappear totally 4–5 days after the onset of menstrual bleeding, the luteal phase has ended, and progesterone as well as allopregnanolone levels have reached their baseline concentrations. During the rest of the follicular and preovulatory phase there is a period of well-being. When the premenstrual decrease in the luteal hormones start, symptom degree has already risen, and thus increases in symptoms in the early luteal phase are not only related to the steroid-withdrawal effect.[1] The seizure pattern during the menstrual cycle in women with petit mal epilepsy is very similar to the pattern of mood changes in PMS. They show an increase in seizure frequency during the luteal phase with an improvement during the follicular phase.[2] In addition, other types of epilepsy can have a similar pattern to the mood changes in PMS.[5]

Despite numerous efforts to identify endocrine disturbances in patients with PMS, there are few consistent findings, and there are no clear-cut peripheral markers of hypothalamus–pituitary–gonadal axis dysfunction in PMS.[63,65] The relationship between symptom development and the increase in progesterone–allopregnanolone serum concentration in the beginning of the luteal phase is obvious, however. The most important finding by far is the necessity of an ovulation and corpus luteum formation for premenstrual symptoms to develop. During anovulatory cycles, spontaneous or induced, a corpus luteum is not formed, allopregnanolone is not produced, and the cyclicity in symptoms disappears.[66–68] When allopregnanolone levels are related to symptom severity in the same individuals, the results support the hypothesis of a biphasic action of allopregnanolone in inducing symptoms in patients.[20] In women with PMDD, an alleviation of symptoms during treatment with the SSRIs sertraline or desipramine was associated with lower allopregnanolone levels even after adjustment for treatment effect.[69] Similar results were obtained with low-dosage GnRH agonist treatment, where improvement of symptoms was related to a decrease in progesterone levels in the same individuals.[70]

EFFECT OF EXOGENOUS OVARIAN HORMONES ON MOOD

Evidence that ovarian hormones and their metabolites are implicated in mood changes is found from sequential hormone replacement therapy (HRT) in postmenopausal women. The estrogen/progestogen sequential replacement therapy resembles the hormonal variations during an ovulatory menstrual cycle, and the estrogen-only treatment is similar to that of an anovulatory cycle. Women receiving sequential HRT respond with a significant deterioration in mood and with physical signs when progestogen is given together with estrogen, but unlike those not on an estrogen-only therapy.[71,72]

There is, however, evidence that a higher estrogen dose in sequential HRT accentuates negative mood and physical symptoms during the progestogen phase, but not in the absence of a progestogen.[73] Moreover, in women with PMS, where ovarian function had been interrupted with GnRH agonists, both estrogen and progesterone induce symptoms.[74] Increased serum estradiol levels during the progestogen phase of HRT treatment, or estradiol treatment during the luteal phase in women with PMS, are both found to be related to more severe symptoms, compared to situations where estradiol levels are lower.[75,76] In women with PMS, studied during two menstrual cycles, cycles with higher serum estradiol levels during the luteal phase, when allopregnanolone and progesterone are high, showed more severe negative mood symptoms than did cycles with lower estradiol levels.[77,78] During the preovulatory phase, allopregnanolone and progesterone levels are very low, but at that time estradiol levels are high. This period coincides with the period when the PMS patients feel their best. Therefore it seems that when estradiol and progesterone/allopregnanolone are acting together, a different response is induced in the central nervous system than when they act separately.

DIFFERENCES IN STEROID SENSITIVITY IN PATIENTS WITH PMS/PMDD COMPARED TO CONTROLS

Studies made show no consistent difference in steroid concentrations between PMS patients and controls.[79] Therefore some other difference must exist between women with PMS and controls. At least two other possibilities exist: either an unknown provoking factor is produced from the corpus luteum in women with PMS or sensitivity in the brain for steroids differs between the patients and controls. Some evidence exists for the latter hypothesis. In a double-blind study of oral contraceptive (OC) effects on mood, it was mainly women with PMS who reacted badly, with negative mood change occurring while on the OCs.[80] Women who had experienced difficulties tolerating OCs reported a greater number of moderate/severe premenstrual changes.[81] In women with premenstrual syndrome who were given a GnRH agonist to inhibit ovarian hormone production, add-back of estradiol or progesterone produced a significant recurrence of symptoms. But no changes in mood occurred in normal women who received the same regimen, or in women with premenstrual syndrome who were given placebo.[74] Postmenopausal women with a history of premenstrual syndrome responded with more negative symptoms on progestogens compared to women without a history of PMS.[72] In PMS/PMDD patients the saccadic eye velocity, controlled by the GABA system, and the sedative response to intravenous pregnanolone was reduced in the luteal phase compared with controls.[26] In addition, patients with severe symptoms were less sensitive to pregnanolone compared to patients with more moderate symptoms.[26] Similar results were obtained when alcohol and benzodiazepines were given intravenously, suggesting that patients with PMS develop tolerance for GABA-A receptor allosteric agonists during the luteal phase.[52,53,82]

INVOLVEMENT OF THE SEROTONIN SYSTEM IN PMDD/PMS

The serotonin transmitter system has also been suggested to be involved in the etiolgy of PMS. The serotonin system is considered mainly because serotonin reuptake inhibitors (SSRIs) are effective treatments for PMS and PMDD. The direct mechanism for this is not known, but many studies indicate a connection between the serotonin system and PMS. Challenge studies have shown blunted responses to serotonergic interventions in PMS patients, but, as this is found over the entire cycle, the change in the serotonin system has been suggested to be a vulnerability trait rather than a state marker of premenstrual syndrome.[83] Tryptophan depletion aggravated premenstrual symptoms, and symptom magnitude was correlated with tryptophan decrease.[84] Altered platelet paroxetine binding in the follicular phase has been found in women with PMDD, compared to controls,[85] and paroxetine binding was normalized by successful treatment of PMDD with a low dose of the GnRH agonist, buserelin.[85] The results are consistent with the hypothesis that changes in serotonergic transmission could be a trait in the premenstrual dysphoric disorder. Connections between the serotonin and GABA-A systems have also been shown as GABA-A receptor subunit composition is changed in knockout mice without the 5HT1A receptor.[86] The same animals are insensitive to benzodiazepines[86] and rats lacking the 5HT1A receptor show increased anxiety.[87] In PMDD patients treated with SSRI the decreased sensitivity towards pregnanolone in the luteal phase normalized in parallel with alleviation of the symptoms.[88]

CONCLUSION

In summary, it is now known that substances produced from the corpus luteum of the ovary induce negative mood changes in sensitive patients. 3alpha-hydroxy-5alpha/beta-steroids (GABA steroids) are strongly implicated in CNS disorders through three mechanisms: (1) direct action; (2) inducing malfunction of the GABA-A system via tolerance induction; and (3) withdrawal effect. Other neurotransmitter systems, like the glutamate and serotonin systems, also seem to be involved.

ACKNOWLEDGMENTS

The work presented here has been supported by the Research Council of Sweden (Proj. 4X-11198), a grant from EU-regional fund, objective 1, Umeå University foundations, Västerbottens läns landsting, and Umeå Kommun.

REFERENCES

1. BÄCKSTRÖM, T. *et al.* 1983. Mood, sexuality, hormones and the menstrual cycle. II. Hormone levels and their relationship to premenstrual syndrome. Psychosom. Med. **45:** 503–507.

2. BÄCKSTRÖM, T. *et al.* 1983 Endocrinological aspects on cyclical mood changes or the premenstrual syndrome. J. Psychosom. Obstet. Gynecol. **2:** 8–20
3. LAIDLAW, J. 1956 Catamenial epilepsy. Lancet **271:** 1235–1237.
4. BÄCKSTRÖM, T 1976. Epileptic seizures in women related to plasma estrogen and progesterone during the menstrual cycle. Acta Neurol. Scand. **54:** 321–347.
5. HERZOG, A.G. *et al.* 1997. Three patterns of catamenial epilepsy. Epilepsia **38:** 1082–1088.
6. MACGREGOR, E.A. 1996. "Menstrual" migraine: towards a definition. Cephalalgia **16:** 11–21.
7. ÖSTERLUND, M.K. *et al.* 2000. The human brain has distinct regional expression patterns of estrogen receptor alpha mRNA isoforms derived from alternative promoters. J. Neurochem. **75:** 1390–1397.
8. ÖSTERLUND, M.K. *et al.* 2000. Estrogen receptor beta (ERbeta) messenger ribonucleic acid (mRNA) expression within the human forebrain: distinct distribution pattern to ERalpha mRNA. J. Clin. Endocrinol. Metab. **85:** 3840–3846.
9. HARRISON, N.L. & M.A. SIMMONDS. 1984. Modulation of the GABA receptor complex by a steroid anaesthetic. Brain Res. **323:** 287–292.
10. MAJEWSKA, M.D. *et al.* 1986. Steroid hormone metabolites are barbiturate-like modulators of the GABA receptor. Science **232:** 1004–1007.
11. MCEWEN, B.S. 1991. Non-genomic and genomic effects of steroids on neural activity. Trends Pharmacol. Sci. **12:** 141–147.
12. MOK, W.M. & N.R. KRIEGER. 1990. Evidence that 5 alpha-pregnan-3 alpha-ol-20-one is the metabolite responsible for progesterone anesthesia. Brain Res. **533:** 42–45.
13. WOOLEY, D.E. & P.S. TIMIRAS. 1962. The gonad-brain relationship: effects of female sex hormones on electro-shock convulsions in the rat. Endocrinology **70:** 196–209.
14. SMITH, S.S. *et al.* 1988. Locally applied estrogens potentiate glutamate-evoked excitation of cerebellar Purkinje cells. Brain Res. **475:** 272–282.
15. WOOLLEY, C.S. *et al.* 1997. Estradiol increases the sensitivity of hippocampal CA1 pyramidal cells to NMDA receptor-mediated synaptic input: correlation with dendritic spine density. J. Neurosci. **17:** 1848–1859.
16. CHAN, A.F. *et al.* 1994. Persistence of premenstrual syndrome during low-dose administration of the progesterone antagonist RU 486. Obstet. Gynecol. **84:**1001–1005.
17. PURDY, R.H. *et al.* 1991. Stress-induced elevations of gamma-aminobutyric acid type A receptor-active steroids in the rat brain. Proc. Natl. Acad. Sci. USA **88:** 4553–4557.
18. BIXO, M. *et al.* 1995. Estradiol and testosterone in specific regions of the human female brain in different endocrine states. J. Steroid Biochem. Mol. Biol. **55:** 297–303.
19. BIXO, M. *et al.* 1997. Progesterone, 5alpha-pregnane-3,20-dione and 3alpha-hydroxy-5alpha-pregnane-20-one in specific regions of the human female brain in different endocrine states. Brain Res. **764:** 173–178.
20. WANG, M. *et al.* 1996. Relationship between symptom severity and steroid variation in women with premenstrual syndrome: Study on serum pregnenolone, pregnenolone sulfate, 5 alpha-pregnane-3,20-dione and 3 alpha-hydroxy-5alpha-pregnan-20-one. J. Clin. Endocrinol. Metab. **81:** 1076–1082.
21. PURDY, R.H. *et al.* 1990. Radioimmunoassay of 3alpha-hydroxy-5alpha-pregnan-20-one in rat and human plasma. Steroids **55:** 290–296.
22. BÄCKSTRÖM, T. *et al.* 1986. The human corpus luteum secretes 5alpha-pregnane-3,20-dione. Acta Endocrinol. (Copenh.) **111:** 116–121.
23. PAUL, S.M. & RH. PURDY. 1992. Neuroactive steroids. FASEB J. **6:** 2311–2322.
24. SUNDSTRÖM, I. *et al.* 1999. Lack of influence of menstrual cycle and premenstrual syndrome diagnosis on pregnanolone pharmacokinetics. Eur. J. Clin. Pharmacol. **55:** 125–130.
25. CARL, P. *et al.* 1990. Pregnanolone emulsion: a preliminary pharmacokinetic and pharmacodynamic study of a new intravenous anaesthetic agent. Anaesthesia 45: 189–197.
26. SUNDSTRÖM, I. 1998. Patients with premenstrual syndrome have a different sensitivity to a neuroactive steroid during the menstrual cycle compared to control subjects. Neuroendocrinology **67:** 126–138.

27. NORBERG, L. *et al.* 1987. The anaesthetic potency of 3 alpha-hydroxy-5 alpha-pregnan-20-one and 3 alpha-hydroxy-5 beta-pregnan-20-one determined with an intravenous EEG-threshold method in male rats. Pharmacol. Toxicol. **61:** 42–47.
28. BITRAN, D. *et al.* 1991. Anxiolytic effects of 3 alpha-hydroxy-5 alpha[beta]-pregnan-20-one: endogenous metabolites of progesterone that are active at the GABAA receptor. Brain Res. **561:** 157–161.
29. LANDGREN, S. *et al.* 1987. The effect of progesterone and its metabolites on the interictal epileptiform discharge in the cat's cerebral cortex. Acta Physiol Scand **131:** 33–42.
30. GASIOR, M. *et al.* 1997. Anticonvulsant and behavioral effects of neuroactive steroids alone and in conjunction with diazepam. J. Pharmacol. Exp. Ther. **282:** 543–553.
31. JOHANSSON, I.M. *et al.* 2002. Allopregnanolone inhibits learning in the Morris water maze. Brain Res. **934:** 125–131.
32. CHEN, S.W. *et al.* 1996. The hyperphagic effect of 3 alpha-hydroxylated pregnane steroids in male rats. Pharmacol. Biochem. Behav. **53:** 777–782.
33. KHISTI, R.T. *et al.* 1998. The neurosteroid 3 alpha-hydroxy-5 alpha-pregnan-20-one induces catalepsy in mice. Neurosci. Lett. **251:** 85–88.
34. BANERJEE, P.K. & O.C. SNERD, III. 1998. Neuroactive steroids exacerbate gamma-hydroxybutyric acid-induced absence seizures in rats. Eur. J. Pharmacol. **359:** 41–48.
35. GRUNEWALD, R.A. *et al.* 1992. Exacerbation of typical absence seizures by progesterone. Seizure **1:** 137–138.
36. FINN, D.A. *et al.* 1997. Rewarding effect of the neuroactive steroid 3 alpha-hydroxy-5 alpha-pregnan-20-one in mice. Pharmacol. Biochem. Behav. **56:** 261–264.
37. WENZEL, R.R. *et al.* 2002. Central-nervous side effects of midazolam during transesophageal echocardiography. J. Am. Soc. Echocardiogr. **15:** 1297–1300.
38. MASIA, S.L. *et al.* 2000. Emotional outbursts and post-traumatic stress disorder during intracarotid amobarbital procedure. Neurology **54:** 1691–1693.
39. MICZEK, K.A. *et al.* 1997. Alcohol, GABAA-benzodiazepine receptor complex, and aggression. Recent Dev. Alcohol **13:** 139–171.
40. SVEINSDOTTIR, H. & T. BÄCKSTRÖM. 2000. Prevalence of menstrual cycle symptom cyclicity and premenstrual dysphoric disorder in a random sample of women using and not using oral contraceptives. Acta Obstet. Gynecol. Scand. **79:** 405–413.
41. GULINELLO, M. *et al.* 2001. Short-term exposure to a neuroactive steroid increases alpha4 GABA(A) receptor subunit levels in association with increased anxiety in the female rat. Brain Res. **910:** 55–66.
42. BEAUCHAMP, M.H. *et al.* 2000 Neurosteroids and reward: allopregnanolone produces a conditioned place aversion in rats. Pharmacol. Biochem. Behav. **67:** 29–35.
43. FISH, E.W. *et al.* 2001. Alcohol, allopregnanolone and aggression in mice. Psychopharmacology (Berl.) **153:** 473–483.
44. MICZEK, K.A. *et al.* 1993. Alcohol, benzodiazepine-GABAa receptor complex and aggression: ethological analysis of individual differences in rodents and primates. J. Stud. Alcohol **11:** 170–179.
45. KURTHEN, M. *et al.* 1991. Severe negative emotional reactions in intracarotid sodium amytal procedures: further evidence for hemispheric asymmetries? Cortex **27:** 333–337.
46. LEE, G.P. *et al.* 1988. Severe behavioral complications following intracarotid sodium amobarbital injection: implications for hemispheric asymmetry of emotion. Neurology **38:** 1233–1236.
47. BJÖRN, I. *et al.* 2002. The impact of different doses of medroxyprogesterone acetate on mood symptoms in sequential hormonal therapy. Gynecol. Endocrinol. **16:** 1–8.
48. ANDRÉEN, L. *et al.* 2003. Progesterone effects during hormone replacement therapy. Eur. J. Endocrinol. **148:** 571–577.
49. YU, R. *et al.* 1996. Down-regulation of the GABA receptor subunits mRNA levels in mammalian cultured cortical neurons following chronic neurosteroid treatment. Brain Res. Mol. Brain Res. **41:** 163–168.
50. MARSHALL, F.H. *et al.* 1997. Development of tolerance in mice to the sedative effects of the neuroactive steroid minaxolone following chronic exposure. Pharmacol. Biochem. Behav. **58:** 1–8.

51. CONCAS, A. *et al.* 1998. Role of brain allopregnanolone in the plasticity of gamma-aminobutyric acid type A receptor in rat brain during pregnancy and after delivery. Proc. Natl. Acad. Sci. USA **95:** 13284–13289.
52. SUNDSTRÖM, I. *et al.* 1997. Reduced benzodiazepine sensitivity in patients with premenstrual syndrome: a pilot study. Psychoneuroendocrinology **22:** 25–38.
53. NYBERG, S. *et al.* 2003. Altered sensitivity to alcohol among patients with premenstrual dysphoric disorder. Psychoneuroendocrinology. In press.
54. GRANT, K.A. *et al.* 1996. Ethanol-like discriminative stimulus effects of the neurosteroid 3 alpha-hydroxy-5 alpha-pregnan-20-one in female *Macaca fascicularis* monkeys. Psychopharmacology **124:** 340–346.
55. CHARETTE, L. *et al.* 1990. Alcohol consumption and menstrual distress in women at higher and lower risk for alcoholism. Alcohol Clin. Exp. Res. **14:** 152–157.
56. MCLEOD, D.R. *et al.* 1994. Family history of alcoholism in women with generalized anxiety disorder who have premenstrual syndrome: patient reports of premenstrual alcohol consumption and symptoms of anxiety, Alcohol Clin. Exp. Res. **18:** 664–670.
57. TOBIN, M.B. *et al.* 1994. Reported alcohol use in women with premenstrual syndrome, Am. J. Psychiatry **151:** 1503–1504.
58. PETURSSON, H. 1994. The benzodiazepine withdrawal syndrome. Addiction **89:** 1455–1459.
59. ANDERBERG, U. *et al.* 1998. Variability in cyclicity affects pain and other symptoms in female fibromyalgia syndrome patients. J. Muscularskeletal Pain **6:** 5–22.
60. MORAN, M.H. *et al.* 1998. Progesterone withdrawal I: pro-convulsant effects, Brain Res. **807:**84–90.
61. SMITH, S.S. *et al.* 1998. GABA(A) receptor alpha4 subunit suppression prevents withdrawal properties of an endogenous steroid. Nature **392:** 926–930.
62. LOGOTHETIS, J. *et al.* 1959. The role of estrogens in catamenial exacerbation of epilepsy. Neurology **9:** 352–360.
63. HALLBREICH, U. *et al.* 1993. Menstrually related disorders: points of consensus, debate, and disagreement. Neuropsychopharmacology **9:**13–15.
64. AMERICAN PSYCHIATRIC ASSOCIATION. 1994. Diagnostic and Statistical Manual of Mental Disorders, 4th edit.: 714–718. U.S. Department of Health and Human Services. Washington, DC.
65. WANG, M. *et al.* 2001. Neuroactive steroids and central nervous system disorders. Int. Rev. Neurobiol. **46:** 421–459.
66. HAMMARBÄCK, S. *et al.* 1991. Spontaneous anovulation causing disappearance of cyclical symptoms in women with the premenstrual syndrome. Acta Endocrinol. **125:** 132–137.
67. HAMARBÄCK, S. & T. BÄCKSTRÖM. 1988. Induced anovulation as treatment of premenstrual tension syndrome: a double-blind cross-over study with GnRH-agonist versus placebo. Acta Obstet. Gynecol. Scand. **67:** 159–166.
68. MUSE, K.N. *et al.* 1984. The premenstrual syndrome: effects of "medical ovariectomy." N. Engl. J. Med. **311:** 1345–1349.
69. FREEMAN, E.W. *et al.* 2002. Allopregnanolone levels and symptom improvement in severe premenstrual syndrome. J. Clin. Psychopharmacol. **22:** 516–520.
70. SUNDSTROM, I. *et al.* 1999. Treatment of premenstrual syndrome with gonadotropin-releasing hormone agonist in a low dose regimen. Acta Obstet. Gynecol. Scand. **78:** 891–899.
71. HAMMARBÄCK, S. *et al.* 1985. Cyclical mood changes as in the premenstrual tension syndrome during sequential estrogen-progestagen postmenopausal replacement treatment. Acta Obstet. Gynecol. Scand. **64:** 393–397.
72. BJÖRN, I. *et al.* 2000. Negative mood changes during hormone replacement therapy: a comparison between two progestogens. Am. J. Obstet. Gynecol. **183:** 1419–1426.
73. BJÖRN, I. *et al.* 2003. Increase of estrogen dose deteriorates mood during progestin phase in sequential hormonal therapy. J. Clin. Endocrinol. Metab. **88:** 2026–2030.
74. SCHMIDT, P.J. *et al.* 1998. Differential behavioral effects of gonadal steroids in women with and in those without premenstrual syndrome. N. Engl. J. Med. **338:** 209–216.

75. DHAR, V. & B.E. MURPHY 1990. Double-blind randomized crossover trial of luteal phase estrogens (Premarin) in the premenstrual syndrome (PMS). Psychoneuroendocrinology **15:** 489–493.
76. KLAIBER, E.L. *et al.* 1997. Relationships of serum estradiol levels. menopausal duration and mood during hormonal replacement therapy. Psychoneuroendocrinology **22:** 549–58.
77. HAMMARBÄCK, S. *et al.* 1989. Relationship between symptom severity and hormone changes in women with premenstrual syndrome. J. Clin. Endocrinol. Metab. **68:** 125–130.
78. SEIPPE,L L. & T. BÄCKSTRÖM. 1998. Luteal phase estradiol relates to symptom severity between patients with premenstrual syndrome. J. Clin. Endocrinol. Metab. **83:** 1988–1892.
79. BÄCKSTRÖM, T. *et al.* 2003. The role of hormones and hormonal treatments in premenstrual syndrome. CNS Drugs **17:** 325–342.
80. CULLBERG, J. 1972. Mood changes and menstrual symptoms with different gestagen/estrogen combinations: a double blind comparison with placebo. Acta Psychiat. Scand. **236**: Suppl. 1–84.
81. GRAHAM, C.A. & B.B. SHERWIN. 1987. The relationship between retrospective premenstrual symptom reporting and present oral contraceptive use. J. Psychosom. Res. **31:** 45–53.
82. SUNDSTRÖM, I. *et al.* 1997. Patients with premenstrual syndrome have reduced sensitivity to midazolam compared to control subjects. Neuropsychopharmacology **17:** 370–381.
83. KOURI, E.M. & U. HALBREICH. 1997. State and trait serotonergic abnormalities in women with dysphoric premenstrual syndromes. Psychopharmacol. Bull. **33:** 767–770.
84. MENKES, D.B. *et al.* 1994. Acute tryptophan depletion aggravates premenstrual syndrome. J. Affect. Disord. **32:** 37–44.
85. BIXO, M. *et al.* 2001. Binding of [3H]paroxetine to serotonin uptake sites and of [3H]lysergic acid diethylamide to 5-HT2A receptors in platelets from women with premenstrual dysphoric disorder during gonadotropin releasing hormone treatment. Psychoneuroendocrinology **26:** 551–564.
86. SIBILLE, E. *et al.* 2000. Genetic inactivation of the serotonin 1α receptor in mice results in downregulation of major GABA-A receptor α subunits: reduction of GABA-A receptor binding, and benzodiazepine-resistant anxiety. J. Neurosci. **20:** 2758–2765.
87. PARKS, C.L. *et al.* 1998. Increased anxiety of mice lacking the serotonin 1α receptor. Proc. Natl. Acad. Sci. USA **95:** 10734–10739.
88. SUNDSTRÖM, I. & T. BÄCKSTRÖM. 1998. Citalopram increases pregnanolone sensitivity in patients with premenstrual syndrome: an open trial. Psychoneuroendocrinology **23:** 73–88.

Estrogen Receptor Gene Expression in Relation to Neuropsychiatric Disorders

HANNA ÖSTLUND,[a] EVA KELLER,[b] AND YASMIN L. HURD[a]

[a]*Department of Clinical Neuroscience, Psychiatry Section, Karolinska Institute, Stockholm, Sweden*

[b]*Department of Forensic Medicine, Semmelweis University, Budapest, Hungary*

ABSTRACT: Compelling evidence now exists for estrogen's involvement in the regulation of mood and cognitive functions. Serum estrogen levels have been shown to play an important role in the expression of psychiatric disorders such as depression and schizophrenia. We have characterized the distribution of the estrogen receptors, ERα and ERβ, in the human brain and showed a preferential limbic-related expression pattern for these transcripts. The ERα mRNA dominates in the amygdala and hypothalamus, suggesting estrogen modulation of autonomic and neuroendocrine as well as emotional functions. In contrast, the hippocampal formation, entorhinal cortex, and thalamus appear to be ERβ-dominant areas, suggesting a role for ERβ in cognition, non-emotional memory, and motor functions. The role of estradiol can also be examined in regard to its relationship to other neurotransmitter systems known to be linked to specific psychiatric disorders. Estradiol has been shown to regulate the serotonin (5-HT) system, which has been strongly implicated in affective disorders. We have studied a genetic animal model of depression, and found altered 5-HT receptor mRNA levels in discrete brain regions; many of the abnormalities are reversed by estradiol treatment, especially for the 5-HT$_{2A}$ receptor subtype. The norepinephrine (NE) system is, similar to serotonin, a target for antidepressant drugs, and projects to mesocorticolimbic structures implicated in mood disorders. We have recently observed that NE neurons in the human locus coeruleus (LC) express moderate levels of both ER transcripts. The possibility of estrogen's regulating LC function has been documented in animal studies. Results from our preliminary experiments have revealed that the ERβ mRNA is decreased in persons committing suicide, a cause of death that is highly linked to affective disorder. Follow-up studies are currently under way with a much larger population to validate these results. Overall, the discrete anatomical organization of the ER mRNAs in the human brain provide evidence as to the specific neuronal populations in which the actions of ERs could modulate mood and thus underlie the neuropathology of psychiatric disorders such as depression.

KEYWORDS: estrogen receptor; anatomical distribution; psychiatric disorders; depression

Address for correspondence: Yasmin Hurd, Karolinska Institute, Department of Clinical Neuroscience, Psychiatry Section, Experimental Psychiatry Laboratory, S-171 76 Stockholm, Sweden. Voice: 468-51772379; fax: 468-346563.

Yasmin.hurd@ks.se

Ann. N.Y. Acad. Sci. 1007: 54–63 (2003). © 2003 New York Academy of Sciences.
doi: 10.1196/annals.1286.006

INTRODUCTION

It is well known that gonadal hormones such as estrogen affect mood and psychiatric disorders including depression and anxiety. The most common mental disorders are affective disorders and these illnesses seem to have pronounced gender differences. The lifetime prevalence rates for major depression, for instance, is approximately 4% in men and 8% in women.[1,2] The higher vulnerability in women is probably due to biological effects, but social situation and expression of distress might also have an influence.[1,2] During the reproductive years there is an increased prevalence of depression and in times of fluctuations of the gonadal hormones it is also more common with affective disorders, such as premenstrual syndrome, and postmenopausal and postpartum depression.[2] These disorders are characterized by low serum levels of estrogens, and hormone replacement therapy has been shown to improve and prevent postnatal[3,4] and postmenopausal depression.[5]

An important role for serum estrogen levels in schizophrenia, as well as in neurological disorders such as Alzheimer's disease, is established. Schizophrenia is equally common in both genders, but the age of onset for men is in the late teens and early twenties, but approximately 4 years later for women.[6–10] Moreover, women show an additional peak of schizophrenia onset at age 45–54, when estrogen levels decline.[6,7,11] There are also gender differences observed in with regard to symptoms. In general, women appear to have a milder form of schizophrenia, better outcome, and shorter hospital stays.[12] Moreover, schizophrenic symptoms vary over the menstrual cycle, where the psychopathology is worsened when estrogen levels are low and improved when they are high.[13–15] These differences have been hypothesized to be due to a protective role of estrogen so that it increases the vulnerability threshold in women.[11]

Estrogen action is mediated by the estrogen receptors (ERs) ERα and ERβ, which are intracellular transcription factors that belong to the nuclear receptor superfamily.[16,17] The pathology of neuropsychiatric disorders has not been elucidated, and consequently the role of estrogen in these diseases is also unclear. However, it is known that estrogen via the ERs affects several neurotransmitter systems, such as serotonin (5-HT), dopamine, and norepinephrine (NE). It has also been documented that ERs are mainly located in several limbic structures suggested to be involved in social behavior, cognition, and emotional interpretation and processing (see Ref. 18).

Characterizing the organization of ERs is an important first step to understanding the potential influence of estrogen in neural functions. We review the evidence of the distribution of ER genes in the human brain and their relevance to psychiatric disorders, and in particular depression.

ANATOMICAL DISTRIBUTION OF ERα AND ERβ mRNA EXPRESSION WITHIN THE HUMAN BRAIN

The ERα and ERβ mRNA distribution has been investigated in the human forebrain, mainly in regions within the temporal lobe because of the significance of the structures within this region for psychiatric disorders and cognitive functions. There is overall a strong degree of anatomical overlap between the human, non-human pri-

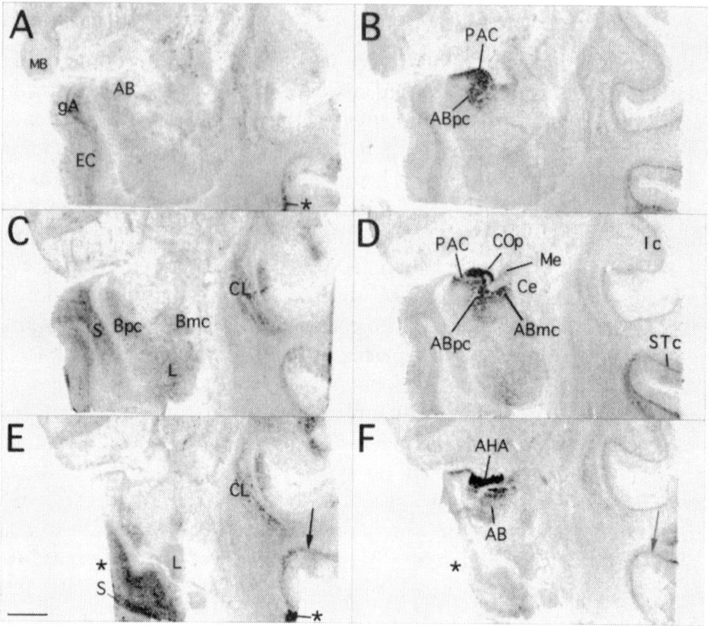

FIGURE 1. Distribution of ERα (**A**, **C**, and **E**) and ERβ (**B**, **D**, and **F**) in three different levels of the human (17-yr-old female) amygdala: rostral (**A** and **B**), middle (**C** and **D**), and caudal (**E** and **F**). Abbreviations: AB, accessory basal nucleus (pc, parvicellular division); AHA, amygdala-hippocampal area; B, basal amygdala nucleus (mc, magnocellular division; pc, parvicellular division); Ce, central amygdala nucleus; CL, claustrum; Cop, posterior cortical amygdala nucleus; EC, entorhinal cortex; gA, gyrus ambiens; Ic, insular cortex; L, lateral amygdala nucleus; MB, mammillary body; Me, medial amygdala nucleus; PAC, periamygdaloid cortex; S, subiculum; STc, superior temporal cortex. *Arrows* indicate hybridization signal in the superior temporal cortex in layers V and VI *(black arrow)* or layer V *(grey arrow)*. *, a tear or fold in the tissue. Scale bar, 5 mm. (Image adapted from Österlund *et al.*[19])

mate, and rodent in the expression pattern of the ER subtypes, but there are some noted significant differences (see Ref. 18). The following sections focus on the human ER mRNA anatomical organization and are based on postmortem *in situ* hybridization studies that are detailed in Refs. 19–21 and reviewed in Refs. 18 and 22.

Amygdala and the Extended Amygdala

The ERα mRNA is predominantly expressed in the more medial nuclei in the amygdaloid complex, throughout the rostral-to-caudal continuum (FIG. 1). The highest levels of ERα are observed in the amygdala-hippocampal area, periamygdaloid cortex, and posterior cortical nucleus. Moderate signals are found in the accessory basal nucleus and the nucleus of the lateral olfactory tract. The accessory basal nucleus is one of the major outputs for projections to the hippocampal formation, perirhinal cortex, and entorhinal cortex,[23] and thus strongly associated with memory. Low ERα labeling is found in the medial and anterior cortical nucleus, lateral nucle-

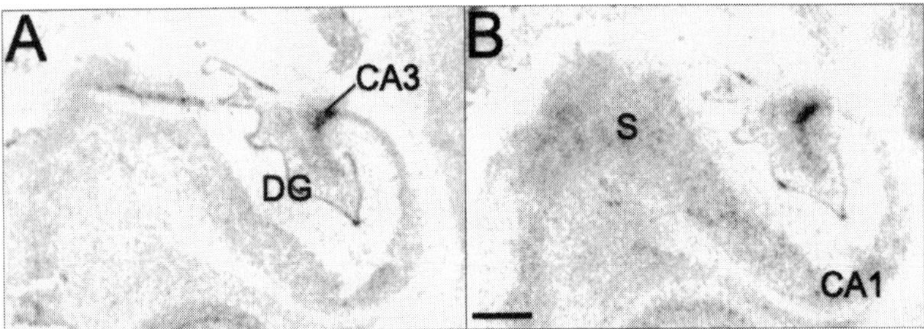

FIGURE 2. Distribution of ERα (**A**) and ERβ (**B**) mRNA expression in adjacent brain sections (coronal) of the human hippocampal formation (17-yr-old female). Abbreviations: DG, dentate gyrus; S, subiculum. Scale bar, 2.5 mm. (Image adapted from Österlund *et al.*[19]).

us, and the magnocellular division of the basal nucleus. However, no ERα signals are present in the basal or lateral nuclei of the primate amygdala. Low ERα signals are also apparent in the bed nucleus stria terminalis and the diagonal band of Broca, key components of the extended amygdala.

The ERβ subtype mRNA expression is very low in the human amygdala and generally not detectable in several of the nuclei (e.g., periamygdaloid cortex, medial, central, and accessory basal nucleus). Low ERβ labeling is detected in the basal and lateral nuclei, with even more reduced expression levels in the amygdala-hippocampal area and posterior cortical nucleus.

Thus, the amygdala appears to be an ERα–dominant area, suggesting primarily the α-subtype to modulate neuronal populations involved in emotional functions and behavioral responses mediated by the amygdala.

Hippocampal Formation

The human hippocampus expresses low ERα mRNA levels (FIG. 2). The signal is primarily detected in the CA3 and the dentate gyrus, with even lower expression in the subiculum and CA1-CA2. In contrast, the ERβ labeling is highest in the subiculum with lower labeling in CA1-CA2 and moderate labeling in CA3 and dentate gyrus. This pattern suggests not only estradiol-mediated regulation of hippocampal input and output signaling in the dentate gyrus and subiculum, but also that this regulation is primarily via the ERβ.

Cerebral Cortex

Both ER subtypes are expressed in the cerebral cortex, but with distinct expression patterns. In the temporal cortex, ERα mRNA is primarily expressed in cortical layer V, whereas ERβ labeling is expressed in both laminae V and VI. Both ERα and ERβ signaling are detected in the entorhinal cortex but with a more pronounced ERβ signal. The entorhinal cortex, origin of the perforant pathway to the hippocampus, and the temporal cortex play a role in memory, and thus the presence of ER mRNA in these regions further supports the notion that the ERs may regulate neuronal populations involved in cognition and declarative memory.

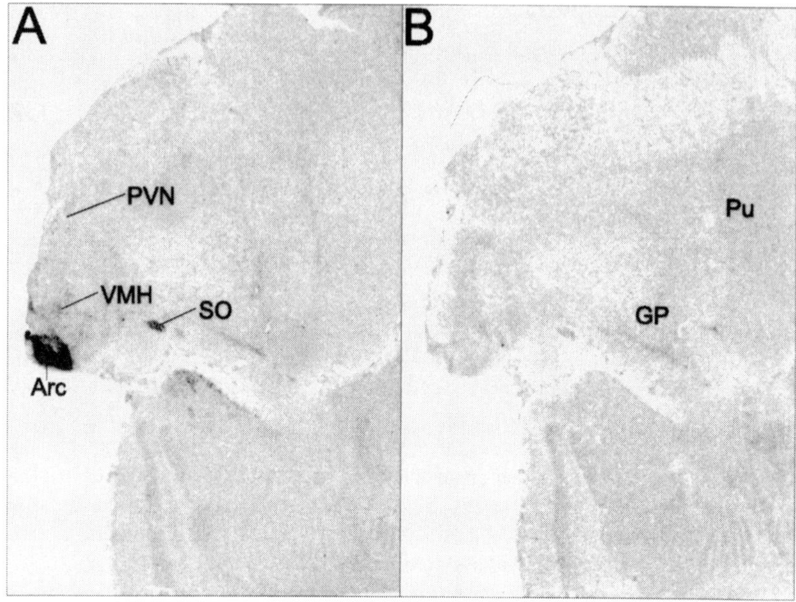

FIGURE 3. Autoradiogram images showing ERα (**A**) and ERβ (**B**) mRNA expression in adjacent brain sections (coronal) of the human hypothalamus (26-yr-old male.) Abbreviations: Arc, arcuate nucleus; GP, globus pallidus; Pu, putamen; PVN, paraventricular nucleus; So, supraoptic nucleus; VMH, ventromedial hypothalamus. Scale bar, 5 mm. (Image adapted from Österlund *et al.*[19])

Hypothalamus

The human hypothalamus expresses high ERα mRNA levels in the supraoptic, arcuate, paraventricular, and periventricular nuclei. Moderate labeling is apparent in the preoptic area, anterior hypothalamic nucleus, and ventromedial hypothalamus (FIG. 3). The ERβ mRNA expression, however, is very low in the human hypothalamic areas studied to date. Low ERβ levels are evident in the supraoptic and paraventricular nuclei, with even lower levels in the arcuate nucleus and ventromedial hypothalamus. Thus, the ERα appears to be the primary mediator of estrogenic hypothalamic regulation of neuroendocrine and autonomic events.

Basal Ganglia and Thalamus

No ERα mRNA expression is detected in the basal ganglia forebrain regions examined (putamen, caudate nucleus, nucleus accumbens, or globus pallidus). The human brain ERβ mRNA expression is also not evident in these structures (but no nucleus accumbens levels was analyzed). A similar lack of ERα labeling is observed in the main body of thalamus, but low to moderate levels of ERβ is found in the ventral lateral nucleus, which provides the major thalamic input to the primary motor cortex. Both ER subtypes show low to moderate hybridization signals in the subthalamic nucleus and claustrum. These results indicate that the ERs are not dominant in motor circuits, but when present it is the ERβ that would most likely mediate estradiol effects on motor behavior.

Distinct Regional Distribution Patterns of ERα mRNA Isoforms Expressed from Alternative Promoters within the Human Brain

One of the major findings regarding the ER genes is that there are distinct regional distribution patterns of alternative ERα gene promoter activity in the human brain.[24] It is known that the human ERα gene can be transcribed from multiple promotors, generating mRNA isoforms with unique 5′ ends in the untranslated region, although translated into identical proteins.[24,25] The brain is a very heterogeneous organ with many diverse cell types and functions, and alternative promoter usage in distinct human brain areas has been revealed using *in situ* hybridization and RT-PCR techniques.[22] The results shows that the proximal A-promoter has low activity in most brain areas examined, whereas the B-promoter activity is more restricted, predominantly localized to the high ERα-expressing mRNA regions, such as the amygdala-hippocampal area, posterior cortical amygdala nucleus, and accessory basal amygdala nucleus. Promoter C transcripts are not present in the brain, although they are evident in peripheral organs. This study shows for the first time that alternative promoters are used to regulate the ERα gene in distinct neuronal populations in the human hypothalamus, amygdala, hippocampus, and cerebral cortex. These findings of alternative ERα promoter activity in distinct neuronal populations suggest that multiple promoter usage is a possible mechanism to achieve differentiated regulation of the ERα expression, dependent on the cell phenotype and consequently the functions mediated by the specific neuron.

ESTROGEN IN RELATION TO PSYCHIATRIC DISORDERS

ER and 5-HT Receptor mRNA Expression and Effects of Estrogen Treatment in the Flinder-line-sensitive Rats, a Genetic Animal Model of Depression

One hypothesis regarding the connection between estrogen and mood disorder is based on the fact that estrogen modulates the serotonergic system, impairment of which has been shown to be highly associated with the etiology of depression and suicidal behavior.[26–28] Moreover, the 5-HT system is a primary target for a great number of antidepressant drugs.[29] The expression of the serotonergic receptors 5-HT_{1A} and 5-HT_{2A} has been extensively investigated in the postmortem human brain of subjects diagnosed with major depression. The results regarding the 5-HT_{2A} receptor are contradictory; some studies indicate a decrease[30,31] of the 5-HT_{2A} densities in the frontal cortex and hippocampus, while others point to an increase[32,33] or no change.[30,34] However, *in vivo* analyses of drug-free depressed patients using positron emission tomography have revealed decreased levels of 5-HT_{2A} receptors in limbic related cortical areas.[35] The results for the 5-HT_{1A} receptor are more in concordance with most studies reporting an increased expression of the receptor in the hippocampus[36] and the cerebral cortex.[37,38] There is also an increased expression of the 5-HT_{1A} receptor in the dorsal raphe nucleus in depressed subjects.[39] Estrogen treatment has interestingly been shown to decrease 5-HT_{1A} receptor mRNA levels in the dorsal raphe nucleus of ovariectomized monkeys, which is consistent with the hypothesis that estrogen is protective in depression disorders.[40] No human studies have been performed to date to determine estradiol effects on 5-HT neural system.

To further investigate the possible link between 5-HT and estrogen in depression, a genetic animal model of depression, the Flinders-sensitive rat (FSL), has been studied.[41]

The mRNA expression levels of the 5-HT_{1A} and the 5-HT_{2A} receptors as well as the ERα, and ERβ were analyzed in limbic brain areas of female ovariectomized FSL and FRL (the corresponding control animals) rats treated with a single dose of 17β-estradiol or vehicle.

No significant differences are evident for the 5-HT_{1A} receptor mRNA levels between the FSL and its control animals in areas examined, such as the cingulate cortex, motor cortex, perirhinal cortex (PRh), piriform cortex (Pir), posteromedial cortical amygdala (PMCo), CA2-3 region in the hippocampus, medial anterodorsal amygdala (MeAD), and the dentate gyrus (DG). Moreover, acute 17β-estradiol treatment equally affects (decreases) the 5-HT_{1A} receptor levels in both strains of animals. In contrast, FSL rats have impaired, primarily reduced, 5-HT_{2A} receptor mRNA expression levels in several of the brain areas examined, for example, PRh, Pir, and MeAD. Acute 17β-estradiol administration to the FSL animal normalizes the 5-HT_{2A} receptor mRNA expression levels in many brain areas, except for the hippocampus.

The abnormal 5-HT_{2A} receptor levels found in several limbic-related structures of the "depressed" FSL rats, indicates that the FSL rats have an imbalance in the 5-HT system, which is counteracted by 17β-estradiol treatment in several brain areas. Thus, the ability of estradiol to regulate the mRNA expression of 5-HT receptors, in particular the 5-HT_{2A} receptor, is a possible underlying mechanism in the link between estrogens and depression.

ER Expression in the Brainstem of Suicide Victims

Another biogenic amine that has been widely implicated in depressive disorders is NE. The NE system is, like the 5-HT system, a target for antidepressant medications. NE neuronal populations are also targets for estrogen in the brain. Distinct subpopulations of brainstem NE neurons in the locus coeruleus express ERs (FIG. 4) and the NE activity is clearly enhanced in response to estrogen. This may be due to the fact that a number of genes expressed by NE neurons are influenced by estrogen, such as transcription factors and co-released neuropeptides.[42] Very limited studies exist as to the expression and regulation of ERs in the NE locus coeruleus (LC) cells in relation to psychiatric disorders.

In the human brainstem, ERs showed the highest expression in the LC; hence this structure may be an important region for gonadal hormones to regulate the noradrenergic system. The NE neurons, localized in the LC, project throughout the forebrain with high levels in the cerebral cortex. Recently we performed a pilot study to examine the potential abnormality in the ER expression in this region. We measured the ERα and ERβ mRNA expression levels in locus coeruleus in human postmortem brains of suicide victims (n = 7) and controls (n = 9) by means of *in situ* hybridization histochemistry. It is well documented that suicide is highly as-

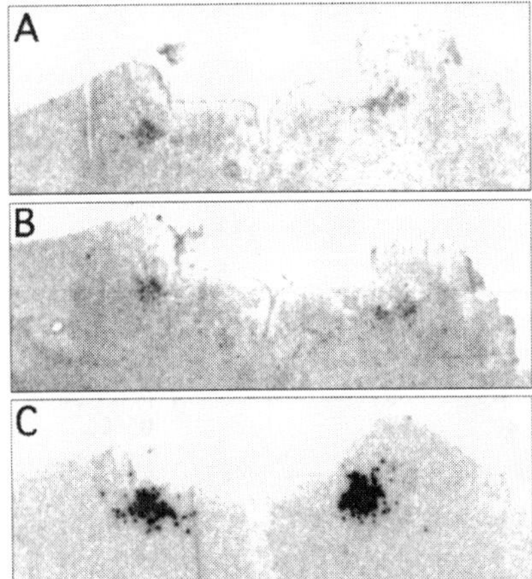

FIGURE 4. ERα (**A**), ERβ (**B**), and NET (**C**) mRNA expression in adjacent brain sections of the human locus coeruleus.

sociated with depression symptoms.[43] Interestingly, we found a significant ($P<0.05$) reduction in ERβ mRNA expression in the LC in the suicide victims (125.3 ± 20 dpm/mg) as compared to control subjects (186.5 ± 19 dpm/mg). There were no significant differences for the ERα levels. A larger study is under way to confirm these preliminary results. Reduced ERs and potentially reduced NE tone would be consistent with decreased NE levels associated with depression disorders.

CONCLUSIONS

The ER mRNA signals are low in the human brain and detected in only a few restricted regions. ERβ is predominantly expressed in the hippocampal formation, entorhinal cortex, thalamus, and claustrum, suggesting a role for ERβ in cognition, non-emotional memory, and motor functions. The ERα subtype on the other hand, dominates in the primate hypothalamus and amygdala, indicating that the α-subtype modulates neuronal cell populations involved in autonomic and reproductive functions as well as emotional expression and mood regulation, which are disturbed in many mental disorders. Moreover, ER expression in the LC suggests that estrogens have the possibility of altering NE function, which is strongly implicated in depressive disorders. These findings further strengthen the association between estrogen and mental diseases, and in particular depression.

ACKNOWLEDGMENTS

This work was supported by the Söderström-Königska Sjukhushem Stiftelse (Y.L.H.), the Karolinska Institute Fond (Y.L.H.), and the Hungarian National Research Foundation (OTKA T32227; E.K.)

REFERENCES

1. PAYKEL, E.S. 1991. Depression in women. Br. J. Psychiatry. (Suppl. 10) **158:** 22–29.
2. PEARLSTEIN, T., K. ROSEN & A.B. STONE. 1997. Mood disorders and menopause. Endocrinol. Metab. Clin. N. Am. **26:** 279–294.
3. SICHEL, D.A., L.S. COHEN, L.M.A. ROBERTSON, *et al.* 1995. Prophylactic estrogen in recurrent postpartum affective disorder. Biol. Psychiatry **38:** 814–818.
4. GREGOIRE, A.J.P., R. KUMAR, B. EVERITT, *et al.* 1996. Transdermal oestrogen for treatment of severe postnatal depression. Lancet **347:** 930–933.
5. BEST, N., M. REES, D. BARLOW & P. COWEN. 1992. Effect of estradiol implant on noradrenergic function and mood in menopausal subjects. Psychoneuroendocrinology **17:** 87–93.
6. HAFNER, H., A. REICHER-RÖSSLER, K. MAURER, *et al.* 1992. First onset and early symptomatology of schizophrenia. Eur. Arch. Psychiatry Clin. Neurosci. **242:** 109–118.
7. HAMBRECHT, M., K. MAURER & H. HÄFNER. 1992. Evidence for a gender bias in epidemiological studies of schizophrenia. Schizophr. Res. **8:** 223–231.
8. GALDOS, P.M., J.J. VAN OS & R.M. MURRAY. 1993. Puberty and the onset of psychosis. Schizophr. Res. **10:** 7–14.
9. FARAONE, S.V., W.J. CHEN, J.M. GOLDSTEIN & M.T. TSUANG. 1994. Gender differences in age at onset of schizophrenia. Br. J. Psychiatry **164:** 625–629.
10. SZYMANSKI, S., J.A. LIEBERMAN, J.M. ALVIR, *et al.* 1995. Gender differences in onset of illness, treatment response, course, and biological indexes in first-episode schizophrenic patient. Am. J. Psychiatry **152:** 698–703.
11. RIECHER-RÖSSLER, A. & H. HÄFNER. 1993. Schizophrenia and oestrogen—is there an association? Eur. Arch. Psychiatry Clin. Neurosci. **242:** 323–328.
12. SEEMAN, M.V. 1986. Current outsome in schizophrenia: women vs men. Acta Psychiatric. Scand. **73:** 609–617.
13. RIECHER-RÖSSLER, A., H. HÄFNER, K. MAURER, *et al.* 1992. Schizophrenic symptomatology varies with serum estradiol levels during menstrual cycle. Schizophr. Res. **6:** 114–115.
14. HALLONQUIST, J., M.V. SEEMAN, M. LANG & N.A. RECTOR. 1993. Variation in symptoms severity over the menstrual cycle of schizophrenics. Biol. Psychiatry **33:** 207–209.
15. GATTAZ, W.F., P. VOGEL, A. RIECHERROSSLER & G. SODDU. 1994. Influence of the menstrual cycle phase on the therapeutic response in schizophrenia. Biol. Psychiatry **36:** 137–139.
16. CARSON-JURICA, M.A., W.T. SCHRADER & B.W. O'MALLEY. 1990. Steroid receptor family: structure and functions. Endocr. Rev. **11:** 201–220.
17. MANGELSDORF, D.J, C. THUMMEL, M. BEATO, *et al.* 1995. The nuclear receptor superfamily: the second decade. Cell **83:** 835–839.
18. M.K. ÖSTERLUND & Y.L. HURD. 2001. Estrogen receptors in the human forebrain and the relation to neuropsychiatric disorders. Prog. Neurobiol. **64:** 251–267.
19. OSTERLUND, M., J-Ý. GUSTAFSSON, E. KELLER & Y.L. HURD. 2000. Estrogen receptor beta (ERbeta) messenger ribonucleic acid (mRNA) expression within the human forebrain: distinct distribution pattern to ERalpha mRNA. J. Clin. Endocrinol. Metab. **85:** 3840–3846.
20. ÖSTERLUND, M.K., E. KELLER & Y.L. HURD. 2000. The human amygdaloid complex is characterized by high expression of the estrogen receptor mRNA. Neuroscience **95:** 333–342.
21. ÖSTERLUND, M.K., K.E. GRANDIEN, E. KELLER & Y.L. HURD. 2000. The human brain has distinct regional expression patterns of estrogen receptor alpha mRNA isoforms derived from alternative promoters. J. Neurochem. **75:** 1390–1397.
22. ÖSTERLUND, M.K. 2002. The role of estrogens in neuropsychiatric disorders. Curr. Opin. Psychiatry **15:** 307–312.
23. GLOOR, P. 1997. The amygdaloid system. *In* The Temporal Lobe and Limbic System. P. Gloor, Ed.: 591–651. Oxford University Press. New York.

24. GRANDIEN, K. 1996. Determination of transcription start sites in the human estrogen receptor gene and identification of a novel, tissue-specific, estrogen receptor-mRNA isoform. Mol. Cell. Endocrinol. **116:** 207–212.
25. FLOURIOT, G., C. GRIFFIN, M. KENEALY, *et al.* 1998. Differentially expressed messenger RNA isoforms of the human estrogen receptor-alpha gene are generated by alternative splicing and promoter usage. Mol. Endocrinol. **12:** 1939–1954.
26. ÅSBERG, M., L. TRÄSKMAN & P. THOREN. 1976. 5-HIAA in the cerebrospinal fluid: a biochemical suicide predictor. Arch. Gen. Psychiatry **33:** 1193–1197.
27. VAN PRAAG, H.M. 1983. Depression, suicide and the metabolites of serotonin in the brain. J. Affective Disord. **4:** 275–290.
28. MELTZER, H.Y. & M.T. LOWY. 1987. The serotonin hypothesis of depression. *In* Psychopharmacology: The Third Generation of Progress. H.Y. Meltzer, Ed.: 513–526. Raven Press. New York.
29. MERSON, S. & P. TYRER. 1991. Physical treatments for depression. *In* Biological Aspects of Affective Disorders. R. Horton & C. Katona, Eds.: 47–68. Academic Press. San Diego, CA.
30. CHEETHAM, S.C., M.R. CROMPTON, C.L.E. KATONA & R.W. HORTON. 1988. Brain 5-HT_2 receptor binding sites in depressed suicide victims. Brain Res. **443:** 272–280.
31. GROSS-ISSEROFF, R., D. SALAMA, M. ISRAELI & A. BIEGON. 1990. Autoradiographic analysis of [^{3}H]ketanserin binding in the human brain postmortem: effect of suicide. Brain Res. **507:** 208–215.
32. STANLEY, M. & J.J. MANN. 1983. Increased serotonin-2 binding site in frontal cortex of suicide victims. Lancet **1:** 214–216.
33. ARORA, R.C. & H.Y. MELTZER. 1989. Serotonergic measures in the brains of suicide victims: 5-HT_2 binding sites in the frontal cortex of suicide victims and control subjects. Am. J. Psychiatry **146:** 730–736.
34. STOCKMEIER, C.A., G.E. DILLEY, B.S. SHAPIRO, *et al.* 1997. Serotonin receptors in suicide victims with major depression. Neuropsychopharmacology **16:** 162–173.
35. BIVER, F., D. WIKLER, F. LOTSTRA, *et al.* 1997. Serotonin 5-HT_2 receptor imaging in major depression: focal changes in orbito-insular cortex. Br. J. Psychiatry **171:** 444–448.
36. MATSUBARA, S., R.C. ARORA & H.Y. MELTZER. 1991. Serotonergic measures in suicide brain: 5-HT1A binding sites in frontal cortex of suicide victims. J. Neural Transm. Gen. Sect. **85:** 181–194.
37. JOYCE, J.N., A. SHANE, N. LEXOW, *et al.* 1993. Serotonin uptake sites and serotonin receptors are altered in the limbic system of schizophrenics. Neuropsychopharmacology **8:** 315–336.
38. ARANGO, V., M.D. UNDERWOOD, A.D. GUBBI & J.J. MANN. 1995. Localized alterations in pre- and postsynaptic serotonin binding sites in the ventrolateral prefrontal cortex of suicide victims. Brain Res. **688:** 121–133.
39. STOCKMEIER, C.A., B.S. SHAPIRO, G.E. DILLEY, *et al.* 1998. Increase in serotonin-1A autoreceptors in the midbrain of suicide victims with major depression-postmortem evidence for decreased serotonin activity. J. Neurosci. **18:** 7394–7401.
40. PECINS-THOMPSON, M. & C.L. BETHEA. 1999. Ovarian steroid regulation of serotonin-1A autoreceptor messenger RNA expression in the dorsal raphe of rhesus macaques. Neuroscience **89:** 267–277.
41. ÖSTERLUND, M., D.H. OVERSTREET & Y.L. HURD. 1999. The Flinders sensitive line rats, a genetic model of depression, show abnormal serotonin receptor mRNA expression in the brain that is reversed by 17β-estradiol. Brain Res. Mol. Brain Res. **10:** 158–166.
42. HERBISON, A.E., S.X. SIMONIAN, N.R. THANKY & R.J. BICKNELL. 2000. Oestrogen modulation of noradrenaline neurotransmission [review]. Novartis Found. Symp. **230:** 74–85; discussion 85–93.
43. HENRIKSSON, M.M., H.M. ARO, M J. MARTTUNEN, *et al.* 1993. Mental disorders and comorbidity in suicide. Am. J. Psychiatry **150:** 935–940.

Neurosteroid Biosynthesis in the Human Brain and Its Clinical Implications

BIRGIT STOFFEL-WAGNER

Department of Clinical Biochemistry, University of Bonn, D-53127 Bonn, Germany

ABSTRACT: This paper summarizes the current knowledge concerning the biosynthesis of neurosteroids in the human brain, the enzymes mediating these reactions, their localization, and the putative effects of neurosteroids. The presence of the steroidogenic enzymes cytochrome $P450_{SCC}$, aromatase, 5α-reductase, 3α-hydroxysteroid dehydrogenase, and 17β-hydroxysteroid dehydrogenase in the human brain has now been firmly established by molecular biological and biochemical studies. Their presence in the cerebral cortex and in the subcortical white matter indicates that various cell types, either neurons or glial cells, are involved in the biosynthesis of neuroactive steroids in the brain. The following functions are attributed to specific neurosteroids: modulation of $GABA_A$, *N*-methyl-D-aspartate (NMDA), nicotinic, muscarinic, serotonin ($5\text{-}HT_3$), kainate, glycine and sigma receptors, neuroprotection and induction of neurite outgrowth, dendritic spines, and synaptogenesis. We still do not know whether and how the steroidogenic enzymes are involved in the pathophysiology of the nervous system. The first clinical investigations in humans produced evidence for an involvement of neuroactive steroids in conditions such as fatigue during pregnancy, premenstrual syndrome, postpartum depression, catamenial epilepsy, and depressive disorders. Further and improved knowledge of the biochemical pathways of neurosteroidogenesis and their actions on the brain may enable new perspectives in the understanding of the physiology of the human brain as well as in the pharmacological treatment of its disturbances.

KEYWORDS: neurosteroid; human brain; 5α-reductase; 3α-hydroxysteroid dehydrogenase; aromatase; 17β-dehydrogenase

INTRODUCTION

Steroid hormones are mainly synthesized in the gonads, the adrenal glands, and the feto-placental unit. The brain is an important target organ of steroid hormones. In the brain, an extensive steroid metabolism occurs. Also, several brain regions are well equipped with enzymes necessary for steroid hormone biosynthesis.[1–4] Development, growth, maturation, and differentiation of the brain are strongly influenced by steroid hormones. As shown in animal studies, steroids synthesized *de novo* in the

Address for correspondence: PD Dr. med. Birgit Stoffel-Wagner, Institut fuer Klinische Biochemie, Universitaet Bonn, Sigmund-Freud-Str. 25, D-53127 Bonn, Germany. Voice: +49-228-2875141; fax: +49-228-2875789

Birgit.Stoffel-Wagner@ukb.uni-bonn.de

Ann. N.Y. Acad. Sci. 1007: 64–78 (2003).
doi: 10.1196/annals.1286.007

central nervous system (i.e., neurosteroids) can affect multiple brain functions (i.e., neuroendocrine and behavioral functions) via intracellular receptors which regulate transcriptionally directed changes in protein synthesis. In addition to the classical genomic actions of steroids, neurosteroids are able to rapidly alter excitability of the central nervous system through binding to neurotransmitter-gated ion channels, thus modulating γ-aminobutyric acid A ($GABA_A$) and *N*-methyl-D-aspartate receptors.[5,6]

In the case of aromatase, the activity of steroidogenic enzymes was identified in human fetal brain tissue 25 years ago.[7] However, the majority of biochemical, physiological, and behavioral studies on aromatase in brain tissue were carried out in rodents or other animal species. For a long time, studies in humans have been precluded owing to the difficulty in obtaining fresh human brain tissue, coupled with presumably low expression or activity of the respective enzymes. This also applies to other steroidogenic enzymes. Steroidogenesis requires a number of sequential enzymatic reactions to convert cholesterol to sex hormones, glucocorticoids, or mineralocorticoids. As the steroids produced within a tissue depend upon the enzymes present in this tissue, only systematic studies on the expression of all relevant steroidogenic enzymes would allow insight into the steroidogenic pathways and the capacity within the respective tissue, that is, the human brain. Reports on the expression and activity of the most important steroidogenic enzymes in the human brain have been published in recent years. The present paper reviews the current knowledge of steroid hormone metabolism within the human brain and the evidence we have for its importance.

SYNTHESIS AND METABOLISM OF STEROIDS IN THE HUMAN BRAIN

Cytochrome $P450_{SCC}$

Expression of P450scc (cytochrome P450scc, CYP11A1), induces *de novo* synthesis of neurosteroids, since it is the single enzyme mediating the conversion of the steroid precursor, cholesterol, to pregnenolone. Human $P450_{SCC}$ is encoded by a single gene on chromosome 15, the CYP11A1 gene.[8] Not only is P450scc present in the adrenal glands and gonads, the major sources of steroid hormone production, but it is also present in the placenta, primitive gut, and brain.[9–11] Once pregnenolone is produced from cholesterol, it may be converted to progesterone and other neuroactive steroids. However, the major role of $P450_{SCC}$ in the brain is probably the regulation of brain neurosteroid levels.[12] We recently investigated the expression of CYP11A1 mRNA in tissue specimens from temporal and frontal neocortex, subcortical white matter from the temporal lobe, and in the hippocampus from patients with medically intractable chronic temporal lobe epilepsy.[13,14] In these brain areas, CYP11A1 mRNA was expressed in significant amounts in all tissue samples investigated, but at a rate ≈ 200 times lower than in adrenal tissue, which is known for highest CYP11A1 expression. Thus, CYP11A1 mRNA expression in the human brain is within the range previously estimated for rat brain in qualitative RT-PCR experiments.[11,12,15] In humans, CYP11A1 mRNA concentrations in the temporal lobe increase markedly during childhood and reach adult levels at puberty.[13] In the temporal and frontal neocortex as well as in the hippocampus of women CYP11A1 mRNA concentrations were significantly higher when compared to those of men.[13,14] An age- and sex-dependent expression of CYP11A1 mRNA in the human brain could be demonstrated with these data for the first time. Few data are available on the relative amount of CYP11A1 mRNA in the brain of male and female animals, but qualitative studies report no obvious sex differences in rats.[11,16] On account of the insensitivity of qualitative RT-PCR in detecting differences in mRNA expression at high cycle numbers, a careful quantitative re-examination of results obtained in rat brain with respect to sex differences of CYP11A1 mRNA expression seems called for. Whereas *in situ* hybridization and cell culture experiments in rat brain demonstrated predominant CYP11A1 expression in the subcortical white matter,[15,17] no such differences could be detected between neocortex and subcortical white matter tissue in the human brain.[13] Evidence that pregnenolone can be produced in the central nervous system is provided by the presence of CYP11A1 mRNA in human brain tissue.

Aromatase

Cytochrome P450 aromatase catalyses the conversion of androgens into estrogens in specific brain areas.[3] It is the product of the CYP19 gene, which has been cloned and sequenced.[18,19]

Only in a few fetal brain specimens has aromatase activity itself been determined.[20–22] Previously published data demonstrated aromatase activity in human temporal and in frontal brain areas.[23] The authors studied biopsy materials removed at autopsy from normal adult control subjects and from patients with Alzheimer's disease. Regardless of sex and/or disease state, temporal aromatase activity was always significantly higher than frontal aromatase activity. This difference was also confirmed by our own studies on the expression of temporal and frontal CYP19 mRNA in fresh brain tissue specimens from adult patients with medically intractable chronic epilepsy undergoing neurosurgery.[24] CYP19 mRNA was not only expressed in temporal and frontal neocortex, but also in the human hippocampus and in subcortical white matter of the temporal lobe.[24,25] No sex-specific differences in CYP19 mRNA expression could be observed in any of these brain areas. In our laboratory, we were able to characterize aromatase activity in the temporal lobe in brain tissue specimens of a similar cohort of patients with epilepsy.[26] We demonstrated a specific, dose-responsive, and competitive inhibition of its activity by atamestane, which is a known specific and competitive inhibitor of placental aromatase activity.[27] Compared to its high activity in the placenta, aromatase activity in the human brain was low. However, rates of aromatase activity in the brain were in the same order of magnitude as in human adipose and testicular tissue.[28,29] Through subsequent experiments with cerebral neocortex and subcortical white matter specimens of children and adults a significantly higher aromatase activity in the cerebral neocortex than in the subcortical white matter was revealed.[26] For CYP19 mRNA expression in the human temporal lobe this difference could not be found.[25] However, in the human temporal neocortex, CYP19 mRNA concentrations were significantly lower in children than in adults.[25] This finding could not be confirmed by measurement of aromatase activity.[26] These contradictory findings indicate that aromatase might be regulated on the post-translational level.

5α-Reductase

Numerous animal studies have shown that, in the brain, progesterone is rapidly metabolized to 5α-dihydroprogesterone (5α-DHP). This is then further reduced to the potent neurosteroid 3α,5α-tetrahydroprogesterone (3α,5αTHP).[6] These conversions are catalyzed by 5α-reductase and 3α-hydroxysteroid dehydrogenase (3α-HSD). In humans, two isozymes of 5α-reductase, which differ in tissue distribution and biochemical characteristics as well as in their responsiveness to specific inhibitors of their enzymatic activity, have been identified.[30,3]

The majority of physiological and biochemical studies on the expression of 5α-reductase in the brain were carried out in rodents and other animal species.[1,2,32,33] However, some investigators documented 5α-reductase activity in human fetal brain.[34–36] Only in a few frontal lobe and temporal lobe tissue specimens was 5α-reductase activity demonstrated in the brain of adults.[37,38]

The predominant expression of 5α-reductase type 1 mRNA in a large series of human temporal neocortex and subcortical white matter as well as hippocampal tissue specimens obtained from patients with medically intractable chronic temporal lobe epilepsy was recently demonstrated by us.[39,40] The expression levels were about 100 times lower than in human liver tissue. 5α-reductase type 2 mRNA was not expressed. Another study reported on 5α-reductase type 1 mRNA expression in a few human cerebellum, hypothalamus, and pons tissue specimens that were collected post mortem.[41] Also, in rat brain, a predominant expression of 5α-reductase type 1 mRNA was found.[2,42]

We also measured 5α-reductase activity in human temporal neocortex and subcortical white matter tissue specimens.[39,43] While enzyme activity was present in all tissue specimens under investigation, the apparent K_m values and the pH profile substantiated the predominant expression of the type 1 isoform. We also investigated the inhibitory effects of MK386, a specific inhibitor of the 5α-reductase type 1 isoform, and of finasteride, a specific inhibitor of the 5α-reductase type 2 isoform on 5α-reductase activity.[43] MK386 was a strong inhibitor of human brain tissue 5α-reductase activity, with an IC50 value of 2.0 nmol/l, whereas finasteride turned out to be a poor inhibitor of the reaction, with an IC50 value of 142.8 nmol/l.[43] Moreover, we observed a potent inhibition of the pH-dependent reaction by MK386, but not by finasteride. An at least predominant activity of the 5α-reductase type 1 isozyme in the human brain is further substantiated by these findings.[43] There were no sex-specific differences in the expression levels of 5α-reductase type 1 mRNA in human brain tissue or in the activity of 5α-reductase.[39,40,43] These findings are consistent with previous animal studies, where no significant sex-specific differences concerning 5α-reductase activity were found in rat brain.[44,45]

3α-Hydroxysteroid Dehydrogenase

Multiple cDNAs encode proteins related to 3α-HSD in humans.[46] However, at least four 3α-HSD isozymes exist which share at least 84% of its amino acid sequence identity.[47–50] These are known as type 1 3α-HSD (AKR1C4), type 2 3α-HSD (AKR1C3), type 3 3α-HSD (AKR1C2), and 20α(3α)-HSD (ACR1C1). This isoform is predominantly a 20α-HSD, and this change in positional specificity implies that it may play an important role in regulating progesterone action.[50]

Penning and co-workers demonstrated that all human 3α-HSD isoforms and the human 20α-HSD act as 3-, 17- and 20-ketosteroid reductases as well as 3-, 17- and 20-hydroxysteroid oxidases.[50]

In a recent study, we could only demonstrate the expression of the mRNA of type 2 and 3 isozyme of 3α-HSD as well as 20α-HSD in the hippocampus and the temporal lobe of patients with temporal lobe epilepsy, whereas the mRNA of the type 1 isozyme of 3α-HSD was not expressed.[40,43] The expression levels of 3α-HSD 2 were about one-fifth of that in liver tissue, those of 3α-HSD 3 about one-tenth of that in liver tissue, and those of 20α-HSD were about 2% percent (≈1/40) of that in liver tissue (own unpublished data). The expression levels of 3α-HSD 2 and 3 as well as 20α-HSD mRNAs did not differ significantly between hippocampal tissue from epileptic men and and hippocampal tissue of women. This is in accordance with data on 3α-HSD activity in the rat brain.[40]

All of these three isoforms, 3α-HSD 2 and 3 and 20α-HSD, are capable of producing the neuroactive tetrahydrosteroids that modulate the $GABA_A$ receptor.[50] Consequently, the meaning of the differential expression of the single isoforms is less established than ever.

17β-Hydroxysteroid Dehydrogenase

Seven human isozymes of 17β-hydroxysteroid dehydrogenase (17β-HSD) have been cloned so far. They all play a major role in the regulation of the biological activity of sex hormones and they are essential for the biosynthesis of the strong androgens and estrogens testosterone and estradiol from their weaker precursors androstenedione and estrone.[51,52] These conversions are reversible and thus can lead to a deactivation of the respective sex hormones.[53] The different isozymes show an individual cell-specific expression and substrate specificity. The ubiquitous distribution of 17β-HSD in peripheral tissues reflects the importance of the 17β-HSD activity in the maintenance of physiological levels of estradiol and testosterone.[54]

17β-HSD activity in the human brain has been reported about 30 years ago.[37,55] However, only very few studies on the expression of the enzyme in the human brain exist to date. Western immunoblot analysis revealed the presence of 17β-HSD 1 in human fetal brain.[56] Recently, we demonstrated the expression of 17β-HSD 1, 3, 4 and 5 mRNA in the human temporal lobe and hippocampus.[57,58] An in-tandem pseudogene of 17β-HSD 1 and 17β-HSD 2 mRNA were not expressed.[57,58] We also characterized androgenic and estrogenic 17β-HSD activity in the human temporal lobe and found the NADPH-dependent reduction of androstenedione and estrone as well as the NAD-dependent oxidation of testosterone and estradiol.[59] Substrate specificity, pH optima, cofactor requirement patterns, and kinetic properties suggest the activity of at least two isozymes, namely, the activating 17β-HSD 3 and the deactivating 17β-HSD 4, in the human brain. The activity of 17β-HSDs and the expression levels of the mRNAs did not differ significantly between the sexes. However, the expression levels of 17β-HSD 3, 4 and 5 mRNAs as well as the conversion of androstenedione, testosterone, estrone, and estradiol were significantly higher in the subcortical white matter than in the cerebral neocortex.[57–59] The predominant expression of 17β-HSD in the subcortical white matter suggests that glial cells could play a role in the biosynthesis and deactivation of sex steroids in the brain. Among a host of potential functions of glia, glial cells are involved in the formation of myelin. This suggests a possible correlation between sex steroids, these enzymatic activities, and the formation or functions of myelin.

In a recent study on the human 17β-HSD 7 gene (*HSD17B7*), its promotor revealed binding sites for brain-specific transcription factors corresponding to expression domains in the developing brain as identified by *in silico* Northern blot.[52] To date, 17β-HSD 8 expression has not been investigated in the human brain.

Other Steroidogenic Enzymes

Other important steroidogenic enzymes are 3β-hydroxysteroid dehydrogenase (3β-HSD), cytochrome $P450c_{17}$, 21-hydroxylase (cytochrome P450c21), 11β-hydroxylase (cytochrome P45011β) and cytochrome P450 aldosterone synthetase (P-450aldo).

3β-HSD catalyzes the conversion of Δ^5-3β-hydroxysteroids into Δ^4-3-ketostreroids (i.e., the conversion of pregnenolone into progesterone). Cytochrome $P450c_{17}$, which possesses both 17α-hydroxylase and 17,20 lyase activity, is responsible for the conversion of C_{21} steroids (pregnenolone, progesterone) into C_{19} steroids (DHEA and androstenedione).

21-hydroxylase converts progesterone to 11-deoxycorticosterone and 17-hydroxyprogesterone to 11-deoxycortisol. These are the substrates required for the production of the main adrenal steroids, corticosterone, aldosterone and cortisol. 11β-hydroxylase (cytochrome P45011β) catalyzes the formation of glucocorticoids (cortisol and corticosterone). Cytochrome P450 aldosterone synthetase (P-450aldo), which exerts three enzyme activities (11β-hydroxylation, 18-hydroxylation, and 18-oxidoreduction), catalyzes the formation of mineralocorticoids (aldosterone).

Only a small number of studies on the expression of 21-hydroxylase in the brain exist to date. In rodents, 21-hydroxylase was detected in the brain stem using the reverse transcription polymerase chain reaction assay and immunohistochemical methods.[60,61] Other investigators could not find 21-hydroxylase mRNA in any extra-adrenal tissue.[62] Since this may be due to the limited sensitivity of the mRNA quantification assay, we investigated the expression of 21-hydroxylase mRNA in the human hippocampus using a highly sensitive nested RT-PCR assay.[63] Our study demonstrated for the first time the expression of 21-hydroxylase mRNA in the human hippocampus. In the hippocampus, the expression levels are approximately 10,000 times lower than in the adrenal gland, which is known for high 21 hydroxylase expression.[63] However, we were unable to measure the enzyme activity of 21-hydroxylase as only small amounts of tissue specimens were available. Although our results clearly demonstrate that 21-hydroxylase mRNA is expressed in small amounts in the human hippocampus, it remains debatable whether hippocampal tissue contains sufficient 21-hydroxylase to produce neuroactive steroid concentrations of physiological or pathophysiological relevance.

The mRNAs of 3β-hydroxysteroid dehydrogenase (3β-HSD) 1 and 2 as well as cytochrome P45011β and cytochrome P450 aldosterone synthetase were neither expressed in the human temporal lobe nor in hippocampus (our own unpublished data). For these investigations a sensitive, nested competitive RT-PCR assay was used. However, several studies demonstrated the expression of 3β-HSD mRNA[15,64,65] and 3β-HSD protein[65] in the rat brain. Data concerning the expression of cytochrome P45011β in rodent brain are conflicting: some authors report the expression throughout the rat brain,[61,66] while others found only low expression levels in rat brain[11,67] or no expression in mouse brain.[61] In various regions of rat brain, including hypothalamus, hippocampus, amygdala and cerebellum, cytochrome P450 aldosterone synthetase expression and activity have been demonstrated.[66,68]

Cytochrome P450c_{17} mRNA was not expressed in the human temporal lobe or hippocampus (our own unpublished data). Previous studies failed to demonstrate 17α-hydroxylase activity or P450c17 mRNA in the adult rat brain.[11,69] However, P450c17 mRNA as well as P450c17 protein were detected in the brain of rat embryos using ribonuclease protection assays and immunocytochemistry.[70] In adults the data reported have been conflicting: Compagnone and co-workers[70] reported expression of P450c17 mRNA only in the peripheral nervous system of rats and mice; others demonstrated the presexnce of P450c17 mRNA in various brain regions of adult rodents.[61]

CLINICAL IMPLICATIONS

The presence of the above-mentioned steroidogenic enzymes cytochrome $P450_{SCC}$, aromatase, 5α-reductase, 3α-hydroxysteroid dehydrogenase, and 17β-hydroxysteroid dehydrogenase in human brain has now been firmly established by molecular biological and biochemical studies. These findings provide evidence that neuroactive steroids can be produced within the human brain. However, the (patho)physiological significance of these findings remains to be elucidated. FIGURE 1 presents a summary of current knowledge and open questions on biochemical pathways of steroid metabolism in the human brain.

Steroid hormone effects on the brain have typically been associated with gene regulation via intracellular steroid receptors. These reproductive and neuroendocrine actions of steroids via intracellular receptors, which regulate transcriptionally directed changes in protein synthesis generally occur within hours or days. In addition to the classic sites of steroid synthesis, neurosteroids can rapidly alter the excitability of the central nervous system by modulating neurotransmitter-gated ion channels such as γ-aminobutyric acid A ($GABA_A$) and *N*-methyl-D-aspartate (NMDA) receptors.[5,6,69]

GABA, a major inhibitory neurotransmitter, mediates fast synaptic inhibition by activating ligand-gated chloride channels. Binding of 3α-reduced neurosteroids to $GABA_A$ receptors results in either inhibition or potentiation of the inhibitory effects of GABA (FIG. 2). Therefore, anticonvulsive, anaesthetic and anxiolytic effects of neuroactive steroids are mediated by their capacity to positively modulate $GABA_A$ receptor function (i.e., these substances act to increase GABA-ergic effects by increasing frequency and duration of chloride channel openings).[5,6] On the other hand, inhibition of $GABA_A$ receptor function, which is mostly documented for the neurosteroids pregenenolone sulfate and DHEAS, produces effects ranging from anxiety and excitability to seizure susceptibility.[71–73]

Other neurosteroid actions have been described in the brain including the inhibition of *N*-methyl-D-aspartate (NMDA) receptor function as well as the modulation of other receptors, such as nicotinic, muscarinic, serotonin (5-HT_3), kainate, glycine and sigma receptors.[74–79] In summary, neurosteroids exert both genomic and nongenomic effects, and regulate neuronal function via their concurrent influence on gene

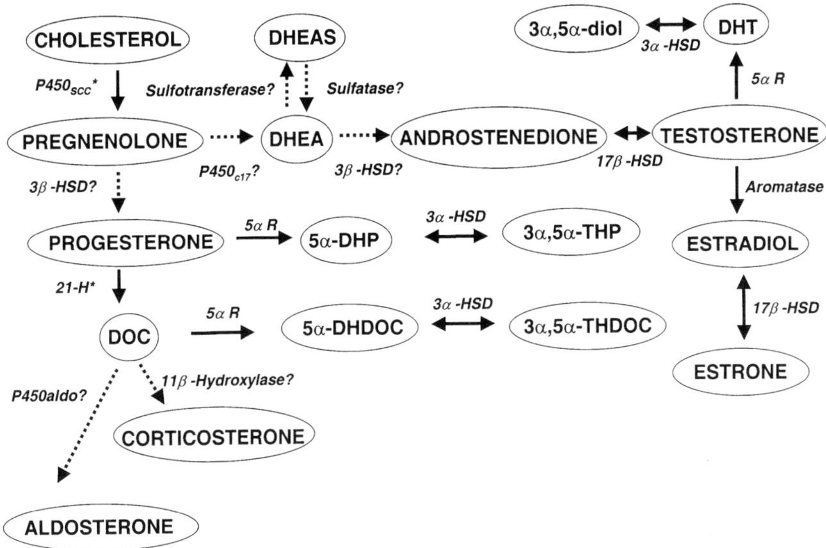

FIGURE 1. Current knowledge and open questions concerning the biochemical pathways of neurosteroidogenesis in the human brain. *Solid arrows* indicate that the activity of the respective enzyme as well as the expression of its mRNA has been documented, with the exception of P450SCC and 21-hydroxylase (marked by an *asterisk*) as here only the expression of its mRNA has been shown. *Dashed arrows* indicate that the occurrence of the enzyme has not yet been found in the nervous system. DOC, deoxicorticosterone; DHT, dihydrotestosterone; 5α-DHP, 5α-dihydroprogesterone; 3α,5α-THP, 3α,5α-tetrahydroprogesterone (allopregnanolone); 5αR, 5α-reductase; 3α-HSD, 3α-hydroxisteroid dehydrogenase; 3β-HSD, 3β-hydroxisteroid dehydrogenase; 17β-HSD, 17β-hydroxisteroid dehydrogenase; 21-H, 21-hydroxylase.

expression and transmitter-gated ion channels. These actions suggest that neurosteroids play a crucial role in mediating many brain functions.

The majority of physiological and behavioral studies have been carried out in rodents or other vertebrate species so far. In recent years, evidence for an intensive neurosteroid formation within the human brain has emerged. Now, the first clinical investigations exist to support the results obtained in preclinical animal studies.

As early as 1941,[80] the potential anaesthetic properties of neuroactive steroids had been suggested. This led to the development of steroid anaesthetics such as alphaxalone.[81] However, side effects have hindered the development of steroid anaesthetics for routine clinical use.[71]

Apparently, the observation that epileptic seizures in cycling women are less frequent in the luteal phase, when circulating levels of progesterone are high, is associated with cyclical variations in the metabolism of progesterone to allopregnanolone in the brain.[6,82,83] Progesterone and 3α-reduced neuroactive steroids have potent anticonvulsant effects.[84,85] Synthetic derivates of neuroactive steroids are under investigation for treatment of epilepsy disorders. Some preliminary investigations in healthy volunteers and in patients with medically intractable epi-

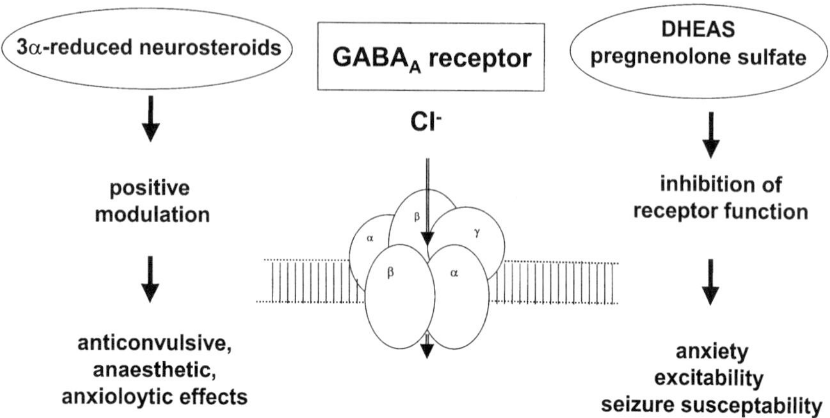

FIGURE 2. Effects of neurosteroids on GABA$_A$ receptor function.

lepsies have already been undertaken. Ganaxolone, for example, showed a promising pharmacokinetic profile and was well tolerated in a trial with healthy volunteers.[86,87] In clinical studies in patients with epilepsy it was also shown to be effective.[88] Although promising, potential side effects call for caution. For example, progesterone and 3α,5α-THP have benzodiazepine-like effects,[84,85] and progesterone withdrawal may lead to an increase in seizure susceptibility.

Through the development of sensitive assays to measure cerebral fluid or blood neurosteroid concentrations researchers have been enabled to document alterations in neurosteroidogenesis in human diseases. Recently, Ströhle and co-workers demonstrated decreased 3α,5α-tetrahydroprogesterone plasma concentrations in patients with major depression compared to healthy control subjects. Also, clinically effective antidepressant treatment was accompanied by an increase of 3α,5α-tetrahydroprogesterone in the plasma of these patients.[89]

Neuroactive steroids may also be involved in physiological conditions where fluctuations of the hormonal balance occur. For example, increased fatigue during pregnancy may be the result of higher concentrations of progesterone and GABA agonistic 3α-reduced neuroactive steroids such as 3α,5α-THP.[90] On the other hand, a rapid decline in these substances may lead to the premenstrual syndrome or postpartum depression.[91,92] Moreover, fluctuations in neuroactive steroid concentrations may in part contribute to the increased risk of developing psychiatric diseases in women at the perimenstrual phase, during pregnancy and the postpartum period, and around menopause.

DHEA and DHEAS are the most abundant circulating steroid hormones in humans. Their concentrations decrease with age and under stress.[93,94] It was hypothezised that DHEA and DHEAS may be neuroprotective agents as both age and stress are associated with neuronal vulnerability to degeneration. Indeed, neuroprotection by DHEA and DHEAS was observed *in vivo* in hippocampal structures.[95] The mechanisms by which DHEA and DHEAS act are still unknown. In patients with Alzheimer's disease and multi-infarct dementia, decreased DHEAS concentrations have also been reported.[96–98] So far trials in which DHEA was administered for a short period of two weeks have failed to demonstrate any benefit of DHEA therapy in cognitive performance.[99–101] However, high-quality trials are required with the duration of DHEA treatment in excess of a few weeks and with a large enough number of participants to detect possible effects. In such trials, the outcome measures must include objective tests of cognitive function.

CONCLUSIONS

It has been firmly established by molecular biological and biochemical studies that several key enzymes of steroidogenesis, namely cytochrome $P450_{SCC}$, aromatase, 5α-reductase, 3α-hydroxysteroid dehydrogenase, and 17β-hydroxysteroid dehydrogenase, are present in human brain (FIG. 1). Whether and how the steroidogenic enzymes are involved in the pathophysiology of the nervous system we still do not know. However, clinical investigations in humans are now providing evidence for an involvement of neuroactive steroids in conditions such as fatigue during pregnancy, premenstrual syndrome, postpartum depression, catamenial epilepsy, and depressive disorders. Results from preclinical and clinical studies strongly support the hypothesis that neuroactive steroids could be useful for therapeutic management of such disorders in the future.

REFERENCES

1. MARTINI, L. & R.C. MELCANGI. 1991. Androgen metabolism in the brain. J. Steroid Biochem. Mol. Biol. **39:** 819–828.
2. LEPHART, E.D. 1993. Brain 5α-reductase: cellular, enzymatic, and molecular perspectives and implications for biological function. Mol. Cell Neurosci. **4:** 473–484.
3. NAFTOLIN, F. 1994. Brain aromatization of androgens. J. Reprod. Med. 39: 257–261.
4. ROBEL, P., M. SCHUMACHER & E.E. BAULIEU. 1999. Neurosteroids: from definition and biochemistry to physiopathologic function. *In* Neurosteroids. A New Regulatory Function in the Nervous System. E.E. Baulieu, P. Robel & M. Schumacher, Eds.: 1–25. Humana Press. Totowa, NJ.
5. MAJEWSKA, M.D. 1992. Neurosteroids: endogenous bimodal modulators of the $GABA_A$ receptor: mechanism of action and physiological significance. Prog. Neurobiol. **38:** 379–395.
6. MELLON, S. 1994. Neurosteroids: biochemistry, modes of action, and clinical relevance. J. Clin. Endocrinol. Metab. **78:** 1003–1008.
7. NAFTOLIN, F., K.J. RYAN, I.J. DAVIES, *et al.* 1975. The formation of estrogens by central neuroendocrine tissues. Rec. Prog. Horm. Res. **31:** 295–319.
8. CHUNG, B.C., K.J. MATTESON, R. VOUTILAINEN, *et al.* 1986. Human cholesterol side-chain cleavage enzyme, P450SCC: cDNA cloning, assignment of the gene to chromosome 15, and expression in the placenta. Proc. Natl. Acad. Sci. USA **83:** 8962–8966.
9. SIMPSON, E.R. & P.C. MACDONALD. 1981. Endocrine physiology of the placenta. Annu. Rev. Physiol. **43:** 163–188.
10. KEENEY, D.S., Y. IKEDA, M.R. WATERMAN, *et al.* 1995. Cholesterol side-chain cleavage cytochrome P450 gene expression in the primitive gut of the mouse embryo does not require steroidogenic factor 1. Mol. Endocrinol. **9:** 1091–1098.
11. MELLON, S. & C.F. DESCHEPPER. 1993. Neurosteroid biosynthesis: genes for adrenal steroidogenic enzymes are expressed in the brain. Brain Res. **629:** 283–292.
12. WARNER, M. & J.-A. GUSTAFSSON. 1995. Cytochrome P450 in the brain: neuroendocrine functions. Front. Neuroendocrinol. **16:** 224–236.

13. WATZKA, M., F. BIDLINGMAIER, J. SCHRAMM, *et al.* 1999. Sex- and age-specific differences in human brain CYP11A1 mRNA expression. J. Neuroendocrinol. **11:** 901–905.
14. BEYENBURG, S., B. STOFFEL-WAGNER, M. WATZKA, *et al.* 1999. Expression of cytochrome P450scc mRNA in the hippocampus of patients with temporal lobe epilepsy. NeuroReport **10:** 3067–3070.
15. SANNE, J.L. & K.E. KRUEGER. 1995. Expression of cytochrome P450 side-chain cleavage enzyme and 3beta-hydroxysteroid dehydrogenase in the rat central nervous system: a study by polymerase chain reaction and in situ hybridization. J. Neurochem. **65:** 528–536.
16. KOHCHI, C., K. UKENA & K. TSUTSUI. 1998. Age- and region-specific expressions of the messenger RNAs encoding for steroidogenic enzymes p450SCC, p450c17 and 3beta-HSD in the postnatal rat brain. Brain Res. **801:** 233–238.
17. HU, Z.Y., E. BOURREAU, I. JUNG-TESTAS, *et al.* 1987. Neurosteroids: oligodendrocyte mitochondria convert cholesterol to pregnenolone. Proc. Natl. Acad. Sci. USA **84:** 8215–8219.
18. CORBIN, J.C., S. GRAHAM-LORENCE, M.J. MCPHAUL, *et al.* 1988. Isolation of a full-length cDNA insert encoding human aromatase system cytochrome P-450 and its expression in non-steroidogenic cells. Proc. Natl. Acad. Sci. USA **85:** 8948–8953.
19. HARADA, N. 1988. Cloning of a comparative cDNA encoding human aromatase: immunochemical identification and sequence analysis. Biochem. Biophys. Res. Commun. **156:** 725–732.
20. NAFTOLIN, F., K.J. RYAN & Z. PETRO. 1971. Aromatization of androstenedione by the diencephalon. J. Clin. Endocrinol. Metab. **33:** 368–370.
21. NAFTOLIN, F., K.J. RYAN & Z. PETRO. 1971. Aromatization of androstenedione by limbic system tissue from human foetuses. J. Endocrinol. **51:** 795–796.
22. DOODY, K.J. & B.R. CARR. 1989. Aromatase in human fetal tissues. Am. J. Obstet. Gynecol. **161:** 1694–1697.
23. WOZNIAK, A., R.E. HUTCHINSON, C.M. MORRIS, *et al.* 1998. Neuroblastoma and Alzheimer's disease brain cells contain aromatase activity. Steroids **63:** 263–267.
24. STOFFEL-WAGNER, B., M. WATZKA, J. SCHRAMM, *et al.* 1999. Expression of CYP19 (aromatase) mRNA in different areas of the human brain. J. Steroid Biochem. Mol. Biol. **70:** 237–241.
25. STOFFEL-WAGNER, B., M. WATZKA, S. STECKELBROECK, *et al.* 1998. Expression of CYP19 (aromatase) mRNA in the human temporal lobe. Biochem. Biophys. Res. Commun. **244:** 768–771.
26. STECKELBROECK, S., D. HEIDRICH, B. STOFFEL-WAGNER, *et al.* 1999 Characterization of aromatase cytochrome P450 activity in the human temporal lobe. J. Clin. Endocrinol. Metab. **84:** 2795–2801.
27. HENDERSON, D., G. NORBISRATH & U. KERB. 1986. 1-Methyl-1,4-androstadiene-3,17-dione (SH 489): characterization of an irreversible inhibitor of estrogen biosynthesis. J. Steroid Biochem. **24:** 303–306.
28. ACKERMAN, G.E., M.E. SMITH, C.R. MENDELSON, *et al.* 1981. Aromatization of androstenedione by human adipose tissue stromal cells in monolayer culture. J. Clin. Endocrinol. Metab. **53:** 412–417.
29. ROWLANDS, M.G., J.H. DAVIES, R.J. SHEARER, *et al.* 1991. Comparison of aromatase activity in human prostatic, testicular and placental tissues. J. Enzyme Inhib. **4:** 307–313.
30. ANDERSSON, S. & D.W. RUSSELL. 1990. Structural and biochemical properties of cloned and expressed human and rat steroid 5α-reductases. Proc. Natl. Acad. Sci. USA **87:** 3640–3644.
31. ANDERSSON, S., D.M. BERMAN, E.P. JENKINS, *et al.* 1991. Deletion of steroid 5α-reductase 2 gene in male pseudohermaphroditism. Nature **354:** 159–161.
32. MARTINI, L. 1982. The 5α-reduction of testosterone in the neuroendocrine structures: biochemical and physiological implications. Endocr. Rev. **3:** 1–25.
33. LI, X., P.J. BERTICS & H.J. KARAVOLAS. 1997. Regional distribution of cytosolic and particulate α-dihydroprogesterone 3α-hydroxysteroid oxidoreductases in female rat brain. J. Steroid Biochem. Mol. Biol. **60:** 311–318.

34. SAITOH, H., K. HIRATO, T. YANAIHARA, *et al.* 1982. A study of 5α-reductase in human fetal brain. Endocrinol. Jpn. **29:** 461–467.
35. SCHINDLER, A.E. 1976. Steroid metabolism in foetal tissues. IV. Conversion of testosterone to 5α-dihydrotestosterone in human foetal brain. J. Steroid Biochem. **7:** 97–100.
36. MICKAN, H. 1972. Metabolism of 4-14C-progesterone and 4-14-C-testosterone in brain of the previable human fetus. Steroids **19:** 659–668.
37. JENKINS, J.S. & C.J. HALL. 1977. Metabolism of [14C]testosterone by human foetal and adult brain tissue. J. Endocrinol. **74:** 425–429.
38. CELOTTI, F., R.C. MELCANGI, P. NEGRI-CESI, *et al.* 1986. A comparative study of the metabolism of testosterone in the neuroendocrine structures of several animal species. Neuroendocrinol. Lett. **5:** 227–236.
39. STOFFEL-WAGNER, B., M. WATZKA, S. STECKELBROECK, *et al.* 1998. Expression of 5α-reductase in the human temporal lobe of children and adults. J. Clin. Endocrinol. Metab. **83:** 3636–3642.
40. STOFFEL-WAGNER, B., S. BEYENBURG, M. WATZKA, *et al.* 2000. Expression of 5α-reductase and 3α-hydroxisteroid oxidoreductase in the hippocampus of patients with chronic temporal lobe epilepsy. Epilepsia **41:** 140–147.
41. THIGPEN, A.E., R.I. SILVER, J.M. GUILEYARDO, *et al.* 1993. Tissue distribution and ontogeny of steroid 5α-reductase isoenzyme expression. J. Clin. Invest. **92:** 903–910.
42. NORMINGTON, K. & D.W. RUSSELL. 1992. Tissue distribution and kinetic characteristics of rat steroid 5α-reductase isozymes. J. Biol. Chem. **267:** 19548–19554.
43. STECKELBROECK, S., M. WATZKA, R. REICHELT, *et al.* 2001. Characterization of the 5α-reductase-3α-hydroxysteroid dehydrogenase complex in the human brain. J. Clin. Endocrinol. Metab. **86:** 1324–1331.
44. MASSA, R., S. JUSTO & L. MARTINI. 1975. Conversion of testosterone into 5a-reduced metabolites in the anterior pituitary and in the brain of maturing rats. J. Steroid Biochem. **19:** 235–239.
45. SELMANOFF, M.K., L.D. BRODKIN, R.I. WEINER, *et al.* 1977. Aromatization and 5α-reduction of androgens in discrete hypothalamic and limbic regions of the male and female rat. Endocrinology **101:** 841–848.
46. QIN, K.N., M.I. NEW & K.C. CHENG. 1993. Molecular cloning of multiple cDNAs encoding human enzymes structurally related to 3α-hydroxysteroid dehydrogenase. J Steroid Biochem. Mol. Biol. **52:** 141–147.
47. KHANNA, M., K.-N. QIN, R.W. WANG, *et al.* 1995. Substrate specificity, gene structure, and tissue-specific distribution of multiple human 3α-hydroxisteroid dehydrogenases. J. Biol. Chem. **270:** 20162–20168.
48. KHANNA, M., K.N. QIN & K.-C. CHENG. 1995. Distribution of 3alpha-hydroxysteroid dehydrogenase in rat brain and molecular cloning of multiple cDNAs encoding structurally related proteins in humans. J. Steroid Biochem. Mol. Biol. **53:** 41–46.
49. PENNING, T.M. 1997. Molecular endocrinology of hydroxisteroid dehydrogenases. Endocr. Rev. **18:** 281–305
50. PENNING, T.M., M.E. BURCZYNSKI, J.M. JEZ, *et al.* 2000. Human 3α-hydroxisteroid dehydrogenase isoforms (AKR1C1-AKR1C4) of the aldo-keto reductase superfamily: functional plasticity and tissue distribution reveals roles in the inactivation and formation of male and female sex hormones. Biochem. J. **351:** 67–77.
51. PELTOKETO, H., V. LUU-THE & J. SIMARD. 1999 17β-hydroxisteroid dehydrogenase (HSD)/17-ketosteroid reductase (KSR) familiy; nomenclature and main characteristics of the 17HSD/KSR enzymes. J. Mol. Endocrinol. **23:** 1–11.
52. KRAZEISEN, A., R. BREITLING, K. IMAI, *et al.* 1999. Determination of cDNA, gene structure and chromosomal localization of the novel 17β-hyxdroxysteroid dehydrogenase type 7. FEBS Lett. **460:** 373–379.
53. LABRIE, F., V. LUU-THE, S.X. LIN, *et al.* 1997. A key role of 17β-hydroxisteroid dehydrogenases in sex steroid biology. Steroids **62:** 148–158.
54. MARTEL, C., M.H. MELNER, D. GAGNÉ, *et al.* 1994. Widespread tissue distribution of steroid sulfatase, 3β-hydroxisteroid dehydrogenase/D5–D4 isomerase (3β-HSD), 17β-HSD, 5α-reductase and aromatase activities in the rhesus monkey. Mol. Cell. Endocrinol. **104:** 103–111.

55. JAFFE, R.B. 1969. Testosterone metabolism in target tissues: hypothalamic and pituitary tissues of the adult rat and human fetus, and the immature rat epiphysis. Steroids **14:** 483–498.
56. MILEWICH, L., B.R. CARR & R.A. FRENKEL. 1990. 17β-hydroxysteroid oxidoreductases of human fetal and adult tissues: immunological cross-reactivity with an anti-human placental cytosolic 17β-hydroxysteroid oxidoreductase antibody. Placenta **11:** 95–108.
57. STOFFEL-WAGNER, B., M. WATZKA, S. STECKELBROECK, *et al.* 1999. D. Expression of 17β-hydroxysteroid dehydrogenase types 1, 2, 3 and 4 in the human temporal lobe. J. Endocrinol. **160:** 119–126.
58. STECKELBROECK, S., M. WATZKA, B. STOFFEL-WAGNER, *et al.* 2001. Expression of 17β-hydroxysteroid dehydrogenase type 5 mRNA in the human brain. Mol. Cell. Endocrinol. **171:** 165–168.
59. STECKELBROECK, S., B. STOFFEL-WAGNER, R. REICHELT, *et al.* 1999. Characterization of 17β-hydroxysteroid dehydrogenase activity in brain tissue: testosterone formation in the human temporal lobe. J. Neuroendocrinol. **11:** 457–464.
60. IWAHASHI, K., Y. KAWAI, H. SUWAKI, *et al.* 1993. A localization study of the cytochrome P-450(21)-linked monooxygenase system in adult rat brain. J. Steroid Biochem. Mol. Biol. **44:** 163–169.
61. STROMSTEDT, M. & M.R. WATERMAN. 1995. Messenger mRNAs encoding steroidogenic enzymes are expressed in rodent brain. Brain Res. Mol. Brain Res. **34:** 75–88.
62. MELLON, S.H. & W.L. MILLER. 1989. Extraadrenal steroid 21-hydroxylation is not mediated by P450c21. J. Clin. Invest. **84:** 1497–1502.
63. BEYENBURG, S., M. WATZKA, H. CLUSMANN, *et al.* 2001. Messenger RNA of steroid 21-hydroxylase (CYP21) is expressed in the human hippocampus. Neurosci. Lett. **308:** 111–114.
64. DUPONT, E., J. SIMARD, V. LUU-THE, *et al.* 1994. Localization of 3beta-hydroxysteroid dehydrogenase in rat brain as studied by in situ hybridization. Mol. Cell. Neurosci. **5:** 119–123.
65. GUENNOUN, R., R.J. FIDDES, M. GOUÉZOU, *et al.* 1995. A key enzyme in the biosynthesis of neurosteroids, 3β-hydroxysteroid dehydrogenase/D5-D4-isomerase (3β-HSD), is expressed in rat brain. Mol. Brain Res. **30:** 287–300.
66. GOMEZ-SANCHEZ, C.E., M.Y. ZHOU, E.N. COZZA, *et al.* 1996. Corticoid synthesis in the central nervous system. Endocr. Res. **22:** 463–470.
67. ERDMANN, B., H. GERST, A. LIPPOLDT, *et al.* 1996. Expression of cytochrome P45011B1 mRNA in the brain of normal and hypertensive transgenic rats. Brain Res. **733:** 73–82.
68. GOMEZ-SANCHEZ, C.E., M.Y. ZHOU & E.N. COZZA. 1997. Aldosterone biosynthesis in the rat brain. Endocrinology **138:** 3369–3373.
69. BAULIEU, E.E. & P. ROBEL. 1990. Neurosteroids: a new brain function? J. Steroid Biochem. Mol. Biol. **37:** 395–403.
70. COMPAGNONE, N.A., A. BUFONE & J.L.R. RUBENSTEIN. 1995. Steroidogenic enzyme P450c17 is expressed in the embryonic central nervous system. Endocrinology **136:** 5212–5223.
71. PAUL, S.M. & R.H. PURDY. 1992. Neuroactive steroids. FASEB J. **6:** 2311–2322.
72. BAULIEU, E.E. 1997. Neurosteroids: of the nervous system, by the nervous system, for the nervous system. Rec. Prog. Horm. Res. **52:** 1–33.
73. BAULIEU, E.E. 1998. Neurosteroids: a novel function of the brain. Psychoneuroendocrinology **23:** 963–987.
74. MENSAH-NYAGAN, A., J.L. DO-REGO, D. BEAUJEAN, *et al.* 1999. Neurosteroids: expression of steroidogenic enzymes and regulation of steroid biosynthesis in the central nervous system. Pharmacol. Rev. **51:** 63–81.
75. RUPPRECHT, R. & F. HOLSBOER. 1999. Neuroactive steroids: mechanism of action and neuropsychopharmacological perspectives. Trends Neurosci. **22:** 410–416.
76. WU, F.S., T.T. GIBBS & D.H. FARB. 1991. Pregnenolone sulfate: a positive allosteric modulator at the N-methyl-D-aspartate receptor. Mol. Pharmacol. **40:** 333–336.
77. PRINCE, R.J. & M.A. SIMMONDS. 1992. Steroid modulation of the strychnine-sensitive glycine receptor. Neuropharmacology. **31:** 201–205.

78. MONNET, F.P., V. MAHÉ, P. ROBEL, *et al.* 1995. Neurosteroids, via σ receptors modulate the [^{3}H]norepinephrine release evoked by N-methyl-D-aspartate in the rat hippocampus. Proc. Natl. Acad. Sci. USA **92:** 3774–3778.
79. LAMBERT, J.J., D. BELELLI, C. HILL-VENNING, *et al.* 1995. Neurosteroids and GABA-A receptor function. Trends Pharmacol. Sci. **16:** 295–303.
80. SELYE, H. 1941. The anesthetic effect of steroid hormones. Proc. Soc. Exp. Biol. Med. **46:** 116–121.
81. RICHARDS, C.D. & T.R. HESKETH. 1975. Implications for theories of anaesthesia of antagonism between anaesthetic and non-anaesthetic steroids. Nature **256:** 179–182.
82. BÄCKSTRÖM, T. 1976. Epileptic seizures in women related to plasma estrogen and progesterone during the menstrual cycle. Acta Neurol. Scand. **54:** 321–347.
83. BÄCKSTRÖM, T. 1975. Epilepsy in women: oestrogen and progesterone plasma levels. Experientia **32:** 248–249.
84. KOKATE, T.G., B.E. SVENSSON & M.A. ROGAWSKI. 1994. Anticonvulsant activity of neurosteroids: Correlation with γ-aminobutyric acid-evoked chloride current potentiation. J. Pharmacol. Exp. Therap. **270:** 1223–1229.
85. BELELLI, D., N.C. LAN & K.W. GEE. 1990. Anticonvulsant steroids and the GABA/benzodiazepine receptor-chloride ionophore complex. Neurosci. Biobehav. Rev. **14:** 315–322.
86. MONAGHAN, E.P., L.A. NAVALTA, L. SHUM, *et al.* 1997. Initial human experience with ganaxolone, a neuroactive steroid with antiepileptic activity. Epilepsia **38:** 1026–1031.
87. MONAGHAN, E.P., S. HARRIS, D. BLUM, *et al.* 1997. Ganaxolone in the treatment of complex partial seizures: a double-blind presurgical design. Epilepsia (Suppl. 8) **38:** S179.
88. SHIELDS, W.D., J.F. KERRIGAN, D.L. BLUESTONE, *et al.* 1997. Ganaxolone in the treatment of refractory infantile spasms. Ann. Neurol. **42:** 503–504.
89. STRÖHLE, A., E. ROMEO, B. HERMANN, *et al.* 1999. Concentrations of 3alpha-reduced neuroactive steroids and their precursors in plasma of patients with major depression and after clinical recovery. Biol. Psychol. **45:** 274–277.
90. BIEDERMANN, K. & P. SCHOCH. 1995. Do neuroactive steroids cause fatigue in pregnancy? Eur. J. Obstet. Gynecol. Reprod. Biol. **58:** 15–18.
91. RUPPRECHT, R. 1997. The neuropsychopharmacological potential of neuroactive steroids. J. Psych. Res. **31:** 297–314.
92. WANG, M., L. SEIPPEL, R.H. PURDY, *et al.* 1996. Relationship between symptom severity and steroid variation in women with premenstrual syndrome: study on serum pregnenolone, pregnenolone sulfate, 5 alpha-pregnane-3,20-dione and 3 alpha-hydroxy 5 alpha-pregnan-20-one. J. Clin. Endocrinol. Metab.. **81:** 1076–1082.
93. ORENTREICH, N., J.L. BRIND, J.H. VOGELMAN. *et al.*1992. Long-term longitudinal measurements of plasma dehydroepiandrosterone sulfate in normal men. J. Clin. Endocrinol. Metab. 75: 1002–1004.
94. GOODYER, I.M., J. HERBERT, P.M. ALTHAM, *et al.* 1996. Adrenal secretion during major depression in 8- to 16-year olds. I. Altered diurnal rhythms in salivary cortisol and dehydroepiandrosterone (DHEA) at presentation. Psychol. Med. **26:** 245–256.
95. KIMONIDES, V.G., N.H. KHATIBI, C.N. SVENDSEN, *et al.* 1998 Dehydroepiandrosterone (DHEA) and DHEA-sulfate (DHEAS) protect hippocampal neurons against excitatory amino acid-induced neurotoxicity. Proc. Natl. Acad. Sci. USA **95:** 1852–1857.
96. NÄSMAN, B., B. OLSSON, T. BÄCKSTRÖM, *et al.* 1991. Serum dehydroepiandrosterone sulfate in Alzheimer's disease and in multiinfarct dementia. Biol. Psychiatry **30:** 684–690.
97. MAGRI, F., F. TERENZI, T. RICCIARDI, *et al.* 2000. Association between changes in adrenal secretion and cerebral morphometric correlates in normal aging and senile dementia. Dement. Geriatr. Cogn. Disord. **11:** 90–99.
98. HILLEN, T., A. LUN, F.M. REISCHIES, *et al.* 2000. DHEA-S plasma levels and incidence of Alzheimer's disease. Biol. Psychiatry **47:** 161–163.
99. WOLF, O.T., O. NEUMANN, D.H. HELLHAMMER, *et al.* 1997. Effects of a two-week physiological dehydroepiandrosterone substitution on cognitive performance and well-being in healthy elderly women and men. J. Clin. Endocrinol. Metab. **82:** 2363–2367.

100. WOLF, O.T., E. NAUMANN, D.H. HELLHAMMER, *et al.* 1998. Effects of dehydroepiandrosterone replacement in elderly men on event-related potentials, memory and well-being. J. Gerontol. A Biol. Sci. Med. Sci. **53:** M385–M390.
101. HUPPERT, F.A., J.K. VAN NIERERK & J. HERBERT. 2000. Dehydroepiandrosterone (DHEA) supplementation for cognition and well-being. Cochrane Database Syst. Rev. **2:** CD000304.

In Vivo Effects of Estrogen on Human Brain

WILLIAM J. CUTTER,[a] MICHAEL CRAIG,[a] RAY NORBURY,[a]
DENE M. ROBERTSON,[a] MALCOLM WHITEHEAD,[b] AND DECLAN G. MURPHY[a]

[a]*Section of Brain Maturation, Department of Psychological Medicine, Institute of Psychiatry, De Crespigny Park, London SE5 8AF, UK*

[b]*Menopause Clinic, King's College Medical School, 100 Denmark Hill, London SE5 9RS, UK*

ABSTRACT: Age-related brain disorders such as Alzheimer's disease (AD) are becoming increasingly prevalent. Estrogen replacement therapy (ERT) has shown potential both as a preventive measure and treatment for such disorders. Good evidence from basic science demonstrates that estrogen has multiple protective effects on neurons and neurotransmitter systems, and the effects of ERT can be demonstrated on the human brain using techniques such as functional neuroimaging. However, the evidence for estrogen's having a clinical role in the treatment and prevention of neuropsychiatric disorders is not well established. In this article we review research into the effects of estrogen on the human brain and we consider the role for ERT as a therapeutic tool.

KEYWORDS: estrogen; cognition; depression; aging; Alzheimer's disease; serotonin; acetylcholine; dopamine; noradrenaline

INTRODUCTION

As the proportion of elderly people worldwide increases, age-related disorders such as Alzheimer's disease (AD) as well as normal age-related cognitive decline will become increasingly prevalent. Any measure that can reduce the incidence and morbidity of such problems will have enormous quality-of-life and financial implications for the individual, their carers, and society in general. One intervention that has shown promise is estrogen replacement therapy (ERT). ERT has measurable protective effects on higher cognitive function in postmenopausal women and is thought to lower the risk for an individual in whom AD develops. Fluctuations in endogenous estrogen are hypothesized to play a role in the etiology of several other neuropsychiatric disorders and estrogen may have some peripheral value in their treatment. Although the biological basis of these effects remains unknown, considerable insight has now been gained into the mechanisms of action of estrogen on the brain. Below we review studies that have contributed to our understanding of the effects and mechanisms of the action of estrogen, and we examine the evidence for ERT as a therapeutic tool.

Address for correspondence: William J. Cutter, Clinical Research Worker, Box P050, Department of Psychological Medicine, Institute of Psychiatry, De Crespigny Park, London, SE5 8AF, UK. Voice: : +44 (0)20 7848 0364; fax: +44 (0)20 7848 0650.
sppmwjc@iop.kcl.ac.uk

**Ann. N.Y. Acad. Sci. 1007: 79–88 (2003). © 2003 New York Academy of Sciences.
doi: 10.1196/annals.1286.008**

NEUROPSYCHOLOGICAL STUDIES

The Effect of Estrogen on Age-Related Memory Impairment

In healthy individuals, there is a global decline in higher cognitive abilities from late middle age.[1] The most frequent finding in postmenopausal women on ERT is that verbal memory decline is prevented.[2,3] This is also true when women undergo surgical menopause[4] and of "add-back" estrogen given after gonadotrophin releasing hormone agonist–induced menopause.[5] Maki *et al.* demonstrated that both immediate and delayed verbal recall were enhanced in women taking ERT,[2] in a sample well controlled for education, thereby controlling for the "healthy user bias" (the tendency for hormone replacement therapy [HRT] users to be healthier than non-users), a potential confounding factor.[6] Not all studies have confirmed a positive effect on verbal memory and the effects on cognition were labelled "small and inconsistent" by one thorough meta-analysis.[7] The variability in findings may be related to issues including differing preparations of HRT, healthy user bias, differing plasma levels of estradiol, and treatment duration.[7] There have been less-well-replicated findings that ERT prevents decline in other cognitive domains, such as visual memory.[8,9] In addition, benefits have been shown on tests of working memory.[10,11] Thus, estrogen replacement therapy may prevent age-related decline in verbal memory (and possibly other aspects of higher cognitive function) in postmenopausal women. Verbal memory is also one of the aspects of neuropsychological functioning severely affected by AD. However, the extent of this protective effect is controversial—larger prospective studies that take into account the shortcomings of earlier studies are needed to determine the true importance of ERT in the prevention of normal cognitive decline.

The Effect of Estrogen on Alzheimer's Disease

Prevention of Alzheimer's Disease

The prevalence of AD in women increases after the menopause and is higher in women than in men, even after adjusting for the greater longevity of women.[12] One possible explanation for this sex difference is the decline in estrogen levels seen after menopause. Early case–control studies of the relationship between use of HRT and the risk of developing AD suggested that taking HRT conveyed no protection on the risk of developing AD.[13,14] Subsequent epidemiological studies found not only a decrease in the relative risk of AD in those taking ERT, but also that the risk was lower both with higher doses of estrogen and longer duration of treatment[15,16] (for review, see Henderson[17]). In two prospective analyses,[18,19] relative risk was reduced to 0.40 and 0.46, respectively, and this was confirmed in two meta-analyses,[7,20] which found relative risks of 0.56 and 0.71, respectively. Thus, ERT appears to lower the risk of developing Alzheimer's disease in postmenopausal women. However, there remain differences between the studies (e.g., differing preparations of ERT and progesterone use). Larger randomized placebo-controlled trials are needed to determine whether estrogen conveys sufficient benefit to warrant its use prophylactically in at-risk or even low-risk individuals.

Treatment of Established Alzheimer's Disease

Initial studies looking at the effectiveness of ERT as a treatment for AD suggested it may be beneficial.[21] Recently, several well-controlled placebo studies have addressed this question in detail.[22–24] Mulnard *et al.* found no benefit on several cognitive outcomes after 12 months on conjugated equine estrogens[22]; indeed placebo was superior to CEE on several outcomes. A temporary improvement on the Mini Mental State Examination at 2 months was seen, however, and in support of this Asthana *et al.* found a benefit of estrogen replacement up to eight weeks with transdermal estradiol.[25] Thus, despite a possible transitory improvement in functioning, recent randomized placebo-controlled trials suggest that ERT taken for 3 months or longer conveys no benefit on established AD. It appears that there may be a "window of opportunity" that is already past when the condition becomes symptomatic. Nevertheless, the only study to use transdermal estradiol was the only positive one, and therefore the type of ERT may be important—an extended study period may yet be warranted. Moreover, in a study examining the benefits of tacrine in AD, women who were established on HRT before starting tacrine had a better outcome than those taking only tacrine.[26] Therefore combining ERT with other treatments for AD may prove beneficial and future studies should address this possibility.

The Effect of Estrogen on Depression

Epidemiological evidence suggests that a vulnerable subgroup of women are more prone to suffer depression at times of reproductive change (e.g. in the postpartum period there is a peak of incidence[27]). This observation has prompted studies examining the effect of estrogen therapy on depression. The small number of studies and methodological difficulties present in many have meant that at present we cannot be sure of the role of estrogen in depression: it may be useful as a prophylaxis against postpartum depression (PPD)[28] and as a treatment for PPD,[29] as well as having a possible adjunctive role in treatment-resistant depression in women.[30] Reports that estrogen may be useful as an antidepressant in the perimenopause[31,32] are difficult to substantiate as estrogen may only be treating menopausal symptoms with the incidental effect of reducing secondary depressive symptoms. ERT is, however, effective in reducing mild depressive symptoms after the menopause.[33] Thus, the extent to which changes in endogenous estrogen are important in the genesis of depression remains unclear. Moreover, estrogen cannot on current evidence be recommended as an antidepressant, except perhaps in circumstances of non-response to standard therapy in women.

The Effect of Estrogen on Schizophrenia

It has been suggested that the later age of onset of schizophrenia in females than males reflects a loss of the antidopaminergic effect of estrogen as levels decline in older age. This hypothesis is partially supported by the observation that psychotic symptoms emerge in some females when estrogen levels are low, for example, during the perimenopausal[34,35] and postpartum periods,[36] and during low estrogen phases of the menstrual cycle.[37] Furthermore, adjunct estrogen treatment has been reported to improve response to antipsychotic medication.[38] Again, however, there is no clear etiologic link between endogenous estrogen and schizophrenia or a therapeutic indication for exogenous estrogen in schizophrenia. Moreover, the relationship between estrogen and dopamine is complex and given acutely may enhance the dopaminergic system (see below).

MECHANISMS OF ACTION OF ESTROGEN ON THE CNS

Animal and in Vitro *Work*

Animal and *in vitro* work has greatly informed our understanding of the basis of observed effects of estrogen on normal aging and neuropsychiatric disorders. For example, ovariectomy in rats leads to a significant decrease in dendritic spine density in the CA1 area of the hippocampus (an area vital for memory function), although estrogen prevents this decline and estradiol levels are significantly related to synaptic spine density.[39] Estrogen is also associated with an increase in *N*-methyl-D-aspartate receptor binding and an increase in the sensitivity of CA1 pyramidal cells to NMDA receptor–mediated synaptic input in rat hippocampal neurons.[40] NMDA is thought to be involved in long-term potentiation, which is a theoretical mechanism for memory formation. Therefore estrogen has biological action on systems and brain areas that are implicated in memory and AD. Estrogen also modulates several processes that are known to form part of the pathology of AD. For example, ovariectomized guinea pigs display increased levels of β amyloid and estradiol treatment significantly reverses this change.[41] Moreover, cultured human microglia show enhanced β amyloid uptake when pre-treated with estrogen.[42] Ovariectomized rats display increased activity of the acetylcholine synthesizing enzyme choline acetyl transferase in the basal forebrain when administered acute estrogen.[43] In addition, estrogen has a number of neuroprotective effects including reducing damage by glutamate.[44] Thus, estrogen displays biological activity in animal and *in vitro* models that is consistent with a protective effect against AD: formation of neural plaques, upregulating the cholinergic system, and decreasing glutamate damage.

Human Studies

A number of studies have provided evidence that ERT modulates neurochemical systems in postmenopausal women. We reported that women treated with ERT show significantly greater growth hormone (GH) response to neuroendocrine challenge with pyridostigmine.[45] In addition, there was a correlation between length of ERT use and GH response. These data provide support to the notion that ERT increases the responsivity of the cholinergic system and that the length of ERT use is related to the integrity of this system. Thus, ERT appears to protect a neurochemical system that is profoundly implicated in AD and memory function, providing a theoretical link between the prophylactic effect of ERT against AD, as well as its protection of verbal memory. We have also reported that central 5-hydroxytryptamine (5-HT) tone (as measured by the prolactin response to *d*-fenfluramine) is similar to that in young women in those taking ERT, but is significantly lower in ERT never-users compared to young women.[46] Therefore the "tone" of the serotonergic system may also be maintained following the menopause in ERT users. Serotonin is also implicated in memory function, is also severely depleted in AD, and is important in mood disorders. Hence, the finding of a protective effect on the serotonergic system is important as it may further help to explain the findings in AD and memory as well as in depression. Dopamine research has reported a significant correlation between plasma estradiol concentration and GH response to apomorphine (a dopamine agonist) in women after estradiol implants.[47] Also, preliminary data from our group suggest that ERT enhances the GH response to apomorphine challenge (Craig *et al.*, unpublished data). Thus the same protective effect of estrogen may also be present in the dopaminergic system, a neurotransmitter system important in schizophrenia.

NEUROIMAGING STUDIES

Structural Studies

There have been two studies that have examined anatomical differences between women on and off ERT. The first of these did not find any differences between the groups in total grey matter, white matter, and lobar brain volumes using a semiautomated technique.[48] However, using voxel-based morphometry, a more sensitive technique that allows the examination of regional differences in grey and white matter volumes, we have found regions where ERT users had a significantly greater volume of grey matter (Robertson *et al.*, unpublished data). These regions were bilateral orbitofrontal cortex, inferior temporal cortices, medial and bilateral cerebellum, right inferior frontal cortex, and left paracentral and right precentral cortices. Thus, ERT may protect grey matter integrity in regions important to higher cognitive functioning and vulnerable to the pathology of AD.

Magnetic Resonance Spectroscopy

Magnetic resonance spectroscopy (MRS) is a technique that allows examination of spectra of energy emitted from regions of interest in the brain. From peaks in this spectrum, we can infer local concentrations of metabolites, such as choline (Cho) (precursor to phosphatidyl choline and hence a measure of membrane turnover) and *N*-acetyl aspartate, a measure of neuronal density. We have used MRS to examine differences in metabolites between ERT users, never-users, and young women.[49] The Cho signal in women who had never taken ERT was significantly higher than that in both young women and ERT users in the hippocampus and parietal lobe, but there was no significant difference between ERT users and young women. In addition, there was a significant association between increased membrane turnover and reduced memory. Therefore, this suggests that the increased membrane catabolism seen with normal aging is reduced by ERT. Furthermore, this membrane catabolism is correlated with visual short-term memory impairment.

Receptor Studies

Advances in neuroimaging and radioligand synthesis now allow us to directly visualize receptor systems in the living human brain. Relatively few studies have capitalized on this technique in the study of the effect ERT on receptor systems. Smith *et al.* studied the effect of estrogen replacement on the brain concentrations of cholinergic synaptic terminals.[50] They found that although there was no overall effect of HRT, there were relationships between cortical terminal concentrations and length of HRT use. However, some subjects were also using progesterone and so it is difficult to distinguish between the effects of estrogen and progesterone. Thus, there are some data to suggest that ERT may have an effect on cholinergic synaptic terminals, but further studies are required to address this question in women who use estrogen-only HRT. Only one published study has examined the effect of ERT on serotonin (5-HT) receptor density. 5-HT2A receptor density was increased in several brain regions (including orbitofrontal cortex and hippocampus) in women who took 8–14 weeks' ERT, followed by the addition of progesterone for 2–6 weeks.[51] This effect cannot be attributed entirely to the estrogen—there was no significant difference between baseline and the first scan in the estrogen-only phase. However, a trend of increased binding potential was present at the culmination of the estrogen-only stage. A more recent study has found an increase in 5HT2A receptor binding among postmenopausal women in several frontal regions after short-term estrogen administration.[52] Therefore, at present, there is some evidence to suggest that ERT affects the 5HT2A receptor density. No studies have directly looked at the effect of ERT on dopamine receptors, although positron emission tomography (PET) studies of age-related differences in the dopaminergic system of human adults report reducing dopamine D2 receptor concentration with increasing age—especially in frontal and basal ganglia regions[53]—and that this decline is more pronounced in women than in men.[54] Women exhibit a linear decline in caudate D2 density, whereas men exhibit a decline best represented by a second-degree polynomial regression with a much steeper fall between 20 and 40 years of age. Thus, although there have been no studies directly examining the effect of ERT on dopamine receptors, there is evidence that women may show a more pronounced decline in dopamine receptor density with age. Therefore, estrogen may play a role in the maintenance of dopamine receptor systems, and studies examining the effect of ERT on dopamine receptor densities would fill this gap in our knowledge.

PET Dynamic Studies

The effect of estrogen replacement can also be demonstrated on cerebral blood flow (CBF), both at rest and during the performance of cognitive tasks. At rest, the results of two studies examining CBF in women on and off ERT are conflicting.[48,55] In the former (cross-sectional) study, no differences were found, but in the latter (longitudinal) study, there were increases in the CBF over 2 years. The discrepancy between the two studies is likely to represent in part methodological differences, as other studies (e.g., Ref. 56) in different groups have shown an increase in CBF in those taking ERT. Regional cerebral glucose metabolism ratios are significantly higher in ERT users than in women with AD, whereas ERT never-users have metabolic ratios that are intermediate to those of the ERT user and AD groups, but not significantly different to women with AD.[57] In studies of PET brain activation during cognitive tasks, ERT affects regional cerebral blood flow. For example, when ERT users were compared to non-users cross-sectionally on a delayed verbal and visual recognition task, they displayed significant differences in relative brain activation patterns.[48] In the verbal task the non-users showed greater activation in the right inferior frontal cortex, whereas ERT users showed greater deactivation in the right parahippocampal gyrus, right precuneus, and right dorsal frontal gyrus. In the figural task, ERT users showed greater relative activation in right inferior parietal lobe and deactivation in right parahippocampal gyrus. In a longitudinal study reported in 2000, Maki and Resnick found that ERT users showed increased cerebral blood flow relative to non-users in the hippocampus, parahippocampal gyrus, and middle temporal gyrus over a two-year period.[55] These brain regions are vital to memory and display decreased blood flow in individuals susceptible to AD. A different approach was taken by Berman *et al.,* who studied the effect of a pharmacologically induced menopause (using Lupron) on rCBF during an executive function task.[58] During treatment with Lupron, there was an attenuated pattern of activity that was restored by adding back both estrogen and progesterone. Thus, ERT can modulate blood flow to brain regions that are important to higher cognitive function and that are implicated in the genesis of AD. In addition, ERT is associated with increased rCBF during cognitive tasks.

Functional Magnetic Resonance Imaging

Functional magnetic resonance imaginf (fMRI) is another tool that can be used to compare differences in brain activity between women who take ERT and never-users. For several reasons, this is likely to become the tool of choice for this kind of study: it gives higher resolution than PET, it does not use radioactivity, and it does not involve cannulation. In a placebo-controlled crossover study using verbal and nonverbal working memory tasks, treatment with CEE increased activation during storage of verbal material in the inferior parietal lobule and when storing nonverbal material decreased activation in the same region.[59] CEE also increased activation in the right superior frontal gyrus during retrieval tasks, with greater left hemisphere activation during encoding. This represents a "sharpening" of the hemisphere encoding/retrieval asymmetry effect. Thus, the only fMRI study to date to examine the effect of ERT on brain activation patterns confirms PET findings that ERT is associated with increased blood flow in brain regions associated with higher cognitive function during cognitive paradigms. This is important, as greater rCBF is an indicator that ERT modulates neuronal activity in these regions.

CONCLUSION

Estrogen has been demonstrated to have an extraordinary complexity and range of actions on the central nervous system, including actions on cellular function, neurotransmitter activity, and macroscopic effects on brain structure and function. From the foregoing evidence, we can conclude that: (1) estrogen has numerous neuroprotective effects on the brain at the cellular, neurochemical, and metabolic levels; (2) ERT may protect aspects of higher cognitive functioning from age-related decline; (3) ERT use may be associated with a lower relative risk for AD; (4) ERT modulates regional cerebral blood flow in regions that are involved in higher cognitive function and implicated in AD; and that (5) the links between (1) and (2)-(4) remain unclear. However, despite these conclusions, the role of estrogen in the treatment of neuropsychiatric disorder such as depression and schizophrenia is not clear. At present, estrogen cannot be recommended as a treatment for AD or as a first-line treatment for any other disorders, such as depression or schizophrenia. However, if ERT proves to have a role in the prevention of AD, the implications for the quality of life of sufferers and financial cost to health care systems would be enormous.

REFERENCES

1. SCHAIE, K.W. 1994. The course of adult intellectual development. Am. Psychol.. **49:** 304–313.
2. MAKI, P.M., A.B. ZONDERMAN & S.M. RESNICK. 2001. Enhanced verbal memory in nondemented elderly women receiving hormone-replacement therapy. Am. J. Psychiatry **158:** 227–233.
3. JACOBS, D.M., M.X. TANG, *et al.* 1998. Cognitive function in nondemented older women who took estrogen after menopause. Neurology **50:** 368–373.
4. PHILLIPS, S.M. & B.B. SHERWIN. 1992. Effects of estrogen on memory function in surgically menopausal women. Psychoneuroendocrinology **17:** 485–95.
5. SHERWIN, B.B. & T. TULANDI. 1996. "Add-back" estrogen reverses cognitive deficits induced by a gonadotropin-releasing hormone agonist in women with leiomyomata uteri. J. Clin. Endocrinol. Metab. **81:** 2545–2549.
6. MATTHEWS, K.A., L.H. KULLER, *et al.* 1996. Prior to use of estrogen replacement therapy, are users healthier than nonusers? Am. J. Epidemiol. **143:** 971–978.
7. HOGERVORST, E., J. WILLIAMS, *et al.* 2000. The nature of the effect of female gonadal hormone replacement therapy on cognitive function in post-menopausal women: A meta-analysis. Neuroscience **101:** 485–512.
8. RESNICK, S.M., E.J. METTER & A.B. ZONDERMAN. 1997. Estrogen replacement therapy and longitudinal decline in visual memory: A possible protective effect? Neurology **49:** 1491–1497.
9. DUKA, T., R. TASKER & J.F. MCGOWAN. 2000. The effects of 3-week estrogen hormone replacement on cognition in elderly healthy females. Psychopharmacology **149:** 129–139.
10. DUFF, S.J. & E. HAMPSON. 2000. A beneficial effect of estrogen on working memory in postmenopausal women taking hormone replacement therapy. Horm. Behav. **38:** 262–276.
11. KEENAN, P.A., W.H. EZZAT, *et al.* 2001. Prefrontal cortex as the site of estrogen's effect on cognition. Psychoneuroendocrinology **26:** 577–590.
12. JORM, A.F., A.E. KORTEN & A.S. HENDERSON. 1987. The prevalence of dementia: A quantitative integration of the literature. Acta Psychiat. Scand. **76:** 465–479.
13. HEYMAN, A., W.E. WILKINSON, *et al.* 1984. Alzheimer's disease: A study of epidemiological aspects. Ann. Neurol. **15:** 335–341.
14. AMADUCCI, L.A., L. FRATIGLIONI, *et al.* 1986. Risk factors for clinically diagnosed Alzheimer's disease: A case-control study of an Italian population. Neurology **36:** 922–931.
15. PAGANINI-HILL, A. & V.W. HENDERSON. 1994. Estrogen deficiency and risk of Alzheimer's disease in women. Am. J. Epidemiol. **140:** 256–261.
16. BRENNER, D.E., W.A. KUKULL, *et al.* 1994. Postmenopausal estrogen replacement therapy and the risk of Alzheimer's disease: A population-based case-control study. Am. J. Epidemiol. **140:** 262–267.
17. HENDERSON, V.W. 1997. The epidemiology of estrogen replacement therapy and Alzheimer's disease. Neurology **48:** S27–S35.
18. TANG, M.X., D. JACOBS, *et al.* 1996. Effect of oestrogen during menopause on risk and age at onset of Alzheimer's disease. Lancet **348:** 429–432.
19. KAWAS, C., S. RESNICK, *et al.* 1997. A prospective study of estrogen replacement therapy and the risk of developing Alzheimer's disease: The Baltimore Longitudinal Study of Aging. Neurology **48:** 1517–1521.
20. YAFFE, K., G. SAWAYA, *et al.* 1998. Estrogen therapy in postmenopausal women: Effects on cognitive function and dementia. JAMA **279:** 688–695.
21. HONJO, H., Y. OGINO & K. NAITOH. 1993. An effect of conjugated estrogen to cognitive impairment in women with senile dementia-Alzheimer's type: a placebo-controlled double-blind study. J. Jpn. Menopause Soc. **1:** 167–171.

22. Mulnard, R.A., C.W. Cotman, *et al.* 2000. Estrogen replacement therapy for treatment of mild to moderate Alzheimer disease: a randomized controlled trial. Alzheimer's Disease Cooperative Study. JAMA **283:** 1007–1015.
23. Henderson, V.W., A. Paganini-Hill, *et al.* 2000. Estrogen for Alzheimer's disease in women: Randomized, double-blind, placebo-controlled trial. Neurology **54:** 295–301.
24. Wang, P.N., S.Q. Liao, *et al.* 2000. Effects of estrogen on cognition, mood, and cerebral blood flow in AD: A controlled study. Neurology **54:** 2061–2066.
25. Asthana, S., L.D. Baker, *et al.* 2001. High-dose estradiol improves cognition for women with AD: results of a randomized study. Neurology **57:** 605–612.
26. Schneider, L.S., M.R. Farlow & J.M. Pogoda. 1997. Potential role for estrogen replacement in the treatment of Alzheimer's dementia. Am. J. Med. **103:** 46S–50S.
27. Kumar, R. & K.M. Robson. 1984. A prospective study of emotional disorders in childbearing women. Br. J. Psychiat. **144:** 35–47.
28. Sichel, D.A., L.S. Cohen, *et al.* 1995. Prophylactic estrogen in recurrent postpartum affective disorder. Biol. Psychiatry **38:** 814–8.
29. Gregoire, A.J.P., R. Kumar, *et al.* 1996. Transdermal oestrogen for treatment of severe postnatal depression. Lancet **347:** 930–933.
30. Klaiber, E.L., D.M. Broverman, *et al.* 1979. Estrogen therapy for severe persistent depressions in women. Arch. Gen. Psychiatry **36:** 550–554.
31. Schmidt, P.J., L. Nieman, *et al.* 2000. Estrogen replacement in perimenopause-related depression: A preliminary report. Am. J. Obstet. Gynecol. **183:** 414–420.
32. Soares, C.N., O.P. Almeida, *et al.* 2001. Efficacy of estradiol for the treatment of depressive disorders in perimenopausal women: a double-blind, randomized, placebo-controlled trial. Arch. Gen. Psychiatry **58:** 529–34.
33. Epperson, C.N., K.L. Wisner & B. Yamamoto. 1999. Gonadal steroids in the treatment of mood disorders. Psychosom. Med. **61:** 676–697.
34. Jablensky, A., N. Sartorius & G. Ernberg. 1992. Schizophrenia: Manifestations, Incidence and Course in Different Cultures. A World Health Organisation Ten-Country Study. Psychological Medicine Monograph 20.
35. Castle, D.J. & R.M. Murray. 1993. The epidemiology of late-onset schizophrenia. Schizophr. Bull. **19:** 691–700.
36. Kendell, R.E., J.C. Chalmers & C. Platz. 1987. Epidemiology of puerperal psychoses. Br. J. Psychiatry **150:** 662–673.
37. Seeman, M.V. & M. Lang. 1990. The role of estrogens in schizophrenia gender differences. Schizophr. Bull. **16:** 185–194.
38. Kulkarni, J., A. Riedel, *et al.* 2001. Estrogen—a potential treatment for schizophrenia. Schizophr. Res. **48:** 137–144.
39. Gould, E, Woolley, C.S., *et al.* 1990. Gonadal steroids regulate dendritic spine density in hippocampal pyramidal cells in adulthood. J. Neurosci. **10:** 1286–1291.
40. Woolley, C.S., N.G. Weiland, *et al.* 1997. Estradiol increases the sensitivity of hippocampal CA1 pyramidal cells to NMDA receptor-mediated synaptic input: Correlation with dendritic spine density. J. Neurosci. **17:** 1848–1859.
41. Petanceska, S.S., V. Nagy, *et al.* 2000. Ovariectomy and 17beta-estradiol modulate the levels of Alzheimer's amyloid beta peptides in brain. Neurology **54:** 2212–2217.
42. Li, R., Y. Shen, *et al.* 2000. Estrogen enhances uptake of amyloid beta-protein by microglia derived from the human cortex. J. Neurochem. **75:** 1447–1454.
43. Luine, V.N. 1985. Estradiol increases choline acetyltransferase activity in specific basal forebrain nuclei and projection areas of female rats. Exp. Neurol. **89:** 484–490.
44. Simpkins, J.W., M. Singh & J. Bishop. 1994. The potential role for estrogen replacement therapy in the treatment of the cognitive decline and neurodegeneration associated with Alzheimer's disease. Neurobiol. Aging **15:** S195–S197.
45. Van Amelsvoort, T., D.G.M. Murphy, *et al.* 2003. Effects of long-term estrogen replacement therapy on growth hormone response to pyridostigmine in healthy postmenopausal women. Psychoneuroendocrinology **28:** 101–112.
46. Van Amelsvoort, T., K.M. Abel, *et al.* 2001. Prolactin response to *d*-fenfluramine in postmenopausal women on and off ERT: Comparison with young women. Psychoneuroendocrinology **26:** 493–502.

47. BEST, N.R., M.P. REES, *et al.* 1992. Effect of oestradiol treatment on 5-HT and dopamine-mediated neuroendocrine response. J. Psychopharmacol. **6:** 483–488.
48. RESNICK, S.M., P.M. MAKI, *et al.* 1998. Effects of estrogen replacement therapy on PET cerebral blood flow and neuropsychological performance. Horm. Behav. **34:** 171–182.
49. ROBERTSON, D.M., T. VAN AMELSVOORT, *et al.* 2001. Effects of estrogen replacement therapy on human brain aging: an in vivo 1H MRS study. Neurology **57:** 2114–2117.
50. SMITH, Y.R., S. MINOSHIMA, *et al.* 2001. Effects of long-term hormone therapy on cholinergic synaptic concentrations in healthy postmenopausal women. J. Clin. Endocrinol. Metabol. **86:** 679–684.
51. MOSES, E.L., W.C. DREVETS, *et al.* 2000. Effects of estradiol and progesterone administration on human serotonin 2A receptor binding: a PET study. Biol. Psychiatry **48:** 854–860.
52. KUGAYA, A., C.N. EPPERSON, *et al.* 2003. Increase in prefrontal cortex serotonin 2A receptors following estrogen treatment in postmenopausal women. Am. J. Psychiatry **160:** 1522–1524.
53. WONG, D.F., H.N. WAGNER, JR., *et al.* 1984. Effects of age on dopamine and serotonin receptors measured by positron tomography in the living human brain. Science **226:** 1393–1296.
54. WONG, D.F., E.P. BROUSSOLLE, *et al.* 1988. In vivo measurement of dopamine receptors in human brain by positron emission tomography: age and sex differences. Ann. N.Y. Acad. Sci. **515:** 203–214.
55. MAKI, P.M. & S.M. RESNICK. 2000. Longitudinal effects of estrogen replacement therapy on PET cerebral blood flow and cognition. Neurobiol. Aging **21:** 373–383.
56. OHKURA, T., Y. TESHIMA, *et al.* 1995. Estrogen increases cerebral and cerebellar blood flows in postmenopausal women. Menopause **2:** 13–18.
57. EBERLING, J.L., B.R. REED, *et al.* 2000. Effect of estrogen on cerebral glucose metabolism in postmenopausal women. Neurology **55:** 875–877.
58. BERMAN, K.F., P.J. SCHMIDT, *et al.* 1997. Modulation of cognition-specific cortical activity by gonadal steroids: A positron-emission tomography study in women. Proc. Natl. Acad. Sci. USA **94:** 8836–8841.
59. SHAYWITZ, S.E., B.A. SHAYWITZ, *et al.* 1999. Effect of estrogen on brain activation patterns in postmenopausal women during working memory tasks. JAMA **281:** 1197–1202.

Neuroprotection by Estrogen in Animal Models of Global and Focal Ischemia

ISTVAN MERCHENTHALER, TAMMY L. DELLOVADE, AND PAUL J. SHUGHRUE

Women's Health Research Institute, Wyeth Research, Collegeville, Pennsylvania 19526, USA

Abstract: Estrogen has been demonstrated to protect against brain injury, neurodegeneration, and cognitive decline. Furthermore, estrogen seems to specifically protect cortical and hippocampal neurons from ischemic injury. Here our data evaluating the neuroprotective effects of estrogens, the selective estrogen receptor modulators (SERMs), and estrogen receptor α- and β-selective ligands in animal models of ischemic injury are discussed. In rats and mice, the middle cerebral artery occlusion (MCAO) model was used as models representing cerebrovascular stroke, while in gerbils the two-vessel occlusion model, resenting acute heart attack, was used. Using focal ischemia in ovariectomized ERαKO, ERβKO, and wild-type mice, we clearly established that the ERα subtype is the critical ER-mediating neuroprotection in mouse focal ischemia. Because of the characteristic blood supply of the gerbil, the gerbil global ischemia model was used to evaluate the neuroprotective effects of estrogen, SERMs, and ERα- and ERβ-selective compounds in the hippocampus. Analysis of neurogranin mRNA, a marker of viability of hippocampal neurons, with *in situ* hybridization, revealed that estrogen treatment resulted in a complete protection in the CA1 regions not only when administered before, but also when given 1 hour after occlusion. Our *in vivo* binding studies with ^{125}I-estrogen in gerbils revealed the presence of nuclear estrogen binding sites primarily in CA1 neurons, but not in the CA3 region, as we saw in rats and mice. Together, these observations demonstrate that estrogen protects from ischemic injury in both the focal and global ischemia models by acting primarily via classical nuclear receptors.

Keywords: stroke; mouse; rat; estrogen receptor; SERM; brain

INTRODUCTION

By now, it is generally accepted that the female sex hormone, estrogen, acts centrally to modulate many aspects of reproduction (sexual differentiation, ovulation and sexual behavior) as well as during neuronal/glial development, growth, differentiation, and maturation. In addition, estrogen has also been proposed to serve as a

Address for correspondence: Istvan Merchenthaler, Women's Health Research Institute, Wyeth Research, 500 Arcola Road, Collegeville, PA 19526. Voice: 484-865-2791; fax: 484-865-9367.

merchei@wyeth.com

Ann. N.Y. Acad. Sci. 1007: 89–100 (2003). © 2003 New York Academy of Sciences.
doi: 10.1196/annals.1286.009

general neurotrophic factor that stabilizes neuronal function, supports viability and prevents neuronal death (for a recent review see Ref. 1).

Several clinical studies have demonstrated that postmenopausal women are more vulnerable than young women to neurodegenerative diseases such as Alzheimer's and Parkinson's disease, stroke, and memory/cognitive dysfunctions. Furthermore, estrogen replacement therapy appears to decrease the risk and/or severity of neurodegenerative conditions and to improve verbal memory and cognition (for recent reviews see Refs. 1–3). Today, women spend a significant proportion of their lifespan in a hypoestrogenic, postmenopausal state. Therefore, it has become increasingly important to understand the cellular and molecular mechanisms that underlie the protective actions of steroidal hormones and to use this information to develop new therapies to prevent and/or treat disorders/dysfunctions associated with hypoestrogenic conditions. In this paper, we summarize our data examining the neuroprotective effects of estrogen in animal models of focal and global ischemia.

ESTROGEN PROTECTS VIA ERα AGAINST PERMANENT FOCAL CEREBRAL ISCHEMIA

We and others have shown that administration of physiological[4–7] or pharmacological[8] levels of 17β-estradiol for one week prior to permanent[6,7] or transient[4] occlusion of the middle cerebral artery leads to a dramatic decrease in the infarct volume when compared to vehicle-treated control rats (FIG. 1) or mice. Interestingly, the neuroprotective effect of estrogen was confined to the cerebral cortex, with no beneficial effect seen in the striatum.

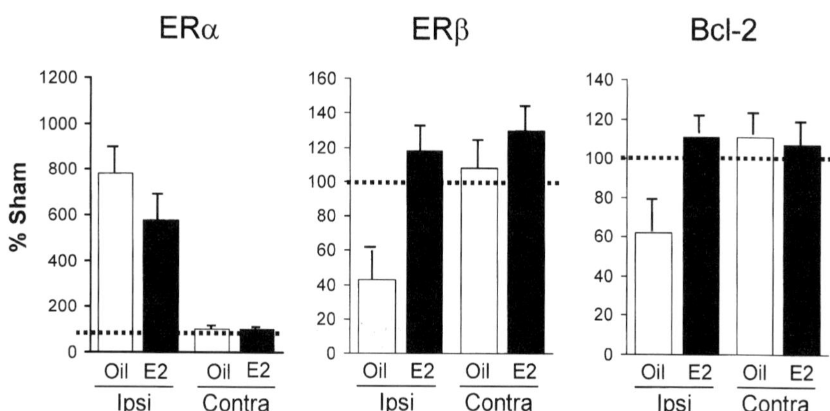

FIGURE 1. Transient focal ischemia upregulates the expression of ERα in the ipsilateral side of the rat cerebral cortex. Estrogen pretreatment does not have a significant effect on ERα expression. The contralateral side does not have ERα. The same lesion downregulates the expression of ERβ in the ipsilateral side of the lesion. Estrogen pretreatment prevents the decrease in ERβ expression. The lesion has no effect on the contralateral side, that is, ERβ is expressed and estrogen does not affect its expression. The ischemic lesion downregulates the expression of *Bcl-2* expression in the ipsilateral side of the lesion and estrogen prevents this decrease in *Bcl-2* expression.

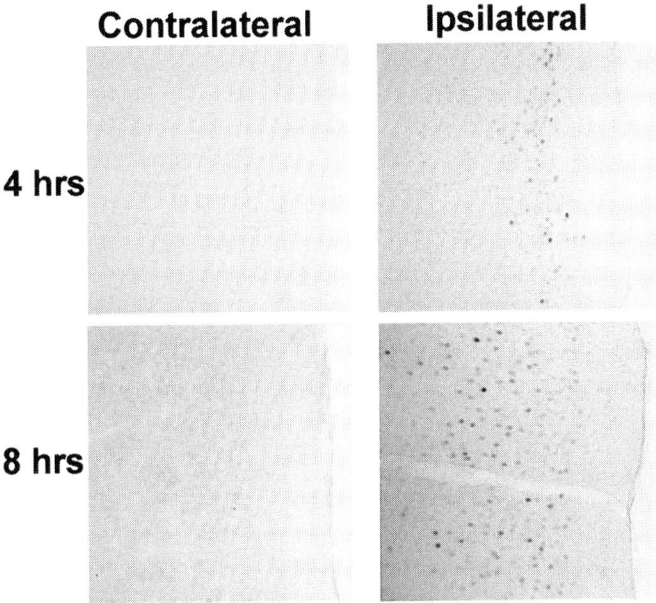

FIGURE 2. Focal ischemic injury upregulates the expression of ERα in the ipsilateral side of the lesion as detected by immunocytochemistry.

Although in most studies estrogen was given several days prior to the ischemic insult, recent studies by Yang *et al.*[9] indicate that estrogen may protect from ischemic stroke in rats even when applied three hours after the onset of injury. These data suggest a potential window for treatment after the occurrence of stroke.

Since there are two major estrogen receptors (ERα and ERβ) in the brain,[10,11] we attempted to identify which one mediates the neuroprotective actions of estrogen. These studies showed that estrogen lessened the ischemia-induced lesion in the cerebral cortex of rats (FIG. 1) and revealed that the penumbra (an area surrounding the ischemic core where the low perfusion rate allows the cells to survive for a few hours) contained a large number of ERα mRNA-expressing and ERα-immunoreactive (FIG. 2) cells in the ipsilateral but not the contralateral side. Interestingly, the number of ERβ mRNA-expressing cells was reduced in the ipsilateral compared to the contralateral cortex. Estrogen pretreatment did not affect the increase in expression of ERα, but it did prevent the drop in the number of ERβ-expressing cells in the rat cortex (FIG. 1)[6] The biological activity of these ERα-expressing cells was confirmed with *in vivo* binding studies[6]: 24 hours after the permanent focal ischemic injury, there were large numbers of cells in the ipsilateral cerebral cortex with nuclear accumulation of ^{125}I-estrogen. Subsequently, ovariectomized, vehicle- and estrogen-treated ERα knockout (ERαKO) and ERβKO mice were used to identify the ER responsible for mediating the protective effect of estrogen. These studies confirmed the critical role of ERα in estrogen-mediated neuroprotection in the cerebral cortex (FIG. 2).[7] Although compelling, these data were surprising since with the exception of the perirhinal cortex, the intact adult mouse cerebral cortex contains only a few, if any cells that bind ^{125}I-estrogen,[12] expresses either ERα[13] or ERβ mRNA[11,14] or cells that contain ERα or ERβ immunoreactivity.[15] However, a major species difference exists between the mouse and rat, that is, while the cerebral cortex of the intact, adult mouse brain practically does not contain either ER, the cortex of the adult rat contains large numbers of ERβ mRNA[11,16] and ERβ-immunoreactive cells.[17] Even more surprising is that after permanent focal ischemia, the number of cells expressing ERα is dramatically increased in both species while the number of ERβ-expressing cells is slightly reduced in the cerebral cortex of the rat.[6] Focal ischemic lesions in the cerebral cortex of the rat therefore were associated with a shift in the expression of ERα vs. ERβ in the cortex. The expression of ERα in the ipsilateral side of the ischemic lesion in the rat cortex resembled that of the developing postnatal rat brain whose cortex also contains large number of ^{125}I-estrogen concentrating cells.[12] Interestingly, these ER-containing cells in the cortex disappear by the end of the first month of life,[12] but reappear after ischemic injury.[6] The "reappearance" of ERα in the mouse cerebral cortex, similar to what is seen during development, following ischemic insult also suggests that the cortex undergoes a dedifferentiation process. Therefore, it is plausible that newly synthesized or upregulation of ERα in cortical cells is associated with neuroprotection by estrogen treatment.

In consequent experiments, we also studied the expression of other genes associated with survival- and death-promoting mechanisms. Cells that die after brain ischemia can be classified as dying of necrosis or apoptosis. Apoptosis may be responsible for as much as 50% of cellular deaths in ischemia[18] and both extra- and intracellular signals that have been reported to initiate this process were identified after brain injury. Since apoptosis, in contrast to necrosis, is a reversible process, therapeutic interventions have been designed to stop and/or reverse the apoptotic process and thus, rescue neurons from cell death.

The mechanisms leading to apoptotic cell death may include several pathways such as an NFκB-dependent pathway, a p53-dependent pathway, and/or activation of inducible pro-apoptotic members of the *bcl* family (*bad, bax*). Induction of these factors leads to the activation of several caspases, including caspase3. Once caspase-3 is activated, it in turn activates DNA braking enzymes, leading eventually to cell death (reviewed in Ref. 19).

Estradiol is known to promote cell survival via activation of *bcl-2* expression in non-neuronal tissues.[20] *Bcl-2* is a survival factor that can block both necrotic and apoptotic cell death that contributes to ischemic injury.[17,18] *Bcl-2* acts upstream to prevent the activation of caspases, inhibits free radical formation, regulates calcium sequestration, and blocks the pro-apoptotic actions of other members of the *bcl-2* family, including *bax* and *bad.*[19]

We have shown that in the rat, estrogen upregulates the expression of *bcl-2* (FIG. 1), but does not modulate the expression of *bax* and *bad* in the lesioned side of the cortex. Other factors such as galanin and nNOS (Dubal, Shughrue, and Merchenthaler, unpublished observations) are also upregulated after lesion, but the regulation of their expression by estrogen treatment is not known. The expression of galanin in the lesioned side is intriguing. In the Alzheimer's disease brain, galanin "hyperinnervates" cholinergic neurons[21] and probably downregulates differentiated

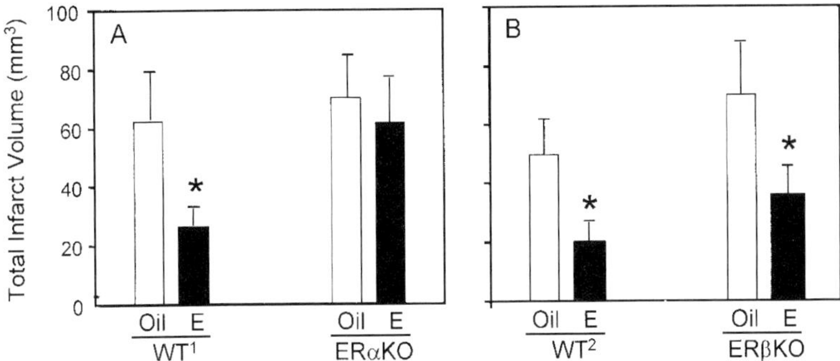

FIGURE 3. Estrogen protects from focal ischemic injury in wild-type (WT) mice of both genetic backgrounds (C57BL6J-129 and 129Sv) and ERβKO mice but not in ERαKO mice, indicating the importance of ERα in mediating the neuroprotective action of estrogen.

and upregulates survival-related functions. It is interesting to hypothesize that elevated galanin expression in the penumbra may also induce de-differentiation of nerve cells as indicated by the "appearance" of ERα-expressing neurons in the ischemic side of the cerebral cortex. Thus, galanin may play a role as a switch to turn genes off and on by turning on those necessary for survival and reparation and turning off those required for differentiated functions.

In addition to inducing the expression of *bcl-2*, and therefore inhibiting the expression of the terminator caspase-3, the beneficial effects of estrogen might include enhancing antioxidant mechanisms, remyelinization, synaptogenesis, and the synthesis of trophic factors and their receptors as well as reducing excitotoxicity, glutamate receptor activity, and inflammation.[19] Moreover, interaction between insulin-like growth factor-I (IGF-I) and estrogen signaling may also promote neuronal survival in response to neuronal injury.[2]

ESTROGEN PROTECTS AGAINST GLOBAL ISCHEMIA: GERBIL HIPPOCAMPUS MODEL

On account of a mutation deficit, gerbils lack the posterior communicating arteries of the circle of Willis at the base of the brain. Because of the incomplete circle, the carotid and vertebral arteries do not communicate. Therefore, transient ligation of the common carotid arteries (two-vessel occlusion model) results in severe global ischemia in the gerbil brain. This model imitates a hypoxic lesion in humans that is associated with cardiac arrest or cardiac surgery. The transient (5-min) ischemia leads to selective and delayed neuronal cell death, particularly in pyramidal neurons of the hippocampal CA1 region.[22] Cell death is most detectable 4–5 days after the 5-min occlusion and may involve necrotic and apoptotic mechanisms.[23–26]

Estrogen has a profound effect on the structure and function of the rodent hippocampus and is therefore thought to play an important role in learning and memory. Interestingly, most of the observed effects of estrogen have been restricted to the pyramidal cells and interneurons of the dorsal hippocampus of the rat and mouse, a region that contains only a few scattered ER-positive (α and β) neurons in these species.[11,17,27]

Hall and colleagues[28] were the first to observe that the degree of neuronal injury after ischemia was abated in the female hippocampus when compared with male gerbils. Subsequent studies[29] in males showed that the chronic infusion of 17β-estradiol into the lateral ventricles reduced the loss of CA1 neurons induced by global ischemia. In addition, estrogen was found to prevent the loss of intact synapses in the male CA1 region, while saline treatment resulted in a 50% reduction in synaptic density.[29] Later studies also showed that the pretreatment of males with a high dose of estrogen (30 mg, i.c.v. or 4 mg/kg i.p.) one hour before ischemic injury was sufficient to protect the hippocampus from injury.[30] Recently, Jover *et al.*[26] showed that even physiological levels of estrogen (17–75 pg/ml) protected male animals from transient global ischemia when administered for several days before and after injury. These authors also demonstrated that the protective effect of estrogen involves the attenuation of the ischemia-induced activation of caspase-3 and p75NTR in CA1 region of the hippocampus. On the basis of the results of these studies, it appeared that exogenous estrogen protected the male hippocampus after an ischemic event and suggested that circulating estrogen may also afford similar protection to females.

Although the gerbil is the most frequently used animal model for studying the mechanism of estrogen-mediated protection in the hippocampus after global ischemia, no information is available on the distribution of ERs in this brain region. The currently available probes for *in situ* hybridization histochemistry do not hybridize with the gerbil mRNA (the gerbil ERs have not been cloned), and antisera against ERα and ERβ do not cross-react with the gerbil ERs. Therefore, we used *in vivo* binding to investigate the presence of ERs in the normal and injured gerbil hippocampus. Ovariectomized (OVX) gerbils with no ischemic injury or 6, 12, or 24 hours

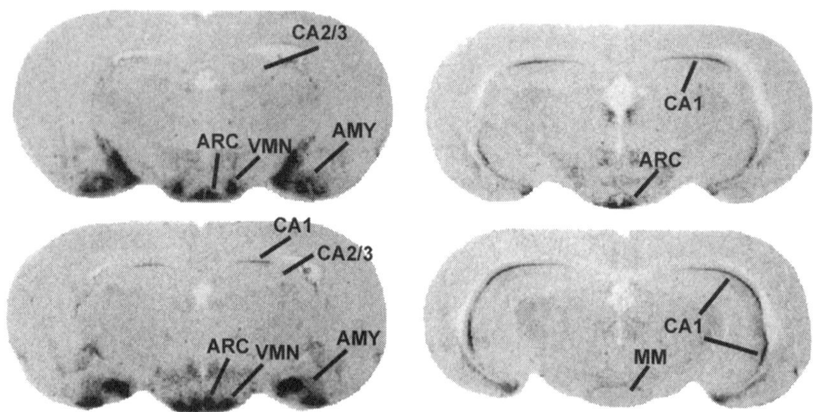

FIGURE 4. Film autoradiograms depicting the distribution ^{125}I-estrogen binding sites in the OVX gerbil brain by *in vivo* autoradiography. Note the localization of nuclear binding sites in the CA1 and, to a lesser extent, in the CA2 but not CA3 region of the hippocampus as well as the arcuate (ARC) and ventromedial (VMN) nuclei of the hypothalamus and amygdala (AMY).

after global ischemia (see above) were subcutaneously injected with ^{125}I-estrogen. Four to six hours after injection of ^{125}I-estrogen, the brains were collected and processed for autoradiographic analysis. These studies clearly showed that the binding pattern (distribution of ERs) in the gerbil hippocampus was different than that seen in mice and rats. In contrast to rats and mice, where the densest accumulation of the radioactively-labeled ligand was seen in CA2-3 areas of the ventral hippocampus, in the gerbil the most dense accumulation of binding was present in ventral CA1 followed by dorsal CA1 areas of the hippocampus (FIG. 4).[31]

To measure the protective effects of estrogen in OVX female gerbils and to evaluate the contribution of ERα and/or ERβ in neuroprotection after transient, global ischemia, instead of counting cell nuclei in the hippocampus, the level of neurogranin hybridization signal in CA1 region was quantitatively evaluated. Neurogranin

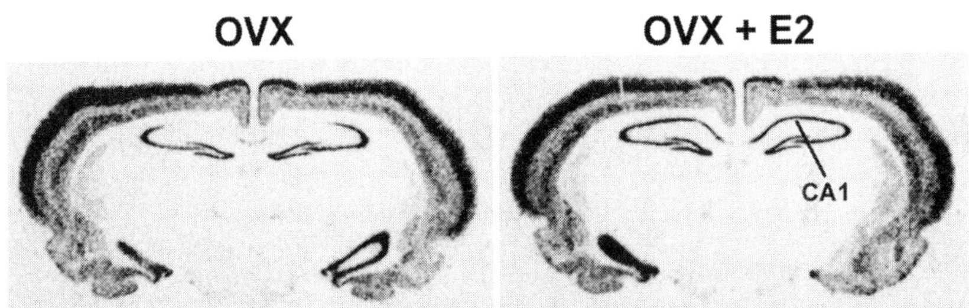

FIGURE 5. Film autoradiograms of neurogranin mRNA in the gerbil hippocampus by *in situ* hybridization. Note the dramatic and selective loss of neurogranin hybridization signal in the CA1 region of placebo-treated animals after injury. In contrast, neurogranin mRNA is still seen in the CA1 region of ovariectomized gerbils treated with 17β-estradiol.

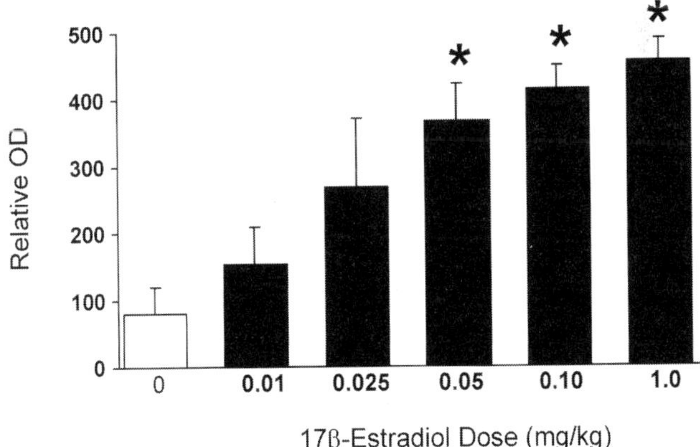

FIGURE 6. Dose–response of 17β-estradiol treatment on neurogranin gene expression (relative OD) in the CA1 region of the hippocampus. Note that 50 and 100 μg/kg and 1.0 mg/kg estradiol provides similar protection.

mRNA was selected for these studies because it is highly expressed in the hippocampal neurons including CA1, but absent in glia and other cell types present in this brain region. Relative optical density measurements of neurogranin hybridization signal were obtained from film autoradiograms with a computer-based image analysis system (C-Imaging Inc., Pittsburgh, PA).

We have found that pretreatment with physiological plasma levels of estrogen provided protection against global ischemia in OVX gerbils (FIGS. 5 and 6).[31] Moreover, ERβ-selective and the ERα-selective compounds also provided protection, although with less efficacy than estrogen (FIG. 7), suggesting that both ERs are present and functional in the gerbil hippocampus. We have also found that a variety of estrogens, such as estrone, and the nonsteroidal estrogenic compound, diethylstilbestrol (DES), also exhibited partial levels of neuroprotection using the same ischemia paradigm.[31] However, tamoxifen[31] and raloxifene (FIG. 8), the partial estrogen receptor agonists/antagonists, or selective estrogen receptor modulators (SERMs), were not effective. Moreover, tamoxifen[31] and raloxifene (FIG. 8) antagonized the neuroprotective effect of estrogen.[31]

Since compounds with a phenolic A ring, including 17β-estradiol, tamoxifen, DES, and estrone, may act as antioxidants to prevent cell death,[32,33] 17α-estradiol (a weak estrogen with a phenolic A ring) and vitamin E (an antioxidant that is not estrogenic) were evaluated in the ischemia model.

Both 17α-estradiol and large doses of vitamin E partially maintained neurogranin mRNA expression,[31] suggesting that the antioxidant nature of these compounds might also contribute to their neuroprotective activity.

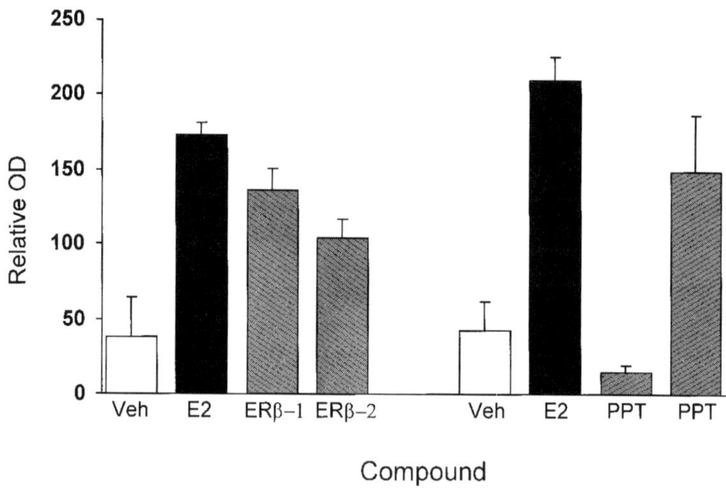

FIGURE 7. Analysis of film autoradiograms reveales that the level of neurogranin hybridization signal is very low in the CA1 region from placebo-treated OVX animals and high in animals treated with 17β-estradiol, the ERβ-selective compounds 1 and 2 and the ERα-selective compound (PPT). However, the ERα-selective compound provides protection only at 15 mg/kg and not at 3.0 mg/kg.

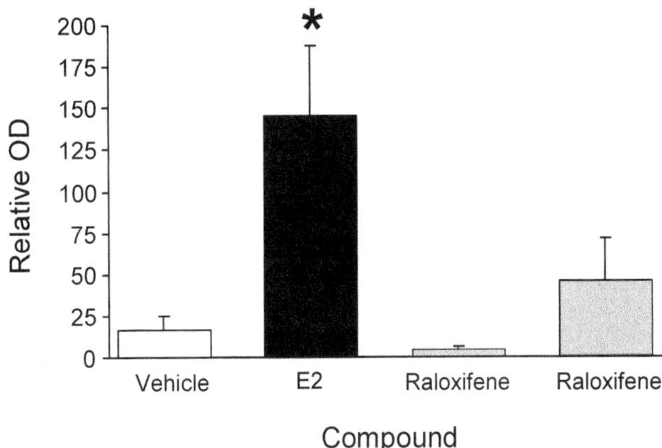

FIGURE 8. Analysis of film autoradiograms reveals that the level of neurogranin hybridization signal is very low in the placebo-treated OVX animals. 17β-estradiol increases the level of neurogranin mRNA in the hippocampus after injury. Raloxifene (up to 20 mg/kg) does not provide protection.

The goal in the treatment of stroke and global ischemia is to identify therapies that can be used following the ischemic event. Therefore, in addition to pretreating OVX gerbils with estrogen, we also administered estrogen to OVX gerbils 0.5, 1.0, 2.0, and 4.0 hours after the transient ischemic insult and we evaluated neurogranin expression in the hippocampus. These studies clearly demonstrated that subcutaneously administered estrogen provided complete protection even when it was administered 1.0 h after the insult (FIG. 9).[34] Estrogen administered 2.0 h after the lesion provided only partial protection. These findings are similar to those observed recently by Yang *et al*,[9] who showed that in the rat focal ischemia model, estrogen treatment reduced the lesion size even when it was administered 3 hours after initiating the occlusion of the middle cerebral artery.

On the basis of these findings, one might speculate that the estrogens, in addition to their action via the classical nuclear receptors, may be acting rapidly via membrane-associated ERs, as already mentioned, or may be acting as antioxidants. However, the finding that tamoxifen and raloxifene, two nonsteroidal anti-estrogens with a phenolic A ring, which is a prerequisite for their anti-oxidant action,[32,33] were unable to protect the hippocampal neurons is at odds with this theory. These conflicting data suggest that estrogens may act via several different mechanisms that are acting in concert. The mechanism might depend on a variety of factors, including estrogen concentration, tissue of action, animal age and the structure of the compound. At high pharmacological concentrations, a variety of estrogen-like compounds appear to act as potent antioxidants, while at more physiological levels they are inactive.[35] In contrast, compounds such as 17β-estradiol may also be very potent modulators at physiological concentrations, acting via ER-dependent pathways. The localization of estrogen binding sites in the gerbil CA1 neurons supports this concept and provides the substrate for which estrogens can act directly after injury. Although these studies do not fully elucidate the mode by which estrogens protect the gerbil hippo-

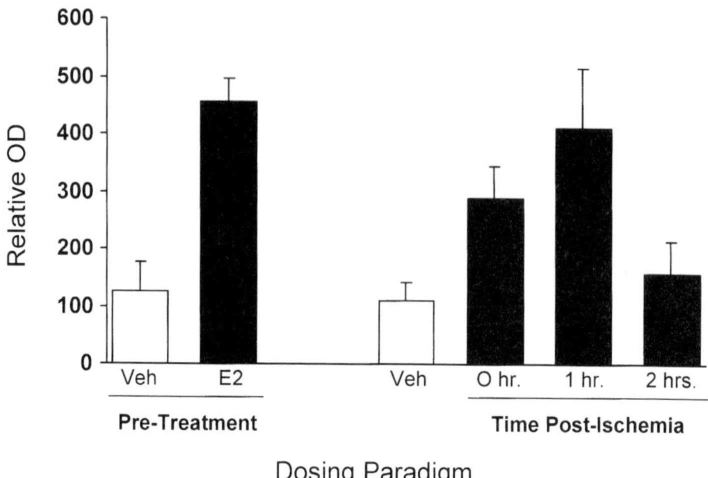

FIGURE 9. Analysis of film autoradiograms depicting the level of neurogranin mRNA in the injured gerbil hippocampus after pretreatment with vehicle or 17β-estradiol (standard paradigm), at the time of the lesioning (0) and 1 h and 2 h after the lesion. Note that 17β-estradiol provides complete protection in the CA1 region of the hippocampus even when administered 1 h after the lesion (occlusion of the common carotid arteries for 5 min).

campus, they do clearly demonstrate that a variety of steroidal and nonsteroidal estrogens are potent neuroprotective agents in this model system.

In summary, estrogens exert their neuroprotective actions probably via a large array of mechanisms including genomic and nongenomic actions. The genomic actions include, among others, the stimulation of the expression of genes involved in survival-promoting mechanisms (*bcl-2*, trophic factors and their receptors, structural proteins, neuropeptides, etc.) and inhibiting death-promoting mechanisms (p75, caspase-3, TNF-α, IL-1 and IL-6, etc.). Estrogens function as antioxidants and enhance antioxidant mechanisms, they reduce excitoxicity and inflammation, and probably they exert rapid membrane ER-associated mechanisms.

ACKNOWLEDGMENTS

We express our sincere gratitude to Malcolm Lane for his excellent technical assistance.

REFERENCES

1. BEHL, C. 2002. Oestrogen as a neuroprotective hormone. Nature Rev. Neurosci. **3:** 433–442.
2. GARCIA-SEGURA, L.M., I. AZCOITIA & L.L. DONCARLOS. 2001. Neuroprotection by estradiol. Progr. Neurobiol. **63:** 29–60.

3. WISE, P.M., D.B. DUBAL, M.E. WILSON, *et al.* 2001. Estrogens: trophic and protective factors in the adult brain. Front. Neuroendocrinol. **22:** 33–66.
4. ALKAYED, N.J., I. HARUKUNI, A.S. KIMES, *et al.* 1998. Gender-linked brain injury in experimental stroke. Stroke **29:** 159–166.
5. DUBAL, D.B., M.L. KASHON, L.C. PETTIGREW, *et al.* 1998. Estradiol protects against ischemic injury. J. Cereb. Blood Flow Metab. **18:** 1253–1258.
6. DUBAL, D.B., P.J. SHUGHRUE, M.E. WILSON *et al.* 1999. Estradiol modulates Bcl-2 in cerebral ischemia: a potential role for estrogen receptors. J. Neurosci. **19:** 6385–6393.
7. DUBAL, D.B., B. ZHU, B. YU, *et al.* 2001. Estrogen receptor-α, not β, is a critical link in estradiol-mediated protection against brain injury. Proc. Natl. Acad. Sci. USA **98:** 1952–1957.
8. SIMPKINS, J.W., G. RAJAKUMAR, Y-Q ZHANG, *et al.* 1997. Estrogens may reduce mortality and ischemic damage caused by middle cerebral artery occlusion in the female rat. J. Neurosurg. **87:** 724–730.
9. YANG, S.H., J. SHI, A.L. DAY & J.W. SIMPKINS. 2000. Estradiol exerts neuroprotective effects when administered after ischemic insult. Stroke **31:** 745–749.
10. KUIPER, G.G.J.M, P.J. SHUGHRUE, I. MERCHENTHALER & J-A. GUSTAFSSON. 1998. The estrogen beta subtype: a novel mediator of estrogen action in neuroendocrine systems. Front. Neuroendocrinol. **19:** 253–286.
11. SHUGHRUE, P.J., M.V. LANE & I. MERCHENTHALER. 1997. The comparative distribution of estrogen receptor-alpha and beta mRNA in the rat central nervous system. J. Comp. Neurol. **388:** 507–525.
12. SHUGHRUE, P.J., W.E. STUMPF, N.J. MACLUSKY, *et al.* 1990. Developmental changes of estrogen receptors in mouse cerebral cortex between birth and postweaning studied by autoradiography with 11beta-methoxy-16alpha[125I]-iodoestradiol. Endocrinology **126:** 1112–1124.
13. SIMERLY, R.B., C. CHANG, M. MURAMATSU & L.W. SWANSON. 1990. Distribution of androgen and estrogen receptor mRNA-containing cells in the rat brain: an in situ hybridization study. J. Comp. Neurol. **294:** 76–95.
14. SHUGHRUE PJ, M.V. LANE & I. MERCHENTHALER. 1999. Biologically active estrogen receptor-alpha: evidence from *in vivo* autoradiographic studies with estrogen receptor alpha-knockout mice. Endocrinology **140:** 2613–2620.
15. DELLOVADE, T. & I. MERCHENTHALER. 2002. Focal ischemic injury in the cerebral cortex of mice induces the expression of estrogen receptor-alpha (ER-alpha): an immunocytochemical analysis. Endocrine Society Abstract: 200. San Francisco.
16. LAFLAMME, N., R.E. NAPPI, G. DROLET, *et al.* 1998. Expression and neuropeptidergic characterization of estrogen receptors (ERalpha and ERbeta) throughout the rat brain: anatomical evidence of distinct roles of each subtype. J. Neurobiol. **36:** 357–378.
17. SHUGHRUE, P.J. & I. MERCHENTHALER. 2001. The distribution of estrogen receptor beta immunoreactivity in the rat central nervous system. J. Comp. Neurol. **436:** 64–81.
18. CHOI, D.W. 1996. Neuronal apoptosis. Ann. Neurol. Curr. Opin. Neurobiol. **6:** 667–672.
19. LEKER, R.R. & E. SHOSAMI. 2002. Cerebral ischemia and trauma. Different etiology yet similar mechanisms: neuroprotective opportunities. Brain. Res. Rev. **39:** 55–73.
20. TEIXEIRA, C., J.C. REED & M.A.C. PRATT. 1995. Estrogen promotes chemotherapeutic drug resistance by a mechanism involving bcl-2 proto-oncogene expression in human breast cancer cells. Cancer Res. **55:** 3902–3907.
21. CHAN-PALAY, V. 1990. Hyperinnervation of surviving neurons of the human basal nucleus of Meynert by galanin in dementias of Alzheimer's and Parkinson's disease. Adv. Neurol. **51:** 253–255.
22. TANAKA, H., S.Y. GROOMS, M.V.L. BENNETT & R.S. ZUKIN. 2000. The AMPAR subunit GluR2: still front, center stage. Brain Res. **886:** 190–207.
23. MACMANUS, J.P. & A.M. BUCHAM. 2000. Apoptosis after experimental stroke: fact or fashion? J. Neurotrauma **17:** 899–914
24. YANAIHARA, T. 2000. Implication of cysteine proteases calpain, cathepsin and caspase in ischemic neuronal death of primates. Prog. Neurobiol. **62:** 272–295.

25. GRAHAM, S.H., & J. CHEN. 2001. Programmed cell death in cerebral ischemia. J. Cereb. Blood Flow Metab. **21:** 99–109.
26. JOVER, T., H.TANAKA, A. CALDERONE, *et al.* 2002. Estrogen protects against global ischemia-induced neuronal death and prevents activation of apoptotic signaling cascades in the hippocampal CA1. J. Neurosci. **22:** 2115–2124.
27. SHUGHRUE, P.J.& I. MERCHENTHALER. 2000. Evidence for novel estrogen binding sites in the rat hippocampus. Neuroscience **21:** 95–101.
28. HALL, E.D., K.E. PAZARA & K.L. LINSEMAN. 1991. Sex differences in postischemic neuronal necrosis in gerbils. J. Cereb. Blood Flow Metab. **11:** 292–298.
29. SUDO. S., T.C. WEN, J. DESAKI, *et al.* 1997. Beta-estradiol protects hippocampal CA1 neurons against transient forebrain ischemia in gerbil. Neurosci. Res. **29:** 345–354.
30. CHEN, J., N. ADACHI, K. LIU & T. ARA. 1998. The effects of 17beta-estradiol on ischemia-induced neuronal damage in the gerbil hippocampus. Neuroscience **87:** 817–822.
31. SHUGHRUE, P. & I. MERCHENTHALER. 2003. Estrogen prevents the loss of CA1 hippocampal neurons in gerbils after ischemic injury. Neuroscience **116:** 851–861.
32. GREEN, P.S., K. GORDON & J.W. SIMPKINS. 1997. Phenolic A ring requirement for the neuroprotective effects of steroids. J. Steroid. Biochem. Mol. Biol. **63:** 229–235.
33. BEHL, C. & F. LEZOUALCH. 1998. Estrogen with an intact phenolic group prevents death of neuronal cells following glutathione depletion. Restor. Neurol. Neurosci. **12:** 127–134.
34. DELLOVADE, T., P SCRIMO & I. MERCHENTHALER. 2001. Estrogen is neuroprotective following transient global ischemia in the gerbil brain. Soc. Neurosci. Abstr. 437.1.
35. MOOSMANN, B. & C. BEHL. 1999. The antioxidant neuroprotective effects of estrogens and phenolic compounds are independent from their estrogenic properties. Proc. Natl. Acad. Sci. USA **96:** 8867–8872.

The Use of Estrogens and Related Compounds in the Treatment of Damage from Cerebral Ischemia

SHAO-HUA YANG,[a] RAN LIU,[b] SAMUEL S. WU,[b] AND JAMES W. SIMPKINS[a]

[a]*Department of Pharmacology and Neuroscience, University of North Texas Health Science Center, Fort Worth, Texas 76107, USA*

[b]*Department of Statistics, College of Medicine, University of Florida, Gainesville, Florida 32601, USA*

ABSTRACT: There are 750,000 new cases of stroke each year in the United States, and brain damage from stroke leads to high health care costs and disabilities. Needed, but currently not available, are therapies that can be administered prior to, during, or after cerebral ischemia that reduce or eliminate neuronal damage from stroke. To address this issue, we began to assess the neuroprotective effects of estrogens and related compounds in stroke neuroprotection to determine whether these compounds had potential for clinical application. First, we demonstrated that 17 β-estradiol (E2) pretreatment exerted potent neuroprotection of the cerebral cortex over a wide dose range and pretreatment interval. Thereafter, we assessed the ability of a variety of non-feminizing estrogens to protect brain tissue from stroke. We observed that pretreatment with 17 α-estradiol, the complete enantiomer of E2 (ENT-E2), 2-adamantylestrone, and the enantiomer of 17-desoxyestradiol, were as effective as E2 in pretreatment protection from stroke damage. These data suggest that non-estrogen receptor mechanisms are involved in brain neuroprotection under our treatment conditions. We then determined whether the observed E2 protection could be extended to times after the onset of the cerebral ischemic event. Using a formulation of E2 that rapidly delivers the steroid, a necessary condition for acute therapy of an ongoing stroke, we demonstrated that 100 μg E2/kg could protect brain tissue for up to 3 h after the onset of the stroke. To determine whether this therapeutic window could be extended with higher doses of the steroid, we conducted a dose–response assessment of E2 when administered at 6 h after the onset of the ischemic event. While the effectiveness of the 100 μg E2/kg was reduced at this time interval, higher doses of E2 were effective. E2, at doses of 500 and 1000 μg/kg, reduced infarct volume by more than 50%, even with this 6-h delay in treatment. Collectively, these data indicate that estrogens could prove to be useful therapies in preventing brain damage from strokes.

KEYWORDS: estrogen; stroke; estrogen receptor; neuroprotection

Address for correspondence: Dr. James W. Simpkins, Department of Pharmacology and Neuroscience, Health Science Center at Fort Worth, University of North Texas, 3500 Camp Bowie Blvd., Fort Worth, TX 76107. Voice: 817-737-2063; fax: 817-737-0485.
jsimpkin@hsc.unt.edu

Ann. N.Y. Acad. Sci. 1007: 101–107 (2003).
doi: 10.1196/annals.1286.010

Stroke ranks as the third leading cause of death and the leading cause of disability in the United States. There are 750,000 new cases of stroke each year in the U.S., and brain damage from stroke leads to high health care costs and disabilities. Stroke patients must not only survive the acute stages of the event, but must then cope with significant physical, mental, and economic stresses associated with neurological damage. Considering the cost both in loss of life and subsequent productivity, the need for effective therapeutic interventions is obvious. The effort to develop effective therapies for stroke achieved several important successes during the past decade. The greatest successes were related to thrombolysis. However, the only federally approved clot-busting medication, tissue plasminogen activator, must be given within 3 hours of a stroke to be effective. Thrombolysis is severely limited by the need for acute administration. For various reasons, only about 2% of the potentially eligible patients are receiving the treatment.[1] Therapeutic methods are desperately needed, but currently not available, that can be administered prior to, during, or after cerebral ischemia that reduce or eliminate neuronal damage from stroke. Neuroprotection, therapeutic interventions that produce enduring benefits by favorably influencing underlying etiology or pathogenesis and thereby forestalling the onset of neuronal damage or decline caused by stroke or other neurodegenerative diseases,[2] can be used alone and as an adjunct to therapies designed to improve cerebral circulation such as thrombolytic agents for cerebral arterial thrombosis.

Neuroprotective agents have been developed and tested for nearly all components of the ischemic cascade. Various strategies include free radical scavengers, anti-excitotoxic agents, apoptosis inhibitors, anti-inflammatory agents, metal ion chelators, ion channel modulators, antisense oligonucleotides, gene therapy, and stem cell transplantation. There various agents aim to prevent the progression of the ischemic cascade therefore reducing brain damage. Some of these intervene at more than one point in the cascade. During the last decade, tremendous effort has been made to develop new neuroprotective agents, including estrogens. The neuroprotective effects of estrogens were first suggested by epidemiologic studies. Sex differences in the incidence and outcome of stroke suggest that hormonal factors may influence the development and outcome of stroke.[3,4] Protective effects of estrogen have been widely reported in different types of neuronal cell against different toxicities, including serum deprivation, oxidative stress, and amyloid β peptide (Aβ)–induced toxicity and excitotoxicity.[5] Additionally, the pathologic mechanisms that are activated during stoke, include oxidative stress, free radical activity, excitotoxicity, inflammatory response, mitochondrial dysfunction, and apoptosis, are antagonized by estrogens.

Since we first demonstrated that estrogens exert neuroprotective effects in a rodent cerebral ischemia reperfusion model in 1997,[6] there is now abundant *in vivo* evidence for neuroprotection by estrogen. The neuroprotective effects of estrogens have been demonstrated in variety of stroke models by different laboratories; these include the transient and permanent middle cerebral artery occlusion model (MCAO),[7–9] subarachnoid hemorrhage model,[10] global forebrain ischemia model,[11–14] photothrombotic focal ischemia model,[15] and glutamate-induced focal cerebral ischemia model.[16] The neuroprotective effects of estrogens have been demonstrated in females as well as males.[17] The neuroprotective effects of estrogens exert in young and in middle-aged females,[18] as well as in reproductively senescent females.[19] Further, these effects of estrogens have been shown despite the presence of diabetes and hypertension.[20,21] This indicates that estrogen could be a valuable candidate for the treatment of stroke, inasmuch as it is effective in both genders and the therapy appears to be resistant to aging, diabetes, and hypertension.

Neuroprotective effects of E2 have been demonstrated over a very large range of concentrations. In *in vitro* studies, the effective concentrations for E2-mediated neuroprotection range from low nanomolar (~0.1 nM) to high micromolar (~50 μM) concentrations.[5] High physiological concentrations (low nM) were sufficient to attenuate toxicity in a variety of cell types,[5] while significantly higher pharmacological concentrations (low μM) were required to lessen glutamate toxicity. Similarly, large concentration ranges of estrogens, from low physiological concentrations to high pharmacological concentration, has been shown to afford their protective effects in stroke model. Increasing evidence has indicated that the neuroprotective effects of estrogens are dose-dependent. No neuroprotection was afford by physiological level of estradiol administered at the time of the onset of ischemia,[9] while neuroprotective effects of estrogens were clearly demonstrated by the acute treatment, even post-treatment, with pharmacological doses of estradiol.[6,17,22,23] The different therapeutic time course for the physiological and pharmacological dose of estrogens also suggest different neuroprotective mechanism afford by different doses.

Many actions of estrogens, including feminizing effects, are mediated by the binding of the steroid to the nuclear estrogen receptor (ER), and the binding of the steroid-receptor complex to the ER response element thereby activating transcriptional events. The feminizing effects of estrogens limit their clinical application as a neuroprotectant in men as well as in some women. However, increasing evidence indicated that estrogens could protect brain tissue from ischemic damage via mechanisms independent of ER-activation. Several lines of *in vitro* evidence suggest that the neuroprotective effects of estrogens do not require ER-dependent gene transcription. First, ER antagonists do not attenuate the protective action of E2 in all models of neurotoxicity.[24,25] Second, neuroprotection of estrogens can occur in the presence of mRNA or protein synthesis inhibitors.[26,27] Third, non-feminizing estrogens, such as 17α-estradiol,[28,29] complete enantiomer of 17β-estradiol,[(30)] and other phenolic compounds[25] have been shown to be neuroprotective and activate signal transduction cascades associated with neurotrophic effects, such as ERKs at the same doses as 17β-estradiol.[31] The receptor-independent non-genomic action of estrogens was also indicated in the *in vivo* studies. The neuroprotective effects of estrogen have also been demonstrated for several nonfeminizing estrogen analogues, such as 17α-estradiol, the enantiomer of 17β-estradiol and 2-adamantylestrone.[6,30,32] These data suggest that non-ER mechanisms are involved in brain neuroprotection under these conditions. On the other hand, an ER-dependent mechanism was also indicated. Dubal *et al.*[33] reported that ERα knockout, but not ERβ knockout, mice were resistant to the neuroprotective effects of 17β-E2 administered chronically at low concentrations and they concluded that ERα is a necessary mediator of estrogen neuroprotection. However, neuroprotective effects of estrogens have been shown in intact ERα knockout females,[34] which have much higher estrogens level than wild-type females.[35] Consistently, McCullough *et al.* later demonstrated neuroprotection in ERα knockout mice using pharmacological doses of the estrogens.[36] Together, these data indicated that estrogens could exert neuroprotective effects through both receptor-dependent and -independent mechanisms depending upon the dose of estro-

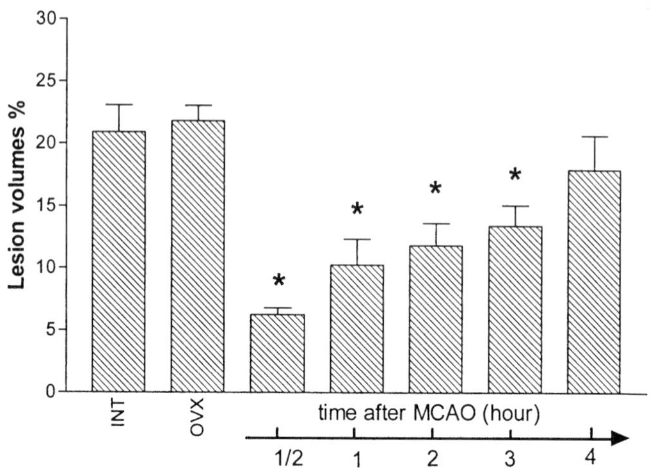

FIGURE 1. Effects of 17β-estradiol treatment on lesion volume after permanent MCAO in ovariectomized rats. Female Charles River Sprague-Dawley rats (225–250g, Wilmington, MA) were maintained in laboratory acclimatization for 3 days prior to ovariectomy. Bilateral ovariectomy was performed under methoxyflurane inhalant anesthesia. The animals were subjected to permanent MCAO 2 weeks after ovariectomy. 17β-estradiol was administered by simultaneous intravenous injection (100 µg E2/kg) and subcutaneous implantation of an E2 pellet at ½ ($n = 8$), 1 ($n = 6$), 2 ($n = 7$), 3 ($n = 6$) or 4 ($n = 9$) hours after MCAO. The animals were decapitated 2 days after MCAO. The brain was sliced and stained with 2,3,5-triphenyltetrazolium chloride for lesion volume analysis. INT = ovary-intact rats; OVX = ovariectomized rats treated with saline and empty pellet implantation. Depicted are the means ± SEM. *$P < 0.05$ vs. OVX & INT. (From Yang *et al.*[22] Reproduced by permission.)

gen administered. The nonfeminizing estrogen analogues with neuroprotective activity, but lacking estrogenic activity in peripheral estrogen-responsive tissues, could be applied in both males and females for whom estrogen therapy is contraindicated.

At pharmacologic doses, neuroprotective effects of estrogens have been demonstrated upon acute pre-treatment, as well as treatments initiated after the onset of the ischemic insult.[6,17,23] We demonstrated that 17β-estradiol exerts neuroprotective effects when administered after an ischemic insult, with a therapeutic window of about 3 hours at the dose of 100 µg/kg (FIG. 1).[22] However, the dose-dependency of estrogen protection after the onset of a stroke is not known. We conducted a dose-response assessment of 17β-estradiol when administered at 6 h after the onset of the ischemic event to determine whether our previously reported 3-h therapeutic window[22] could be extended with higher doses of the steroid. Encouragingly, 17β-estradiol treatment at 500 µg/kg and 1000 µg/kg still exert neuroprotective effects against the cerebral ischemic damage when administered 6 hours after permanent middle cerebral artery occlusion (FIG. 2). Given the effectiveness of thrombolysis and the neuroprotective effectiveness of estrogen for both the ischemic and reperfusion phases, combination of reperfusion-enhancing agents with estrogens could greatly improve the outcome of stroke. The potential approach to prolonging the

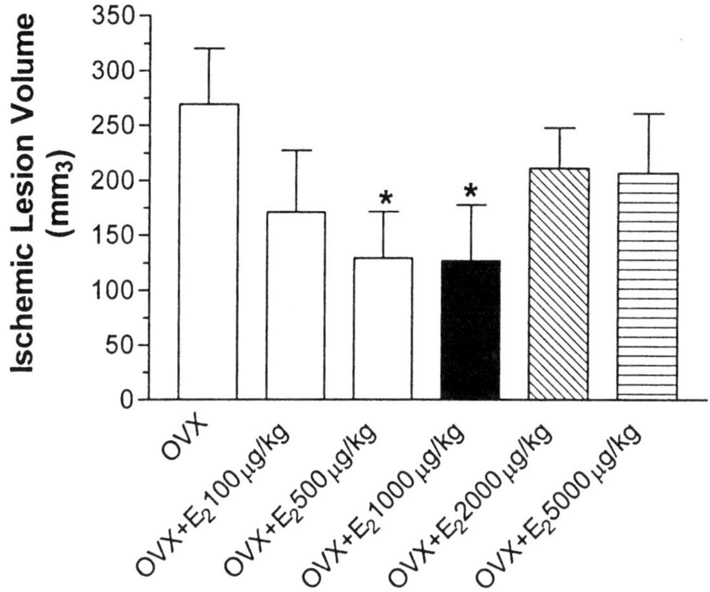

FIGURE 2. Dose-dependent neuroprotection of 17β-estradiol when administered at 6 h after permanent MCAO. Female Charles River Sprague-Dawley rats (250g, Wilmington, MA) were maintained in laboratory acclimatization for three days prior to ovariectomy. Bilateral ovariectomy was performed using halothane anesthesia. The animals were subjected to permanent MCAO 2 weeks after ovariectomy. 17β-estradiol formulated in sesame oil was administered by subcutaneous injection at 6 hours after MCAO at the dose of 100 ($n = 9$), 500 ($n = 10$), 1000 ($n = 10$), 2000 ($n = 9$), or 5000 µg/kg ($n = 9$), respectively. OVX animals received sesame oil as control ($n = 10$). The animals were decapitated 24 h after MCAO. The brain was sliced and stained with 2,3,5-triphenyltetrazolium chloride for lesion volume analysis. Depicted are the means ± SEM. *$P < 0.05$ vs. OVX.

therapeutic time window for successful thrombolysis would be to give estrogen as a neuroprotectant before, during, or after thrombolytic therapy. It is likely that this combination therapy will restore blood flow, halt or reverse the cascade of neuronal damage, and will be used to achieve effective stroke care in the future.

Although the application of estrogens for treatment of stroke require further clinical studies, a plethora of data support a direct neuroprotective role for estrogens. Given the proven clinical safety of this steroid, estrogen therapy may be useful in treating acute cerebral ischemia. Further, the efficacy of non-feminizing estrogen analogues suggest that these compounds may be clinically useful for prevention of cerebral damage in men or women for whom estrogen therapy is contraindicated. However, one cannot assume that estrogen administration will always improve outcome in cerebral ischemia. The neuroprotective effects of estrogens are both dose-dependent and severity-of-damage–dependent. The mechanisms that contribute to the loss of neuroprotection at the high dose of 17β-estradiol (FIG. 2) are not clear. It is likely that some side effects were induced by these very high doses of 17β-estradiol, which abolish or mask its neuroprotective actions.

ACKNOWLEDGMENTS

This work was supported by NIH Grant AG 10485, AG 22550, U.S. Army Grant DAMD 17-19-1-9473, and by MitoKor, Inc.

REFERENCES

1. ZIVIN, J.A. 1999. Thrombolytic stroke therapy: past, present, and future. Neurology **53:** 14–19.
2. SHOULSON, I. 1998. DATATOP: a decade of neuroprotective inquiry. Parkinson Study Group. Deprenyl and tocopherol antioxidative therapy of parkinsonism. Ann. Neurol. **44:** S160–166.
3. THORVALDSEN, P. *et al.* 1995. Stroke incidence, case fatality, and mortality in the WHO MONICA project: World Health Organization monitoring trends and determinants in cardiovascular disease. Stroke **26:** 361–367.
4. STEGMAYR, B. *et al.* 1997. Stroke incidence and mortality correlated to stroke risk factors in the WHO MONICA Project: An ecological study of 18 populations. Stroke **28:** 1367–1374.
5. GREEN, P.S. & J.W. SIMPKINS. 2000. Neuroprotective effects of estrogens: potential mechanisms of action. Int. J. Dev. Neurosci. **18:** 347–358.
6. SIMPKINS, J.W. *et al.* 1997. Estrogens may reduce mortality and ischemic damage caused by middle cerebral artery occlusion in the female rat. J. Neurosurg. **87:** 724–730.
7. ZHANG, Y.Q. *et al.* 1998. Effects of gender and estradiol treatment on focal brain ischemia. Brain Res. **784:** 321–324.
8. ALKAYED, N.J. *et al.* 1998. Gender-linked brain injury in experimental stroke. *Stroke* **29:** 159–165; discussion 166.
9. DUBAL, D.B. *et al.* 1998. Estradiol protects against ischemic injury. J. Cereb. Blood Flow Metab. **18:** 1253–1258.
10. YANG, S.H. *et al.* 2001. 17-beta estradiol can reduce secondary ischemic damage and mortality of subarachnoid hemorrhage. J. Cereb. Blood Flow. Metab. **21:** 174–181.
11. SUDO, S. *et al.* 1997. Beta-estradiol protects hippocampal CA1 neurons against transient forebrain ischemia in gerbil. Neurosci. Res. **29:** 345–354.
12. CHEN, J. *et al.* 1998. The effects of 17beta-estradiol on ischemia-induced neuronal damage in the gerbil hippocampus. Neuroscience **87:** 817–822.
13. HE, Z. *et al.* 2002. Proestrus levels of estradiol during transient global cerebral ischemia improves the histological outcome of the hippocampal CA1 region: perfusion-dependent and-independent mechanisms. J. Neurol. Sci. **193:** 79–87.
14. JOVER, T. *et al.* 2002. Estrogen protects against global ischemia-induced neuronal death and prevents activation of apoptotic signaling cascades in the hippocampal CA1. J. Neurosci. **22:** 2115–2124.
15. FUKUDA, K. *et al.* 2000. Ovariectomy exacerbates and estrogen replacement attenuates photothrombotic focal ischemic brain injury in rats. Stroke **31:** 155–160.
16. MENDELOWITSCH, A. *et al.* 2001. 17beta-Estradiol reduces cortical lesion size in the glutamate excitotoxicity model by enhancing extracellular lactate: a new neuroprotective pathway. Brain Res. **901:** 230–236.
17. TOUNG, T.J. *et al.* 1998. Estrogen-mediated neuroprotection after experimental stroke in male rats. Stroke **29:** 1666–1670.
18. WISE, P.M. & D.B. DUBAL. 2000. Estradiol protects against ischemic brain injury in middle-aged rats. Biol. Reprod. **63:** 982–985.
19. ALKAYED, N.J. *et al.* 2000. Neuroprotective effects of female gonadal steroids in reproductively senescent female rats. Stroke **31:** 161–168.
20. TOUNG, T.K. *et al.* 2000. Estrogen decreases infarct size after temporary focal ischemia in a genetic model of type 1 diabetes mellitus. Stroke **31:** 2701–2706.
21. CARSWELL, H.V. *et al.* 2000. Estrogen status affects sensitivity to focal cerebral ischemia in stroke-prone spontaneously hypertensive rats. Am. J. Physiol. Heart Circ. Physiol. **278:** H290–294.

22. YANG, S.H. *et al.* 2000. Estradiol exerts neuroprotective effects when administered after ischemic insult. Stroke **31:** 745-749; discussion 749–750.
23. MCCULLOUGH, L.D. *et al.* 2001. Postischemic estrogen reduces hypoperfusion and secondary ischemia after experimental stroke. Stroke **32:** 796–802.
24. WEAVER, C.E., JR. *et al.* 1997. 17beta-Estradiol protects against NMDA-induced excitotoxicity by direct inhibition of NMDA receptors. Brain Res. **761:** 338–341.
25. MOOSMANN, B. & C. BEHL. 1999. The antioxidant neuroprotective effects of estrogens and phenolic compounds are independent from their estrogenic properties. Proc. Natl. Acad. Sci.. USA **96:** 8867–8872.
26. SAWADA, H. *et al.* 1998. Estradiol protects mesencephalic dopaminergic neurons from oxidative stress-induced neuronal death. J. Neurosci. Res. **54:** 707–719.
27. REGAN, R.F. & Y. GUO. 1997. Estrogens attenuate neuronal injury due to hemoglobin, chemical hypoxia, and excitatory amino acids in murine cortical cultures. Brain Res. **764:** 133–140.
28. BEHL, C. *et al.* 1997. Neuroprotection against oxidative stress by estrogens: structure-activity relationship. Mol. Pharmaco.l **51:** 535–541.
29. GREEN, P.S. *et al.* 1997. 17 alpha-estradiol exerts neuroprotective effects on SK-N-SH cells. J. Neurosci. **17:** 511–515.
30. GREEN, P.S. *et al.* 2001. The nonfeminizing enantiomer of 17beta-estradiol exerts protective effects in neuronal cultures and a rat model of cerebral ischemia. Endocrinology **142:** 400–406.
31. SINGH, M. *et al.* 2000. Estrogen-induced activation of the mitogen-activated protein kinase cascade in the cerebral cortex of estrogen receptor-alpha knock-out mice. J. Neurosci. **20:** 1694–1700.
32. LIU, R. *et al.* 2002. Neuroprotective effects of a novel non-receptor-binding estrogen analogue: in vitro and in vivo analysis. Stroke **33:** 2485–2491.
33. DUBAL, D.B. *et al.* 2001. Estrogen receptor alpha, not beta, is a critical link in estradiol-mediated protection against brain injury. Proc. Natl.. Acad. Sci. USA **98:** 1952–1957.
34. SAMPEI, K. *et al.* 2000. Stroke in estrogen receptor-alpha-deficient mice. Stroke **31:** 738-743; discussion 744.
35. COUSE, J.F. & K.S. KORACH. 1999. Estrogen receptor null mice: what have we learned and where will they lead us? Endocr. Rev. **20:** 358–417.
36. MCCULLOUGH, L.D. *et al.* 2001. Estrogen protects ischemic brain of ERα and ERβ-knockout mice [abstract]. The Physiologist **44:** 269.

An ICI 182,780-Sensitive, Membrane-Related Estrogen Receptor Contributes to Estrogenic Neuroprotective Actions against Amyloid-Beta Toxicity

R. MARIN,[a] B. GUERRA,[a] A. MORALES,[a] M. DÍAZ,[b] AND R. ALONSO[a]

[a]*Laboratory of Cellular Neurobiology, Department of Physiology, University of La Laguna, School of Medicine, 38071 Sta. Cruz de Tenerife, Spain*

[b]*Laboratory of Animal Physiology, Department of Animal Biology, Faculty of Biology, 38206 Sta. Cruz de Tenerife, Spain*

Abstract: Although estrogen (E2)-related neuroprotection has been repeatedly demonstrated in different models, the involvement of non-classical estrogen receptors (ERs) in this activity remains unclear. Using SN56 murine cholinergic cell line from the basal forebrain, we present evidence indicating that an ER associated with the plasma membrane participates in estrogen-dependent reduction of neuronal death induced by amyloid-β peptide (Aβ) toxicity. Exposure to either E2 or estradiol-horseradish peroxidase (E-HRP) for 15 min significantly reduced Aβ-induced cell death. This effect was decreased by the ER antagonist ICI 182,780 as well as by MC-20 antibody directed to a region neighboring the ligand-binding domain of ERα. Using MC-20 antibody in unpermeabilized SN56 cells, we detected a protein at the plasma membrane region. The binding of impermeant forms of E2, E-HRP, and E-BSA-FITC to specific sites of SN56 plasma membrane was blocked by pre-incubation with E2, ICI 182,780, and MC-20 antibody in a concentration-dependent manner. Thus, a membrane-related ER that shares some structural homologies with ERα may participate in estrogen-mediated neuroprotection.

Keywords: estrogen; estrogen receptor; β-amyloid; neuroprotection; SN56 cell line

INTRODUCTION

Estrogen has been traditionally thought to act by binding nuclear estrogen receptors (ERs), which act as transcription factors and regulate gene expression. However, emerging data have implicated alternative mechanisms of estrogen (E2) action often initiated at the cell membrane, which can trigger within minutes multiple signal transduction pathways.[1]

Address for correspondence: Dr. R. Marin, Laboratory of Cellular Neurobiology, Department of Physiology, University of La Laguna, School of Medicine, 38071 Sta. Cruz de Tenerife, Spain. Voice: 34 922 319311; fax: 34 922 648457
rmarin@ull.es

**Ann. N.Y. Acad. Sci. 1007: 108–116 (2003). © 2003 New York Academy of Sciences.
doi: 10.1196/annals.1286.011**

In vitro paradigms that imitate some aspects of Alzheimer's disease (AD) pathology have demonstrated that estrogen has the ability to prevent neuronal death from amyloid-beta peptide (Aβ) accumulation with the involvement of classic ERs.[2] However, it remains unexplored in neurons whether these estrogen preventive actions could be regulated by membrane receptors. So far, a single report[3] in transfected hippocampal-derived cells (HT22) has reported the involvement of ERs in rapid preventive actions of estrogen against Aβ-induced toxicity, although the possible participation of a plasma membrane-related ER (mER) counterpart still has not been documented.

Using murine SN56 cell line from the basal forebrain, we present here evidence of estrogen neuroprotective actions against Aβ-induced injury that may be modulated by a putative plasma membrane-associated ER.

RESULTS AND DISCUSSION

Short-term Exposure to Either E2 or E-HRP Reduces SN56 Cell Death during Aβ Injury, an Effect That is Attenuated by the Antiestrogen ICI 182,780

Exposure of SN56 cells to 5 μM $A\beta_{1-40}$ for 24 h induced 65% cell death as compared to vehicle-treated cultures (FIG. 1). Cell viability was quantified by the trypan

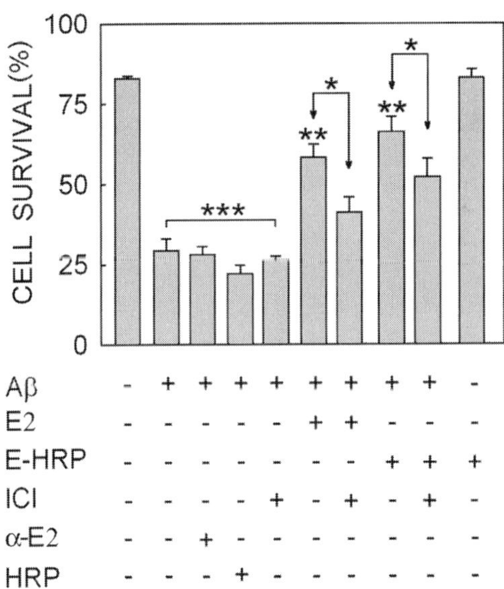

FIGURE 1. Neuroprotective effects of short exposures to E2 or the membrane-impermeant E-HRP against $A\beta_{1-40}$-induced toxicity. SN56 cultures were incubated with 10 nM E2 or E-HRP for 15 min prior to $A\beta_{1-40}$ (5 μM). For ICI 182,780 treatments, cells were preincubated for 2 h with an excess (10 μM) of the antiestrogen. Cell viability was measured after 24 h. Vehicle-treated cells were used as an experimental control (*first bar on the left*). (*) $P < 0.05$; (**) $P < 0.001$ vs. Aβ; (***) $P < 0.0001$ vs. vehicle-treated cells. Number of assays per group = 5.

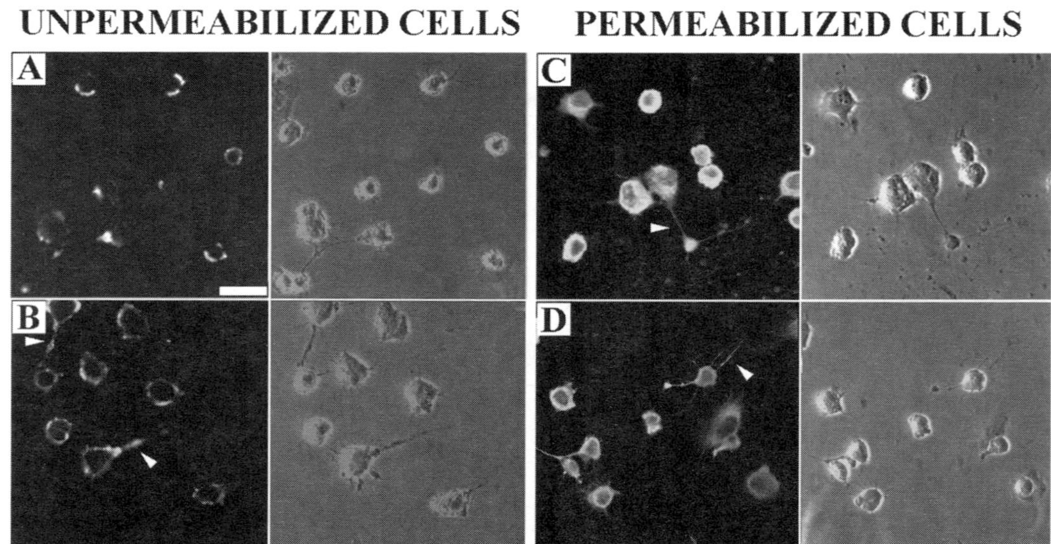

FIGURE 2. Membrane-related immunostaining of ERα in this model of toxicity. Either non-permeabilized [2% paraformaldehyde, 1% glutaraldehyde, and 120 mM sucrose in PBS pH 7.4 for 30 min at room temperature] (**A** and **B**) or detergent-permeabilized [2% paraformaldehyde, 1% glutaraldehyde, 120 mM sucrose, and 0.5% NP-40 in PBS pH 7.4 for 1 min] (**C** and **D**) SN56 cultures were labeled with MC-20 anti-ERα antibody and goat biotinylated anti-goat antibody linked to Cy2-conjugated streptavidin. **A** and **C** correspond to vehicle-treated (0.001% ethanol for E2 and 0.05% acetic acid) cells; and **B** and **D** to 10 nM estrogen and 5 μM $A\beta_{1-40}$ co-treated cells for 24 h. Matched brightfields are shown on the right of each image. Notice the staining in neurites (*arrowheads*). Number of assays per group = 4. Bar: 50 μm.

blue exclusion method.[4] Pre-incubation with 10 nM E2 or the impermeable form of E2, estradiol coupled to horseradish peroxidase (E-HRP), for 15 min reduced cell death to 25–30%, suggesting that estrogen-mediated neuroprotection may be promoted by alternative pathways initiated at the plasma membrane. These preventive effects were partially reversed (in about 35%) by 2-h treatment with the ER antagonist ICI 182,780 (10 μM), whereas ICI 182,780 or HRP alone did not alter Aβ-induced cell death. No significant neuroprotective effect was observed in the presence of 10 nM of biologically inactive 17α-estradiol under similar experimental conditions. E-HRP did not modify cell viability in unstressed conditions.

Immunolocalization of an ERα-like Receptor Associated with the Plasma Membrane

The potential existence of a mER-like receptor was explored in cultures treated with 10 nM E2 and 5 μM $A\beta_{1-40}$ and fixed under either non-permeabilizing or detergent-permeabilizing conditions. As observed by confocal microscopy, unpermeabilized cells incubated with MC-20 antibody directed to the carboxy-terminal region of ERα showed some immunostaining at the cell surface (FIG. 2A and B). A strong staining at the cytoplasmic and nuclear levels was observed in permeabilized cells (FIG. 2C and D).

Neuroprotective Membrane-Related Effects of E2 are Modulated by MC-20 Antibody

We next exposed SN56 cultures to MC-20 anti-ERα antibody (4 ng/μL) for 2 h at 37°C, prior to either E2 or E-HRP exposure. This treatment reduced the neuropro-

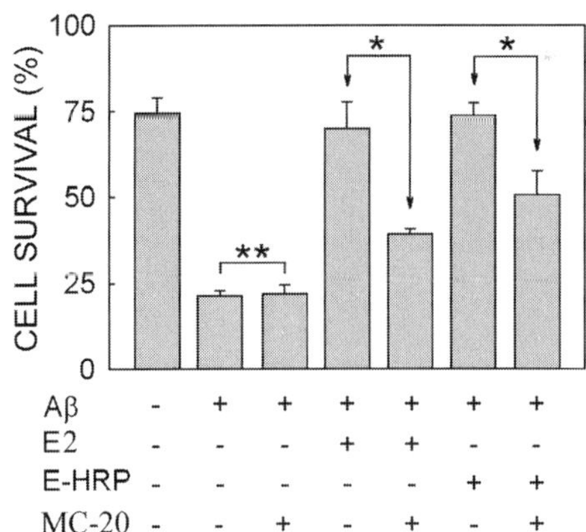

FIGURE 3. MC-20 antibody inhibits neuroprotective effects of E2 and E-HRP. SN56 cultures were pre-incubated with the specific anti-ERα antibody (1:50) prior to treatment with either form of steroid for 15 min. Cells were then exposed to 5 μM $A\beta_{1-40}$ for 24 h and viability was measured. For comparative purposes, other cultures were concomitantly exposed to the same treatments without the antibody. Both cells exposed to free antibody during injury and vehicle-treated cells were used as controls of viability. (*) $P < 0.01$; (**) $P < 0.0001$ vs. vehicle-treated cells. Number of assays per group = 5.

tective effect of both steroids (35–50%) (FIG. 3), whereas the antibody alone did not provoke any effect on cell survival. Altogether, these data support the idea that estrogen is able to prevent Aβ_{1-40}-induced SN56 cell death by acting through a potential membrane form of ER that shares some structural similarities with ERα. Although the existence of a mER has been previously reported in other cell models,[5] to our knowledge this is the first demonstration of the involvement of an endogenous ER at the plasma membrane in estrogenic neuroprotection against Aβ injury.

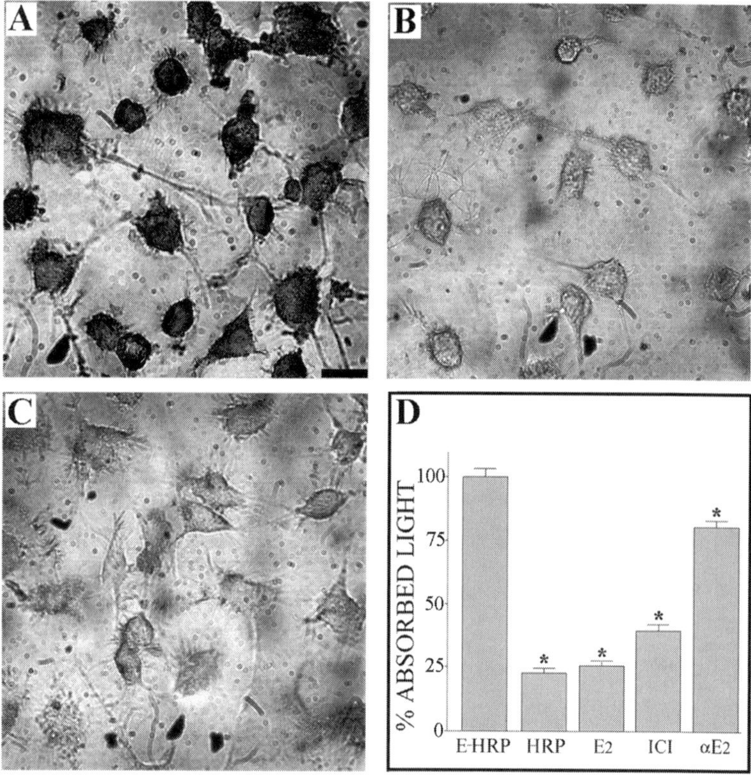

FIGURE 4. E-HRP binding assay in SN56 cells. Cultures were fixed under non-permeabilizing conditions and incubated with 100 nM E-HRP overnight at 4°C. For double-binding assays, cells were previously exposed to an excess of E2 or ICI 182,780. (**A**) Staining with 100 nM E-HRP in unpermeabilized SN56 cells; (**B** and **C**) E-HRP labeling blockade with 30 μM E2 (**B**) and ICI 182,780 (**C**). (**D**) Quantification of competition of E-HRP binding by 30 μM of E2 (E2), ICI 182,780 (ICI) and 17α-estradiol (αE2), as compared to the maximal absorbed light obtained with E-HRP binding alone (E-HRP). Number of cells per group = 90. (*) $P < 0.0001$ vs. E-HRP. Bar: 10 μm.

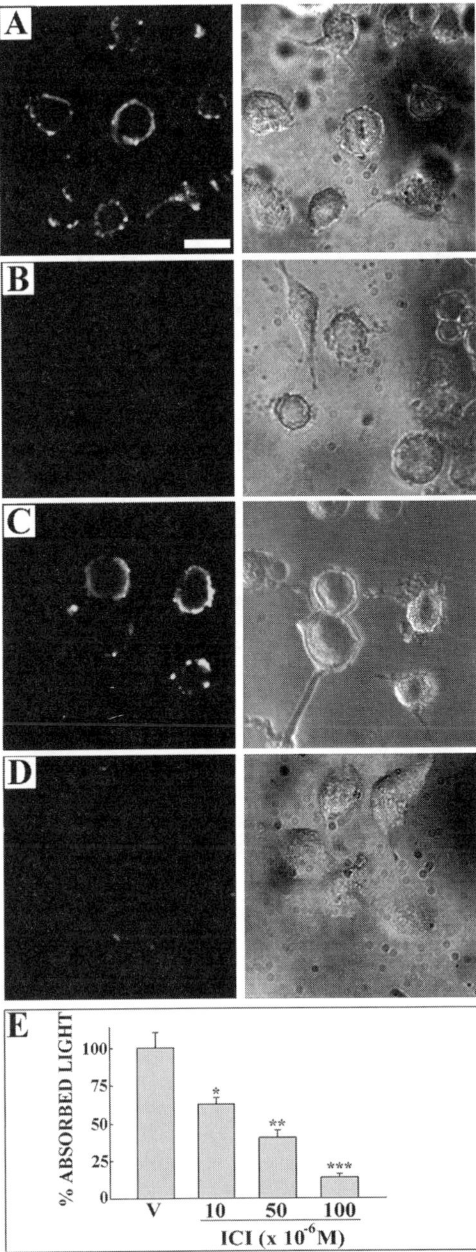

FIGURE 5. E-BSA-FITC binding of SN56 cells and competition with ICI 182,780. (**A**) Specific fluorescence staining at the surface of SN56 cells with 10 μM E-BSA-FITC. This labeling was competed off with a 10-fold excess of E2 (**B**), but remained unaffected with a 10-fold excess of BSA (**C**). Staining was blocked with 100 μM ICI 182,780 (**D**). (**E**) Quantification of ICI 182,780 competition at the different doses used. Values are referred to the percentage of absorbed light in vehicle-treated cells used as a control. Corresponding transmission images of the different cultures are shown on the right. Number of cells per group = 80. (*) $P < 0.001$ vs. V; (**) $P < 0.001$ vs. 10; (***) $P < 0.001$ vs. 50. Bar: 30 μm.

Both Impermeant Conjugates, E-HRP and E-BSA-FITC, Bind to Specific Sites of SN56 Cell Plasma Membrane that are Recognized by E2, ICI 182,780 and MC-20 Antibody

We further studied the existence of specific plasma membrane binding sites in SN56 cells using two impermeant compounds, E-HRP and E-BSA-FITC. SN56 cells were exposed to 100 nM E-HRP overnight at 4°C, and then HRP reaction was developed with DAB-based primary product of peroxidase reaction. As revealed by confocal microscopy, E-HRP binding (FIG. 4A) was competed off by a 300-fold excess of

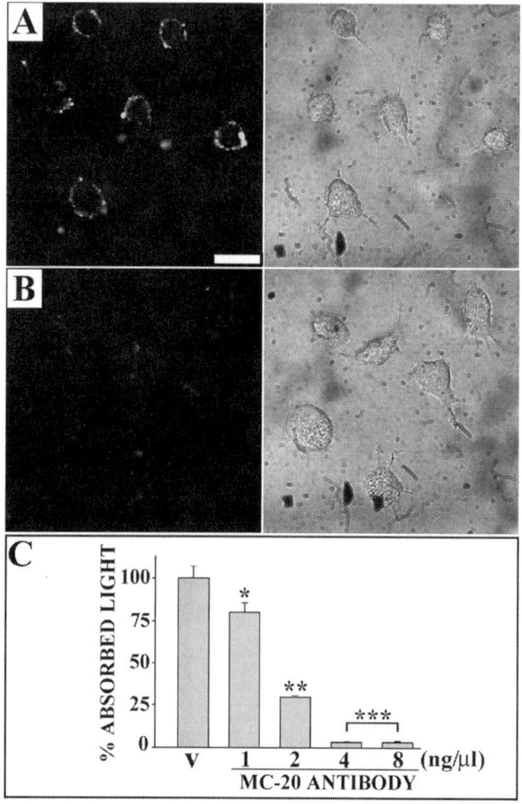

FIGURE 6. Blockade of E-BSA-FITC binding with MC-20 anti-ERα antibody in SN56 cells. (**A**) Specific fluorescence staining at the surface of SN56 cultures incubated with 10 μM E-BSA-FITC used as a control. This binding was competed off by increasing concentrations of MC-20 antibody that progressively displaced steroid labeling. Staining was inhibited when cultures were pre-incubated with 8 ng/μL of the antibody (**B**). (**C**) Quantification of E-BSA-FITC staining in the presence of different concentrations (1–8 ng/μL) of the antibody. Values are referred to the percentage of absorbed light in vehicle-treated cells used as a control. Corresponding transmission images of the different cultures are shown on the right of each immunofluorescence image. Number of cells per group = 60. (*) $P < 0.05$ vs. V; (**) $P < 0.001$ vs. 1; (***) $P < 0.001$ vs. 2. Bar: 50 μm.

either unlabeled E2 (Fig. 4B) or ICI 182,780 (FIG. 4C). Incubation with 17α-estradiol only exerted a slight effect (15%) (FIG. 4D). In another group of experiments, SN56 cells were incubated with 10 μM E-BSA-FITC showing fluorescent staining at the outer cell membrane (FIG. 5A). Labeling was blocked by a 10-fold excess of E2 (FIG. 5B), but it was not affected by 10-fold excess of BSA (FIG. 5C). A complete blockade of immunostaining was obtained with 100 μM ICI 182,780 (FIG. 5D). Quantification of percentage of emitted light revealed a dose-dependent reduction of labeling with ICI 182,780 (FIG. 5E). A decrease in E-BSA-FITC-related fluorescence was also obtained in the presence of MC-20 (FIG. 6B), as compared to control cultures incubated with the fluorescent complex alone (FIG. 6A). The inhibitory effect of MC-20 at different doses (2–8 ng/μL) was quantified by confocal microscopy (FIG. 6C). These data support the idea that estrogen specifically binds to a mER that shares some homologies with the ligand binding domain (LBD) of classic ERα.

Previous data in different estrogen-targeted cells have substantiated that mER originates from classic ER, and translocates to the membrane to participate in several estrogenic actions.[6,7] Interestingly, a recent work in neocortical explants has proposed the existence of a novel mER that has homology with ERα LBD and is associated with estrogen-induced activation of the MAPK cascade.[8] However, other alternative mechanisms may also be involved depending on cell origin and type of injury.

In summary, our results show that estrogen can exert rapid neuroprotective effects against Aβ-induced toxicity in a cell line derived from septal cholinergic neurons by acting at the plasma membrane. This action may be triggered after estrogen binding to a membrane-associated ER which could be coordinated with more delayed intracellular responses mediated by activation of nuclear ERs. Further understanding of multiple mechanisms of estrogen to induce neuroprotection may provide alternative strategies for preventing or treating AD-related neurodegeneration.

ACKNOWLEDGMENTS

This work was supported by Grant SAF2001-3614-C03-01/02 from the Ministry of Science and Technology, Spain. Additional financial support was received from Lilly S.A. and Astra-Zeneca.

REFERENCES

1. NADAL, A., M. DÍAZ & M.A. VALVERDE. 2001. The estrogen trinity: membrane, cytosolic, and nuclear effects. News Physiol. Sci. **16:** 251–255.
2. KIM, H., O.Y. BANG, M.W. JUN, *et al.* 2001. Neuroprotective effects of estrogen against beta-amyloid toxicity are mediated by estrogen receptors in cultured neuronal cells. Neurosci. Lett. **302:** 58–62.
3. FITZPATRICK, J.L., A.L. MIZE, C.B. WADE, *et al.* 2002. Estrogen-mediated neuroprotection against beta-amyloid toxicity requires expression of estrogen receptor alpha or beta and activation of the MAPK pathway. J. Neurochem. **82:** 674–682.
4. BLACK, L. & M.C. BERENBAUM. 1964. Factors affecting the dye exclusion test for cell viability. Exp. Cell Res. **35:** 9–13.
5. PIETRAS, R.J., I. NEMERE & C.M. SZEGO. 2001. Steroid hormone receptors in target cell membranes. Endocrine **14:** 417–427.

6. Razandi, M., A. Pedram, G.L. Greene, *et al.* 1999. Cell membrane and nuclear estrogen receptors (ERs) originate from a single transcript: studies of ERalpha and ERbeta expressed in Chinese hamster ovary cells. Mol. Endocrinol. **13:** 307–319.
7. Russell, K.S., M.P. Haynes, D. Sinha, *et al.* 2000. Human vascular endothelial cells contain membrane binding sites for estradiol, which mediate rapid intracellular signalling. Proc. Natl. Acad. Sci. USA **97:** 5930–5035.
8. Toran-Allerand, C.D., X. Guan, N.J. MacLusky, *et al.* 2002. ER-X: A novel, plasma membrane-associated, putative estrogen receptor that is regulated during development and after ischemic brain injury. J. Neurosci. **22:** 8391–8401.

Neurosteroids in the Retina

Neurodegenerative and Neuroprotective Agents in Retinal Degeneration

P. GUARNERI,[a] C. CASCIO,[a] D. RUSSO,[a] S. D'AGOSTINO,[a] G. DRAGO,[a] G. GALIZZI,[a] G. DE LEO,[b] F. PICCOLI,[c] M. GUARNERI,[d] AND R. GUARNERI[a]

[a]*Istituto di Biomedicina e Immunologia Molecolare–CNR,*
[b]*Sezione Biologia e Genetica, Dipartimento Biopatologia e Metodologie Biomediche,*
[c]*Istituto di Neuropsichiatria,* [d]*Facoltà di Medicina e Chirurgia, Università di Palermo, 90146 Palermo, Italy*

ABSTRACT: Steroids may have a powerful role in neuronal degeneration. Recent research has revealed that steroids may influence the onset and progression of some retinal disorders as well as neurodegenerative diseases and, as in brain, they accumulate in the retina via a local synthesis (neurosteroids) and metabolism of blood-circulating steroid hormones. Their crucial role as neurodegenerative and neuroprotective agents has been also upheld in a retinal excitotoxic paradigm. These findings are reviewed especially from the emerging perspective that after an insult local changes in steroidogenic responses and consequent neurosteroid availability might turn out to be offensive or defensive cellular adaptations for the potentiation or prevention of neuronal death.

KEYWORDS: pregnenolone sulfate; 17β-estradiol; DHEA; DHEAS; neurodegeneration; neuroprotection; retina

INTRODUCTION

Neuronal degeneration is the fatal consequence in acute and chronic neurodegenerative diseases and in various primary and secondary retinal disorders.[1–3] Although much has been learned over the last decade, the neuropathological mechanisms leading to progressive dysfunction and death of neurons remain still elusive. Any central nervous system (CNS) insult is accomplished by an array of processes, involving intra- and intercellular environment of neurons and their dialogue with glial and vascular cells; consequently, many damaging neurochemical modulators lead to the amplification and progression of death signal. Initiating factors, such as excitotoxicity, oxidative stress, growth factor withdrawal, cytokines, and toxins, are often interrelated in order to elaborate mechanisms usually linked to an apoptotic cell death or a mixed form of necrosis and apoptosis. It is now widely held that an insult generates not only

Address for correspondence: Dr. Patrizia Guarneri, Istituto di Biomedicina e Immunologia Molecolare, CNR, Via Ugo La Malfa, 153, 90146-Palermo, Italy. Voice: 39-91-6809541/6809519; fax: 39-91-6809548.
pguarneri@ibim.pa.cnr.it

Ann. N.Y. Acad. Sci. 1007: 117–128 (2003). © 2003 New York Academy of Sciences.
doi: 10.1196/annals.1286.012

negative but also positive responses, resulting in stimulation of neuronal defenses; thus, some neurons succumb sooner than others while certain neurons are never affected.[1,3–6] In this context, the steroidal environment of the CNS is considered of great importance in that it varies as a function of the life cycle and as a component of stress- and illness-activated circuits, thus having effects on CNS integrity, functionality, and resistance to toxic attacks.[7–12] Evidence suggests a close relationship among steroid availability, neuronal susceptibility, and rate of occurrence of seizures, ischemic and traumatic injury, Alzheimer's disease, and also the likelihood of cognitive aging,[10–13] and finally some ophthalmic diseases such as age-related macular degeneration, and retinal ischemic conditions.[14–17] Certain steroids have clear neuroprotective effects in several experimental paradigms shaping the biochemical and metabolic changes linked to these diseases. Thus, prevention is observed in oxidative stress, mitochondrial dysfunction, and glutamate toxicity.[7–12,17] However, detrimental effects may also be promoted with steroid levels elevated to toxic concentrations, depending upon the type of injury and/or the region affected.[7,9,11] Progress has been made in the search for the mechanisms through which steroids interfere with neurodegenerative processes. Our research has recently brought to light the possibility that neurosteroids other than steroids of an endocrine source contribute to neuronal cell death. We have focused on the role served by neurosteroids synthesized in the retina as neurodegenerative or neuroprotective agents in the course of excitotoxic cell death. These results will be reviewed herein, together with new insights into the influence of steroids on ocular diseases and on the characterization of the retina and other ocular structures as targets of steroids; the retina as a site of steroid production that strongly corroborates their role in the visual physiology and pathophysiology by nongenomic and genomic actions will also be studied.

Steroids in the Retina: Basic and Clinical Observations

The retina is part of the CNS; like the cerebral and cerebellar cortices, the neural retina develops into a layered array of different neuronal types. The layers include the light- and color-sensitive photoreceptor cells, the cell bodies of ganglion cells, and the bipolar interneurons that transmit electrical stimuli from photoreceptors to ganglion cells. The ganglion cells are the output neurons extending their axons to target areas within the brain through the optic nerve whose myelination is provided by oligondendrocytes. Numerous Müller glial cells are necessary for the retinal integrity, and amacrine and horizontal neurons for the transmission of electrical impulses in the plane of the retina. Nearness interactions occur in two plexiform layers. Of relevance to retinal homeostasis is the retinal pigment epithelium (RPE) which lies over photoreceptors and down Bruch's membrane and contributes to the blood–ocular barrier, phagocytosis, nutritional and solute support. The vast majority of retinal synapses use glutamate for the light transmission along retinal layers, and GABA and glycine for the lateral inhibition; Ach and dopamine in amacrine cells and several neuropeptides also cooperate in the control of the visual pathway.

As with the brain, the retina is a target of steroids and a site of steroid production. The endocrine influence on visual processing was originally proposed in the late 1970s based on the evidence that susceptibility of retinal cells to light damage occurred concomitantly with sexual maturation in both male and female animals.[18] However, recent advances in research have proved the existence of hormone steroid receptors, steroid enzymes for the formation of *ex novo* steroids or neurosteroids, and their involvement in the physiology and pathology of visual function.

Hormone Steroid Receptors

Evidence now suggests that ocular tissues express androgen, estrogen, and progesterone receptors that might be responsible for hormone actions in the structural and functional organization of the visual system, as well as in the altered visual function that occurs during the mestrual cycle, menopause, and pregnancy.[14–16,19] The epidemiological studies point also to a possible role of estrogens in age- and gender-associated variations in ocular disease. A greater prevalence of these diseases is described in elderly and in postmenopausal women in particular, and estrogen replacement therapy has been associated with a reduction in the incidence of glaucoma, age-related macular degeneration (AMD), and cataract.[14,15,20] The precise biological mechanisms of hormone receptor activities still remain to be elucidated. Two subtypes of estrogen receptors, ERα and ERβ, have been recently identified in ocular tissues and their expression correlated with sex, age, and tissue specificity. ERα is seen in the retina and RPE of young human female eyes, but not in the eye of men and postmenopausal women.[14] In the retina, ERα is present in the outer and inner nuclear layers, in the outer plexiform layer, and in some nuclei of the ganglion cell layer. ERα is also expressed in ciliary body, iris and epithelium of the lens. In contrast, ERβ is primarily located at the ganglion cell layer and choroid of human eyes of both sexes and at all ages.[16] The functional consequence of the different ER distribution is presently unknown. The distribution of ERα matches that of estrogen-responsive genes involved in cell proliferation, differentiation, physiology, and development—e.g., progesterone receptors, cathepsin D, α2-macroglobulin, cytochrome P450aromatase, c-fos, c-myc, heat-shock protein 27, TNF-α, pS2, and different neurotrophic factors—thus being exposed to a possible estrogen influence in the architectural and functional organization of the eye.[14] A recent observation of Salyer *et al.* reveals that estradiol formed by the aromatization of testosterone in the RPE where ERα are located may really play a role in the development of retinal thickness and likely influence sexually dimorphic changes in visual processing occurring in rodents and humans.[21] Changes in the expression of estrogen-responsive genes, such as the aspartic protease cathepsin D and apolipoprotein E (apoE), in patients affected by AMD have been suggested to account for the presumed estrogen influence in the outcome of the disease.[16] The understanding of the role of hormone receptors is still in its infancy, and certainly more research is needed for its definition in the retinal function and dysfunction. As will be discussed later, hormone receptor-mediated transcription of survival factors might presumably explain progesterone- or estrogen-induced neuroprotection against retinal excitotoxicity.

Glucocorticoid receptors are also an important component in the homeostasis of the eye; they are distributed in all cell types of ocular tissues, including all retinal cells and particularly in Müller glial cells.[22] Glucocorticoids (GR) have several effects in ocular tissues as well as in brain, and their administration is one of the most important ophthalmologic treatments.[23] In the retina, two prominent actions may have possible neuroprotective effects: first, GR-mediated induction of glutamine synthase, a key enzyme co-located with GR receptors in Müller glial cells, which may be involved in neuronal defensive mechanisms because it transforms glutamate into glutamine and blocks deleterious effects of excess glutamate;[24] second, the inhibition of AP-1 activity and resistance of photoreceptors to light damage through elevation in GR levels via metabolic stress or administration of dexamethasone.[25] However, excessive local GR concentrations, such as those that occur after GR treatment, may provoke deleterious effects in some disorders. Chronic topical or systemic administration of dexamethasone and other synthetic GR are frequently a cause of elevation in intraocular pressure referred as to "steroid glaucoma."[23] Elevation in intraocular pressure is also associated with the excessive production of endogenous GR in patients affected of Cushing's syndrome; central serous chorioretinopathy leading to retinal detachment develops in conditions such as pregnancy, stress, and type A personality characterized by endogenous hypercortisolism.[23] Although mechanisms underlying GR-mediated detrimental effects are still unclear, these observations provide important information on the probable role of GR as an inviting or precipitating factor for the development of some ocular disorders.

Neurosteroid Synthesis in the Retina

Consistent with the definition of a steroidogenic tissue, the retina is capable of transforming cholesterol into pregnenolone; then in progestens, corticosteroids and sex steroids, the retina is an authentic steroidogenic structure of the CNS in which steroid synthesis is integrated in its circuits for a conceivable role in the visual function. Most cholesterol is synthesized in neural retina and transported to membranes of rod outer segments of photoreceptors where it is required for continuous renewal during life.[2] The renewal process also involves RPE where cholesterol is additionally provided from an extracellular source through LDL receptors and the apolipoprotein E (ApoE) synthesized locally.[27] ApoE is also formed in retinal Müller glial cells and/or internalized by ganglion cells from which it can be rapidly transported into the optic nerve and brain.[27] Recently, high cholesterol in RPE, changes in ApoE expression by Müller glia of the human retina, and the apolipoprotein polymorphism have been suggested to increase the risk of AMD, the impairment of visual function during aging, and the progression of glaucoma.[27–29] It is intriguing that similar changes in cholesterol homeostasis and ApoE are known to be crucial in the onset and progression of some neurodegenerative and mental diseases; yet estrogens influence the outcome of brain as well as eye disorders.

Cholesterol is also used for retinal steroidogenesis in the adult rat. The transformation of cholesterol into pregnenolone appears to occur at ganglion cells and in some cells in the inner nuclear layer, the amacrine cells, where the cytochrome P450 cholesterol side-chain cleavage (P450scc) is located.[30] In brain and peripheral nerves, the cytochrome P450scc is mainly expressed in glial cells;[31] the only exception is that of cerebellar Purkinje cells and hippocampal neurons which, like the retina, provide a neuronal-type pregnenolone synthesis.[32] This raises the possibility that diverse regulatory mechanisms could exist to control the enzyme expression and activity at different locations. As a matter of fact, retinal pregnenolone synthesis is stimulated by $GABA_A$ receptors that are also localized at amacrine and ganglion cells where they exert a control in the output of visual stimuli to brain regions.[33] Adaptation to darkness by rats enhances $GABA_A$ receptor-mediated stimulation of retinal steroidogenesis, suggesting a high requirement of neurosteroids in the dark.[34] Consistently, levels of deoxycorticosterone and tetrahydrodeoxycorticosterone

(THDOC), which are known to act as positive allosteric modulator of $GABA_A$ receptors, increase in dark-adapted retinas; also, the diurnal variations of retinal neurosteroid levels endorse their functional role.[34] How neurosteroids contribute to retinal physiology is unknown. Feedback inhibition from amacrine cells provided by GABAergic transmission contributes to light-induced transient responses; blocking this feedback prolongs the responses of transient ganglion cells which convey information about motion and edge detection. The interplay between $GABA_A$ receptors and neurosteroid synthesis and action could provide an additional loop for the modulation of these responses. It is also unclear how $GABA_A$ receptors may activate the transformation of cholesterol into pregnenolone. Hyperpolarization by $GABA_A$ receptor-activated Cl^- conductance could induce environmental changes affecting steroidogenic activity, i.e., changes in intracellular pH. Similarly, in testicular Leydig and ovarian granulosa cells, Cl^- channels influence steroidogenesis. Recently, reduction in 3β-hydroxysteroid dehydrogenase (3β-HSD) and 17α-hydroxylase ($P450_{C17}$) enzyme activities by $GABA_A$ receptors has been reported in hypothalamic neurons of frog.[35] These results are certainly intriguing in that they emphasize the existence of a quick regulation of neurosteroid availability for a rapid response to neuronal demands. They suggest the possibility that modulation of $GABA_A$ receptors could accumulate pregnenolone, its sulfate ester, 7α-pregnenolone, and other unknown metabolites upon upregulation of P450scc or downregulation of 3β-HSD and $P450_{C17}$ activities. As will be pointed out in the next section, retinal $GABA_A$ receptor activation also stimulates the formation of pregnenolone sulfate (PS), which has several biological properties, including those at $GABA_A$ receptors as a negative modulator and those at NMDA receptors through which it may work as an excitotoxin. Therefore, on a specific cell requirement, the *ex novo* formation of neurosteroids could be part of regulatory loop(s) of inhibitory or excitatory transmission.

In the retina, as well as in brain and peripheral steroidogenic tissues, pregnenolone synthesis is also modulated by cAMP and peripheral-type benzodiazepine receptors, both promoting cholesterol transport to mitochondria where the synthesis occurs.[30,33,34] Several types of amacrine and ganglion cells have been identified in the retina; therefore, it is possible that diverse retinal cells expressing cytochrome P450scc enzyme may account for different regulatory mechanisms. However, it cannot be excluded that a synergism among these regulatory elements takes place in order to exert a strict control of the neurosteroid availability at different steps of its synthesis.

Steroids such as 17α-hydroxypregnenolone, 17α-hydroxyprogesterone, dehydroepiandrosterone (DHEA), dehydroepiandrosterone sulfate (DHEAS), progesterone, 5α-dihydroprogesterone, 3α-hydroxy-5α-dihydroprogesterone, deoxycorticosterone, THDOC, 5α-androstenedione, androsterone, testosterone, 5α-dihydrotestosterone, androstenediol, estrone, and estradiol have been detected in the retina of mammals, including humans.[30,34] Data on the identification of steroidogenic enzymes and/or the transformation of steroid precursors now indicate their local synthesis. $P450_{C17}$ and steroid sulfatase enzymes are found in the inner nuclear layer, probably in amacrine cells, of embryonic mouse retina.[32] Recently, the 3β-HSD enzyme has been noticed at a subset of ganglion and amacrine cells in the retina of zebrafish[36] and the aromatase enzyme in RPE of embryonic rat and in the retina of teleost fish.[21,37] Whereas the presence of enzymes such as 5α-reductase and 3α-hydroxysteroid dehydrogenase in the adult retina has been indirectly proved by the conversion of progesterone, androstenedione, and testosterone in 5α-reduced and 3α-hydroxy dehydrogenated compounds.[34] Preliminary data obtained from our laboratory reveal that expression and activity of P450c17, 3β-HSD, and aromatase (other than those of P450scc) are maintained in the retina of adult rats; P450c17 and 3β-HSD are almost exclusively located at the outer and inner nuclear layers, while P450scc at the ganglion cell layer and in some amacrine cells in the inner nuclear layer.

Retinal Steroids: the Impact —Pro and Con—on Excitotoxic-Mediated Neuronal Demise

Excitotoxicity is regarded as crucial to the pathogenesis of ischemic conditions linked to retinal artery occlusion, diabetes mellitus, glaucoma, and optic neuropathy, and to the progression of retinal damage in some forms of inherited disorders such as retinitis pigmentosa characterized by a massive glutamate release.[2,3]

It is widely accepted that in excitotoxicity NMDA receptor-induced Ca^{2+} overload accounts for a series of deleterious events; some of these events are now thought to be adaptive cellular responses with the precise intent to reduce the spreading of damage.[1,3–6] Our research has recently suggested that in retinal excitotoxicity, neurosteroid synthesis may result in a critical event in that it might address life-or-death decisions in retinal cells.

Pregnenolone Sulfate as a Neurotoxin in Retinal Excitotoxicity

Pregnenolone sulfate (PS), the sulfate ester of pregnenolone, is one of the most abundant neurosteroids in brain and in retina that has the potential to exert widespread control of CNS functions. PS inhibits $GABA_A$, glycine, and AMPA/kainate receptors and voltage-gated Ca^{2+} currents via a G-protein mechanism, and reduces GABA, dopamine, and acetylcholine release;[38–41] but, it also stimulates glutamate release and NMDA receptor-gated channel currents and the subsequent increase in intracellular Ca^{2+}.[39,42] The findings gathered thus far reveal that endogenously its concentration rates, ranging from nanomolar to micromolar concentrations, may vary in specific circumstances, e.g., sex recognition, circadian variations, and dark adaptation, or in conditions of altered CNS functions such as stress and aggressiveness, and more recently in excitotoxic insult;[31,34,43] exogenously, neurosteroid concentrations in the micromolar range provide a predominant action at NMDA receptors.[39,44] Recently, it has been observed that NMDA receptor subunit composition, which differs among CNS structures and during development or seizure activity or still in ischemia, may determine the nature of PS interaction as the neurosteroid enhances or inhibits responses mediated by NR1/NR2A and NR1/NR2B receptors and by NR1/NR2C and NR1/NR2D receptors, respectively;[39] the rate of PS-induced prolongation of deactivation of NMDA responses is larger in the presence of NR1a/NR2A than of NR1a/NR2B.[45] A peculiar $GABA_A$ receptor subunit composition appears also to favor the antagonism by PS[38]. Consequently, dose and site of action and the specific receptor subunit composition might shape a typical PS-mediated response. We have demonstrated that exposure of retinal explant to NMDA induces PS synthesis before retinal cell death occurs.[43,46,47] In contrast, blockade of PS synthesis results in a delay of retinal excitotoxicity, thus suggesting production of PS as an important process in a positive circuit for autocrine and/or paracrine induction, amplification, and propagation of death signal.[43] Studies clearly show that PS may act as a neurotoxic agent with agonist actions at NMDA receptors in retinal neurons. Consistently, NR2A and NR2B subunits which, as mentioned above, favor a positive PS action at the receptors, are indicated as responsible for signaling events leading to retinal cell death.[48] When the retinal explant is challenged with PS or NMDA or both, the intensity of exposure establishes the neuronal demise in a necrotic or apoptotic fashion. A continuous application of PS potentiates NMDA-induced cell death and causes toxicity in itself by a nonspecific breakdown of cellular homeostasis and subsequent necrotic/lytic cell death.[44] A brief pulse of 10–50 μM PS and 50 μM NMDA triggers delayed retinal cell death in a slowly evolving apoptotic fashion characterized by a cycloheximide-sensitive program downstream of ROS generation and lipid peroxidation.[48] Apoptogenic factors are involved in the pre- and post-commitment phases of apoptotic death, so that a caspase-3-dependent pathway is activated in response to cytochrome c and requires caspase-2 activation and a late cytochrome c release in specific cellular subsets of retinal layers.[47] Of critical importance with regard to the effective toxic doses of PS, low concentrations of PS (0.1–10 μM), which themselves do not affect retinal survival, are capable of exacerbating a mild retinal cell damage evoked by a low NMDA dose (10 μM).[43,46]

The role of PS as an excitotoxin is not confined to the retina but extends to cortical and hippocampal neurons where an increase in PS synthesis and consequent cell death have also been recently found to follow NMDA receptor stimulation.[49,50] In the retinal explant, where the structural and functional integrity of a heterogeneous cell population is maintained, an NMDA receptor-mediated increase in the neurosteroid synthesis occurs throughout activation of $GABA_A$ receptors.[43] This observation, together with evidence that shows potentiation in excitotoxic-mediated retinal cell death by blocking $GABA_A$ receptors, indicates an intricate transmembrane mechanism in which stimulation rather than inhibition of $GABA_A$ receptor activity, as well as a predominant PS formation and action at NMDA receptors, play a role in retinal excitotoxicity. Interestingly, activation of $GABA_A$ receptors by treatment with the endogenous neurosteroid (3α,5α)-3-hydroxypregnan-20-one causes hippocampal death.[51]

Neuroprotective Neurosteroids in Retinal Excitotoxicity

During the last decade, a significant amount of evidence has been accumulated with respect to the neuroprotective actions played by steroids such as DHEA, DHEAS, progesterone, testosterone, and estradiol.[8,10–13] It has been shown that steroids may prevent neuronal cell death triggered by different stimuli including excitotoxicity, and changes in steroidal environment may influence the neuronal fate in various neurological and mental disorders. Decreased levels of DHEA during aging make neurons more vulnerable to damage.[8] Progesterone and estrogen influence the outcome of ischemic and traumatic injury in female and male brain, and in different ways they promote reduction in the consequences of the injury cascade.[10,12,13] Testosterone as a survival factor for axotomized motor neurons promotes regeneration;[10] estrogens prevent or delay the onset of Alzheimer's disease and cognitive deficit.[10,12] Also, in the peripheral nervous system, local progesterone synthesis promotes myelin formation during regenerating processes of injured peripheral nerves.[8] Similar knowledge is now emerging in some forms of primary or secondary retinal degeneration. As mentioned above, estrogen is thought to have a role in age- and gender-associated ocular diseases and to prevent retinal ischemia reperfusion injury.[14–17,20] Our recent data also provide evidence for the capability of DHEA, DHEAS, progesterone, 17β-estradiol, and 3α5βS to protect against retinal excitotoxicity.[46,47] Cell death in retinas exposed to NMDA or PS used at toxic concentrations is reduced by progesterone and DHEA/DHEAS, and is completely blocked by 3α5βS and 17β-estradiol. The mechanisms underlying neuroprotection still remain to be defined. All these steroids possess antioxidant properties; differences, however, in their efficacy seem to indicate the possible existence of different mechanisms. With the exception of the neurosteroid 3α5BS, which acts as an NMDA receptor antagonist,[39] these steroids collectively are known to attenuate neuronal damage by reducing glutamate receptor activity, lessening immune inflammation, providing neurotrophic factors, enhancing synaptogenesis and dendritic arborization, through both genomic and nongenomic actions.[9–13] The antiglucocorticoid actions, as well as conversion into estrogens and androgens of DHEA/DHEAS, are also possible alternative devises for neuroprotection.[52] Of interest, complete protection against retinal cell death is promoted by 17β-estradiol but not by caspase inhibitors. Whether both estrogen receptor-mediated or receptor-independent mechanisms may be involved in retinal neuroprotection is still an open question.

As mentioned previously, DHEA/DHEAS, progesterone, testosterone, and estradiol may be synthesized by the retina; thus, fluctuations in their concentrations might affect retinal survival. Interestingly, retinal cells appear vulnerable to the excitotoxic insult in different ways, and preliminary data from our laboratory show a diverse distribution of 3β-HSD, $P450_{C17}$, and P450aromatase involved in the synthesis of neuroprotective neurosteroids and of P450scc, which synthesizes PS, acting as a neurodegenerative agent. On the other hand, in the retinal explant exposed to NMDA, the inhibition of pregnenolone and PS formation by aminoglutethimide reduces cell death in the ganglion cell layer, but not in the outer and inner nuclear layers where neuroprotective steroids are likely produced.[43]

CONCLUDING REMARKS

It is now widely held that variations in circulating steroid levels may alter cell vulnerability to adverse insults, thereby having a profound impact on the onset and/or delay of degenerating processes that characterize neurodegenerative diseases and, more recently, some ocular disorders. New evidence is indeed emerging on the possibility that among the cellular events following an insult, local changes in steroidogenic enzyme expression and activity contribute to form native steroid products (neurosteroids) that may act as harmful or healthful agents, thus increasing the likelihood of neuronal death or decreasing the spread of damaging signals. For instance, high P450scc mRNA expression is reported in the hippocampus of patients with temporal lobe epilepsy;[53] an increased aromatase expression in brain injured by kainic acid likely results in a cellular defensive response because of its involvement in producing neuroprotective estrogens and androgens.[10] This review specifically points out changes in retinal steroidogenic responses during excitotoxicity. Findings

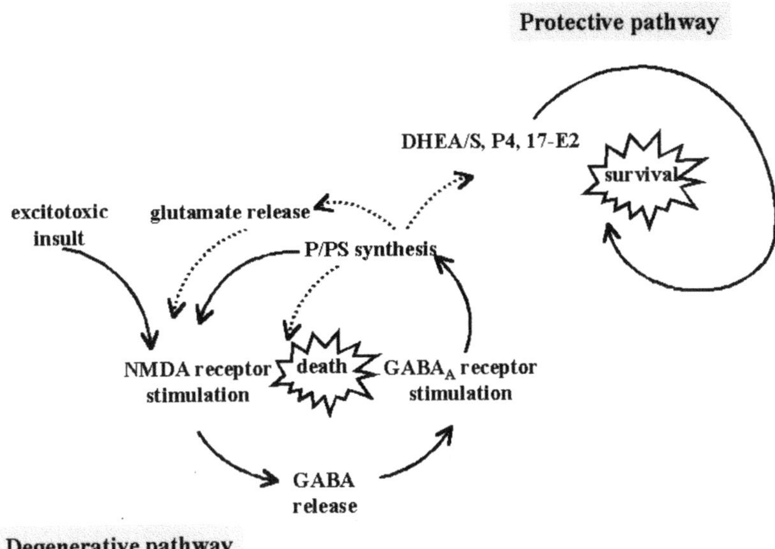

FIGURE 1. Schematic diagram depicting a neurodegenerative circuit in which NMDA-mediated pregnenolone (P) and pregnenolone sulfate (PS) formation concurs to the induction and amplification of retinal neurodegeneration, and a possible neuroprotective circuit in which formation of dehydroepiandrosterone (DHEA), dehydroepiandrosterone sulfate (DHEAS), progesterone (P4), and 17β-estradiol (17β-E2) might cooperate in the survival of specific retinal cell populations.

clearly show that, in the retinal excitotoxic paradigm, *de novo* formation of PS occurs as a result of NMDA-mediated activation of GABA$_A$ receptors and that it is a crucial event in a neurodegenerative circuit in which principal actions of PS as an agonist of NMDA receptors, and likely as a promoter of glutamate release,[42] are instrumental in the induction, amplification, and propagation of retinal neuronal death (FIG. 1). Given the capability of specific retinal cell populations to synthesize DHEA/DHEAS, progesterone, and estradiol, and the pivotal role of these neurosteroids as neuroprotective agents, a potential neuroprotective circuit might be also compatible with a reduction in cell vulnerability to toxic assault and consequential increase in the survival of peculiar retinal cells (FIG. 1). Therefore, during a toxic insult, retinal neurosteroidogenesis could result in a cellular offensive response by potentiating excitotoxic-mediated cell death; in a cellular defensive response by preventing damaging processes. This assumption certainly brings new elements to the understanding of neurodegenerative events. The definition of the interplay between neurosteroid expression and function and neurodegeneration could reveal ways to discern the diverse susceptibility of neurons capable of injury.

REFERENCES

1. JELLINGER, K.A. 2001. Cell death mechanisms in neurodegeneration. J. Cell. Mol. Med. **5:** 1–17.
2. LEVIN, L.A. & L.K. GORDON. 2002. Retinal ganglion cell disorders: types and treatments. Prog. Retinal Eye Res. **21:** 465–484.
3. YOLES, E. & M. SCHWARTZ. 1998. Elevation of intraocular glutamate levels in rats with partial lesion of the optic nerve. Arch. Ophthalmol. **116:** 906–910.
4. SAPOLSKY, R. 2001. Cellular defenses against excitotoxic insults. J. Neurochem. **76:** 1601–1611.
5. KIPNIS, J., E. YOLES, H. SCHORI, *et al.* 2001. Neuronal survival after CNS insult is determined by a genetically encoded autoimmune response. J. Neurosci. **21:** 4564–4571.
6. CLARKE, G., R.A. COLLINS, B.R. LEAVITT, *et al.* 2000. A one-hit model of cell death in inherited neuronal degenerations. Nature **406:** 195–199.
7. SAPOLSKY, R.M., L.M. ROMERO & A.U. MUNCK. 2000. How do glucocorticoids influence the stress-response? Integrating permissive, suppressive, stimulatory and preparative actions. Endocr. Rev. **21:** 55–78.
8. SCHUMACHER, M., Y. AKWA, R. GUENNOUN, *et al.* 2000. Steroid synthesis and metabolism in the nervous system: trophic and protective effects. J. Neurocytol. **29:** 307–326.
9. GUBBA, E.M., C.M. NETHERTON & J. HERBERT. 2000. Endangerment of the brain by glucocorticoids : Experimental and clinical evidence. J. Neurocytol. **29:** 439–449
10. GARCIA-SEGURA, L.M., I. AZCOITIA & L.L. DONCARLOS. 2001. Neuroprotection by estradiol. Prog. Neurobiol. **63:** 29–60.
11. MCEWEN, B.S. 2002. Sex, stress and the hippocampus: allostasis, allostatic load and the aging process. Neurobiol. Aging **23:** 921–939.
12. WISE, P.M., D.B. DUBAL, M.E. WILSON, *et al.* 2001. Minireview: neuroprotective effects of estrogen-new insights into mechanisms of action. Endocrinology **142:** 963–973.
13. STEIN, D.G. 2001. Brain damage, sex hormones and recovery: a new role for progesterone and estrogen? Trends Neurosci. **24:** 386–391.
14. OGUETA, S.B., S.D. SCHWARTZ, C.K. YAMASHITA, *et al.* 1999. Estrogen receptor in the human eye: influence of gender and age on gene expression. Invest. Ophthalmol. Visual Sci. **40:** 1906–1911.
15. WICKHAM, L.A., J. GAO, I. TODA, *et al.* 2000. Identification of androgen, estrogen and progesterone receptor mRNAs in the eye. Acta Ophthalmol. Scand. **78:** 146–153.
16. MUNAUT, C., V. LAMBERT, A. NOEL, *et al.* 2001. Presence of oestrogen receptor type β in human retina. Br. J. Ophthalmol. **85:** 877–882.
17. NONAKA, A., J. KIRYU, A. TSUJIKAWAM *et al.* 2000. Administration of 17beta-estradiol attenuates retinal ischemia-reperfusion injury in rats. Invest. Ophthalmol. Visual Sci. **41:** 2689–2696.
18. O'STEEN, W.K. & K.V. ANDERSON. 1974. Photoreceptor degeneration in albino rats: dependency on age. Invest. Ophthalmol. **13:** 334–339.
19. KOBAYASHI, K., H. KOBAYASHI, M. UEDA, *et al.* 1998. Estrogen receptor expression in bovine and rat retinas. Invest. Ophthalmol. Visual Sci. **39:** 2105–2110.
20. SATOR, M.O., E.A. JOURA, P. FRIGO, *et al.* 1997. Hormone replacement therapy and intraocular pressure. Mauritas **28:** 55–58.
21. SALYER, D.L., T.D. LUND, D.E. FLEMING, *et al.* 2001. Sexual dimorphism and aromatase in the rat retina. Dev. Brain Res. **126:** 131–136.
22. GOROVITS, R., I. BEN-DROR, L.E. FOX, *et al.* 1994. Developmental changes in the expression and compartmentalization of the glucocorticoid receptors in the embryonic retina. Proc. Natl. Acad. Sci. USA **91:** 4786–4790.
23. CARTIER, A., J.L. MALO, D. GAUTRIN, *et al.* 1997. Glucocorticoid use and risks of ocular hypertension and glaucoma. JAMA **277:** 19929–1930.
24. GOROVITS, R., A. YAKIR, L.E. FOX, *et al.* 1996. Hormonal and non-hormonal regulation of glutamine synthetase in the developing neural retina. Mol. Brain Res. **43:** 321–329.

25. WENZEL, A., C. GRIMM, M.W. SEELIGER, *et al.* 2001. Prevention of photoreceptor apoptosis by activation of the glucocorticoid receptor. Invest. Ophthalmol. Visual Sci. **42**: 1653–1659.
26. FLIESLER, S.J., R. FLORMAN & R.K. KELLER 1995. Isoprenoid lipid metabolism in the retina: dynamics of squalene and cholesterol incorporation and turnover in frog rod outer segment membranes. Exp. Eye Res. **60:** 57–69.
27. ONG, J.M., N.C. ZORAPAPEL, K.A. RICH, *et al.* 2001. Effects of cholesterol and apolipoprotein E on retinal abnormalities in ApoE-deficient mice. Invest. Ophthalmol. Visual Sci. **42:** 1891–1900.
28. SEN, K., A. MISRA, A. KUMAR, *et al.* 2002. Simvastatin retards progression of retinopathy in diabetic patients with hypercholesterolemia. Diabetes Res. Clin. Pract. **56:** 1–11.
29. ANDERSON, D.H., S. OZAKI, M. NEALON, *et al.* 2001. Local cellular sources of apolipoprotein E in the human retina and retinal pigmented epithelium: implications for the process of drusen formation. Am. J. Ophthalmol. **131:** 767–781.
30. GUARNERI, P., R. GUARNERI, C. CASCIO, *et al.* 1994. Neurosteroidogenesis in rat retina. J. Neurochem. **63:** 86–96.
31. BAULIEU, E.E. 1997. Neurosteroids: of the nervous system, by the nervous system, for the nervous system. Recent Prog. Horm. Res. **52:** 1–32.
32. COMPAGNONE, N. A. & S. H. MELLON. 2000. Neurosteroids: biosynthesis and function of these novel neuromodulators. Front. Neuroendocrinol. **21:** 1–56.
33. GUARNERI, P., R. GUARNERI, C. CASCIO, *et al.* 1995. γ-Aminobutyric acid type A/benzodiazepine receptors regulate rat retina neurosteroidogenesis. Brain Res. **683:** 65–72.
34. GUARNERI, P. 1996. Neurosteroids in retina: synthesis and neuronal function. *In* . The Brain: Source and Target for Sex Steroid Hormones. A.R. Genazzani, F. Petraglia & R.H. Purdy, Eds.: 63–81. The Parthenon Publishing Group. New York.
35. DO-REGO, J.L., G.A. MENSAH-NYAGAN, D. BEAUJEAN, *et al.* 2000. γ-Aminobutyric acid, acting through γ-aminobutyric acid type A receptors, inhibits the biosynthesis of neurosteroids in the frog hypothalamus. Proc. Natl. Acad. Sci. USA **97:** 13925–13930.
36. SAKAMOTO, H., K. UKENA & K. TSUTSUI. 2001. Activity and localization of 3β-hydroxysteroid dehydrogenase/δ^5-δ^4-isomerase in the zebrafish central nervous system. J. Comp. Neurol. **439:** 291–305.
37. CALLARD, G.V., M. DRYGAS & D. GELINAS. 1993. Molecular and cellular physiology of aromatase in the brain and retina. J. Steroid Biochem. Mol. Biol. **44:** 541–547.
38. ZHU, W.J., J.F. WANG, K.E. KRUEGER, *et al.* 1996. Delta subunit inhibits neurosteroid modulation of GABAA receptors. J. Neurosci. **16:** 6648–6656.
39. MALAYEV, A., T.T. GIBBS & D.H. FARB. 2002. Inhibition of the NMDA response by pregnenolone sulphate reveals subtype selective modulation of NMDA receptors by sulphated steroids. Br. J. Pharmacol. **135:** 901–909.
40. BARROT, M., M. VALLEE, M.A. GINGRAS, *et al.* 1999. The neurosteroid pregnenolone sulphate increases dopamine release and the dopaminergic response to morphine in the rat nucleus accumbens. Eur. J. Neurosci. **11:** 3757– 3760.
41. DARNAUDERY, M., M. KOEHL, P.V. PIAZZA, *et al.* 2000. Pregnenolone sulfate increases hippocampal acetylcholine release and spatial recognition. Brain Res. **852:** 1733–179.
42. MEYER, D.A., M. CARTA, L.D. PARTRIDGE, *et al.* 2002. Neurosteroids enhance spontaneous glutamate release in hippocampal neurons. Possible role of metabotropic sigma like receptors. J. Biol Chem. **277:** 28725–28732.
43. GUARNERI, P., D. RUSSO, C. CASCIO, *et al.* 1998. Induction of neurosteroid synthesis by NMDA receptors in isolated rat retina: a potential early event in excitotoxicity. Eur. J. Neurosci. **10:** 1752–1763.
44. GUARNERI, P., D. RUSSO, C. CASCIO, *et al.* 1998. Pregnenolone sulfate modulates NMDA receptors, inducing and potentiating acute excitotoxicity in isolated retina. J. Neurosci. Res. **54:** 787–797.
45. CECCON, M., G. RUMBAUGH & S. VICINI. 2001. Distinct effect of pregnenolone sulfate on NMDA receptor subtypes. Neuropharmacology **40:** 491–500.

46. Cascio, C., R. Guarneri, D. Russo, *et al.* 2000. Pregnenolone sulfate, a naturally-occurring excitotoxin involved in delayed retinal cell death. J. Neurochem. **74:** 2380–2391.
47. Cascio, C., R. Guarneri, D. Russo, *et al.* 2002. A caspase-3-dependent pathway is predominantly activated by the excitotoxin pregnenolone sulphate and requires early and late cytochrome c release and cell-specific caspase-2 activation in the retinal cell death. J. Neurochem. **83:** 1358–1371.
48. Goebel, D.J. & M.S. Poosch. 2001. Transient down-regulation of NMDA receptor subunit gene expression in the rat retina following NMDA-induced neurotoxicity is attenuated in the presence of the non-competitive NMDA receptor antagonist MK-801. Exp. Eye Res. **72:** 547–558.
49. Shirakawa, H., H. Katsuki, T. Kume, *et al.* 2002. Regulation of *N*-methyl-D-aspartate cytotoxicity by neuroactive steroids in rat cortical neurons. Eur. J. Pharmacol. **454:** 165–175.
50. Kimoto, T., T. Tsurugizawa, Y. Ohta, *et al.* 2001. Neurosteroid synthesis by cytochrome P450-containing systems localized in the rat brain hippocampal neurons: *N*-methyl-D-aspartate and calcium-dependent synthesis. Endocrinology **142:** 3578–3589.
51. Xu, W., R. Cormier, T. Fu, *et al.* 2000. Slow death of postnatal hippocampal neurons by $GABA_A$ receptor overactivation. J. Neurosci. **20:** 3147–3156.
52. Kimonides, V.G., M.G. Spillantini, M.V. Sofroniew, *et al.* 1999. Dehydroepiandrosterone antagonizes the neurotoxic effects of corticosterone and stress-activated protein kinase 3 in hippocampal primary cultures. Neuroscience **89:** 429–436
53. Beyenburg, S., B. Stoffel-Wagner, M. Watzka, *et al.* 1999. Expression of cytochrome P450scc mRNA in the hippocampus of patients with temporal lobe epilepsy. Neuroreport **10:** 3067–3070.

In Vitro Paradigms for the Study of GnRH Neuron Function and Estrogen Effects

VALÉRIE MATAGNE, MARIE-CHRISTINE LEBRETHON, ARLETTE GÉRARD, AND JEAN-PIERRE BOURGUIGNON

Developmental Neuroendocrinology Unit, Research Center of Cellular and Molecular Neurosciences (CNCM), University of Liège, CHU, Sart-Tilman, B-4000 Liège, Belgium

ABSTRACT: The elaboration of *in vitro* paradigms has enabled direct study of GnRH secretion and the regulation of this process. Common findings using different models are the pulsatile nature and calcium-dependency of GnRH secretion, the excitatory effect of glutamate, and the inhibitory or excitatory effect of GABA. Among the different paradigms, the fetal olfactory placode cultures exhibit the unique property of migration *in vitro* and may retain the capacity to undergo maturational changes *in vitro*. The short-term incubation of hypothalamic explants obtained at different ages enables one to study developmental changes as well. Estrogens may have important roles in the regulation of GnRH function and can act indirectly via the neighboring neuronal/glial apparatus and directly on GnRH neurons at the cell body and terminal levels. A direct effect is supported by the recent localization of ERα and ERβ transcripts in GnRH neurons using most paradigms. Discrepant effects of estrogens on GnRH neurons were observed since GnRH biosynthesis is inhibited while GnRH secretion can be either stimulated, unaffected, or reduced. It is likely that the regulatory role of sex steroids including estradiol is very complex since it could involve direct and indirect effects on GnRH neurons through genomic and/or non-genomic mechanisms.

KEYWORDS: GnRH secretion; estradiol

INTRODUCTION

The hypothalamus is involved in basic survival functions including regulation of food intake and reproduction through the secretion of gonadotropin-releasing hormone (GnRH), which is also named LHRH (LH-releasing hormone). GnRH is typically secreted in a pulsatile manner by a specific population of hypothalamic neurons. Immunocytochemical studies indicated that the GnRH neurons were widely scattered in the hypothalamus,[1] thus hindering the study of the mechanisms involved in direct regulation of the GnRH neuron function. In the anterior pituitary gland, GnRH stimulates the synthesis and secretion of the gonadotropins, LH and

Address for correspondence: Jean-Pierre Bourguignon, M.D., Ph.D., Division of Pediatric and Adolescent Medicine, CHU Sart-Tilman, B-4000 Liège, Belgium. Voice: 00 32 4 366 7247; fax: 00 32 4 366 7246.
jpbourguignon@ulg.ac.be

**Ann. N.Y. Acad. Sci. 1007: 129–142 (2003). © 2003 New York Academy of Sciences.
doi: 10.1196/annals.1286.013**

FSH, which will in turn stimulate the secretion of sex steroids by the gonads. The GnRH neuronal system is modulated by afferences from the neighboring hypothalamic areas as well as by hormones secreted by the gonads, including estradiol. This steroid accounts for a negative feedback (inhibitory) control of GnRH and the gonadotropins in both sexes at different developmental stages. In the mature female, a so-called positive feedback is also exerted by estradiol and leads to the preovulatory GnRH and gonadotropin surge.[2,3]

In general, estrogen action on the GnRH neurons was thought to be indirectly mediated since the estrogen receptors could not be co-localized with GnRH transcripts or peptide in neither the rat,[4] the ewe,[5] nor the monkey.[6] However, after the discovery of a new subtype of estrogen receptor (ER) named ERβ[7] and with the improvement of detection methods, rat GnRH neurons were reported to contain the classical receptor (ERα) immunoreactivity,[8] whereas others found that rat GnRH neurons expressed ERβ mRNA and were immunoreactive for ERβ[9–12] (for review see Herbison *et al.*[13]). In addition to the *in vivo* paradigms, various *in vitro* models allowing the study of GnRH neurons and/or their secretion were established from the early 1980s. Here, we aim at reviewing these different models and their response to estradiol.

IN VITRO MODELS AND CHARACTERISTICS

TABLE 1 summarizes the different *in vitro* paradigms used to study GnRH neurons and their characteristics. Mouse GnRH cell lines immortalized through coupling of the GnRH promoter with the SV40 oncogene were available since the early 1990s.[14,15] Among these "tumorized" cell lines, the GT-1 cells have been the most widely studied. The advantage of this model is the involvement of a single cell line which could be used in different research laboratories, to which the cells were made available by Drs. P. Mellon and R. Weiner and their colleagues. Some limits come from the tumoral nature of the cells and their immature functional characteristics since neoplastic transformation occurred at an embryonic stage. In addition, there is some heterogeneity among different cultured batches, which is perhaps related to the number of passages.[16]

Primary cultures were obtained from the fetal olfactory placode from which the GnRH neurons migrate during intrauterine life.[17–19] Such cultures use the opportunity of the high density of GnRH neurons in the olfactory placode, while they will subsequently be widespread along their migratory pathway between the olfactory placode and the mediobasal hypothalamus. This model was successfully set up using monkey[20] and mouse[21] material initially, and rat[22] and sheep[23] material more recently. A unique feature of this paradigm is that the GnRH neurons retain *in vitro* their migratory capacity.[20–23] These neurons, however, are also obtained at an embryonic stage, resulting in immature functional characteristics possibly different from the postnatal phenotype. As opposed to the immortalized cell lines, these neurons may not be definitively arrested at an immature stage since their pattern of GnRH release/expression changes with the incubation period,[20] indicating a maturational process possibly related to that occurring *in vivo.*[24,25] Primary cultures were also prepared from the neonatal[26] and adult[27,28] rat hypothalamus or rat hypothalamic slices,[29] but these two paradigms were only scarcely used.

The short-term incubation of rat hypothalamic explants has been the first *in vitro* model used to study GnRH secretion.[30] The explants were prepared from the rat,[31–33] guinea pig,[31] monkey,[34] quail,[35] and human[36] hypothalamus and were used often as whole piece of tissue or sometimes cut into slices.[32,35] The advantages of the explant model involve the preserved structural and functional architecture of the neuronal/glial apparatus which regulates GnRH secretion. Moreover, this system enables one to study separately or together different parts of the GnRH neurons: the nerve endings and their glial cell environment in the median eminence, the afferent neurons in the arcuate nucleus/mediobasal hypothalamus which converge to the median eminence area or the GnRH cell bodies and, finally, the GnRH cell bodies and the neighboring network in the preoptic area/anterior hypothalamus.

Such a paradigm has been extensively used in our laboratory, based on a static incubation system with sampling and renewal of the incubation medium every 7.5 min,[33] while others used perifusion systems. Under our conditions, hypothalamic explants containing the preoptic area or the retrochiasmatic part of the rat hypothalamus, where GnRH cell bodies are absent, can secrete GnRH in a pulsatile manner, while the median eminence cannot.[37] This model is consistent with the existence of a GnRH pulse generator extrinsic to the GnRH neurons. The occurrence of GnRH secretory pulses *in vitro* is dependent on glucose and calcium.[38] GnRH secretion can be evoked nonspecifically by depolarization using veratridine[38,39] or specifically by glutamate and glutamate receptor agonists such as kainate, NMA, or quisqualate.[40] The sensitivity to these secretagogues changes with age and is maximal using NMA at 25 days.[41] Spontaneous pulsatile GnRH secretion changes as well throughout development in rats of both sexes, with an increase in pulse frequency between early postnatal life (one pulse/90 min at 5 days) to the age of 25 days (1 pulse/30 min), with no further change until adulthood in the male.[33,41,42] Using hypothalamic explants of adult female rats, the amplitude of GnRH secretory pulses is increased in the afternoon of proestrus.[43]

The developmental acceleration of GnRH pulse frequency, which occurs prior to the onset of puberty, was found to involve an increase in glutaminase activity, that is, the enzyme responsible for the glutamate biosynthesis from glutamine[44] as well as a reduction in prolylendopeptidase activity accounting for a decreased sensitivity to an inhibitory autofeedback mediated by $GnRH_{1-5}$ through an interaction at NMDA receptor.[45,46] The increase in GnRH pulse frequency also involved reduction in GABAergic inhibitory control together with the increase in glutamatergic stimulatory control.[47] This *in vitro* paradigm was also used to show the involvement of orexigenic (NPY) and anorexigenic (leptin and CART) peptides in the hypothalamic mechanism controlling pulsatile GnRH secretion before puberty[48] and in adult life in both sexes.[43]

A most recently developed system consists of hypothalamic slices from transgenic mice carrying reporter genes linked to the GnRH promoter and thus specifically expressed in GnRH neurons. The two major reporter genes linked to the GnRH promoter were sequences coding for the green fluorescent protein (GFP) obtained from the jellyfish *Acquorea victoria,*[49,50] or β-galactosidase (β-Gal) incorporated in the Lac-Z gene of *E. coli.*[51] Other less frequently used transgenes were luciferase and β-lactamase (for review see Spergel *et al.*[52]). Immunocytochemical studies showed expression of GFP[49] or enhanced GFP[50] in most of the GnRH immunoreactive neurons, whereas β-Gal was expressed not only by immunoreactive GnRH neu-

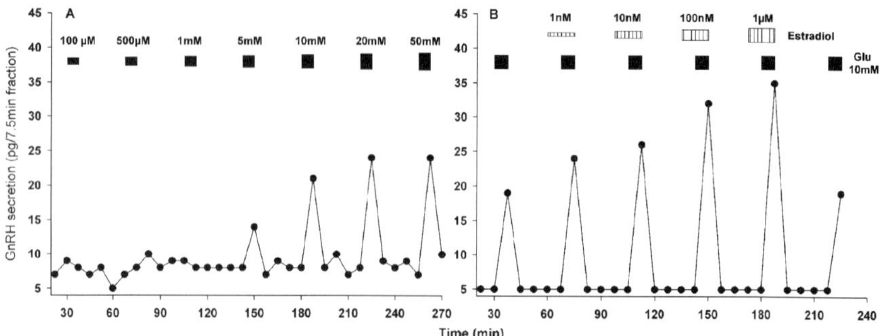

FIGURE 1. Representative profiles of GnRH secretion obtained using individual hypothalamic explants (from 50-day-old male rat) which were incubated with increasing concentrations of glutamate for 7.5 min at 37.5-min intervals (**A**) or with 10 mM glutamate and increasing concentrations of estradiol added for two 7.5-min fractions, before and together with glutamate (**B**). GnRH was measured by RIA and the limit of detection was 5 pg/fraction.

rons, but also by other cell populations expressing GnRH at an embryonic stage but not later in life.[53] This model provides a novel opportunity to identify and study directly the GnRH neurons *in situ*, in their original setting, particularly using electrophysiological techniques.[49–51,54–58] A transgenic rat model expressing enhanced GFP in GnRH neurons has been developed as well,[59] and the GnRH neurons identified in such conditions express different types of calcium channel, including the developmentally regulated P/Q- and L-type channels.

The GnRH secretion has been studied using the various paradigms and appeared to be evoked by various secretagogues, including KCl and glutamate receptor agonists in all conditions, including immortalized GnRH neurons,[60–63] primary cultures of hypothalamic neurons,[26] or olfactory placodes[20,24,64] and explant systems.[34,40,60,65,66] Some authors, however, found that the GT1-7 neurons expressed few or no glutamate receptor subtypes and did not respond to glutamate.[16] The dose–response effect of glutamate using the explant paradigm in our conditions is illustrated in FIGURE 1A. A spontaneous pulsatile pattern of GnRH secretion was observed using GnRH cell lines[60,67] and primary cultures of hypothalamic neurons[26,27,60] as well as using primary cultures of olfactory placodes from monkey,[20,68] sheep,[25] and rat,[22] or by using hypothalamic explants.[31,33,34,60] Thus, the capacity to release GnRH in a pulsatile manner appears to be an intrinsic property of the GnRH neurons. This, however, does not exclude the possibility of an extrinsic pulse generator, as suggested by the occurrence of pulsatile GnRH secretion using rat retrochiasmatic hypothalamic explants, where no GnRH cell bodies could be identified,[37] or by using median eminence explants from rat[69] and human fetal hypothalamus.[36] Quite logically, intermittent secretory activity should be coupled to calcium movements and/or variations in electrophysiological activity. The spontaneous firing pattern of the GT-1 cells are associated with waves in calcium influx.[70] The pulsatile secretion of GnRH by neurons cultured from the olfactory placode of the monkey are synchronized with calcium waves.[68] The studies in the primate also indicate that the synchronized calcium movements occur in non-neuronal cells distinct from the GnRH neurons,[71] in contrast to the explanted mouse olfactory placode, where the GnRH neurons seem to be the only neurons directly involved in intracellular calcium oscillations.[72] The frequency of GnRH secretory episodes is relatively similar using the different paradigms. GnRH pulse frequency may vary on account of possibly physiologically relevant factors such as species or age. The time since starting cell culture may result in change in GnRH pulse frequency caused by a maturational process, as suggested for the olfactory placode cultures,[20,24] but may also depend on loss of differentiation of hypothalamic neurons. Using the explant system, we showed that technical conditions, that is, the interval of medium sampling, was affecting frequency due to the inhibitory autofeedback effect of GnRH on its secretion.[73] The influence of the GABAergic pathway on the GnRH neurons has been widely studied and GnRH neurons were reported to be responsive to GABA in the different systems. The effect of GABA, however, may be inhibitory or stimulatory, the latter being particularly observed with fetal or immature GnRH neurons[24,64,74] (for review see Moguilevsky[75]). Using our static incubation system, we found that the changes in glutamatergic and GABAergic control of GnRH secretion played a crucial developmental role in the neuroendocrine mechanism of GnRH secretion.[47,76]

ESTROGEN AND GnRH NEURONS

As summarized in TABLE 1, direct effect on GnRH neurons through ER is possible since both α and β subtypes were found to be expressed in the different paradigms. Using GT-1 cells or cultures of hypothalamic slices, an inhibition of GnRH synthesis by estradiol is suggested by the reduced mRNA expression.[77–79] Equivocal data have been obtained regarding GnRH secretion, which can be either unaffected or stimulated.[28,34,80,81] The K^+-evoked secretion was found to be increased by estradiol, whereas the norepinephrine (NE)-evoked secretion was stimulated, depending on short or prolonged exposure to estradiol.[32,35] Early *in vivo* studies reported effects on GnRH secretion several hours or days after estradiol treatment.[82–84] These *genomic* or *long term effects of estrogens* provide the basic mechanism of the positive and negative feedback controls (for review see Herbison[85]). It is now agreed that estradiol can also act on the CNS in a rapid manner,[86,87] through activation of ER or an estrogen membrane binding site.[88] Only few studies reported a rapid action of estradiol on GnRH secretion evoked by KCl[32] or NE.[35] Using rat hypothalamic explants, we found that estradiol could rapidly increase the glutamate-evoked GnRH secretion (FIG. 1B). Using median eminence explants, Prevot *et al.* also observed that estradiol could increase the NO release within 2 minutes as well as the GnRH secretion within 10 minutes.[80] Taken together, these data indicate that estradiol can rapidly increase the secretion of GnRH through different mechanisms.

The generation of GFP-GnRH mice has facilitated studies about estradiol effect on GnRH neurons. Using these mice, estradiol was reported to alter electrophysiological properties of GnRH neuron through a phosphorylation process.[55] Estradiol also increased the interval between the firing pattern displayed by GnRH neurons.[57,58] These results were obtained after long-term treatment of the animals with estradiol and a direct action of estradiol on GnRH neurons is not proven so far. It

TABLE 1. Characteristics of different *in vitro* systems used to study the GnRH neurons/neurosecretion

Systems	Immortalized Cell Line Culture	Primary Cultures of Fetal Olfactory Placode	Primary Cultures of Hypothalamic Neurons	Cultures of Tumoral Cell Lines from Olfactory Placode	Short-term Incubation of Hypothalamic Explants or Slices	Hypothalamic Slices with Reporter Transgenes
Species	Mouse GT1[14] GN[15]	Mouse[31,89] Monkey[20] Sheep[23] Rat[22]	Rat[26,28]	Human[90] FNC-B4[81]	Rat[32,33] Guinea pig[31] Human[36] Quail[35]	Mouse • lac Z reporter[51] • GFP reporter[49,50] Rat • GFP reporter[59]
GnRH secretion	• KCl-evoked[60,91,92] • Pulsatile[60,62,67]	• KCl-evoked[20,24] • Pulsatile[22,25,68]	• KCl-evoked[26] • Pulsatile[26,,60]		• KCl-evoked[34,35,93,94] • Pulsatile[31,33,,60,69]	
Interpulse interval	20–35 min	30–50 min (depending on species and time *in vitro*[22,25,68])	20–80 min (depending on time *in vitro*[26,27,60])		20–90 min (depending on species) and age)	
Electro-physiology	Spontaneous firing pattern[98]	Spontaneous firing pattern[64]				Spontaneous firing pattern[50,54,56]
Calcium dependency	• GnRH secretion[60,96,97] • Firing[70] • Ca^{2+} influx waves[67,92]	• GnRH secretion[24,68] • Ca^{2+} influx waves[50,99]	• GnRH secretion[60]		• GnRH secretion[40,69]	• L-, N-, and R-type calcium channels[59] • P/Q- and T-type developmentally regulated
Amino acid neurotransmission	• Glutamate+[62,63,67,100] • GABA+/–[92,101] • GABA+[98]	• Glutamate-induced depolarization[64] • GABA+[24,64] • GABA–[102]			• Glutamate+[40,66,103,104] • GABA+/–[76]	• Glutamate+[49,56] • GABA–[49]

+, stimulating effect; –, inhibitory effect.

TABLE 1. Characteristics of different *in vitro* systems used to study the GnRH neurons/neurosecretion (*continued*)

Systems	Immortalized Cell Line Culture	Primary Cultures of Fetal Olfactory Placode	Primary Cultures of Hypothalamic Neurons	Cultures of Tumoral Cell Lines from Olfactory Placode	Short-term Incubation of Hypothalamic Explants or Slices	Hypothalamic Slices with Reporter Transgenes
Developmental changes		• Modulation of GnRH secretion • Maturational change in GnRH content[24]			• GnRH secretion[33,93] • Glutamate and GABA effects[75]	• GABA+/− effects
Migratory capacity		Yes (in all tested species)				
Signaling	• Protein kinase[105,106] • NO[100, 107–109]				NO[107,110]	
Estrogen receptor	• ERα mRNA[77,111] • ERβ mRNA[77]	• ERβ mRNA[11]		• ERβ mRNA, protein[81] • ERα mRNA, protein[81]	• ERα mRNA[8] • ERβ mRNA[9,10]	• ERβ mRNA[12,13]
Estrogen effects	• ↓GnRH mRNA[77,79]		• ↑GnRH secretion not affected	• GnRH basal secretion not affected[81] • ↑GnRH secretion when co-treated with progesterone[81]	• ↑basal GnRH secretion[80] • ↑K^+ or NE-evoked GnRH secretion[32,35]	Modulation of spontaneous firing patterns in GnRH neurons[55,57,58]

+, stimulating effect; −, inhibitory effect.

could be interesting to study whether GnRH neurons and GnRH secretion could be directly influenced by short-term estradiol treatment in this particular model.

CONCLUSION

Depending on the condition of preparation (age, species, genetic manipulation, dissociation from the neighboring neuronal/glial network), the *in vitro* paradigms using GnRH neurons account for specific advantages and also some limits in the direct study of GnRH neuron function. We have elected to use a model of static incubation of hypothalamic explants which is offering the possibility of studying developmental changes in pulsatile GnRH secretion and GnRH secretion evoked by glutamate receptor agonists. In addition, we can study the involvement of different parts of the GnRH neuron including or not the cell bodies in the preoptic area and the afferent neuronal/glial network in the mediobasal hypothalamus/median eminence. The effects of estradiol on GnRH neurons should be further studied with particular emphasis on localization, receptor involvement, intracellular signaling and developmental variations.

ACKNOWLEDGMENTS

This study was supported by the French Community of Belgium (ARC 99/04-241), FRSM (3.4515.01), the Faculty of Medicine at the University of Liege, and the Belgian Study Group for Pediatric Endocrinology.

REFERENCES

1. Silverman, A.J., L.C. Krey & E.A. Zimmerman. 1979. A comparative study of the luteinizing hormone releasing hormone (LHRH) neuronal networks in mammals. Biol. Reprod. **20:** 98–110.
2. Terasawa, E. 2001. Luteinizing hormone-releasing hormone (LHRH) neurons: mechanism of pulsatile LHRH release. Vitam. Horm. **63:** 91–129.
3. Levine, J.E. 1997. New concepts of the neuroendocrine regulation of gonadotropin surges in rats. Biol. Reprod. **56:** 293–302.
4. Shivers, B.D., R.E. Harlan, J.I. Morrell & D.W. Pfaff. 1983. Absence of oestradiol concentration in cell nuclei of LHRH-immunoreactive neurones. Nature **304:** 345–347.
5. Lehman, M.N. & F.J. Karsch. 1993. Do gonadotropin-releasing hormone, tyrosine hydroxylase-, and beta-endorphin-immunoreactive neurons contain estrogen receptors? A double-label immunocytochemical study in the Suffolk ewe. Endocrinology **133:** 887–895.
6. Herbison, A.E., T.L. Horvath, F. Naftolin & C. Leranth. 1995. Distribution of estrogen receptor-immunoreactive cells in monkey hypothalamus: relationship to neurones containing luteinizing hormone-releasing hormone and tyrosine hydroxylase. Neuroendocrinology **61:** 1–10.
7. Mosselman, S., J. Polman & R. Dijkema. 1996. ER beta: identification and characterization of a novel human estrogen receptor. FEBS Lett. **392:** 49–53.
8. Butler, J.A., M. Sjoberg & C.W. Coen. 1999. Evidence for oestrogen receptor alpha-immunoreactivity in gonadotrophin-releasing hormone-expressing neurones. J. Neuroendocrinol. **11:** 331–335.

9. HRABOVSZKY, E., P.J. SHUGHRUE, I. MERCHENTHALER, *et al.* 2000. Detection of estrogen receptor-beta messenger ribonucleic acid and 125I-estrogen binding sites in luteinizing hormone-releasing hormone neurons of the rat brain. Endocrinology **141:** 3506–3509.
10. HRABOVSZKY, E., A. STEINHAUSER, K. BARABAS, P., *et al.* 2001. Estrogen receptor-beta immunoreactivity in luteinizing hormone-releasing hormone neurons of the rat brain. Endocrinology **142:** 3261.
11. SHARIFI, N., A.E. REUSS & S. WRAY. 2002. Prenatal LHRH Neurons in nasal explant cultures express estrogen receptor beta transcript. Endocrinology **143:** 2503–2507.
12. SKYNNER, M.J., J.A. SIM & A.E. HERBISON. 1999. Detection of estrogen receptor alpha and beta messenger ribonucleic acids in adult gonadotropin-releasing hormone neurons. Endocrinology **140:** 5195–5201.
13. HERBISON, A.E. & J.R. PAPE. 2001. New evidence for estrogen receptors in gonadotropin-releasing hormone neurons. Front. Neuroendocrinol. **22:** 292–308.
14. MELLON, P.L., J.J. WINDLE, P.C. GOLDSMITH, *et al.* 1990. Immortalization of hypothalamic GnRH neurons by genetically targeted tumorigenesis. Neuron **5:** 1–10.
15. RADOVICK, S., S. WRAY, E. LEE, *et al.* 1991. Migratory arrest of gonadotropin-releasing hormone neurons in transgenic mice. Proc. Natl. Acad. Sci. USA **88:** 3402–3406.
16. MAHESH, V.B., P. ZAMORANO, L. DE SEVILLA, *et al.* 1999. Characterization of ionotropic glutamate receptors in rat hypothalamus, pituitary and immortalized gonadotropin-releasing hormone (GnRH) neurons (GT1-7 cells). Neuroendocrinology **69:** 397–407.
17. WRAY, S., P. GRANT & H. GAINER. 1989. Evidence that cells expressing luteinizing hormone-releasing hormone mRNA in the mouse are derived from progenitor cells in the olfactory placode. Proc. Natl. Acad. Sci. USA **86:** 8132–8136.
18. RONNEKLEIV, O.K. & J.A. RESKO. 1990. Ontogeny of gonadotropin-releasing hormone-containing neurons in early fetal development of rhesus macaques. Endocrinology **126:** 498–511.
19. RAIKOKU-ISHIDO, H., Y. OKAMURA, N. YANAIHARA & S. DAIKOKU. 1990. Development of the hypothalamic luteinizing hormone-releasing hormone-containing neuron system in the rat: in vivo and in transplantation studies. Dev. Biol. **140:** 374–387.
20. TERASAWA, E., C.D. QUANBECK, C.A. SCHULZ, *et al.* 1993. A primary cell culture system of luteinizing hormone releasing hormone neurons derived from embryonic olfactory placode in the rhesus monkey. Endocrinology **133:** 2379–2390.
21. FUESHKO, S. & S. WRAY. 1994. LHRH cells migrate on peripherin fibers in embryonic olfactory explant cultures: an in vitro model for neurophilic neuronal migration. Dev. Biol. **166:** 331–348.
22. FUNABASHI, T., S. DAIKOKU, K. SHINOHARA & F. KIMURA. 2000. Pulsatile gonadotropin-releasing hormone (GnRH) secretion is an inherent function of GnRH neurons, as revealed by the culture of medial olfactory placode obtained from embryonic rats. Neuroendocrinology **71:** 138–144.
23. DUITTOZ, A.H., M. BATAILLER & M. CALDANI. 1997. Primary cell culture of LHRH neurones from embryonic olfactory placode in the sheep (*Ovis aries*). J. Neuroendocrinol. **9:** 669–675.
24. MOORE, J.P.J. & S. WRAY. 2000. Luteinizing hormone-releasing hormone (LHRH) biosynthesis and secretion in embryonic LHRH. Endocrinology **141:** 4486–4495.
25. DUITTOZ, A.H. & M. BATAILLER. 2000. Pulsatile GnRH secretion from primary cultures of sheep olfactory placode explants. J. Reprod. Fertil. **120:** 391–396.
26. KRSMANOVIC, L.Z., A.J., K.K. ARORA, N. MORES, *et al.* 1999. Autocrine regulation of gonadotropin-releasing hormone secretion in cultured hypothalamic neurons. Endocrinology **140:** 1423–1431.
27. MELROSE, P., L. GROSS, I. CRUSE & M. RUSH. 1987. Isolated gonadotropin-releasing hormone neurons harvested from adult male rats secrete biologically active neuropeptide in a regular repetitive manner. Endocrinology **121:** 182–189.
28. MELROSE, P. & L. GROSS. 1987. Steroid effects on the secretory modalities of gonadotropin-releasing hormone release. Endocrinology **121:** 190–199.
29. WRAY, S., B.H. GAHWILER & H. GAINER. 1988. Slice cultures of LHRH neurons in the presence and absence of brainstem and pituitary. Peptides **9:** 1151–1175.

30. DePaolo, L.V. & A. Negro-Vilar. 1982. Neonatal monosodium glutamate treatment alters the response of median eminence luteinizing hormone-releasing hormone nerve terminals to potassium and prostaglandin E2. Endocrinology **110:** 835–841.
31. McKibbin, P.E. & P.E. Belchetz. 1986. Prolonged pulsatile release of gonadotropin-releasing hormone from the guinea pig hypothalamus in vitro. Life Sci. **38:** 2145–2150.
32. Drouva, S.V., E. Laplante, J.P. Gautron & C. Kordon. 1984. Effects of 17 beta-estradiol on LH-RH release from rat mediobasal hypothalamic slices. Neuroendocrinology **38:** 152–157.
33. Bourguignon, J.P. & P. Franchimont. 1984. Puberty-related increase in episodic LHRH release from rat hypothalamus in vitro. Endocrinology **114:** 1941–1943.
34. Levine, J.E., C.L. Bethea & H.G. Spies. 1985. In vitro gonadotropin-releasing hormone release from hypothalamic tissues of ovariectomized estrogen-treated cynomolgus macaques. Endocrinology **116:** 431–438.
35. Li, Q., L. Tamarkin, P. Levantine & M.A. Ottinger. 1994. Estradiol and androgen modulate chicken luteinizing hormone-releasing hormone-I release in vitro. Biol. Reprod. **51:** 896–903.
36. Rasmussen, D.D., M. Gambacciani, W. Swartz, *et al.*. 1989. Pulsatile gonadotropin-releasing hormone release from the human mediobasal hypothalamus in vitro: opiate receptor-mediated suppression. Neuroendocrinology **49:** 150–156.
37. Purnelle, G., A. Gerard, V. Czajkowski & J.P. Bourguignon. 1997. Pulsatile secretion of gonadotropin-releasing hormone by rat hypothalamic explants without cell bodies of GnRH neurons. Neuroendocrinology **66:** 305–312.
38. Bourguignon, J.P., A. Gerard, G. Debougnoux, *et al.* 1987. Pulsatile release of gonadotropin-releasing hormone (GnRH) from the rat hypothalamus in vitro: calcium and glucose dependency and inhibition by superactive GnRH analogs. Endocrinology **121:** 993–999.
39. Bourguignon, J.P., A. Gerard & P. Franchimont. 1984. Age-related differences in the effect of castration upon hypothalamic LHRH content in male rats. Neuroendocrinology **38:** 376–381.
40. Bourguignon, J.P., A. Gerard & P. Franchimont. 1989. Direct activation of gonadotropin-releasing hormone secretion through different receptors to neuroexcitatory amino acids. Neuroendocrinology **49:** 402–408.
41. Bourguignon, J.P., A. Gerard, J. Mathieu, *et al.* 1990. Maturation of the hypothalamic control of pulsatile gonadotropin-releasing hormone secretion at onset of puberty. I. Increased activation of N-methyl-D-aspartate receptors. Endocrinology **127:** 873–881.
42. Bourguignon, J.P., A. Gerard & P. Franchimont. 1990. Maturation of the hypothalamic control of pulsatile gonadotropin-releasing hormone secretion at onset of puberty: II. Reduced potency of an inhibitory autofeedback. Endocrinology **127:** 2884–2890.
43. Parent, A.S., M.C. Lebrethon, A. Gerard, *et al.* 2000. Leptin effects on pulsatile gonadotropin releasing hormone secretion from the adult rat hypothalamus and interaction with cocaine and amphetamine regulated transcript peptide and neuropeptide Y. Regul. Pept. **92:** 17–24.
44. Bourguignon, J.P., A. Gerard, G.M. Alvarez, *et al.* 1995. Endogenous glutamate involvement in pulsatile secretion of gonadotropin-releasing hormone: evidence from effect of glutamine and developmental changes. Endocrinology **136:** 911–916.
45. Bourguignon, J.P., G.M. Alvarez, A. Gerard & P. Franchimont. 1994. Gonadotropin releasing hormone inhibitory autofeedback by subproducts antagonist at N-methyl-D-aspartate receptors: a model of autocrine regulation of peptide secretion. Endocrinology **134:** 1589–1592.
46. Yamanaka, C., M.C. Lebrethon, E. Vandersmissen, *et al.* 1999. Early prepubertal ontogeny of pulsatile gonadotropin-releasing hormone (GnRH) secretion: I. Inhibitory autofeedback control through prolyl endopeptidase degradation of GnRH. Endocrinology **140:** 4609–4615.
47. Bourguignon, J.P., A. Gerard, G. Purnelle, *et al.* 1997. Duality of glutamatergic and GABAergic control of pulsatile GnRH secretion by rat hypothalamic explants:

II. Reduced NR2C- and GABAA-receptor-mediated inhibition at initiation of sexual maturation. J. Neuroendocrinol. **9:** 193–199.

48. LEBRETHON, M.C., E. VANDERSMISSEN, A. GERARD, *et al.* 2000. Cocaine and amphetamine-regulated-transcript peptide mediation of leptin stimulatory effect on the rat gonadotropin-releasing hormone pulse generator in vitro. J. Neuroendocrinol. **12:** 383–385.
49. SPERGEL, D.J., U. KRUTH, D.F. HANLEY, *et al.* 1999. GABA- and glutamate-activated channels in green fluorescent protein- tagged gonadotropin-releasing hormone neurons in transgenic mice. J. Neurosci. **19:** 2037–2050.
50. SUTER, K.J., W.J. SONG, T.L. SAMPSON, *et al.* 2000. Genetic targeting of green fluorescent protein to gonadotropin-releasing hormone neurons: characterization of whole-cell electrophysiological properties and morphology. Endocrinology **141:** 412–419.
51. HAN, S.K., I.M. ABRAHAM & A.E. HERBISON. 2002. Effect of GABA on GnRH neurons switches from depolarization to hyperpolarization at puberty in the female mouse. Endocrinology **143:** 1459–1466.
52. SPERGEL, D.J., U. KRUTH, D.R. SHIMSHEK, *et al.* 2001. Using reporter genes to label selected neuronal populations in transgenic mice for gene promoter, anatomical, and physiological studies. Prog. Neurobiol. **63:** 673–686.
53. SKYNNER, M.J., R. SLATER, J.A. SIM, *et al.*. 1999. Promoter transgenics reveal multiple gonadotropin-releasing hormone-I-expressing cell populations of different embryological origin in mouse brain. J. Neurosci. **19:** 5955–5966.
54. SUTER, K.J., J.P. WUARIN, B.N. SMITH, *et al.* 2000. Whole-cell recordings from preoptic/hypothalamic slices reveal burst firing in gonadotropin-releasing hormone neurons identified with green fluorescent protein in transgenic mice. Endocrinology **141:** 3731–3736.
55. DEFAZIO, R.A. & S.M. MOENTER. 2002. Estradiol feedback alters potassium currents and firing properties of gonadotropin-releasing hormone neurons. Mol. Endocrinol. **16:** 2255–2265.
56. KUEHL-KOVARIK, M.C., W.A. POULIOT, G.L. HALTERMAN, *et al.* 2002. Episodic bursting activity and response to excitatory amino acids in acutely dissociated gonadotropin-releasing hormone neurons genetically targeted with green fluorescent protein. J. Neurosci. **22:** 2313–2322.
57. NUNEMAKER, C.S., R.A. DEFAZIO & S.M. MOENTER. 2002. Estradiol-sensitive afferents modulate long-term episodic firing patterns of GnRH neurons. Endocrinology **143:** 2284–2292.
58. NUNEMAKER, C.S., M. STRAUME, R.A. DEFAZIO & S.M. MOENTER. 2003. Gonadotropin-releasing hormone neurons generate interacting rhythms in multiple time domains. Endocrinology **144:** 823–831.
59. KATO, M., K. UI-TEI, M. WATANABE & Y. SAKUMA. 2003. Characterization of voltage-gated calcium currrents in gonadoptropin-releasing hormone neurons tagged with green fluorescent protein in rats. Endocrinology **144:** 5118–5125.
60. KRSMANOVIC, L.Z., S.S. STOJILKOVIC, F. MERELLI, *et al.* 1992. Calcium signaling and episodic secretion of gonadotropin-releasing hormone in hypothalamic neurons. Proc. Natl. Acad. Sci. USA **89:** 8462–8466.
61. JUNG, N., W. SUN, H. LEE, *et al.* 1998. Gonadotropin-releasing hormone (GnRH) gene regulation by N-methyl-D-aspartic acid in GT1-1 neuronal cells: differential involvement of c-fos and c-jun protooncogenes. Brain Res. Mol. Brain Res. **61:** 162–169.
62. MAHACHOKLERTWATTANA, P., J. SANCHEZ, S.L. KAPLAN & M.M. GRUMBACH. 1994. N-methyl-D-aspartate (NMDA) receptors mediate the release of gonadotropin-releasing hormone (GnRH) by NMDA in a hypothalamic GnRH neuronal cell line (GT1-1). Endocrinology **134:** 1023–1030.
63. SPERGEL, D.J., L.Z. KRSMANOVIC, S.S. STOJILKOVIC & K.J. CATT. 1995. L-type Ca2+ channels mediate joint modulation by gamma-amino-butyric acid and glutamate of [Ca2+]i and neuropeptide secretion in immortalized gonadodropin-releasing hormone neurons. Neuroendocrinology **61:** 499–508.
64. KUSANO, K., S. FUESHKO, H. GAINER & S. WRAY. 1995. Electrical and synaptic properties of embryonic luteinizing hormone-releasing hormone neurons in explant cultures. Proc. Natl. Acad. Sci. USA **92:** 3918–3922.

65. CHAPPELL, P.E., J.P. LYDON, O.M. CONNEELY, *et al.* 1997. Endocrine defects in mice carrying a null mutation for the progesterone receptor gene. Endocrinology **138:** 4147–4152.
66. SORTINO, M.A., G. ALEPPO, U. SCAPAGNINI & P.L. CANONICO. 1996. Different responses of gonadotropin-releasing hormone (GnRH) release to glutamate receptor agonists during aging. Brain Res. Bull. **41:** 359–362.
67. NUNEZ, L., C. VILLALOBOS, F.R. BOOCKFOR & L.S. FRAWLEY. 2000. The relationship between pulsatile secretion and calcium dynamics in single, living gonadotropin-releasing hormone neurons. Endocrinology **141:** 2012–2017.
68. TERASAWA, E., K.L. KEEN, K. MOGI & P. CLAUDE. 1999. Pulsatile release of luteinizing hormone-releasing hormone (LHRH) in cultured LHRH neurons derived from the embryonic olfactory placode of the rhesus monkey. Endocrinology **140:** 1432–1441.
69. RASMUSSEN, D.D. 1993. Episodic gonadotropin-releasing hormone release from the rat isolated median eminence in vitro. Neuroendocrinology **58:** 511–518.
70. VAN GOOR, F., L.Z. KRSMANOVIC, K.J. CATT & S.S. STOJILKOVIC. 1999. Coordinate regulation of gonadotropin-releasing hormone neuronal firing patterns by cytosolic calcium and store depletion. Proc. Natl. Acad. Sci. USA **96:** 4101–4106.
71. RICHTER, T.A., K.L. KEEN & E. TERASAWA. 2002. Synchronization of Ca(2+) oscillations among primate LHRH neurons and nonneuronal cells in vitro. J. Neurophysiol. **88:** 1559–1567.
72. MOORE, J.P.J., E. SHANG & S. WRAY. 2002. In situ GABAergic modulation of synchronous gonadotropin releasing hormone-1 neuronal activity. J. Neurosci. **22:** 8932–8941.
73. BOURGUIGNON, J.P., A. GERARD, M.L. ALVAREZ-GONZALEZ, *et al.* 1995. The role of excitatory amino acids in triggering the onset of puberty. *In* The Neurobiology of Puberty. T.M. Plant & P.A. Lee, Eds.: 129–138. Society of Endocrinology. Bristol.
74. HORI, Y. & T. NAKAYAMA. 1982. Temperature sensitivity of the preoptic and anterior hypothalamic neurons in organ culture. Tohoku. J. Exp. Med. **136:** 79–87.
75. MOGUILEVSKY, J.A. & W. WUTTKE. 2001. Changes in the control of gonadotrophin secretion by neurotransmitters during sexual development in rats. Exp. Clin. Endocrinol. Diabetes **109:** 188–195.
76. BOURGUIGNON, J.P., A. GERARD, G. PURNELLE, *et al.* 1997. Duality of glutamatergic and GABAergic control of pulsatile GnRH secretion by rat hypothalamic explants. I.: Effects of antisense oligodeoxynucleotides using explants including or excluding the preoptic area. J. Neuroendocrinol. **9:** 183–191.
77. ROY, D., N.L. ANGELINI & D.D. BELSHAM. 1999. Estrogen directly respresses gonadotropin-releasing hormone (GnRH) gene expression in estrogen receptor-alpha (ERalpha)- and ERbeta-expressing GT1-7 GnRH neurons. Endocrinology **140:** 5045–5053.
78. WRAY, S., R.T. ZOELLER & H. GAINER. 1989. Differential effects of estrogen on luteinizing hormone-releasing hormone gene expression in slice explant cultures prepared from specific rat forebrain regions. Mol. Endocrinol. **3:** 1197–1206.
79. BOWE, J., X.F. LI, D. SUGDEN, J.A. KATZENELLENBOGEN, *et al.* 2003. The effects of the phytoestrogen, coumestrol, on gonadotropin-releasing hormone (GnRH) mRNA expression in GT1-7 GnRH neurones. J. Neuroendocrinol. **15:** 105–108.
80. PREVOT, V., D. CROIX, C.M. RIALAS, *et al.* 1999. Estradiol coupling to endothelial nitric oxide stimulates gonadotropin- releasing hormone release from rat median eminence via a membrane receptor. Endocrinology **140:** 652–659.
81. BARNI, T., M. MAGGI, G. FANTONI, *et al.* 1999. Sex steroids and odorants modulate gonadotropin-releasing hormone secretion in primary cultures of human olfactory cells. J. Clin. Endocrinol Metab **84:** 4266–4273.
82. ANDREWS, W.W., G.J. MIZEJEWSKI & S.R. OJEDA. 1981. Development of estradiol-positive feedback on luteinizing hormone release in the female rat: a quantitative study. Endocrinology **109:** 1404–1413.
83. DLUZEN, D.E. & V.D. RAMIREZ. 1986. In vivo LH-RH output of ovariectomized rats following estrogen treatment. Neuroendocrinology **43:** 459–465.
84. EVANS, N.P., G.E. DAHL, D. MAUGER & F.J. KARSCH. 1995. Estradiol induces both qualitative and quantitative changes in the pattern of gonadotropin-releasing hor-

mone secretion during the presurge period in the ewe. Endocrinology **136:** 1603–1609.
85. HERBISON, A.E. 1998. Multimodal influence of estrogen upon gonadotropin-releasing hormone neurons. Endocr. Rev. **19:** 302–330.
86. MCEWEN, B. 2002. Estrogen actions throughout the brain. Recent Prog. Horm. Res. **57:** 357–384.
87. KELLY, M.J. & O.K. RONNEKLEIV. 2002. Rapid membrane effects of estrogen in the central nervous system. *In* Hormones, Brain and Behavior.: 361–379. Elsevier. San Diego.
88. KELLY, M.J. & E.R. LEVIN. 2001. Rapid actions of plasma membrane estrogen receptors. Trends Endocrinol. Metab. **12:** 152–156.
89. WRAY, S., S. KEY, R. QUALLS & S.M. FUESHKO. 1994. A subset of peripherin positive olfactory axons delineates the luteinizing hormone releasing hormone neuronal migratory pathway in developing mouse. Dev. Biol. **166:** 349–354.
90. VANNELLI, G.B., F. ENSOLI, R. ZONEFRATI, *et al.* 1995. Neuroblast long-term cell cultures from human fetal olfactory epithelium respond to odors. J. Neurosci. **15:** 4382–4394.
91. GALLO, F., M.C. MORALE, C. TIROLO, *et al.* 2000. Basic fibroblast growth factor priming increases the responsiveness of immortalized hypothalamic luteinizing hormone releasing hormone neurones to neurotrophic factors. J. Neuroendocrinol. **12:** 941–959.
92. SUN, W., H. JARRY, W. WUTTKE & K. KIM. 1997. Gonadotropin releasing hormone modulates gamma-aminobutyric acid-evoked intracellular calcium increase in immortalized hypothalamic gonadotropin releasing hormone neurons. Brain Res. **747:** 70–77.
93. LACAU-MENGIDO, I.M., I.A. GONZALEZ, G. DIAZ-TORGA, *et al.* 1998. Effect of stage of development and sex on gonadotropin-releasing hormone secretion in in vitro hypothalamic perifusion. Proc. Soc. Exp. Biol. Med. **217:** 445–449.
94. BURNS, K.H. & M.M. MATZUK. 2002. Minireview: genetic models for the study of gonadotropin actions. Endocrinology **143:** 2823–2835.
95. KRSMANOVIC, L.Z., N. MORES, C.E. NAVARRO, *et al.* 2003. An agonist-induced switch in G protein coupling of the gonadotropin-releasing hormone receptor regulates pulsatile neuropeptide secretion. Proc. Natl. Acad. Sci. USA **100:** 2969–2974.
96. WETSEL, W.C., M.M. VALENCA, I. MERCHENTHALER, *et al.* 1992. Intrinsic pulsatile secretory activity of immortalized luteinizing hormone-releasing hormone-secreting neurons. Proc. Natl. Acad. Sci. USA **89:** 4149–4153.
97. MARTINEZ, D.L.E., A.L. CHOI & R.I. WEINER. 1992. Generation and synchronization of gonadotropin-releasing hormone (GnRH) pulses: intrinsic properties of the GT1-1 GnRH neuronal cell line. Proc. Natl. Acad. Sci. USA **89:** 1852–1855.
98. FUNABASHI, T., K. SUYAMA, T. UEMURA, *et al.* 2001. Immortalized gonadotropin-releasing hormone neurons (GT1-7 cells) exhibit synchronous bursts of action potentials. Neuroendocrinology **73:** 157–165.
99. TERASAWA, E., W.K. SCHANHOFER, K.L. KEEN & L. LUCHANSKY. 1999. Intracellular Ca(2+) oscillations in luteinizing hormone-releasing hormone neurons derived from the embryonic olfactory placode of the rhesus monkey. J. Neurosci. **19:** 5898–5909.
100. MAHACHOKLERTWATTANA, P., S.M. BLACK, S.L. KAPLAN, *et al.* 1994. Nitric oxide synthesized by gonadotropin-releasing hormone neurons is a mediator of N-methyl-D-aspartate (NMDA)-induced GnRH secretion. Endocrinology **135:** 1709–1712.
101. MARTINEZ-DE LA ESCALERA, A.L. CHOI & R.I. WEINER. 1994. Biphasic gabaergic regulation of GnRH secretion in GT1 cell lines. Neuroendocrinology **59:** 420–425.
102. FUNABASHI, T., S. DAIKOKU, K. SUYAMA, *et al.* 2002. Role of gamma-aminobutyric acid neurons in the release of gonadotropin-releasing hormone in cultured rat embryonic olfactory placodes. Neuroendocrinology **76:** 193–202.
103. BOURGUIGNON, J.P., A. GERARD, J. MATHIEU, *et al.* 1989. Pulsatile release of gonadotropin-releasing hormone from hypothalamic explants is restrained by blockade of N-methyl-D,L-aspartate receptors. Endocrinology **125:** 1090–1096.
104. CARBONE, S., B. SZWARCFARB, D. RONDINA, *et al.* 1996. Differential effects of the N-methyl-D-aspartate and non-N-methyl-D-aspartate receptors of the excitatory amino

acids system on LH and FSH secretion: its effects on the hypothalamic luteinizing hormone releasing hormone during maturation in male rats. Brain Res. **707:** 139–145.

105. MARTINEZ-DE LA ESCALERA, A.L. CHOI & R.I. WEINER. 1995. Signaling pathways involved in GnRH secretion in GT1 cells. Neuroendocrinology **61:** 310–317.
106. WETSEL, W.C., S.A. ERALY, D.B. WHYTE & P.L. MELLON. 1993. Regulation of gonadotropin-releasing hormone by protein kinase-A and -C in immortalized hypothalamic neurons. Endocrinology **132:** 2360–2370.
107. MORETTO, M., F.J. LOPEZ & A. NEGRO-VILAR. 1993. Nitric oxide regulates luteinizing hormone-releasing hormone secretion. Endocrinology **133:** 2399–2402.
108. SORTINO, M.A., G. ALEPPO, U. SCAPAGNINI & P.L. CANONICO. 1994. Involvement of nitric oxide in the regulation of gonadotropin-releasing hormone release from the GT1-1 neuronal cell line. Endocrinology **134:** 1782–1787.
109. CLAYTON, R.N. 1993. Regulation of gonadotrophin subunit gene expression. Hum. Reprod. **8:** 29–36.
110. BHAT, G.K., V.B. MAHESH, C.A. LAMAR, *et al.* 1995. Histochemical localization of nitric oxide neurons in the hypothalamus: association with gonadotropin-releasing hormone neurons and co-localization with N-methyl-D-aspartate receptors. Neuroendocrinology **62:** 187–197.
111. SHEN, E.S., E.H. MEADE, M.C. PEREZ, *et al.*1998. Expression of functional estrogen receptors and galanin messenger ribonucleic acid in immortalized luteinizing hormone-releasing hormone neurons: estrogenic control of galanin gene expression. Endocrinology **139:** 939–948.

Steroid Regulation of GnRH Neurons

SUZANNE M. MOENTER, R. ANTHONY DEFAZIO, MARTIN STRAUME, AND CRAIG S. NUNEMAKER

Departments of Medicine and Cell Biology, University of Virginia Health System, Charlottesville, Virginia 22908, USA

ABSTRACT: GnRH neurons form the final common pathway for regulating fertility. Estradiol feedback controls GnRH release, but the cellular mechanisms are unknown. Targeted extracellular recordings were used to examine the firing rate of GFP-identified GnRH neurons in a model for estradiol negative feedback (OVX vs. OVX+E). Episodes of increased firing rate occurred in both groups with intervals consistent with hormone secretion; estradiol more than doubled this interval. Spectral analysis identified additional rhythmic activity that was grouped by period: bursts (<100 s), clusters (100–1000 s), or episodes (>1000 s). Bursts were trains of action currents. Estradiol did not alter burst characteristics, but rather changed the patterning of inter-burst intervals to increase the period of the low-frequency episode rhythm. To change inter-burst-interval, estradiol might alter conductances in GnRH neurons, such as potassium currents. Whole-cell voltage-clamp revealed that estradiol affected the amplitude, decay time, and the voltage dependence of A-type potassium currents in GnRH neurons. Blockade of protein kinases reversed some but not all effects of estradiol. Consistent with changes in the A-current, estradiol increased excitability in GnRH neurons. Estradiol thus targets multiple mechanisms to alter GnRH neuron firing patterns, and the balance of stimulatory and inhibitory actions determines whether the integrated response is to increase or to decrease release.

KEYWORDS: GnRH; LHRH; estradiol; patch-clamp; potassium channel; feedback; burst; rhythm

INTRODUCTION

The final common pathway for the central control of reproduction is through the neurons that synthesize and secrete gonadotropin-releasing hormone (GnRH). GnRH neurons populate a midventral continuum that extends caudally from the diagonal band of Broca past the optic chiasm and into the medial basal hypothalamus.[1] Their axons project to the external layer of the median eminence, where GnRH is released near the pituitary portal vessels. GnRH stimulates synthesis[2,3] and secretion[4] of the pituitary gonadotropins and through this action activates the gonadal functions of ga-

Address for correspondence: Suzanne Moenter, Ph.D., Associate Professor of Internal Medicine, Division of Endocrinology and Metabolism, Departments of Medicine and Cell Biology, University of Virginia Health System, P.O. Box 800578, Charlottesville, VA 22908. Voice: 434-982-0076; fax: 434-982-0088.
smm4n@virginia.edu

**Ann. N.Y. Acad. Sci. 1007: 143–152 (2003). © 2003 New York Academy of Sciences.
doi: 10.1196/annals.1286.014**

metogenesis and steroidogenesis. Steroid hormones feed back to regulate both the secretion of GnRH and pituitary response to this hormone.[5–9]

Of the steroid hormones, estradiol is particularly interesting, as it has both negative and positive actions on GnRH release. When estradiol levels are increased from a basal level to a late follicular phase, or proestrous level, there is a biphasic response in terms of GnRH release.[6,10] Initially, GnRH pulse amplitude and sometimes frequency are suppressed in what is termed negative feedback. Several hours later, there is a massive increase in GnRH release such that levels in portal blood are continuously elevated. This GnRH surge, which is initiated by estradiol is the neural pre-requisite for ovulation in most species. Our long-term goal is to understand the neurobiological mechanisms that underlie the effects of estradiol on GnRH neurons. This report summarizes our findings to date using a model for estradiol negative feedback.

MODEL AND APPROACHES

To identify living GnRH neurons, we use transgenic mice in which expression of the jellyfish reporter gene green fluorescent protein or GFP is targeted to GnRH neurons.[11] To study the cells, slices are made through the preoptic area and hypothalamus, and a combination of the fluorescent GFP signal and infrared-differential interference contrast microscopy is used to target a patch pipette to a GnRH neuron. Two types of recordings were used. Targeted extracellular recordings detect the action currents that occur during action potential firing and thus provide information on firing pattern of GnRH neurons over time.[12] This is thus a measure of the integrated response of GnRH neurons to the applied treatment. Whole-cell recordings were made to study specific properties of GnRH neurons, in this case potassium currents and firing properties, that might contribute to the integrated response of the cell.[13]

For the animal model, a fixed feedback signal was chosen. Adult (>42 days) female GnRH-GFP mice were ovariectomized (OVX) and half were implanted with an estradiol capsule that produces a physiological level of the steroid in circulation (OVX+E).[13] The animals were studied one week later to avoid transient effects of steroid manipulation as well as any effects of chronic steroid deprivation. At the time brain slices were prepared, LH levels were suppressed in the OVX+E group, presumably due at least in part to an inhibition of GnRH neuron function, demonstrating this a model for estradiol negative feedback.[13]

ESTRADIOL ALTERS THE PATTERN OF GnRH NEURON FIRING

We began by monitoring the effect of this estradiol regimen on the long-term firing pattern using the targeted extracellular approach.[14] In GnRH neurons from both OVX and OVX+E mice, the firing of GnRH neurons was intermittent (FIG. 1A). In other neuroendocrine systems, firing rate is correlated with hormone release,[15,16] and thus intermittent firing is what might be predicted from a neuron that releases hormone in a pulsatile fashion. Consistent with this hypothesis, significant increases in firing rate in GnRH neurons detected by the Cluster7 pulse detection algorithm[17]

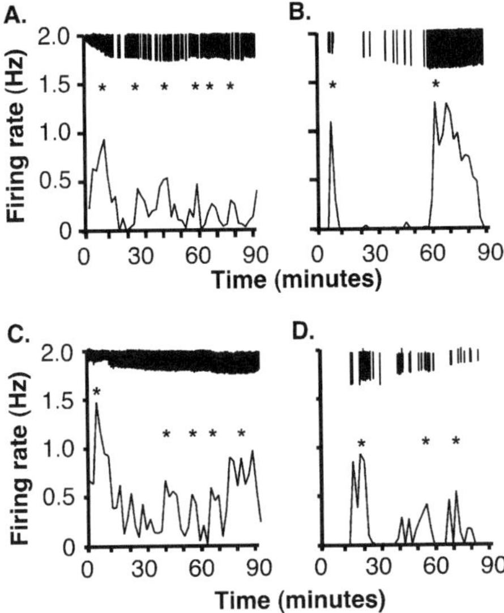

FIGURE 1. Estradiol lengthens the interval between episodes of increased firing rate. Representative examples are shown of firing patterns of a GnRH neuron from OVX (**A**) and from OVX+E (**B**) mice. Blockade reverses estradiol effects in a substantial population of GnRH neurons from OVX+E mice. Representative examples of firing patterns are shown for a GnRH neuron from an OVX+E mouse that responded (**C**) to receptor antagonists (20 μM bicuculline, 20 μM CNQX, and 50 μM APV blockade) and a GnRH neuron from an OVX+E mouse that did not respond (**D**) to receptor antagonists. (**A**–**D**) Data are plotted as mean firing rate at 2-min intervals. *Vertical lines* at the top of each graph illustrate timing of individual action currents detected. *Asterisks* (*) indicate episodes of increased firing rate detected by Cluster7. (Adapted from Nunemaker *et al.*[14] by permission of The Endocrine Society.)

occurred at intervals that are consistent with the frequency of GnRH release in rodents, suggesting that these episodes of increased firing rate may be associated with secretory activity. Estradiol more than doubled the interval between these episodes (Fig. 1B). These observations indicate that *in vivo* estradiol treatment produces a change in the firing pattern of GnRH neurons consistent with the reduction in LH release. This was important to establish as brain slices are prepared a couple of hours in advance of recording. During this resting period, steroids are not present, and thus it was possible that any effects would dissipate.

An important question to address is where estradiol acts to bring about these changes in GnRH neuron firing pattern. Historically there has been an assumption that steroid feedback occurred through action on presynaptic neurons that are estradiol-sensitive, but recent work in several labs has suggested that the beta isoform of the estradiol receptor is expressed in GnRH neurons,[18,19] raising the possibility of direct action. To start addressing this question, the major forms of fast synaptic transmission were inhibited in slices before recording by including drugs to block AMPA and NMDA glutamatergic receptors and $GABA_A$ receptors. This treatment had no effect on episodic firing in GnRH neurons from ovariectomized mice. This is evidence that neither ionotropic glutamatergic nor GABAergic inputs drive episodic activity. In contrast, this treatment reversed the effects of estradiol on firing pattern in about half of the cells tested, so that increases in firing rate occurred more frequently than was typical of GnRH neurons from estradiol-treated animals (FIGS. 1C and D). Interestingly, GnRH neurons in the midventral preoptic area were more sensitive to effects transmitted by GABA and/or glutamate. Cells outside this region, either more rostral, caudal, or lateral typically did not respond to the antagonists. This may be an artifact of slice preparation in that neurons in this central core may have properties preserved that others do not. Or it may be an indication that either estradiol does act directly on some cells or that the phenotype of synaptic input conveying estradiol negative feedback actions differs from region to region.

During the characterization of firing patterns of GnRH neurons from OVX and OVX+E mice, rhythmic activity was observed in these cells that extended beyond the low-frequency changes in firing rate being characterized; specifically, repetitive higher-frequency firing activity also occurred. This sort of high-frequency rhythm had been observed in both immortalized GT1 cells[20,21] and also in cultured embryonic GnRH neurons.[22] This raised two questions. Is the high-frequency activity related to low-frequency activity associated with secretory patterns? Does estradiol also affect high-frequency activity in GnRH neurons?

To investigate this, the firing rate data from the previous study were subjected to spectral analysis by fast Fourier transform.[23] In this analysis, the pattern of events is fit to sinusoidal waveforms of different frequencies, each representing a different periodicity in the original firing pattern. In this way, patterns could be detected in many time domains. This analysis revealed multiple rhythms in GnRH neurons that were arbitrarily divided on the basis of period for further analysis. Rhythms with a period of less than 100 s were termed bursts, those with periods from 100 to 1000 s were termed clusters, and those with a period greater than 1000 s were termed episodes. For reference, 1000 s is 16.67 min; episodes thus have a period similar to that we associate with neurosecretion in this system.

Typically GnRH neurons exhibited rhythms in two or all three of these time frames. Bursts consisted of trains of action currents alternating with quiescence, and were observed in ~90% of GnRH neurons. The composition of bursts varied from cell to cell in terms of the number of spikes/burst, duration, and interval between bursts. Clusters and episodes both consisted of multiple bursts in rapid succession, resulting in phases of increased firing rate. Examination of the underlying change in burst firing pattern suggests that the interval between bursts, rather than the composition of the burst itself, is changed in order to produce peaks and nadirs in firing.

To better quantify this observation, five-minute segments of recordings were examined at both peak and nadir phases of episode activity as determined by Cluster7 analysis. Three characteristics of burst firing that could result in changes in mean firing rate were measured. Events/burst and burst duration were similar between peaks and nadirs in low-frequency firing. In contrast, there was a clear and profound difference in burst interval between peak and nadir phases of activity. This suggests that bursts are a fundamental or quantal unit of activity in GnRH neurons. Low-frequency rhythms arise when the production of these units is cyclically increased and decreased.

Because estradiol has an impact on the low-frequency firing rhythm, the possibility exists that it does so by altering rhythms in the high-frequency time domain. Us-

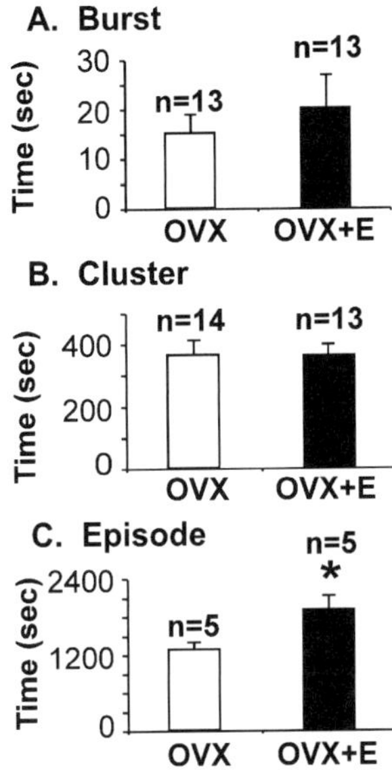

FIGURE 2. Estradiol's effects on mean spectral periods are confined to the episode time domain. Mean (± SEM) interval identified by spectral analysis in firing patterns of GnRH neurons recorded from OVX and OVX+E mice are seen in the range of (**A**) bursts (0–100 s), (**B**) clusters (100–1000 s), and (**C**) episodes (>1000 s) over the entire recording period. Estradiol increased the interval between episodes by 50% (*, $P<0.05$), but did not affect mean burst or cluster intervals. The number of cells exhibiting patterns in each time domain is indicated above the respective column in each graph. Note that this analysis of overall period does not reveal the changes in period that occur *within* recordings for bursts, as shown in FIGURE 3. (From Nunemaker *et al.*[23] Reproduced by permission of The Endocrine Society.)

ing the Fourier spectral analysis results, the effects of estradiol on the periodicity of patterns in all three time domains were compared between OVX and OVX+E groups. The only significant change in period was in the low-frequency episode time domain, which was increased by estradiol (FIG. 2). There were no significant changes in GnRH neuron firing patterns in either the burst or cluster time domain due to estradiol treatment. Estradiol also did not affect other characteristics of the high-frequency burst firing rhythm. Estradiol did, however, alter the spacing between phases of increased burst interval (FIG. 3). Specifically, transitions occur less frequently between long burst intervals (during nadirs in the low-frequency rhythm) and short burst intervals (during peaks in the low-frequency rhythm). These data are consistent with the hypothesis that estradiol acts on a low-frequency rhythm to increase the interval between episode peaks.

ESTRADIOL AFFECTS POTASSIUM CURRENTS AND EXCITABILITY OF GnRH NEURONS

One mechanism by which estradiol may bring about the above changes is through altering conductances intrinsic to GnRH neurons and thereby affecting their excitability. We began investigating this idea by examining voltage-gated potassium currents in GnRH neurons from OVX vs. OVX+E mice.[13]

Voltage-gated potassium currents in GnRH neurons from the ovariectomized animal had two main components. The dominant current was a rapidly inactivating current with characteristics of an A-type potassium current (I_A). In addition, there

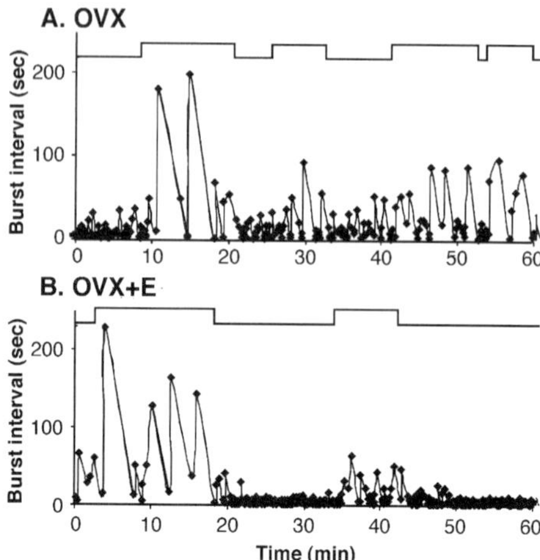

FIGURE 3. Estradiol changes burst interval pattern. Representative examples of burst interval patterns are shown for GnRH neurons from an OVX (**A**) and OVX+E (**B**) mouse. Burst interval (*y*-axis, s) is plotted vs. time of occurrence (*x*-axis, min). Significant shifts between higher and lower burst interval detected by Cluster7 are indicated by the lines at the top of each graph. (From Nunemaker *et al.*[23] Reproduced by permission of The Endocrine Society.)

was a slowly inactivating current (I_K). Estradiol altered both components; both were reduced in amplitude and decayed, or inactivated, more slowly (FIG. 4). In addition, the voltage-dependence of inactivation of I_A was depolarized by estradiol. That these estradiol-induced changes are targeted to GnRH neurons was suggested by the observation that these currents were unaffected by estradiol treatment in magnocellular neurons of the paraventricular hypothalamus.

To alter potassium currents in GnRH neurons, estradiol may alter the level or type of potassium channels expressed in GnRH neurons through traditional genomic mechanisms.[24] Estradiol could also change phosphorylation of channels[25,26] due either to direct action on GnRH neurons, or secondary to a change in synaptic drive. Inclusion of the kinase inhibitor, H7, in the recording pipette to block PKA, PKC, and PKG reversed the effects of estradiol on amplitude and decay time, but interestingly not on voltage-dependence of inactivation for I_A. These data suggest estradiol alters potassium channels through more than one mechanism, and that one of these involves changing the phosphorylation state of these proteins.

We next examined how the estradiol-induced changes in I_A in GnRH neurons would affect the firing properties of these cells. I_A can increase latency to firing by fighting depolarization of the membrane to threshold.[27] I_A can also reduce spike width by increasing the rate of repolarization.[28] At threshold, there is more than twice as much I_A available in GnRH neurons from OVX mice. In contrast, at the peak, the availability of I_A is only slightly more in cells from estradiol-treated mice. On this basis, we would expect latency to action potential firing to be longer in GnRH neurons from ovariectomized mice. This is indeed the case. In cells from estradiol-treated mice, action potentials were initiated with short latency, whereas ac-

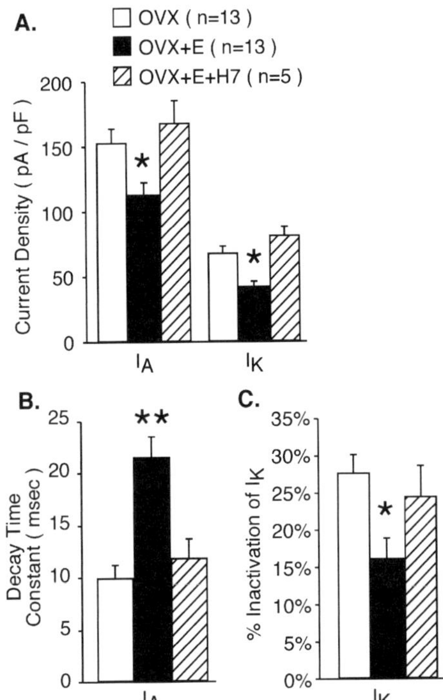

FIGURE 4. Summary of estradiol and H7 effects on K^+ currents in GnRH neurons. (**A**) Estradiol decreased the current density of I_A and I_K. (**B**) I_A decay time constant obtained from single exponential fit of isolated I_A (see FIGURE 5). (**C**) Percent inactivation of I_K during the 500-ms test pulse. *$P < 0.05$, ** $P < 0.01$. (Adapted from DeFazio and Moenter[13] by permission of The Endocrine Society.)

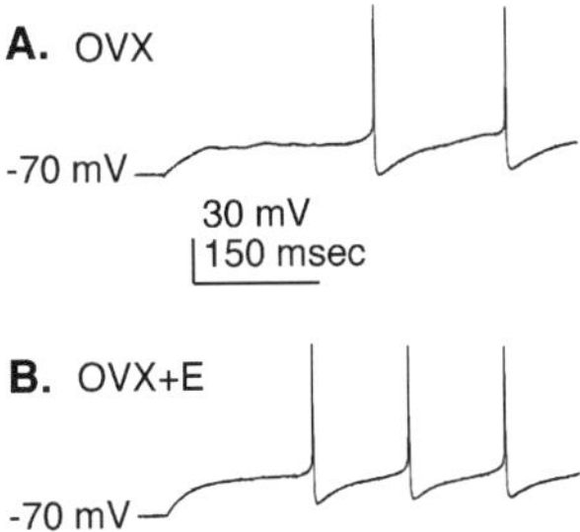

FIGURE 5. Estradiol-induced changes in I_A affect the firing properties of GnRH neurons. Latency was significantly decreased in neurons from OVX+E mice. Traces were truncated to emphasize differences in latency. (Adapted from DeFazio and Moenter[13] by permission of The Endocrine Society.)

tion potential generation was quite delayed in cells from OVX mice. Estradiol also hyperpolarized the threshold for firing, making it closer to the resting potential. Together these changes in latency and threshold would make it easier for GnRH neurons from OVX+E mice than those from OVX mice to fire in response to the same stimulus. That is, GnRH neurons from the estradiol negative feedback model are more excitable. This is contrary to what would be predicted in a model of negative feedback, if indeed negative and positive feedback are mutually exclusive. Of interest in this regard, an analogous effect of estradiol has been reported for GnRH release in sheep. Specifically, estradiol increases basal GnRH release that occurs between pulses, while at the same time blunting the pulses themselves.[29]

SUMMARY

Our electrophysiological investigations into mechanisms underlying estradiol feedback on GnRH neurons are in their early stages. Nonetheless, intriguing results have emerged that are sculpting our future studies. In a model for negative feedback, the integrated response of the GnRH neuron was suppressed as measured by episodic increases in firing rate that occur on the time scale of hormone release from this system in rodents. This appears to be due in part to changes in synaptic drive induced by estradiol as blockade of the major forms of fast synaptic transmission within the brain slice reversed this effect in a substantial subpopulation of GnRH neurons from OVX+E mice. Changes in intrinsic properties of GnRH neurons were also observed in this model. In this case, however, the data were the opposite of what we expected in that an estradiol "negative" feedback signal changed potassium currents in a way that increased, rather than decreased, the excitability of GnRH neurons.

Together these findings have adjusted how we consider estradiol feedback. The terms "negative" and "positive" arose from measurements largely of gonadotropin release, which reports the integrated response of the hypothalamo-pituitary axis. The robust change in GnRH release that occurs at the start of the preovulatory surge gives the appearance of an all-or-none event. Now that we have access to the mechanistic underpinnings leading to the switch from negative to positive feedback, the many levels at which estradiol acts are becoming evident. Some of these may be exclusively negative, others exclusively positive, and still others alternating between negative and positive impact on GnRH release. This model suggests that it is an adjustment in the balance of these effects, rather than a complete shift from negative to positive actions, that brings about initiation of the GnRH surge. Although our mechanistic picture is far from complete, we believe this approach is forcing the GnRH neuron to yield its secrets, and will eventually provide an integrated model for the negative and positive feedback effects of estradiol.

REFERENCES

1. Silverman, A.J. 1994. The gonadotropin-releasing hormone (GnRH) neuronal systems: immunocytochemistry and in situ hybridization. Physiol. Reprod. **1:** 1683–1709.
2. Haisenleder, D.J. *et al.* 1988. Influence of gonadotropin-releasing hormone pulse amplitude, frequency, and treatment duration on the regulation of luteinizing hormone (LH) subunit messenger ribonucleic acids and LH secretion. Mol. Endocrinol. **2:** 338–343.

3. KAISER, U.B. *et al.* 1997. Differential effects of gonadotropin-releasing hormone (GnRH) pulse frequency on gonadotropin subunit and GnRH receptor messenger ribonucleic acid levels in vitro. Endocrinology **138:** 1224–1231.
4. WEINER, R.I. *et al.* 1972. Changes in serum luteinizing hormone folowing intraventricular and intravenous injections of luteinizing hormone-releasing hormone in the rat. Neuroendocrinology **10:** 261–272.
5. KASA-VUBU, J.Z. *et al.* 1992. Progesterone blocks the estradiol-induced gonadotropin discharge in the ewe by inhibiting the surge of gonadotropin-releasing hormone. Endocrinology **131:** 208–212.
6. MOENTER, S.M., A. CARATY & F.J. KARSCH. 1990. The estradiol-induced surge of gonadotropin-releasing hormone in the ewe. Endocrinology **127:** 1375–1384.
7. CLARKE, I.J. & J.T. CUMMINS. 1984. Direct pituitary effects of estrogen and progesterone on gonadotropin secretion in the ovariectomized ewe. Neuroendocrinology **39:** 267–274.
8. LEIPHEIMER, R.E., A. BONA-GALLO & R.V. GALLO. 1984. The influence of progesterone and estradiol on the acute changes in pulsatile luteinizing hormone release induced by ovariectomy on diestrus day 1 in the rat. Endocrinology **114:** 1605–1612.
9. LEVINE, J.E. *et al.* 1985. In vivo gonadotropin-releasing hormone release and serum luteinizing hormone measurements in ovariectomized, estrogen-treated rhesus macaques. Endocrinology. **117:** 711–721.
10. CARATY, A., A. LOCATELLI & G.B. MARTIN. 1989. Biphasic response in the secretion of gonadotrophin-releasing hormone in ovariectomized ewes injected with oestradiol. J. Endocrinol. **123:** 375–382.
11. SUTER, K.J. *et al.* 2000. Genetic targeting of green fluorescent protein to gonadotropin-releasing hormone neurons: characterization of whole-cell electrophysiological properties and morphology. Endocrinology **141:** 412–419.
12. NUNEMAKER, C.S., R.A. DEFAZIO & S.M. MOENTER. 2003. A targeted extracellular approach for recording long-term firing patterns of excitable cells: a practical guide. Biological Procedures Online **5:** 53–62.
13. DEFAZIO, R.A. & S.M. MOENTER. 2002. Estradiol feedback alters potassium currents and firing properties of gonadotropin-releasing hormone neurons. Mol. Endocrinol. **16:** 2255–2265.
14. NUNEMAKER, C.S., R.A. DEFAZIO & S.M. MOENTER. 2002. Estradiol-sensitive afferents modulate long-term episodic firing patterns of GnRH neurons. Endocrinology **143:** 2284–2292.
15. DUTTON, A. & R.E. DYBALL. 1979. Phasic firing enhances vasopressin release from the rat neurohypophysis. J. Physiol. **290:** 433–440.
16. NORDMANN, J.J. & E.L. STUENKEL. 1986. Electrical properties of axons and neurohypophysial nerve terminals and their relationship to secretion in the rat. J. Physiol. **380:** 521–539.
17. VELDHUIS, J.D. & M.L. JOHNSON. 1986. Cluster analysis: a simple versatile, and robust algorithm for endocrine pulse detection. Am. J. Physiol. **250:** E486–E493.
18. HRABOVSZKY, E. *et al.* 2000. Detection of estrogen receptor-beta messenger ribonucleic acid and 125I-estrogen binding sites in luteinizing hormone-releasing hormone neurons of the rat brain. Endocrinology **141**: 3506–3509.
19. SKYNNER, M.J., J.A. SIM & A.E. HERBISON. 1999. Detection of estrogen receptor alpha and beta messenger ribonucleic acids in adult gonadotropin-releasing hormone neurons. Endocrinology **140:** 5195–5201.
20. CHARLES, A.C. & T.G. HALES. 1995. Mechanisms of spontaneous calcium oscillations and action potentials in immortalized hypothalamic (GT1-7) neurons. J. Neurophysiol. **73:** 56–64.
21. VAN GOOR, F. *et al.* 1999. Coordinate regulation of gonadotropin-releasing hormone neuronal firing patterns by cytosolic calcium and store depletion. Proc. Natl. Acad. Sci. USA **96:** 4101–4106.
22. TERASAWA, E. *et al.* 1999. Intracellular Ca(2+) oscillations in luteinizing hormone-releasing hormone neurons derived from the embryonic olfactory placode of the rhesus monkey. J. Neurosci. **19:** 5898–5909.

23. NUNEMAKER, C.S., M. STRAUME, R.A. DEFAZIO & S.M. MOENTER. 2003. Gonadotropin-releasing hormone neurons generate interacting rhythms in multiple time domains. Endocrinology **144**.
24. NILSSON, S., S. MAKELA, E. TREUTER, *et al.* 2001. Mechanisms of estrogen action. Physiol Rev. **81:** 1535–1565.
25. KELLY, M.J. *et al.* 1999. Rapid effects of estrogen to modulate G protein-coupled receptors via activation of protein kinase A and protein kinase C pathways. Steroids **64:** 64–75.
26. LAGRANGE, A.H., O.K. RONNEKLEIV & M.J. KELLY. 1997. Modulation of G protein-coupled receptors by an estrogen receptor that activates protein kinase A. Mol. Pharmacol. **51:** 605–612.
27. LUTHER, J.A. & J.G. TASKER. 2000. Voltage-gated currents distinguish parvocellular from magnocellular neurones in the rat hypothalamic paraventricular nucleus. J. Physiol. **523:** 193–209.
28. MAGEE, J.C. & M. CARRUTH. 1999. Dendritic voltage-gated ion channels regulate the action potential firing mode of hippocampla CA1 pyramidal neurons. J. Neurophysiol. **82:** 1895–1901.
29. EVANS, N.P. *et al.* 1995. Estradiol induces both qualitative and quantitative changes in the pattern of gonadotropin-releasing hormone secretion during the presurge period in the ewe. Endocrinology **136:** 1603–1609.

Ovarian Steroid and Growth Factor Regulation of Female Reproductive Function Involves Modification of Hypothalamic α_1-Adrenoceptor Signaling

ANNE M. ETGEN

Department of Neuroscience, Albert Einstein College of Medicine, Bronx, New York 10461, USA

ABSTRACT: The ovarian steroids estradiol (E_2) and progesterone (P) act on target neurons in the hypothalamus and preoptic area to coordinate the expression of female reproductive behaviors with the timing of the preovulatory luteinizing hormone (LH) surge. This chapter will summarize evidence that E_2 and P facilitation of the receptive component of female reproductive behavior, lordosis, involves changes in both the expression of and intracellular signal transduction pathways engaged by α_1-adrenergic receptors in the hypothalamus and preoptic area. The α_1-adrenoceptors are thought to mediate the facilitatory effects of the catecholamine neurotransmitter norepinephrine on both lordosis behavior and LH release. E_2 first induces the expression of the α_{1B}-adrenergic receptor subtype in the hypothalamus and preoptic area. P then acts in an E_2-dependent manner to promote linkage of hypothalamic α_1-adrenoceptors to an intracellular signaling pathway involving nitric oxide and cyclic GMP. This chapter will also describe recent findings that implicate brain insulin-like growth factor-I (IGF-I) receptors as obligatory co-mediators of hormonal regulation of hypothalamic α_1-adrenoceptors and female neuroendocrine function. Additional studies suggest that E_2 and IGF-I facilitate lordosis behavior by activating kinases traditionally associated with growth factor signal transduction (mitogen-activated protein kinases and phosphatidlyinositol-3-kinases). These molecular events are proposed to help coordinate the timing of ovulation with the expression of sexual receptivity, thereby maximizing reproductive success.

KEYWORDS: estradiol; progesterone; insulin-like growth factor-I; hypothalamus; female reproductive function; signal transduction

INTRODUCTION

The long-term objective of this research is to understand how the ovarian steroids, estradiol (E_2) and progesterone (P), act in the brain to govern female reproductive physiology. To accomplish this goal, we study specific biochemical and behavioral

Address for correspondence: Anne Etgen, Ph.D., Department of Neuroscience, Albert Einstein College of Medicine, 1300 Morris Park Avenue, Bronx, NY 10461. Voice: 718-430-3662; fax: 718-430-8654.

etgen@aecom.yu.edu

Ann. N.Y. Acad. Sci. 1007: 153–161 (2003).
doi: 10.1196/annals.1286.015

effects of E_2 and P in the hypothalamus and preoptic area. In rodents and a variety of other mammals, expression of the female receptive posture (lordosis behavior) depends on sequential exposure of neurons in the hypothalamus and preoptic area to E_2 and P.[1–3] It should be emphasized that hormones do not simply "elicit"or "activate" lordosis; rather, the hormonal milieu determines the probability that animals display the behavior in response to appropriate sensory stimulation.[4] Thus, E_2 and P must alter synaptic transmission in hypothalamic neural circuits underlying lordosis. Ovarian steroids also work in these brain areas to determine the timing and magnitude of the preovulatory luteinizing hormone (LH) surge,[5] ensuring that females are behaviorally receptive when the likelihood of fertilization is high. A major goal of our research is to delineate how E_2 and P modulate neurotransmission in the hypothalamic and preoptic area neurons to coordinate the timing of reproductive behavior, especially lordosis, with preovulatory LH secretion.

Others and we have shown that hormone treatments that are sufficient to reinstate mating behavior and LH surges in ovariectomized animals alter the release of a variety of neurotransmitters and neuromodulatory peptides in the hypothalamus and preoptic area (see Etgen[6]). Nonetheless, it is apparent that one cannot attribute hormonal regulation of female reproductive function solely to changes in transmitter release. None of the neurotransmitters and neuropeptides whose release changes in association with reproductive behavior or gonadotropin release can induce either receptive behavior or LH secretion unless the relevant neurons have first been exposed to E_2 and/or P. For example, the catecholamine neurotransmitter norepinephrine (NE), which has been the focus of much of our work, has no effect on mating behavior and actually inhibits LH release when administered to ovariectomized animals. However, ovariectomized females primed with physiologically relevant doses of E_2 exhibit robust LH surges and lordosis behavior in response to NE.[5–8] Therefore, we have explored the cellular and molecular mechanisms by which ovarian hormones alter the behavioral and neuroendocrine responses to NE. This article focuses on evidence that E_2 and P regulate both the expression of a specific NE receptor subtype, the α_{1B}-adrenoceptor, in the hypothalamus and preoptic area and the linkage of hypothalamic α_1-adrenoceptors to specific intracellular signal transduction pathways. We will also describe recent findings that implicate brain insulin-like growth factor-I (IGF-I) receptors as obligatory co-mediators of hormonal regulation of hypothalamic α_1-adrenoceptors and female neuroendocrine function.

E_2 AND P MODULATION OF α_1-ADRENERGIC RECEPTOR EXPRESSION AND SIGNAL TRANSDUCTION

E_2 Increases the Expression and Function of α_{1B}-Adrenergic Receptors in Hypothalamus and Preoptic Area

Behavioral and neuroendocrine studies implicate α_1-adrenergic receptors as the mediators of NE facilitation of both lordosis behavior and LH release.[8–15] As noted above, NE stimulates LH secretion and enhances lordosis responding only in E_2-exposed animals. Hence it is reasonable to hypothesize that ovarian steroids might regulate α_1-adrenergic receptor expression in the hypothalamus and preoptic area. Early studies that used ligand binding methods to quantify α_1-adrenergic receptor levels as a function of hormone treatment yielded inconsistent results (see Refs. 6 and 8 for reviews). Our initial studies using the antagonist ligand ^{3}H-prazosin to assess α_1-adrenergic receptor levels in hypothalamic and preoptic area membranes detected small but statistically significant (e.g., 30%) increases in the density of α_1-adrenergic binding sites in these two brain areas two days after E_2 was administered to ovariectomized rats.[16] However, with the availability of pharmacological tools that could distinguish between two receptor subtypes, the α_{1A}- and the α_{1B}-adrenoceptor, we were able to demonstrate that E_2 selectively regulated the α_{1B}-adrenoceptor.[17] In ovariectomized control rats, the predominant α_1-adrenergic receptor expressed in both the hypothalamus and preoptic area is the α_{1A}-adrenoceptor, and its levels are unchanged by estrogen treatment. By contrast, α_{1B}-adrenoceptors are expressed at extremely low levels in ovariectomized rats, and their density increases markedly in response to two days of E_2 priming. P neither increases nor decreases the density of either receptor subtype when given alone or after estrogen treatment. Later studies showed that the increased density of α_{1B}-adrenoceptor binding sites correlated with increased levels of α_{1B}-adrenoceptor mRNA in the hypothalamus and preoptic area.[18] We have also used an antibody selective for the α_{1B}-adrenoceptor to characterize the distribution of these receptors in the hypothalamus of female rats.[19]

The findings summarized above suggest that enhanced expression of a specific NE receptor subtype represents one important mechanism by which E_2 alters the responses of hypothalamic neurons to NE. We have also evaluated α_1-adrenoceptor signal transduction by measuring the generation of second messengers in response to pharmacological activation of these receptors in brain slices from hormone-treated animals. The α_1-adrenergic receptors couple primarily to $G\alpha_q$, thereby stimulating phospholipase C to generate diacylglycerol (DAG) and inositol triphosphate (IP_3). DAG can activate protein kinase C, which in a number of brain regions can potentiate adenylyl cyclase-mediated cyclic AMP synthesis (see Petitti and Etgen[20]), while IP_3 interacts with receptors on the endoplasmic reticulum to mobilize intracellular calcium. We observed that α_1-adrenoceptor potentiation of cyclic AMP accumulation markedly increases in hypothalamic and preoptic area slices from E_2-primed females.[21] However, when P is administered to estrogen-primed rats, it reconfigures hypothalamic α_1-adrenergic signaling, abolishing augmentation of adenylyl cyclase and attenuating phospholipase C-dependent synthesis of IP_3.[22,23] Yet as noted above, it is clear that in animals treated with both E_2 and P, α_1-adrenergic receptors are functional and mediate the facilitatory actions of NE on lordosis behavior and LH release. Therefore, we next determined which intracellular signaling pathways are activated upon ligand binding to α_1-adrenoceptors in the hypothalamus and preoptic area of E_2- and P-treated rats. Specifically, we tested the hypotheses (1) that α_1-adrenoceptors enhance lordosis by activating the nitric oxide (NO)/cyclic GMP signaling pathway, and (2) that coupling of α_1-adrenoceptors to this signal transduction pathway is hormone-dependent.

In E_2-Primed Rats, P Promotes Linkage of α_1-Adrenergic Receptor Activation to the NO/cGMP Pathway

Brain slice experiments showed that basal levels of cyclic GMP were significantly higher in hypothalamus and preoptic area from animals treated with E_2 and P when compared to ovariectomized controls or females treated with only E_2 or P. When slices from ovariectomized female rats were incubated with NE or the α_1-adrenoceptor agonist phenylephrine, cyclic GMP accumulation was observed only in slices derived from females treated with both E_2 and P prior to experimentation. To verify that α_1-adrenoceptor stimulation induces cyclic GMP synthesis by activation of NO synthase (NOS), some slices were incubated with NOS inhibitors. The NOS inhibitors not only blocked NE-stimulated cyclic GMP formation in hypothalamic/preoptic area slices, but they also significantly reduced basal levels of cyclic GMP. The latter finding suggests that most of the cellular cyclic GMP in the hypothalamus and preoptic area is derived from NO stimulation of soluble guanylyl cyclase. We also conducted behavioral studies demonstrating that intracerebroventricular infusion of the cyclic GMP analogue, 8-br-cyclic GMP, reverses the inhibitory effects of the α_1-adrenoceptor antagonist prazosin on lordosis behavior in E_2 and P-treated female rats.[24,25] Thus, our data suggest that the NO/cyclic GMP pathway mediates the facilitatory effects of α_1-adrenoceptors on lordosis behavior in female rats, and that prior exposure of the hypothalamus and preoptic area to both E_2 and P is required to link α_1-adrenoceptors to this pathway.

FUNCTIONAL INTERACTIONS AMONG E_2, INSULIN-LIKE GROWTH FACTOR-I (IGF-I), AND α_1-ADRENOCEPTORS

Because there is considerable evidence that growth factors, which often signal by activation of tyrosine kinases, can engage in "cross-talk" with G protein–coupled receptor signal transduction,[25–28] we began to explore this interaction in brain slices. We were particularly interested in examining whether IGF-I might influence NE receptor signaling. A possible role for IGF-I in estrogen action in the hypothalamus was first proposed by Toran-Allerand and colleagues, who showed that E_2 and insulin have synergistic effects on neurite outgrowth in fetal hypothalamic explants, probably via interactions with IGF-I receptors.[29] Since then, several laboratories have reported that concurrent activation of estrogen receptors and IGF-I receptors is required for the effects of E_2 and IGF-I on neuronal survival,[30–33] neurite outgrowth in cultured neurons,[34,35] and synaptic and glial plasticity in the adult hypothalamus.[36–38] Our initial findings raised the possibility that IGF-I and α_1-adrenergic receptors may interact in the hypothalamus and preoptic area during the period of behavioral receptivity and the LH surge. When we preincubated hypothalamic slices with IGF-I for 15 minutes, we observed a significant enhancement of NE stimulation of cyclic AMP synthesis, but only if the slices were prepared from females treated with E_2 for two days before experimentation.[39] Interestingly, pharmacological studies showed that IGF-I potentiates cyclic AMP responses to NE by modifying α_1-adrenoceptor augmentation of adenylyl cyclase activity. IGF-I facilitation of the cyclic AMP response to NE was blocked by application of the specific IGF-I receptor antagonist JB-1 onto the slices, indicating that the acute effect of the growth factor on α_1-adrenergic receptor function was mediated by IGF-I receptors.

There are at least two possible explanations for the E_2-dependence of the IGF-I/α_1-adrenoceptor interaction. The density of IGF-I binding sites in the hypothalamus and preoptic area was modestly but significantly increased by estrogen treatment.[39] Thus, increased expression of IGF-I receptors may be necessary to support cross-talk between the growth factor and the NE receptor signal transduction machinery. Alternatively, it may be that IGF-I specifically targets the α_{1B}-adrenoceptor subtype, whose expression is estrogen-regulated.[17] When we examined the intrahypothalamic distribution of α_{1B}-adrenoceptor immunostaining in female rats, we noted the intense labeling of fibers in the arcuate-median eminence. The arcuate nucleus also demonstrated some cell body labeling.[19] These regions of the hypothalamus are critically involved in gonadotropin-releasing hormone release and represent sites of E_2 action in regulation of the preovulatory LH surge, a neuroendocrine event that involves activation of α_1-adrenergic receptors. Garcia-Segura and colleagues have also demonstrated E_2- and IGF-I-dependent synaptic remodeling in this area.[37,40,41]

INVOLVEMENT OF BRAIN IGF-I RECEPTORS IN REPRODUCTIVE ACTIONS OF E_2 IN THE HYPOTHALAMUS

These observations led us to hypothesize that brain IGF-I receptors may be involved in E_2 induction of α_{1B}-adrenoceptor expression in reproductively relevant brain regions. Therefore, we infused the selective IGF-I receptor antagonist JB-1 or saline vehicle into the third ventricle of ovariectomized female rats at 12-h intervals, beginning 1 hour before the first of two E_2 injections.[42] Ligand binding studies showed that blockade of IGF-I receptors during the period of estrogen priming abolishes E_2 induction of α_{1B}-adrenoceptor binding in the hypothalamus and preoptic area. Because α_1-adrenoceptors mediate NE enhancement of female reproductive behavior and LH release, we then determined whether brain IGF-I receptor signaling is also necessary for E_2 facilitation of lordosis behavior and gonadotropin release. Indeed we found that i.c.v. infusion of the IGF-I receptor antagonist during the two-day estrogen priming period completely eliminated hormone-dependent LH release and significantly attenuated lordosis behavior. Reproductive behavior was restored by i.c.v. infusion of 8-bromo-cyclic GMP, the second messenger implicated in α_1-adrenergic facilitation of lordosis. IGF-I receptor blockade inhibited lordosis if JB-1 was infused throughout the two-day estrogen treatment period but not if it was administered only during the first or last 12 hours of estrogen treatment or just prior to P administration. These data document the existence of a novel mechanism by which IGF-I participates in the remodeling of NE receptor signaling in the hypothalamus and preoptic area following E_2 treatment. Moreover, we can speculate that these molecular events may help coordinate the timing of ovulation with the expression of sexual receptivity.

We are now attempting to identify downstream signal transduction pathways that underlie the E_2/IGF-I facilitation of lordosis behavior. Both E_2 and IGF-I can act independently or synergistically to stimulate serine-threonine kinases associated with growth factor action.[43–47] The two most intensely studied pathways are those involving mitogen-activated protein kinase (MAPK), especially the p42/44 MAPKs, and phosphatidylinositol-3-kinase (PI3K). Therefore, we utilized i.c.v. infusion of MAPK and PI3K inhibitors during a two-day estrogen priming period to test the hypothesis that one or both of these signal transduction pathways mediates E_2 facilitation of lordosis. When infused individually during estrogen priming, PI3K inhibitors (wortmannin and LY294002) and MAPK inhibitors (PD98059 and U0126) partially attenuate lordosis behavior. None of these drugs modifies lordosis if it is infused only once, during the last 12 hours of estrogen treatment. When both wortmannin and PD98059 are infused together during E_2 priming, lordosis is completely abolished.[48] These data suggest that activation of both PI3K and MAPK by E_2 and IGF-I may be required for hormonal facilitation of lordosis behavior.

HOW DO E_2 AND IGF-I INTERACT?

The requirement for ongoing brain IGF-I receptor activity to support the priming effects of E_2 on hypothalamic neurons involved in female reproductive function points to either common downstream targets of E_2 and IGF-I receptors, or some mechanism whereby one receptor regulates the activity of the other. Although the precise molecular mechanisms by which E_2 and IGF-I interact are unclear, recent studies provide direct evidence for the formation of a supramolecular complex involving estrogen receptor-α (ERα), the IGF-I receptor and PI3K *in vitro* and *in vivo*. Application of E_2 to mammalian cells expressing ERα (but not ERβ) promotes rapid phosphorylation of endogenous IGF-I receptors and p42/44 MAPKs. In addition, estrogen promotes rapid binding of ERα to the IGF-I receptor.[49] It is well known that ERs and IGF-I receptors are coexpressed in neurons throughout the brain.[50] Systemic administration of E_2 to ovariectomized female rats promotes formation of a supramolecular complex involving ERα, IGF-I receptor, the p85 subunit of PI3K and insulin receptor substrate-1 in the hypothalamus.[51] Moreover, E_2 and IGF-I act synergistically to induce prolonged increases in phosphorylation of the PI3K substrate Akt in the hypothalamus.[45]

Previous studies of cross-talk between IGF-I receptors and ERα were unable to determine whether these receptors interact within individual neurons, through communication between neurons, or via neuronal-glial interactions. Glia have been implicated in estrogen-induced neurite outgrowth,[36,52–54] but it is not clear whether this is the only mechanism through which IGF-I receptors and ERs interact. Therefore, we used PC12 cells to examine these interactions in the absence of glia. PC12 cells are commonly used for studying neurite outgrowth, and Lustig *et al.* [55] previously showed that PC12 cells stably transfected with ERα elaborate neurites in response to E_2. We replicated this finding and also showed that IGF-I promotes neurite outgrowth in these cells. Moreover, inhibition of ERα with the antagonist ICI-182,780 blocks the neurite-promoting effects of both E_2 and IGF-I. Likewise, inhibition of IGF-I receptor with the antagonist JB-1 blocks the neurite-promoting effects of both IGF-I and E_2 (Topalli and Etgen, in review). Thus, concurrent activation of both receptors is necessary to induce neurite outgrowth in PC12 cells, and receptor cross-talk within a single cell is sufficient for hormone-dependent neurite formation and outgrowth.

SUMMARY AND SPECULATIONS

We speculate that E_2 and IGF-I may work together to promote biochemical (and perhaps anatomical) synaptic remodeling in reproductively relevant hypothalamic neural circuits that utilize NE as a neurotransmitter. Modulation of hypothalamic NE signal transduction by IGF-I and E_2 involves changes in both NE receptor expression (i.e., induction of α_{1B}-adrenoceptors) and signal transduction. Moreover, our data suggest that sequential exposure of hypothalamic neurons to E_2 followed by P reconfigures the biochemical responses of these neurons to α_1-adrenergic receptor activation. These molecular events are proposed to help coordinate the timing of ovulation with the expression of sexual receptivity, thereby maximizing reproductive success.

ACKNOWLEDGMENTS

This work was supported by DHHS Grants R37 MH41414 and R01 HD29856 and by the Department of Neuroscience, Albert Einstein College of Medicine. Drs. Maricedes Acosta-Martinez, Hsiao-Pai Chu, and Arnulfo Quesada carried out much of the work described in this article. Experiments with PC12 cells were conducted by Ilir Topalli. The technical assistance of Jun (Alice) Shu in carrying out some of the behavioral studies is gratefully acknowledged. Recombinant IGF-I was provided by Dr. Arthur Parlow and the National Hormone and Pituitary Program, NIDDK.

REFERENCES

1. Barfield, R.J. *et al.* 1982. Sites of action of ovarian hormones in the regulation of oestrous responsiveness in rats. *In* Hormones and Behaviour in Higher Vertebrates. J. Balthazart, E. Prove & R. Gilles, Eds.: 2–18. Springer-Verlag. Berlin.
2. Whalen, R.E. 1974. Estrogen-progesterone induction of mating in female rats. Horm. Behav. **5:** 157–162.
3. Pfaff, D.W. *et al.* 1994. Cellular and molecular mechanisms of female reproductive behaviors. *In* The Physiology of Reproduction, Vol. 2. E. Knobil & J. D. Neill, Eds.: 107–220. Raven Press. New York.
4. Etgen, A.M. *et al.* 1999. Hormonal integration of neurochemical and sensory signals governing female reproductive behavior. Behav. Brain Res. **105:** 93–103.
5. Freeman, M.E. 1994. The neuroendocrine control of the ovarian cycle in the rat. *In* The Physiology of Reproduction. E. Knobil & J.D. Neill, Eds.: 613–658. Raven Press. New York.
6. Etgen, A.M. 2002. Estrogen regulation of neurotransmitter and growth factor signaling in the brain. *In* Hormones, Brain and Behavior, Vol. 3. D.W. Pfaff *et al.*, Eds.: 381–440. Academic Press. San Diego, CA.
7. Taleisnik, S. & C.H. Sawyer. 1986. Activation of the CNS noradrenergic system may inhibit as well as facilitate pituitary luteinizing hormone release. Neuroendocrinology **44:** 265–268.
8. Etgen, A.M., S. Ungar & N. Petitti. 1992. Estradiol and progesterone modulation of norepinephrine neurotransmission: implications for the regulation of female reproductive behavior. J. Neuroendocrinology. **31:** 799–807.
9. Barraclough, C.A. & P.M. Wise. 1982. The role of catecholamines in the regulation of pituitary luteinizing hormone and follicle-stimulating hormone secretion. Endocr. Rev. **3:** 91–119.
10. Chappel, S.C. 1985. Neuroendocrine regulation of luteinizing hormone and follicle stimulating hormone: a review. Life Sci. **36:** 97–103.
11. Etgen, A.M. 1990. Intrahypothalamic implants of noradrenergic antagonists disrupt lordosis behavior in female rats. Physiol. Behav. **48:** 31–36.
12. Kow, L.M. & D.W. Pfaff. 1995. Functional analyses of α_1-adrenoceptor subtypes in rat hypothalamic ventromedial nucleus neurons. Eur. J. Pharmacol. **282:** 199–206.
13. Rosie, R., B.E. Sumner & G. Fink. 1994. An α_1 adrenergic mechanism mediates estradiol stimulation of LHRH mRNA synthesis and estradiol inhibition of POMC mRNA synthesis in the hypothalamus of the prepubertal female rat. J. Steroid Biochem. Mol. Biol. **49:** 399–406.

14. WEESNER, G.D., L.C. KREY & D.W. PFAFF. 1993. α_1 adrenergic regulation of estrogen-induced increases in luteinizing hormone-releasing hormone mRNA levels and release. Brain Res. Mol. Brain Res. **17:** 77–82.
15. YANG, S.P. *et al.* 1998. Attenuation of gonadotropin-releasing hormone reflex to coitus by α_1-adrenergic receptor blockade in the rabbit. Proc. Soc. Exp. Biol. Med. **218:** 204–209.
16. ETGEN, A.M. & G.B. KARKANIAS. 1990. Estradiol regulates the number of α_1- but not β- or α_2-noradrenergic receptors in hypothalamus of females rats. Neurochem. Int. **16:** 1–9.
17. PETITTI, N., G.B. KARKANIAS & A.M. ETGEN. 1992. Estradiol selectively regulates α_{1B} -noradrenergic receptors in the hypothalamus and preoptic area. J. Neurosci. **12:** 3869–3876.
18. KARKANIAS, G.B., M.A. ANSONOFF & A.M. ETGEN. 1996. Estradiol regulation of α_{1b}-adrenoceptor mRNA in female rat hypothalamus-preoptic area. J. Neuroendocrinol. **8:** 449–455.
19. ACOSTA-MARTINEZ, M. *et al.* 1999. Localization of α_{1B}-adrenergic receptor in female rat brain regions involved in stress and neuroendocrine function. Neurochem Int. **35:** 383–391.
20. PETITTI, N. & A.M. ETGEN. 1991. Protein kinase C and phospholipase C mediate α_1- and β-adrenoceptor intercommunication in rat hypothalamic slices. J. Neurochem. **56:** 628–635.
21. PETITTI, N. & A.M. ETGEN. 1990. α_1-adrenoceptor augmentation of β-stimulated cAMP formation is enhanced by estrogen and reduced by progesterone in rat hypothalamic slices. J. Neurosci. **10:** 2842–2849.
22. PETITTI, N. & A.M. ETGEN. 1992. Progesterone promotes rapid desensitization of α_1-adrenergic receptor augmentation of cAMP formation in rat hypothalamic slices. Neuroendocrinology **55:** 1–8.
23. KARKANIAS, G.B., N. PETITTI & A.M. ETGEN. 1995. Progesterone attenuation of α_1-adrenergic receptor stimulation of phosphoinositol hydrolysis in hypothalamus of estrogen-primed female rats. Endocrinology **136:** 1993–1999.
24. CHU, H.P. & A.M. ETGEN. 1999. Ovarian hormone dependence of α_1-adrenoceptor activation of the nitric oxide-cGMP pathway: relevance for hormonal facilitation of lordosis behavior. J. Neurosci. **19:** 7191–7197.
25. KAROOR, V. *et al.* 1996. Regulating expression and function of G-protein-linked receptors. Prog. Neurobiol. **48:** 555–568.
26. LIEBMANN, C. *et al.* 1996. Tyrosine phosphorylation of GSα and inhibition of bradykinin-induced activation of the cyclic AMP pathway in A431 cells by epidermal growth factor receptor. J. Biol. Chem. **271:** 31098–31105.
27. WILLIAMS, N.G., H. ZHONG & K.P. MINNEMAN. 1998. Differential coupling of α_1-, α_2- and β-adrenergic receptors to mitogen-activated protein kinase pathways and differentiation in transfected PC12 cells. J. Biol. Chem. **273:** 24624–24632.
28. MURGA, C. *et al.* 1998. Activation of Akt/protein kinase B by G protein-coupled receptors. A role for α and $\beta\gamma$ subunits of heterotrimeric G proteins acting through phosphatidylinositol-3-OH kinaseγ. J. Biol. Chem. **273:** 19080–19085.
29. TORAN-ALLERAND, C.D., L. ELLIS & K.H. PFENNINGER. 1988. Estrogen and insulin synergism in neurite growth enhancement in vitro: mediation of steroid effects by interactions with growth factors? Brain Res. **469:** 87–100.
30. CARDONA-GOMEZ, G.P. *et al.* 2001. Interactions of estrogens and insulin-like growth factor-I in the brain: implications for neuroprotection. Brain Res. Brain Res. Rev. **37:** 320–334.
31. GARCIA-SEGURA, L.M. *et al.* 1996. Interaction of the signalling pathways of insulin-like growth factor-I and sex steroids in the neuroendocrine hypothalamus. Horm. Res. **46:** 160–164.
32. AZCOITIA, I., A. SIERRA & L.M. GARCIA-SEGURA. 1999. Neuroprotective effects of estradiol in the adult rat hippocampus: interaction with insulin-like growth factor-I signalling. J. Neurosci. Res. **58**: 815–822.
33. GARCIA-SEGURA, L.M. *et al.* 2000. Insulin-like growth factor-I receptors and estrogen receptors interact in the promotion of neuronal survival and neuroprotection. J. Neurocytol. **29:** 425–437.

34. CAMBIASSO, M.J., J.A. COLOMBO & H.F. CARRER. 2000. Differential effect of oestradiol and astroglia-conditioned media on the growth of hypothalamic neurons from male and female rat brains. Eur. J. Neurosci. **12:** 2291–2298.
35. AGRATI, P. *et al.* 1997. SK-ER3 neuroblastoma cells as a model for the study of estrogen influence on neural cells. Brain Res. Bull. **44:** 519–523.
36. FERNANDEZ-GALAZ, M.C. *et al.* 1997. Role of astroglia and insulin-like growth factor-I in gonadal hormone-dependent synaptic plasticity. Brain Res. Bull. **44:** 525–531.
37. FERNANDEZ-GALAZ, M.C., F. NAFTOLIN & L. M. GARCIA-SEGURA. 1999. Phasic synaptic remodeling of the rat arcuate nucleus during the estrous cycle depends on insulin-like growth factor-I receptor activation. J. Neurosci. Res. **55:** 286–292.
38. CARDONA-GOMEZ, G.P. *et al.* 2000. Estrogen receptors and insulin-like growth factor-I receptors mediate estrogen-dependent synaptic plasticity. Neuroreport **11:** 1735–1738.
39. QUESADA, A. & A.M. ETGEN. 2001. Insulin-like growth factor-1 regulation of α_1-adrenergic receptor signaling is estradiol dependent in the preoptic area and hypothalamus of female rats. Endocrinology **142:** 599–607.
40. GARCIA-SEGURA, L.M., D. BAETENS & F. NAFTOLIN. 1986. Synaptic remodelling in arcuate nucleus after injection of estradiol valerate in adult female rats. Brain Res. **366:** 131–136.
41. GARCIA-SEGURA, L.M. *et al.* 1994. Gonadal hormones as promoters of structural synaptic plasticity: cellular mechanisms. Prog. Neurobiol. **44:** 279–307.
42. QUESADA, A. & A.M. ETGEN. 2002. Functional interactions between estrogen and insulin-like growth factor- I in the regulation of α_{1B}-adrenoceptors and female reproductive function. J. Neurosci. **22:** 2401–2408.
43. LEROITH, D. *et al.* 1995. Molecular and cellular aspects of the insulin-like growth factor I receptor. Endocr Rev. **16**: 143–163.
44. TORAN-ALLERAND, C.D. 2000. Novel sites and mechanisms of oestrogen action in the brain. *In* Neuronal and Cognitive Effects of Oestrogens. D. Chadwick & J. Goode, Eds.: 56–73. John Wiley. West Sussex, England.
45. CARDONA-GOMEZ, G.P., P. MENDEZ & L.M. GARCIA-SEGURA. 2002. Synergistic interaction of estradiol and insulin-like growth factor-I in the activation of PI3K/Akt signaling in the adult rat hypothalamus. Brain Res. Mol. Brain Res. **107:** 80–88.
46. SINGH, M. 2001. Ovarian hormones elicit phosphorylation of Akt and extracellular-signal regulated kinase in explants of the cerebral cortex. Endocrine **14:** 407–415.
47. WATTERS, J.J. *et al.* 1997. Rapid membrane effects of steroids in neuroblastoma cells: effects of estrogen on mitogen activated protein kinase signalling cascade and c-fos immediate early gene transcription. Endocrinology **138:** 4030–4033.
48. ETGEN, A.M. & M. ACOSTA-MARTINEZ. 2003. Participation of growth factor signal transduction pathways in estradiol facilitation of female reproductive behavior. Endocrinology **144:** 3828–3835.
49. KAHLERT, S. *et al.* 2000. Estrogen receptor α rapidly activates the IGF-1 receptor pathway. J. Biol. Chem. **275:** 18447–18453.
50. CARDONA-GOMEZ, G.P., L. DONCARLOS & L.M. GARCIA-SEGURA. 2000. Insulin-like growth factor I receptors and estrogen receptors colocalize in female rat brain. Neuroscience **99:** 751–760.
51. MENDEZ, P., I. AZCOITIA & L.M. GARCIA-SEGURA. 2003. Estrogen receptor α forms estrogen-dependent multimolecular complexes with insulin-like growth factor receptor and phosphatidylinositol 3-kinase in the adult rat brain. Brain Res. Mol. Brain Res. **112:** 170–176.
52. MELCANGI, R.C., L. MARTINI & M. GALBIATI. 2002. Growth factors and steroid hormones: a complex interplay in the hypothalamic control of reproductive functions. Prog. Neurobiol. **67:** 421–449.
53. MUDD, L. M. *et al.* 1998. Effects of growth factors and estrogen on the development of septal cholinergic neurons from the rat. Brain Res. Bull. **45**: 137–142.
54. GARCIA-SEGURA, L.M. *et al.* 1999. Role of astroglia in estrogen regulation of synaptic plasticity and brain repair. J. Neurobiol. **40:** 574–584.
55. LUSTIG, R.H. *et al.* 1994. An in vitro model for the effects of estrogen on neurons employing estrogen receptor-transfected PC12 cells. J. Neurosci. **14:** 3945–3957.

Steroid Hormones and Growth Factors Act in an Integrated Manner at the Levels of Hypothalamic Astrocytes

A Role in the Neuroendocrine Control of Reproduction

MARIARITA GALBIATI, SIMONA SAREDI, AND ROBERTO C. MELCANGI

Department of Endocrinology and Center of Excellence on Neurodegenerative Diseases, Via Balzaretti 9, 20133, Milan, Italy

ABSTRACT: Several growth factors (e.g., transforming growth factors beta and alpha, basic fibroblast growth factor), produced by hypothalamic astrocytes, participate in the control of hypothalamic gonadotrophin-releasing hormone (GnRH) neurons. On this basis, we have hypothesized that steroid hormones, like estrogens and progestagens, influence the GnRH neurons by modulating in glial cells the synthesis and the release of these growth factors. Data reported here indicate that the expression of transforming growth factor beta 1 is modulated in hypothalamic astrocytes by a progesterone derivative (i.e., dihydroprogesterone), while estrogens modulate that of basic fibroblast growth factor. Moreover, it is interesting to highlight that the effect of estrogens on basic fibroblast growth factor is mediated by another growth factor (i.e., transforming growth factor alpha). Altogether, the present findings support the concept that steroid hormones and growth factors act in an integrated manner at the level of hypothalamic astrocytes, thus adding a further piece of knowledge in the understanding of the mechanisms controlling GnRH neurons.

KEYWORDS: hypothalamus; GnRH; estrogen; progesterone; astrocyte; TGFβ; TGFα; bFGF

INTRODUCTION

Hypothalamic gonadotrophin-releasing hormone (GnRH) neurons represent a key factor in the regulation of the reproductive functions. They belong to a complex system called the "GnRH network" that also comprises glial cells and other neurons, and which integrates all internal and external factors regulating the reproductive functions.

Among the molecules involved in the control of GnRH neurons, steroid hormones certainly have a pivotal role because they may provide either positive or negative feedback signals modulating the synthesis and release of GnRH. The mechanisms

Address for correspondence: Mariarita Galbiati, Department of Endocrinology and Center of Excellence on Neurodegenerative Diseases, Via Balzaretti 9, 20133, Milan, Italy. Voice: +39-02-50318237; fax: +39-02-50318204.
rita.galbiati@unimi.it

Ann. N.Y. Acad. Sci. 1007: 162–168 (2003). © 2003 New York Academy of Sciences. doi: 10.1196/annals.1286.016

through which gonadal steroids exert their modulatory actions on the GnRH network are not completely clear. Three hypotheses may be considered: (1) a direct effect on steroid receptors present in GnRH neurons themselves; (2) an indirect effect via interneuronal systems possessing steroid receptors and transferring the information via classical neurotransmitters or neuropeptides; and (3) an indirect effect on glial cell via the activation of glial steroid receptors. Among these, only the second hypothesis is well established,[1] while the first (i.e., whether GnRH neurons express steroid receptors) is still controversial despite recent studies that have provided consistent evidence for the expression of estrogen receptors in GnRH neurons of rodents.[2] Regarding the third hypothesis, many observations obtained in our and in other laboratories indicate that glial cells may modulate the activity of GnRH neurons in two different manners: (1) changing their ensheathment around GnRH neurons and consequently the synaptic inputs to these neurons[3] and (2) releasing different growth factors, such as transforming growth factor β1 (TGFβ1) and β2 (TGFβ2), transforming growth factor (TGFα), and basic fibroblast growth factor (bFGF).[4,5]

These growth factors influence GnRH neurons in many different ways. For instance, it has been demonstrated that TGFβ may act directly on native GnRH neurons and on GT1-1 cells (a line of hypothalamic immortalized GnRH-secreting neurons) via the interaction with its specific receptors modulating the synthesis and the release of GnRH.[6–9] Also, bFGF acts directly on these neurons, promoting the neuronal differentiation and facilitating the conversion of GnRH prohormone into the mature decapeptide.[10] In contrast, TGFα acts in an indirect manner. In particular, it stimulates the secretion of GnRH via the activation of receptors not located on GnRH neurons, but rather on glial cells.[5,11] Activation of these receptors induces the production and the secretion of prostaglandin E2, which then binds to specific receptors on GnRH neurons to facilitate the decapeptide secretion.[5,12]

On the basis of the observations mentioned thus far, we have taken into consideration the hypothesis that the feedback control exerted by steroid hormones on GnRH neurons might be mediated, at the level of astrocytes, by growth factors (i.e., TGFβ1 and bFGF). This hypothesis is also supported by the fact that astrocytes possess both classical (e.g., estrogen and progesterone receptors) and nonclassical (e.g., $GABA_A$ receptor) steroid receptors and consequently may be considered a target for the action of steroids.[13]

Effect of Progesterone and Its Derivatives on Growth Factors at the Level of Hypothalamic Astrocytes

The first experimental approach to test the above hypotheses has been to verify whether progesterone (P) and/or its 5α- and 3α-5α-derivatives (respectively, DHP and THP) are able to modulate the gene expression of TGFβ1 and bFGF in glial cells. To this purpose, we have evaluated the gene expression of TGFβ1 in type 1 astrocytes, which represent the major component of mixed glial cultures obtained from neonatal rat hypothalamus, after treatment with P or its derivatives. The results obtained indicate that after 6 h of exposure not only P, but also DHP and THP, is able to stimulate the mRNA levels of TGFβ1. On the contrary, on longer exposure (24 h), only DHP and THP may increase the gene expression of TGFβ1.[14] These observations suggest that the effect of P might be ascribed to its conversion into DHP and into THP. DHP, like

TABLE 1. Effect of treatment with THP or muscimol for 6 and 24 h on TGFβ1 gene expression in hypothalamic type 1 astrocyte cultures

	TGFβ1 mRNA/28S rRNA (% of control)	
	6 h	24 h
Controls	100 ± 3 (8)	100 ± 6 (6)
THP (10 nM)	165 ± 25* (6)	145 ± 12* (7)
Muscimol (1 mM)	95 ± 10 (4)	81 ± 8 (4)

Quantitative data (after normalization with 28S rRNA) are expressed as percent vs. the levels found in control cultures and represent the mean ± SEM of the determinations performed (numbers in parentheses). *P <0.05 vs. controls.

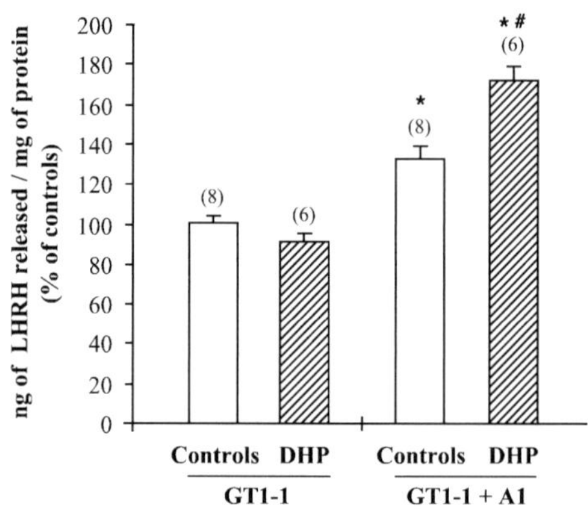

FIGURE 1. Effect of DHP on GnRH release from GT1-1 cells alone or in co-culture with type 1 astrocytes (A1). The GnRH released in the culture medium was measured by RIA after 8 h of exposure to DHP. Values are expressed as percent vs. the levels found in GT1-1 control cultures. Each bar represents the mean ± SEM of determinations performed (numbers in the parentheses). *P <0.01 vs. GT1-1 control cultures. #P <0.01 vs. co-culture controls.

P, is able to bind to the P receptor (PR), while THP is a well-known ligand of the $GABA_A$ receptor.[13] Moreover, because the conversion of DHP into THP is a reversible process, THP may also be retroconverted into DHP, with a consequent binding to PR. In order to evaluate whether $GABA_A$ receptor may be involved in the effect of THP on TGFβ1 expression, we have exposed type 1 astrocytes to muscimol, a $GABA_A$ receptor agonist, and we have evaluated the mRNA levels of TGFβ1 by Northern blot analysis. As shown in TABLE 1, it is evident that, at variance to what was observed with THP, muscimol does not modulate the gene expression of TGFβ1. These findings suggest that the effects of DHP on TGFβ1 expression, as well as those of THP (after its retroconversion into DHP), might be ascribed to the interaction with PR.

The effects of P derivatives in type 1 astrocytes are peculiar for TGFβ1 gene expression because they are not able to affect the gene expression of bFGF in this kind of cells.[14]

To support the concept that the feedback control of progestagens—and in particular of DHP—on GnRH neurons might be mediated by glial cells, we have analyzed the effect of this steroid on GnRH secretion from GT1-1 cells in the presence or absence of hypothalamic type 1 astroctyes (FIG. 1). The data obtained indicate that DHP does not influence directly the release of GnRH from GT1-1 cells, but when applied in the presence of glial cells it is able to significantly intensify the stimulatory effect of the co-culture on GnRH secretion.

Altogether, this set of experiments indicates that progestagens, and in particular DHP, may influence the release of GnRH from GT1-1 cells acting in an indirect manner (i.e., inducing, via the P receptor, the synthesis of TGFβ1 in astrocytes). This hypothesis seems to be in line with a model proposed by Herbison and colleagues, in which P and DHP are supposed to act on GnRH neurons with an indirect trans-synaptic mechanism.[15]

Effect of 17β-Estradiol on the Synthesis of Growth Factors in Type 1 Astrocytes

Recent observations have indicated that estrogens are able to affect TGFβ1 secretion in the medium of cultured hypothalamic astrocytes,[16] while no information is available on the effects of estrogens on bFGF at the level of hypothalamic astrocytes. To this purpose, we decided to evaluate the effects of 17β-estradiol on the synthesis of bFGF in hypothalamic type 1 astrocytes. As shown in FIGURE 2, 17β-estradiol, both at concentrations of 10^{-9} and 10^{-10} M, proved able to increase the mRNA levels of bFGF measured by RNase protection assay. These observations are in agreement with our previous *in vivo* studies indicating that a single treatment of 17β-estradiol for 48 h is able to increase the messenger levels of bFGF in the hypothalamus of ovariectomized rats.[17] The observations obtained *in vitro* also indicate that the effects of estrogen on bFGF need 24 h to become evident; consequently, we have taken into consideration the possibility that the effects of 17β-estradiol on bFGF synthesis might be indirect. In particular, as a possible mediator, we considered another growth factor, the TGFα, because it is known to be produced by hypothalamic astrocytes under the influence of estrogens and it is able to stimulate the synthesis and release of GnRH from hypothalamic neurons.[5] We analyzed first the synthesis of bFGF in type 1 astrocytes after the exposure to TGFα. As shown in FIGURE 3, TGFα is able to induce the gene expression of bFGF at all times of exposure considered. At this point, we directly evaluated whether TGFα may be the mediator of the effect of 17β-estradiol on bFGF. We exposed hypothalamic type 1 astrocytes to 17β-estradiol in the presence or absence of an antibody raised against the TGFα receptor.[18] The results obtained have indicated that, after the blockade of the TGFα receptor, 17β-estradiol is no longer able to increase mRNA levels of bFGF (TABLE 2). Altogether, this set of experiments indicates that at the level of hypothalamic astrocytes the effects of 17β-estradiol on the synthesis of bFGF are mediated by TGFα.

It is important to remember that bFGF is not directly involved in the control of GnRH release, but that it is able to enhance the processing of the GnRH prohormone;[10] and furthermore that our previous *in vivo* observations[17] have indicated a peak of the gene expression of this growth factor in the late phase of the proestrus when the secretion of the gonadotrophins has already been initiated. For these rea-

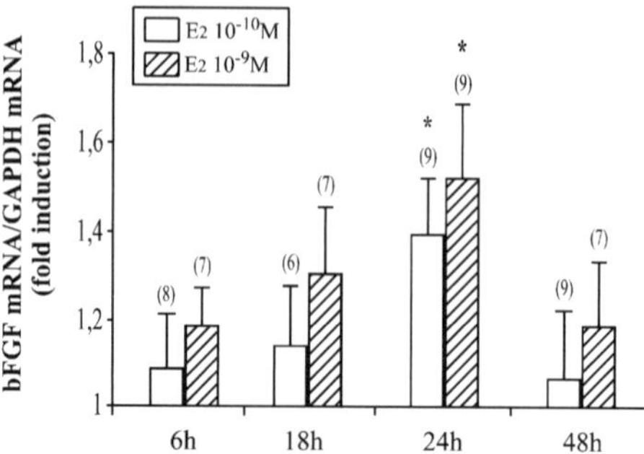

FIGURE 2. Effect of treatment of female rat hypothalamic type 1 astrocytes cultures with 17β-estradiol (E2) at different concentrations (10^{-9} M and 10^{-10} M) for 6, 18, 24, and 48 h on bFGF mRNA levels. Quantitative data (after normalization with GAPDH mRNA) are expressed as mean ± SEM of the fold induction relative to the controls. Numbers in the parentheses represent the number of determinations performed. *P <0.05 vs. controls.

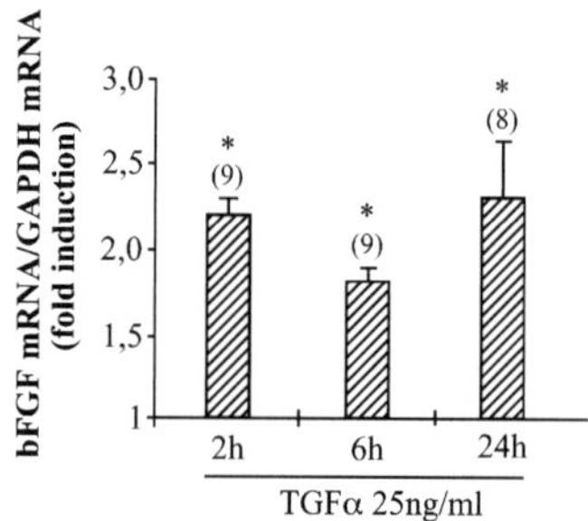

FIGURE 3. Effect of treatment of female rat hypothalamic type 1 astrocytes cultures with TGFα for 2, 6, and 24 h on bFGF mRNA levels. Quantitative data (after normalization with GAPDH mRNA) are expressed as mean ± SEM of the fold induction relative to the controls. Numbers in the parentheses represent the number of determinations performed. *P <0.05 vs. controls.

TABLE 2. Effect of treatment with 17β-estradiol (E2) on bFGF gene expression in hypothalamic type 1 astrocyte cultures in the presence or absence of an antibody raised against TGFα receptor

	bFGF mRNA/GAPDH mRNA (% of control)
Controls	100 ± 10 (7)
E2 10^{-9} M	143 ± 7* (6)
Anti TGFα-R	90 ± 22 (5)
E2 + Anti TGF-R	102 ± 10 (7)

Quantitative data (after normalization with GAPDH mRNA) are expressed as percent vs. the levels found in control cultures and represent the mean ± SEM of the determinations performed (numbers in parentheses). *P <0.05 vs. controls.

sons and on the basis of *in vitro* observations discussed previously, we are tempted to propose that bFGF plays a role in the control of replenishment of GnRH in hypothalamic neurons when the stores of the hormone have been depleted after the peak secretion of luteinizing hormone and follicle-stimulating hormone.

CONCLUSIONS

The present data further suggest that steroids deriving from peripheral glands are able to control GnRH neurons, also modulating the activity of the surrounding glial cells. In these cells, and in particular in hypothalamic astrocytes, steroid hormones are able to affect the synthesis of different growth factors (i.e., TGFα, TGFβ1, and bFGF), which then are able to modulate the synthesis and the release of GnRH.

ACKNOWLEDGMENTS

Financial support from MURST "FIRST—Special Project" and the Commission of the European Communities, specific RTD program (Quality of Life and Management of Living Resources, contract QLK6-CT-2000-00179) is gratefully acknowledged.

REFERENCES

1. Herbison, A.E. 1998. Multimodal influence of estrogen upon gonadotropin-releasing hormone neurons. Endocr. Rev. **19:** 302–330.
2. Herbison, A.E. & J.-R. Pape. 2001. New evidence for estrogen receptors in gonadotropin-releasing hormone neurons. Front. Neuroendocrinol. **22:** 292–308.
3. Silverman, A., I. Livne & J.W. Witkin. 1994. The gonadotrophin releasing hormone (GnRH) neuronal systems: immunocytochemistry and in situ hybridization. *In* The Physiology of Reproduction. E. Knobil & J.D. Neill, Eds.: 1683–1706. Raven Press. New York.
4. Melcangi, R.C., L. Martini & M. Galbiati. 2002. Growth factors and steroid hormones: a complex interplay in the hypothalamic control of reproductive functions. Prog. Neurobiol. **67:** 421–449.
5. Ojeda, S.R. & Y.J. Ma. 1999. Glial-neuronal interactions in the neuroendocrine control of mammalian puberty: facilitatory effects of gonadal steroids. J. Neurobiol. **40**: 528–540.
6. Melcangi, R.C., M. Galbiati, E. Messi, *et al.* 1995. Type 1 astrocytes influence luteinizing hormone-releasing hormone release from the hypothalamic cell line GT1-1: is transforming growth factor-β the principle involved? Endocrinology **136**: 679–686.
7. Galbiati, M., M. Zanisi, E. Messi, *et al.* 1996. Transforming growth factor-β and astrocytic conditioned medium influence luteinizing hormone-releasing hormone gene expression in the hypothalamic cell line GT1. Endocrinology **137:** 5605–5609.
8. Messi, E., M. Galbiati, V. Magnaghi, *et al.* 1999. TGFβ2 is able to modify mRNA levels and release of luteinizing hormone releasing hormone in a immortalized hypothalamic cell line (GT1-1). Neurosci. Lett. **270:** 165–168.
9. Prevot, V., S. Bouret, D. Croix, *et al.* 2000. Evidence that members of the TGFα superfamily play a role in regulation of the GnRH neuroendocrine axis: expression of a type I serine-threonine kinase receptor for TGFα and activin in GnRH neurones and hypothalamic areas of the female rat. J. Neuroendocrinol. **12:** 665–670.

10. WETSEL, W.C., D.F. HILL & S.R. OJEDA. 1996. Basic fibroblast growth factor regulates the conversion of pro-luteinizing hormone releasing hormone (pro-LHRH) to LHRH in immortalized hypothalamic neurons. Endocrinology **137:** 2606–2616.
11. MA, Y.J., K. BERG-VON DER EMDE, F. RAGE, *et al.* 1997. Hypothalamic astrocytes respond to transforming growth factor alpha with secretion of neuroactive substances that stimulate the release of luteinizing hormone releasing hormone. Endocrinology **138:** 19–25.
12. RAGE, F., D.F. HILL, M. SENA-ESTEVES, *et al.* 1997. Targeting transforming growth factor alpha expression to discrete loci of the neuroendocrine brain induces female sexual precocity. Proc. Natl. Acad. Sci. USA **94:** 2735–2740.
13. MELCANGI, R.C., V. MAGNAGHI, M. GALBIATI, *et al.* 2001. Glial cells: a target for steroid hormones. Prog. Brain Res. **132:** 31–40.
14. MELCANGI, R.C., I. CAVARRETTA, V. MAGNAGHI, *et al.* 2001. Interactions between growth factors and steroids in the control of LHRH neurons. Brain Res. Rev. **37:** 223–234.
15. SIM, J.A., M.J. SKYNNER & A.E HERBISON. 2001. Direct regulation of postnatal GnRH neurons by the progesterone derivative allopregnanolone in the mouse. Endocrinology **142:** 4448–4453.
16. BUCHANAN, C.D., V.B. MAHESH & D.W. BRANN. 2000. Estrogen-astrocyte-luteinizing hormone-releasing hormone signaling: a role for transforming growth factor β1. Biol. Reprod. **62:** 1710–1721.
17. GALBIATI, M., V. MAGNAGHI, L. MARTINI, *et al.* 2001. Hypothalamic transforming growth factor β1 and basic fibroblast growth factor mRNA expression is modified during the rat oestrous cycle. J. Neuroendocrinol. **13:** 483–489.
18. GALBIATI, M., L. MARTINI & R.C. MELCANGI. 2002. Oestrogens, via transforming growth factor alpha, modulate basic fibroblast growth factor synthesis in hypothalamic astrocytes: in vitro observations. J. Neuroendocrinol. **14:** 829–835.

Seasonal Regulation of Reproductive Activity in Sheep

Modulation of Access of Sex Steroids to the Brain

JEAN-CLAUDE THIERY AND BENOIT MALPAUX

Neurobiologie et Maîtrise des Fonctions Saisonnières, UMR 6073 INRA/CNRS/Université de Tours, 37380 Nouzilly, France

ABSTRACT: Sheep in temperate latitudes are seasonal breeders. In female sheep, ovarian activity decreases during the anestrous period due to modification of secretion of luteinizing hormone (LH). The seasonal changes in the hormonal LH pattern mainly reflect an increase in the brain responsiveness to the negative feedback exerted by estradiol during long days (LD) on the frequency of pulsatile LH secretion, under neurohormonal GnRH control. The resulting seasonal inhibition of LH secretion mainly involves the activation of dopaminergic systems by E2, which in turn inhibits the GnRH cells from the preoptico-hypothalamic structures. The increased responsiveness of the brain during LD could lead to increased expression of central E2 receptors. In addition, our study shows that steroid access to the brain could be modulated by photoperiodism, thus increasing the availability of steroids to the nervous structures during LD.

KEYWORDS: female sheep; progesterone; estradiol; brain; blood–brain barrier

INTRODUCTION

The ewe is a seasonal breeder. The breeding season (a succession of 16–18 day-long estrous cycles) begins at the end of summer and finishes in late winter or at the very beginning of spring. This is followed by the anestrous period that shows no ovarian cyclicity.[1] In males, seasonal modulation is also clearly observed not as an all-or-nothing condition, but quantitatively with a decrease in quality and quantity of sperm output.[2] These seasonal changes depend on photoperiod variations and can be mimicked under an artificial light regimen of constant long days (LD: 16 h of light/8 h of darkness) or short days (SD: 8 h of light/16 h of darkness). Day-length is translated into a hormonal signal by secretion of melatonin from the pineal gland during the dark period (see Ref. 3 for review). After a number of predominantly unidentified intermediate stages, the change in reproductive status is controlled by modifications in the activity of the gonadotrophic axis through variations in secretion of pulsatile

Address for correspondence: Jean-Claude Thiery, Neurobiologie et Maîtrise des Fonctions Saisonnières, UMR 6073 INRA/CNRS/Université de Tours, 37380 Nouzilly, France. Voice: 33 2 47427976; fax: 33 2 47427743.
thiery@tours.inra.fr

Ann. N.Y. Acad. Sci. 1007: 169–175 (2003). © 2003 New York Academy of Sciences.
doi: 10.1196/annals.1286.017

luteinizing hormone (LH), which in turn controls gonadal activity. This has been demonstrated in the model of ovariectomized ewes with a subcutaneous 17b-E2 implant that releases a constant amount of this hormone throughout the year. In this experimental situation, LH pulse frequency is reduced during the anestrous period of intact females or during constant LD.[4,5] Thus, the variation in seasonal inhibition of LH pulsatility results mainly from an increase of brain sensitivity to the negative E2 feedback on the LH pulse frequency during the LD of spring and summer. Similarly, a moderate increase in progesterone negative feedback is observed at that time.[4]

SEASONAL REGULATION OF HYPOTHALAMIC GnRH ACTIVITY

Since LH secretion depends on pulsatile stimulation by the hypothalamic gonadotropin-releasing hormone, GnRH, the photoperiodic control of sexual activity in the ewe results from the control of the neurons that release this neuropeptide. Even though E2-receptors (ER) of β type (ERβ) on the GnRH cells from the mouse and rat have been demonstrated, the paucity of data in sheep does not allow a similar direct action to be assumed in sheep.[3] The anterior part of the hypothalamus, whose destruction blocks the anestrous period,[6] contains A15 and A14 dopaminergic nuclei of the retrochiasmatic area. In ovariectomized ewes supplemented with a subcutaneous E2 implant and in intact ewes during the anestrous season, lesions in the dopaminergic A15 nuclei and A14 nuclei stimulate LH pulsatile secretion.[3] During LD, the use of an intracranial implantation of E2 shows that this steroid acts directly on the lateral retrochiasmatic area, probably in the A15 nucleus, to control LH pulsatile secretion.[7] Thus, dopamine from the A15 nucleus is an intermediate in the E2 negative feedback loop that decreases LH pulsatility in ewes during LD. However, the molecular mechanism involved in the action of E2 on dopaminergic cells remains unknown. There is an expression of mRNA for the ERα and ERβ in the A15 nucleus in female and male sheep, but the receptors themselves have not been identified yet, although their presence has been clearly demonstrated in other hypothalamic nuclei.[3] Several studies indicate that dopamine acts on GnRH in the median eminence involving D2 receptors.[8–11] In addition, recent data[12] have shown a link between the A15 nucleus and the GnRH cell bodies from the mediobasal hypothalamus, a group of cells potentially involved in regulating pulsatile secretion.[13] Thus, the inhibition of GnRH cell activity during anestrous could depend on actions in the terminals from the median eminence as well as at the level of the cell bodies. Other studies have investigated neurotransmitters in relation to the seasonal control of reproduction in sheep, but in less detail. Noradrenaline could interact with the negative feedback effect of E2 on LH secretion in the hypothalamus, while serotonin could also be involved in the inhibition of LH secretion during long days, but in an E2-independent mechanism. Inhibitory or excitatory amino acids could also play a role in the seasonal control of reproduction in the ewe, but their site of action in the brain remains unidentified.[3] In addition, it has been shown that GnRH cells from the preoptic area (POA) undergo morphological changes in relation to the season. Indeed, a greater number of dendritic processes occur during the anestrous season,[14] as well as an increase in the innervation of preoptic GnRH elements during the breeding season.[15] Furthermore, the expression of the polysialylated form of neural cell adhesion molecule (PSA-NCAM) associated with GnRH neurons changes seasonally. This suggests a possible seasonal plasticity in adult GnRH neurons.[16]

POSSIBLE MECHANISMS INVOLVED IN THE SEASONAL SHIFT IN RESPONSIVENESS TO STEROIDS

Few reports deal with the mechanism responsible for the seasonal shift in responsiveness to steroids. Photoperiodic change in the distribution of ER has been investigated in female sheep under various photoperiodic regimens. In the POA, a larger number of ERa have been observed during LD than SD.[17] More recently, a population of neurons showing specific ERα immunoreactivity has been identified in ewes in the ventral POA close to the organum vasculosum of the lamina terminalis.[18] These neurons are activated, as seen by the stimulation of Fos protein expression, by subcutaneous implantation of E2 in ovariectomized ewes only during the seasonal anestrous period. Moreover, implantation of E2 in the POA induces an inhibition of LH pulses during LD[19] in a similar way to that in the A15 nucleus.[7]

Apart from the changes in expression of steroid receptors, our laboratory has suggested another mechanism that could also be involved in the photoperiodic shift in steroid responsiveness. In the literature, an active participation of the blood–brain barrier in the physiological regulation of energy metabolism[20,21] and an increased permeability of the blood–brain barrier in nonpathological aging, have been suggested.[22,23] It is therefore tempting to speculate that subtle modifications of the blood–brain barrier permeability modulate the action of peripheral factors at the level of the brain in physiological situations. In addition to the alterations that have been observed in neurons bearing steroid receptors during these periods of increased brain responsiveness,[17,18] it is possible that an increased availability of the steroids in the brain is involved (FIG. 1). As a consequence, we tested the hypothesis that photoperiodicity can modulate the passage of sex steroids through the blood–brain barrier.

First, we showed that in ovariectomized ewes the content of progesterone (P) in the tissues of POA was higher in LD than in SD after the same peripheral treatment (chronic release of physiological levels delivered by intravaginal device, termed "CIDR," InterAg, Hamilton, New Zealand). In contrast, its metabolites 5α-dihydroprogesterone and 3α-hydroxy-5α-pregnane-20-one were not different in relation to the photoperiod in the same structure. Thus, our data suggest a modification of uptake from the brain rather than a change in metabolism within the brain. Furthermore, in ewes equipped with an intracerebral cannula for *in vivo* collection of cerebrospinal fluid (CSF), we saw that injection into the carotid artery of a massive dose of hydrosoluble, cyclodextrin-P (10 mg) resulted in detectable P in the CSF only during LD.[24] Finally, we showed that a physiological amount of P given by CIDR could also generate a threefold higher concentration of P in CSF during LD than during SD, while the concentration of the steroid in blood plasma was equal in LD and SD females.

Second, we extended the study to E2 passage from the peripheral blood stream to the CSF. We compared the E2 concentrations in the CSF between ovariectomized ewes bred during LD and ewes bred during SD, before E2 substitutive treatment, and 21 h after receiving a 2-cm subcutaneous E2 implant and 21 h after receiving a 4-cm additional subcutaneous E2 implant. The concentrations of E2 during the control pe-

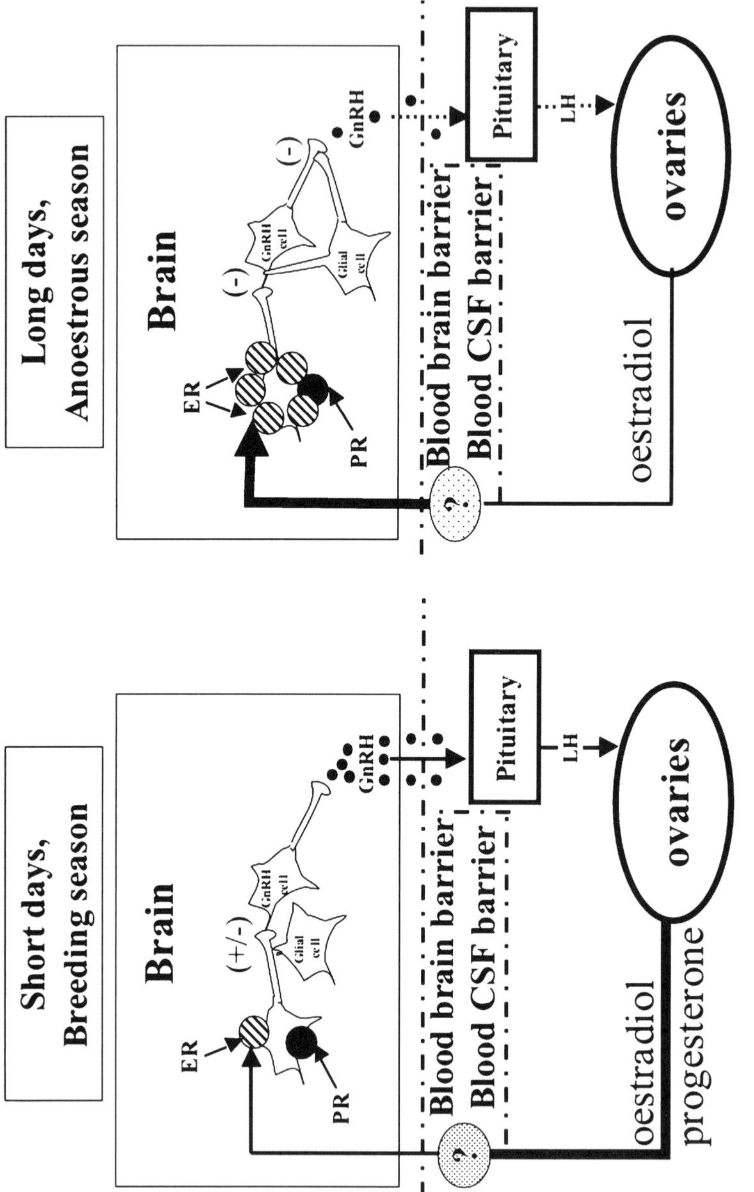

FIGURE 1. *See following page for legend.*

riod did not differ during the first hour. The E2 concentration after 21 h with a 2-cm implant that yielded an estimated plasma concentration of about 2 pg/mL became significantly higher in LD than in SD ewes. The difference in concentration of E2 again increased in LD ewes after 21 h with a 6-cm implant yielding an estimated plasma concentration of about 15 pg/mL, similar to the preovulatory concentration of E2 during the estrous cycle.

Third, we compared a group of ovariectomized ewes with a group of castrated rams, both bearing a subcutaneous E2 implant. The CSF from females and males were sampled during LD and after a shift in the light regimen to SD—after 10 SD and 25 SD (when LH is inhibited), respectively, and after 70 SD in females or 55 SD in males (when LH is stimulated). In females, E2 in CSF fell from 43.3 ± 17.9 pg/mL during LD to 3.7 ± 0.7 pg/mL, 8.5 ± 3.2 pg/mL, and 7 ± 1.4 pg/mL after 10, 25, and 70 SD, respectively. In males, during LD, E2 in the CSF (9.2 ± 2.6 pg/mL) was lower than in females and did not change significantly during SD (8.1 ± 2.6 pg/mL, 6.1 ± 1.5 pg/mL, and 7.4 ± 1.9 pg/mL for 10, 25, and 55 SD, respectively).

CONCLUSION

The results obtained with P and E2 taken together demonstrated an effect of day-length on the access of sex steroids to the brain in ovariectomized ewes. This phenomenon could play a role in the photoperiodic changes in brain responsiveness to steroids. The effect appears to be limited to females. Further experiments are required to demonstrate the physiological impact of a modulating brain supply of sex steroids in nongonadectomized sheep. Due to their lipophilic nature, steroids penetrate the brain easily, but recent results have shown that active transporters in the blood–brain barrier can limit the access of steroids from peripheral vasculature.[25,26] In our model, the putative transporters and hormonal intermediates involved in the photoperiodic modulation of access of sex sterioids to the brain remain to be identified.

REFERENCES

1. Ortavant, R., J. Pelletier, J.P. Ravault, *et al.* 1985. Photoperiod, main proximal and distal factor of the circannual cycle of reproduction in farm animal. Oxford Rev. Reprod. Biol. **7:** 562–571.
2. Dacheux, J.L., C. Pisselet, M.R. Blanc, *et al.* 1981. Seasonal variations in rete testis fluid secretion and sperm production in different breeds of ram. J. Reprod. Fertil. **61:** 363–371.

FIGURE 1. Diagram representing mechanisms involved in the photoperiodic regulation of reproductive activity in female sheep. During the breeding season in short days, estradiol and progesterone from the ovaries act on their respective receptors (ER and PR) in the brain to control positively and negatively (+/–) the GnRH-producing cells. During the anestrous season in long days, there is no progesterone due to the lack of corpus luteum that results from absence of ovulation. Estradiol acts on an increased number of receptors to stimulate the structures inhibiting GnRH cells (–).[17,18] Glial-cell plasticity at that time also could modulate the control of GnRH cells.[16] Higher blood–brain barrier permeability during long days could also increase the estradiol availability for its receptors, thus amplifying the negative feedback effect.

3. THIERY, J.C., P. CHEMINEAU, S. HERNANDEZ, *et al.* 2002. Neuroendocrine interactions and seasonality. Dom. Anim. Endocr. **23:** 87–100.
4. GOODMAN, R.L., E.L. BITTMAN, D.L. FOSTER & F.J. KARSCH. 1982. Alterations in the control of luteinizing hormone pulses frequency underlie the seasonal variation in estradiol negative feedback in the ewe. Biol. Reprod. **27:** 580–589.
5. MARTIN, G.B., R.J. SCARAMUZZI & J.D. HENSTRIDGE. 1983. Effects of oestradiol, progesterone and androstenedione on the pulsatile secretion of luteinizing hormone in ovariectomized ewes during spring and autumn. J. Endocrinol. **96:** 181–193.
6. PRZEKOP, F. 1978. Effect of anterior deafferentation of the hypothalamus on the release of luteinizing hormone (LH) and reproduction in sheep. Acta Physiol. Pol. **29:** 293–307.
7. GALLEGOS-SANCHEZ, J., B. DELALEU, A. CARATY, *et al.* 1997. Estradiol acts locally within the retrochiasmatic area to inhibit pulsatile luteinizing-hormone release in the female sheep during anestrus. Biol. Reprod. **56:** 1544–1549.
8. THIERY, J.C. 1991. Monoamine content of the stalk-median eminence and hypothalamus in adult female sheep as affected by daylength. J. Neuroendocrinol. **3:** 407–411.
9. VIGUIE, C., S. PICARD, J.C. THIERY & B. MALPAUX. 1998. Blockade of tyrosine hydroxylase activity in the median eminence partially reverses the long day-induced inhibition of pulsatile LH secretion in ewe. J. Endocrinol. **10:** 551–558.
10. HAVERN, R.L., C.S. WHISNANT & R.L. GOODMAN. 1991. Hypothalamic sites of catecholamine inhibition of luteinizing hormone in the anestrous ewes. Biol. Reprod. **44:** 476–482.
11. BERTRAND, F., C. VIGUIE, S. PICARD & B. MALPAUX. 1998. Median eminence dopaminergic activation is critical for the early long-day inhibition of luteinizing hormone secretion in the ewe. Endocrinology **139:** 5094–5102.
12. COOLEN, L.M., H.T. JANSEN, R.L. GOODMAN, *et al.* 1999. A new method for simultaneous demonstration of anterograde and retrograde connections in the brain: co-injections of biotinylated dextran amine and the beta subunit of cholera toxin. J. Neurosci. Methods **91:** 1–8.
13. BOUKHLIQ, R., R.L. GOODMAN, S.J. BERRIMAN, *et al.* 1999. A subset of gonadotropin-releasing hormone neurons in the ovine medial basal hypothalamus is activated during increased pulsatile luteinizing hormone secretion. Endocrinology **140:** 5929–5536.
14. LEHMAN, M.N., J.E. ROBINSON, F.J. KARSCH & A.J. SILVERMAN. 1986. Immunocytochemical localization of luteinizing hormone-releasing hormone (LHRH) pathways in the sheep brain during anoestrus and the mid-luteal phase of the estrous cycle. J. Comp. Neurol. **244:** 19–35.
15. XIONG, J.J., F.J. KARSCH & M.N. LEHMAN. 1997. Evidence for seasonal plasticity in the gonadotropin-releasing hormone (GnRH) system of the ewe: changes in synaptic inputs onto GnRH neurons. Endocrinology **138:** 1240–1250.
16. VIGUIE, C., H.T. JANSEN, J.D. GLASS, *et al.* 2001. Potential for polysialylated form of neural cell adhesion molecule-mediated neuroplasticity within the gonadotropin-releasing hormone neurosecretory system of the ewe. Endocrinology **142:** 1317–1324.
17. SKINNER, D.C. & A.E. HERBISON. 1997. Effects of photoperiod on estrogen receptor, tyrosine hydroxylase, neuropeptide Y, and beta-endorphin immunoreactivity in the ewe hypothalamus. Endocrinology **138:** 2585–2595.
18. STEFANOVIC, I., B. ADRIAN, H.T. JANSEN, *et al.* 2000. The ability of estradiol to induce fos expression in a subset of estrogen receptor-alpha-containing neurons in the preoptic area of the ewe depends on reproductive status. Endocrinology **141:** 190–196.
19. ANDERSON, G.M., J.M. CONNORS, S.L. HARDY, *et al.* 2001. Oestradiol microimplants in the ventromedial preoptic area inhibit secretion of luteinizing hormone via dopamine neurones in anoestrous ewes. J. Neuroendocrinol. **13:** 1051–1058.
20. BANKS, W.A., A. MOINUDDIN & J.E. MORLEY. 2001. Regional transport of TNF-alpha across the blood-brain barrier in young ICR and young and aged SAMP8 mice. Neurobiol. Aging **22:** 671–676.
21. KASTIN, A.J. & V. AKERSTROM. 2001. Glucose and insulin increase the transport of leptin through the blood-brain barrier in normal mice but not in streptozotocin-diabetic mice. Neuroendocrinology **73:** 237–242.

22. McLay, R.N., A.J. Kastin & J.E. Zadina. 2000. Passage of interleukin-1-beta across the blood-brain barrier is reduced in aged mice: a possible mechanism for diminished fever in aging. Neuroimmunomodulation **8:** 148–153.
23. Preston, J.E. 2001. Ageing choroid plexus-cerebrospinal fluid system. Microsc. Res. Technol. **52:** 31–37.
24. Thiery, J.C., P. Robel, S. Canepa, *et al.* 2003. Passage of progesterone into the brain changes with photoperiod in the ewe. Eur. J. Neurosci. **18:** 895–901.
25. Nishino, J., H. Suzuki, D. Sugiyama, *et al.* 1999. Transepithelial transport of organic anions across the choroid plexus: possible involvement of organic anion transporter and multidrug resistance-associated protein. J. Pharmacol. Exp. Ther. **290:** 289–294.
26. Schinkel, A.H., E. Wagenaar, L. van Deemter, *et al.* 1995. Absence of the mdr1a P-glycoprotein in mice affects tissue distribution and pharmacokinetics of dexamethasone, digoxin, and cyclosporin-A. J. Clin. Invest. **96:** 1698–1705.

Two Perspectives on the Origin of Sex Differences in the Brain

ARTHUR P. ARNOLD,[a] EMILIE F. RISSMAN,[b] AND GEERT J. DE VRIES[c]

[a]*Department of Physiological Science, and Laboratory of Neuroendocrinology of the Brain Research Institute, University of California, Los Angeles, California 90095, USA*

[b]*Department of Biochemistry & Molecular Genetics, University of Virginia, Charlottesville, Virginia 22908, USA*

[c]*Center for Neuroendocrine Studies, University of Massachusetts, Amherst, Massachusetts 01003, USA*

Abstract: Most sex differences in brain function are attributed to sex differences in the effects of gonadal secretions. In addition, however, male and female cells differ because of differential effects of sex chromosome genes expressed within the cells themselves. The latter conclusion comes from numerous studies in which sexual phenotype appears to be insensitive to the effects of sex hormones during development or cases in which sex differences develop before the onset of sex-specific patterns of gonadal secretions. Recently, mouse models have become available in which the genetic sex of brain cells is independent of the gonadal type (testes vs. ovaries), which allows a test of the role of sex chromosome genes in brain development. This paper reviews the evidence that genetic sex of brain cells influences their sexual phenotype, and critically discusses the relative advantages of various experimental approaches to study this effect.

Keywords: sex chromosomes; sexual differentiation; Y chromosome; X chromosome; songbird; genetic models

TWO VIEWS OF SEXUAL DIFFERENTIATION

Almost a century ago, Lillie[1] and Keller and Tandler[2] published observations on freemartin cattle, suggesting strongly that the sexual phenotype of reproductive tissues develops under control of endocrine secretions carried in the blood. Female freemartin calves share their fetal blood supply with a male twin, resulting in masculinization of some of their reproductive tissues (genitals, gonads, etc.). The humoral masculinizing factors, they concluded, derived from the male. The same factors likely were responsible for determining the masculine phenotype of the normal male's own reproductive organs. These ideas were conclusively supported by the classic experiments of Jost in the late 1940s,[3] who manipulated gonadal secretions

Address for correspondence: Arthur P. Arnold, Department of Physiological Science, UCLA, 641 Charles Young Drive South, Room 4117, Los Angeles, California 90095-1606, USA. Voice: 310-825-2169; fax: 310-825-8081.
arnold@ucla.edu

**Ann. N.Y. Acad. Sci. 1007: 176–188 (2003). © 2003 New York Academy of Sciences.
doi: 10.1196/annals.1286.018**

prenatally to prove that fetal secretion of testosterone from the testes was responsible for masculine (male-typical) differentiation of the genitalia (penis, scrotum) and Wolffian ducts. Jost also inferred the existence of a testicular Müllerian inhibiting hormone that causes involution of the Müllerian structures in males.[4] In 1959, Young and colleagues suggested that testicular secretions also induce masculine differentiation of the brain because they found that female guinea pigs given testosterone during fetal life displayed more masculine behavior and less feminine behavior than normal females.[5] These classic experiments, and many others performed subsequently, gave rise to the important conclusion that many tissues of the body are sexually differentiated permanently by the action of gonadal hormones, especially testosterone and its metabolite estradiol.[6–8] The effects of gonadal hormones are impressive, and thus the study of sexual differentiation has appropriately focused on the mechanisms of hormonal action. Moreover, the dominant effects of gonadal hormones suggested that other factors need not be invoked to explain sexual differentiation. For example, because XX and XY individuals both develop a masculine phenotype if they are exposed to testicular secretions during fetal or neonatal periods of development, it appears that an XX or XY genotype is not a pervasive determinant of phenotypic sex.

In its extreme form, the dogma of gonadal origin of somatic sexual differentiation has a corollary, usually implicit, that XX and XY cells are functionally equivalent unless gonadal secretions act on them in a sex-specific fashion. This corollary conflicts with another perspective that emerged from studies of genes encoded on the sex chromosomes. Starting around the turn of the twentieth century, various investigators linked phenotypic sex to the sex chromosomes in several invertebrate organisms. By 1920, for example, the sex of *Drosophila* was found to be related to the number of X chromosomes, not the presence or absence of the Y chromosome, because XO flies are male.[9] Similarly, a mechanism that measures X gene dosage determines sex in the nematode *Caenorhabditis elegans.*[10] Not until 1959 was it established that the mammalian Y chromosome plays a dominant male-determining role (XO humans and mice have ovaries and XXY individuals have testes).[11] The testis-determining gene on the mammalian Y chromosome is *Sry*, which is necessary and sufficient to cause the formation of testes in mice.[12] The *Sry* gene is transiently expressed in the undifferentiated gonadal ridge of XY embryos, where it acts to initiate a complex cascade of molecular and cellular events that lead to formation of the testis. Thus, cell-autonomous sexual differentiation, caused by an unequal effect of sex chromosome genes, occurs in numerous unrelated animal species, either because of the male-specific action of Y genes or the difference in dose of X genes.

What features of the X and Y chromosomes influence our thinking about their potential to differentiate XX and XY cells? Could X gene dosage contribute to the difference in XX and XY cells in mammals, as in flies and *C. elegans*? In each of these species, mechanisms exist to reduce the effect of the sex difference in X gene dosage, presumably because the balance of X gene dose to autosomal gene dose is important for healthy functioning of individuals of both sexes. That balance would be disrupted in one sex if the X genes were expressed at a much higher level in females than in males. In mammals, dosage compensation is accomplished by X-inactivation, in which one of the two X chromosomes is transcriptionally silenced in each nongermline cell.[13] X-inactivation is incomplete and imperfect, however, because some X genes escape inactivation,[14] and thus XX cells probably are not equivalent to XY cells in dosage of all X genes. The mammalian Y chromosome is small and heterochromatic.[15] The human Y chromosome encodes only 27 different proteins.[16] In mice, only 12 Y-linked genes have been identified to date. Eight Y genes are expressed in the brain of males and could have a male-specific effect on the brain (discussed further in Refs. 17 and 18). Finally, dosage of X and Y genes is not the only difference between XX and XY cells attributed to the sex chromosomes. XX cells contain an X chromosome that received a paternal genomic imprint, whereas XY cells do not. These differences in genomic imprinting could contribute to cell-autonomous differences in male and female cells.[19,20]

This discussion highlights the inherent nonequivalence of XX and XY cells, at least in some tissues and at specific times of development. Accordingly, studies of the sex chromosomes and genetics of sex determination evoke a different attitude towards sexual differentiation of the brain than do studies coming from the endocrine tradition. Although no one doubts the strong effect of testosterone to cause masculine development of the brain and other tissues, one might wish to stop short of pronouncing XX and XY brain cells functionally equivalent. The question then becomes, how are XX and XY cells different, and does this difference have any effect on sex differences in phenotype of the brain? To discuss this question, we briefly review previous research suggesting that sex differences are caused by cell-autonomous action of sex chromosome genes in mammals and birds. These cases are grouped according to the experimental paradigms used, to illustrate the strengths and weaknesses of specific approaches.

Sex Differences in Phenotypes That Resist Sex Reversal by Manipulations of Gonadal Steroid Hormones

Zebra-finch males sing a courtship song that females cannot sing. Accordingly, the brain regions controlling courtship song are much larger in males than in females.[21] Attempts to test the role of gonadal steroids in sexual differentiation have met with mixed results. Treating neonatal females with testosterone or estradiol causes significant masculinization of the brain circuit and as adults such females sing,[22] suggesting that the male is normally masculinized by his own testicular secretions. Although numerous hormonal treatment regimes have been used in a variety of studies, the neural song circuit of steroid-masculinized females is only about half as masculine as that of a normal male (e.g., Refs. 23 and 24). Moreover, attempts to prevent masculine development in males, by blocking androgen or estrogen action *in vivo,* have often been unsuccessful[25] (but see Refs. 26 and 27). Similarly, the dramatic sex difference in plumage of zebra finches is not sex reversed by a wide variety of manipulations of gonadal steroids at various times of life. Although one is tempted to invoke other factors to explain sexual differentiation when steroid-induced sex reversal is incomplete,[24,28] the lack of an hormonal effect is not strong evidence favoring cell-autonomous actions of sex chromosome genes.[25] In each case, the failure of the sex steroid treatment is potentially attributed to use of the wrong dose, wrong treatment period, or an ineffective drug, etc. Experiments that manipulate steroid hormones test a role for those hormones, but do not provide a strong test for the role of other factors.

In zebra finches, it has been possible to manipulate the phenotype of the gonad in genetic females to compare brain phenotype in females with ovaries and females with testes. Because ovarian development in birds requires the action of estrogen at early stages of gonadal development, females are induced to develop testes if they are treated as embryos with an inhibitor of aromatase, the synthetic enzyme for estrogen. This treatment typically causes development of a testis on the right side of the animal and an ovotestis on the left side. Despite the presence of a large quantity of testicular tissue in some of these birds, the neural song circuit is masculinized little or not at all.[29] This result raises doubts about the importance of testicular secretions in the development of a masculine song circuit.

Sex Differences Detected prior to Gonadal Differentiation

In some cases, sex differences can be observed in nongonadal tissues prior to the time of gonadal differentiation and/or sex-specific gonadal secretions. For example, XY embryos grow faster than XX embryos in mice, rats, cattle, and humans[30,31] even before gonads have developed. In mice, both the dosage of X gene(s) and male-specific action of Y gene(s) participate in this sex difference.[32,33] In tammar wallabies, the scrotum begins to differentiate in XY males, and mammary tissue begins to differentiate in XX females, prior to gonadal differentiation.[34] X dosage is implicated because XXY wallabies have feminine phenotype in these tissues.

Reisert, Pilgrim, and colleagues have investigated the differences in the *in vitro* phenotype of XX and XY brain cells harvested from rat and mouse embryos, just after gonadal differentiation but prior to the stage at which large sex differences in plasma levels of steroid hormones have been detected.[35,36] For example, when mesencephalic or diencephalic cells are harvested from day 14 rat embryos, then dissociated and grown under identical conditions *in vitro*, XX cultures differ from XY cultures in several respects, including the number of tyrosine hydroxylase immunoreactive neurons, the size or neuritic length of dopamine neurons, the effects of neurotoxin, or the number of prolactin immunoreactive neurons. These investigators conclude that the difference in XX and XY cells is not the result of the action of gonadal hormones, but rather is caused by cell-autonomous factors, presumably those on the sex chromosomes. This conclusion is also supported by recent experiments using a different experimental approach discussed below.

Studies of Genetic Anomalies in Which Genetically Male and Female Cells Are Exposed to a Common Gonadal Hormone Environment

It is experimentally difficult to compare XX and XY cells that are exposed to an identical hormonal environment in order to determine the role of the sex chromosomes in specific traits. Infrequently, nature performs this experiment for us, as in the case of bilateral gynandromorphs. Recently, Agate *et al.*[37] studied a gynandromorphic zebra finch in which the right half of the body was genetically male, and the left half genetically female. The plumage on the right half was typical of males, with an orange cheek patch, zebra stripes and a black bar on the breast, and white spots under the wing. On the left half of the body, the plumage lacked these characteristics and was gray, typical of females. The right gonad was a testis, and the left gonad an ovary. These findings suggest that the genetic mechanisms responsible for sexual differentiation of plumage and gonadal phenotype, both of which are thought to be caused by cell-autonomous action of sex chromosome genes, were lateralized with female determinants on the left and male determinants on the right. In birds, the sex chromosomes of females are ZW and ZZ in males. Analysis of the gynandromorph's genomic DNA showed that W genes were present at a higher level on the left than on the right. Moreover, the expression of W genes was largely restricted to the left half of the brain, and a Z gene was expressed higher in the right brain, suggesting that the brain was genetically female on the left and male on the right. Because the two halves of the brain would have been exposed throughout life to the same levels of gonadal hormones, the sexual phenotype of the two sides of the brain would be expected to be the same if gonadal hormones were the only factors responsible for sexual differentiation. In contrast, if the genetic sex of cells in the brain contributes to sex differences in brain phenotype, then the genetically male right side of the brain would be expected to be more masculine than the genetically female left side. The neural circuit for song was found to be more masculine on the right than on the left, supporting the idea that sex chromosome genes act cell-autonomously to influence sexual differentiation. However, because both sides of the gynandromorph's brain were more masculine than those in females, diffusible factors such as gonadal hormones (or masculinizing hormones from the male half of the brain) apparently also played a role. The gynandromorphic male is reminiscent of a half-male, half-female wallaby.[38,39] In this wallaby, the male side had a hemi-scrotum and the female side had a hemipouch, again confirming the cell-autonomous action of sex chromosome genes.

Behavioral Differences in Strains of Mice That Differ Only in the Allelic Composition of the Y Chromosome

Maxson compared aggressive behavior in congenic mouse strains that are genetically identical except for the alleles present on the Y chromosome.[40] DBA/1 males are more aggressive than C57BL/10 males when they are tested in encounters with males of the same strain. When the C57BL/10 Y chromosome is crossed onto a DBA/1 background (by crossing C57BL/10 males with DBA/1 females and backcrossing each successive generation of males to DBA/1 females), the resulting males (DBA1.C57BL10Y) differ genetically from DBA/1 males only in the nonpseudoautosomal region of their Y chromosomes. (The nonpseudoautosomal region does not recombine with the X chromosome and therefore contains genes specific to the Y chromosome.) DBA/1 males (with a DBA/1 Y chromosome) are more aggressive than DBA1.C57BL10Y males (with a C57BL/10 Y chromosome). Thus, allelic differences in the Y chromosome lead to differences among males in their aggressive behavior. Numerous other studies performed on different mouse strains and using different paradigms of testing indicate that the Y chromosome contains genes that influence aggression.[41] If Y genes differ in their influence on aggression, it is logical to assume that the presence or absence of Y genes (when comparing males and females) might also contribute to sex differences in aggression.

These classic techniques of behavioral genetics demonstrate the Y linkage of a behavioral trait. They are designed to test the importance of different Y alleles, but are not designed to test the importance of gonadal hormones in sexual differentiation. For example, in the congenic mouse strains, Y genes could increase the secretion of testosterone by the gonads or adrenals, either at the time of testing of the gonadally intact males used in these studies, or during other times of life such as perinatal critical periods of sexual differentiation.[42,43] Measurements of plasma hormone levels suggest that strain differences in hormone levels may occur at specific ages.[44,45] In general, however, even when no difference in the level of hormones is found, the evidence does not rule out differences in hormone levels at other ages.

Two strategies can be followed to attempt to resolve whether Y-linkage implies a cell-autonomous action of Y genes in the brain, or whether the Y effect is explained by an hormonal or some other effect. The best method is to determine which Y genes(s) is responsible for the effect, and to determine where in the brain or body the expression of the Y gene(s) impacts aggressive behavior. This could involve, for example, manipulation of Y gene expression in specific tissues such as the brain cells using transgenic or other methods. Another approach is to attempt to eliminate the hormonal differences between the congenic strains, to determine whether the Y effect persists in mice that have similar hormonal profiles. For example, one might test the aggressive behavior of animals that are gonadectomized and treated with equivalent levels of testosterone, to determine whether the Y effect is found when testosterone levels are eliminated as a potential contributing variable at the time of testing. Alternatively, perinatal animals may be treated equivalently with gonadal steroids or steroid hormone antagonists in an attempt to ensure that the strains receive the same gonadal steroid effects during development. Although such studies can help suggest whether steroids do or do not mediate the Y gene effect, they are not completely satisfactory because it is experimentally impossible to make two different strains hormonally equivalent.

Comparison of Mice with Similar Gonads but Different Sex Chromosomes: XX Males vs. XY Males and XX Females vs. XY Females

To investigate the role for X and Y genes, one must vary the action of those genes and observe the effect on the phenotype. One particularly promising approach has been developed by Burgoyne and Lovell-Badge and colleagues.[46–48] This involves the comparison of mice in which the complement of sex chromosomes (XX or XY) is made independent of the phenotype of the gonads. In these mice, a 12-kb region of the Y chromosome is deleted, removing the *Sry* gene. This "Y$^-$" chromosome no longer causes differentiation of testes; thus, XY$^-$ mice have ovaries and are female (defining sex by gonadal phenotype). Some mice carry an *Sry* transgene inserted into an autosome, so that XY$^-$*Sry* mice are fully reproductive males. When one crosses XY$^-$*Sry* males with XX females, four types of progeny are produced: XY$^-$*Sry* males, XX*Sry* males, XY$^-$ females, and XX females. These four genotypes allow a 2X2 comparison of mice with different gonadal phenotypes (testes vs. ovaries) and with different complements of sex chromosomes (XX vs. XY$^-$). When one compares animals with the same gonadal type but with different sex chromosomes (XY$^-$*Sry* males vs. XXSry males, or XY$^-$ females vs. XX females), differences between groups can be attributed to an effect of sex chromosome complement. When one compares animals with the same complement of sex chromosomes but different gonadal type (XY$^-$*Sry* males vs. XY$^-$ females, or XX*Sry* males vs. XX females), differences in phenotype can be attributed to an effect of the *Sry* transgene. Because the main known effect of *Sry* is to induce differentiation the testes, the *Sry* effect is probably mediated mainly by differences in gonadal secretions. However, the *Sry* transgene is also expressed in nongonadal tissues such as the brain; thus, the hormonal

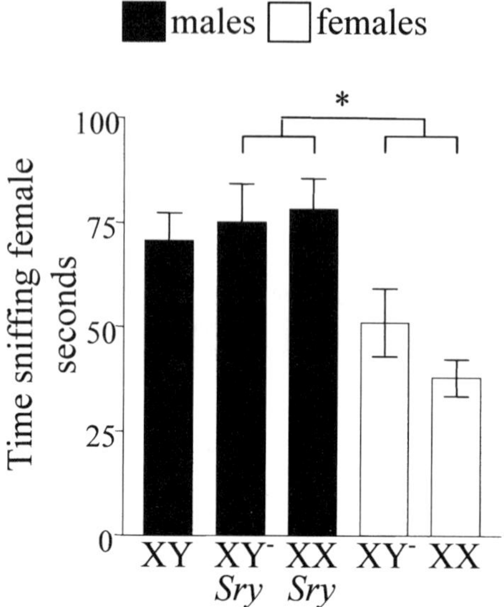

FIGURE 1. Sexual differentiation of social exploration. Five genotypes of mice were compared in a choice paradigm in which they could sniff an anesthetized male or female mouse in a 10-min social exploration test (means ± SEM). The graph shows the amount of time spent sniffing the female. Males (*black bars*) spent more time sniffing the stimulus female than did females (*clear bars*, $P < 0.0005$), suggesting that gonadal secretions control sexual differentiation of this trait. The complement of sex chromosomes (XY^- vs. XX) did not have a significant effect. (Data from De Vries *et al.*[49])

differences between these groups are confounded potentially by *Sry* effects in the brain itself. Using the two-way ANOVA, one can test the separate effects of sex chromosome complement and gonadal type, and their interaction.

De Vries *et al.*[49] and Markham *et al.*[50] compared these four genotypes by measuring numerous brain structures and behaviors that were predicted or known to be sexually dimorphic in mice. These variables included measures of male copulatory behavior and social exploration, and structural traits in the lateral septum, anterior hypothalamus, cerebral cortex, and lumbar spinal cord. Prior to behavioral testing, all animals were gonadectomized and treated equally with Silastic capsules containing testosterone. By holding testosterone levels constant in between-group comparisons, any differences between groups could be attributed to factors other than levels of gonadal secretions at the time of testing (i.e., "activational" effects). On most measures, male mice (those with *Sry*) were different than female mice (those without *Sry*), independent of sex chromosome complement (FIG. 1). For example, males showed more masculine copulatory behavior than females, and their complement of sex chromosomes (XX vs. XY^-) had no effect. Thus, for these variables gonadal secretions during development appear to be the primary determinant of sexual phenotype, as predicted by the strong differentiating role of testosterone in many previous studies in which sexual phenotype is reversed by altering testosterone or estradiol action in the period around birth in rodents. In the lateral septum, males also had a higher density of vasopressin fibers than females, but, in addition, the complement of sex chromosomes had an effect (FIG. 2). Thus, XY^{-}*Sry* males had a higher density of vasopressin fibers than XX*Sry* males, and when females from all female litters were compared, XY^{-} females had a higher density than XX females. The results indicate that the genetic sex of cells (XY^{-} vs. XX) influences this trait. When the complement of sex chromosomes is similar to that possessed by normal XY males, the trait is more masculine than when the complement of sex chromosomes is similar to that of normal XX females.

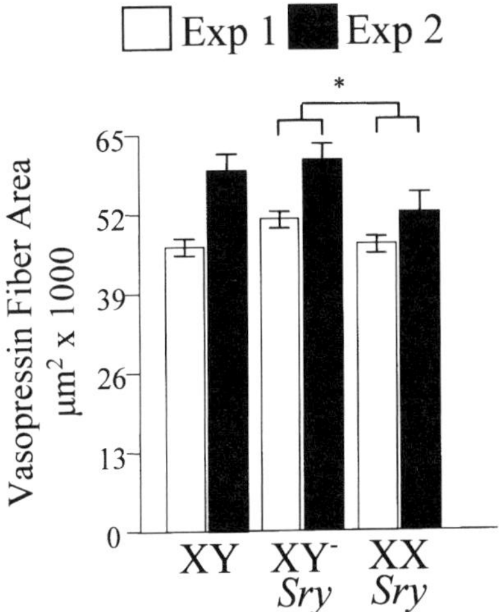

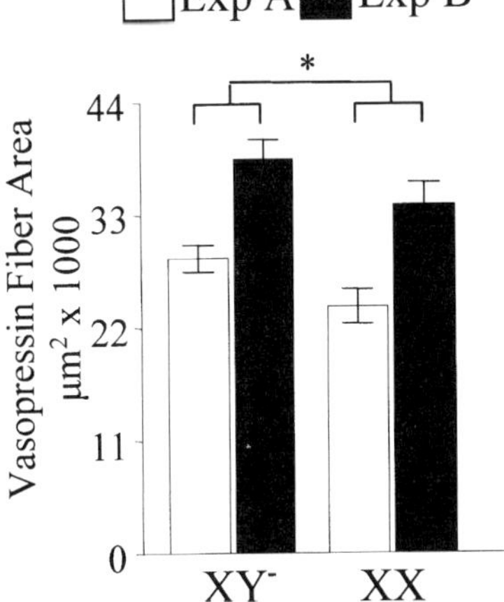

FIGURE 2. (**A**) The density of vasopressin immunoreactive fibers in the lateral septum of male genotypes (means ± SEM). *Black* and *clear bars* represent the results from two different experiments. XY^{-}*Sry* males had a higher density than did XX*Sry* males ($P < 0.05$), showing an effect of sex chromosome complement on this trait. (**B**) Vasopressin fiber density in females from all-female litters shows the same effect of sex chromosome complement because XY^{-} females had a higher density than XX females in two experiments ($P < 0.02$). (Data from De Vries *et al.*[49])

Does this finding prove that sex chromosome genes act within cells in the brain to contribute to sex differences in phenotype? If so, does it contradict the classic idea that sex differences in brain phenotype are caused by gonadal steroid hormones? The conservative answer is that the finding shows an effect of sex chromosome complement, but does not answer where or how the effect is mediated. It is possible that the action of X and Y genes is outside of the brain. For example, one may question whether XY⁻*Sry* males and XX*Sry* males, or XX and XY⁻ females, are hormonally equivalent. In both cases, the gonads are functionally different. For example, XX*Sry* males lack Y genes necessary to make sperm; therefore their testes are smaller than those of XY⁻*Sry* males. XY⁻ females are subfertile. Despite these apparent differences in functional capacity of the gonads, the two male groups are phenotypically similar in their brains and behavior, as are the two female groups. Furthermore, XX animals were probably not exposed to different levels of gonadal hormones than XY⁻ animals because such a difference should have influenced several of the brain phenotypes measured, which are all barometers of hormonal action. However, because the experiment primarily involved manipulation of the sex chromosomes, not manipulation of hormonal secretions, the results primarily bear on the role of X and Y genes. As discussed above, comparisons of animals with different genotypes are aimed at a strong answer to the question of which genes are involved, not at resolving the possibility of hormonal mediation.

How can one answer the interesting question of whether the sex chromosome effect is mediated by hormonal or other mechanisms? The best approach is to determine which X or Y genes are involved, and determine where and how they act to contribute to a phenotypic difference. If XX and XY⁻ animals differ in phenotype, then one can narrow down the genes responsible to the X or Y chromosome, for example, by comparing XO vs. XX (varying X dose independent of Y dose) and XO vs. XY (varying Y dose independent of X dose), as was done when measuring effects on mouse embryo size.[32,33] If a specific gene can be implicated, then varying the dose of that gene is feasible, for example by transgenic insertion of Y genes into XX mice.[47] Once a specific gene is implicated, its sites of expression and mechanisms of action can be studied to determine whether it acts via a hormonal intermediate or via direct action on the brain.

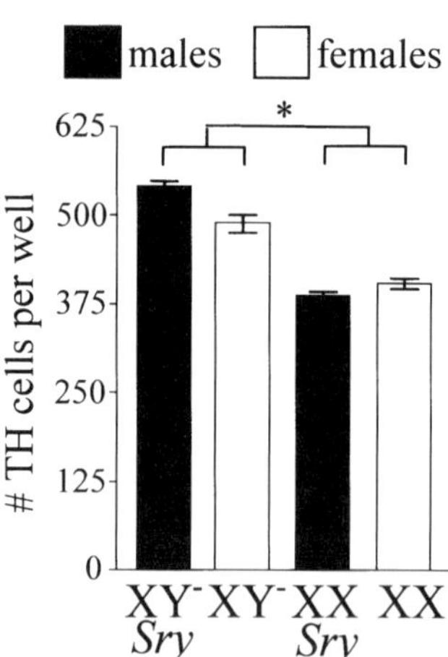

FIGURE 3. Effect of sex chromosome complement on neuronal phenotype *in vitro*. Mesencephalic cells were harvested from day 14 embryos, dissociated, and plated out. When measured 6 days later, cultures derived from XY⁻ embryos (either XY⁻*Sry* males or XY⁻ females) contained more tyrosine hydroxylase immunoreactive neurons than did XX cultures (derived from XX*Sry* males or XX females) ($P < 0.00001$). The primary determinant of this sex difference *in vitro* is the complement of sex chromosomes. (Data from Carruth *et al.*[51])

The four genotypes described above have also been used to study the sex difference in phenotype of XX and XY mesencephalic cells *in vitro*. Using the paradigm pioneered by Reisert and colleagues, Carruth *et al.*[51] dissociated mesencephalic cells from mouse embryos on embryonic day 14. These cells were grown under identical conditions for 6 or 11 days before their phenotype was measured. The XY cultures, harvested from male (XY^{-}*Sry*) or female (XY^{-}) embryos, developed more tyrosine hydroxylase immunoreactive neurons than XX cultures harvested from embryos of either sex (XX*Sry* or XX) (FIG. 3). The sex chromosome effect was specific to TH-immunoreactive neurons, since the total number of neurons was not different between groups. Thus, for this phenotype *in vitro*, sex chromosome complement is the primary determinant of the differences observed, not any gonadal hormones that might circulate as early as embryonic day 14.

CONCLUSION

Because the field of neuroendocrinology has long focused on the dominant differentiating role of testosterone in sexual differentiation of the brain, based on abundant evidence supporting this role for many sexually dimorphic traits, there is understandable resistance to the view that the genetic sex of brain cells might also contribute to differences in XX and XY brains. Viewed from the perspective of sex chromosome geneticists, however, the equivalence of XX and XY brain cells is doubtful, but the evidence to date does not indicate how different these cells are, or how the difference interacts with testosterone's role in sexual differentiation. In part, the absence of information is the result of the paucity of experimental models in which XX and XY brains can be compared under conditions in which gonadal hormone levels are similar or equivalent. Fortunately, at least in mice, the ability to dissociate sex chromosome complement from gonadal phenotype now offers opportunities for further measurement of sex chromosome effects. The first results using these models suggest that the genetic sex of brain cells plays a role in sexual differentiation. Other mouse models may also be useful, for example, mice in which gonadal development is prevented by deletion of steroid factor 1 or other genes critical for gonadal development.[52] In quail, the genetic sex of the brain has been altered recently by transplanting genetically male brain tissue into the body of a female host and vice versa.[53] Under these conditions a genetically female quail brain appears unable to sustain normal tesiticular development, adding support to the importance of the sex chromosomes in determining sexual phenotype. We are optimistic that future studies will lead to identification of specific sex-chromosome genes that impact brain development and behavior in a sex-specific fashion.

ACKNOWLEDGMENTS

We thank Paul Burgoyne, Robin Lovell-Badge, and Amanda Swain, who have taught us a great deal about the sex chromosomes and methods to investigate sex chromosome effects on neural and behavioral development. This work was supported by National Institutes of Health grants MH59268 and NS43196.

REFERENCES

1. LILLIE, F.R. 1916. The theory of the freemartin. Science **43:** 611–613.
2. KELLER, K. & J. TANDLER. 1916. Über des Verhalten der Eihäute bei der Zwillingsssträchtigkeit des Rindes. Untersuchungen über die Entstehungsursache der geschlectlichen Unterentwicklung von weiblichen Zwillingskälbern, welche neben einem männlichen Kalbe zur Entwicklung gelangen. Wien Tierärztliche Wehnscrift **3:** 513.
3. JOST, A., B. VIGIER, J. PREPIN & J.P. PERCHELLET. 1973. Studies on sex differentiation in mammals. Rec. Prog. Horm. Res. **29:** 1–41.
4. BEHRINGER, R.R. 1994. The in vivo roles of Müllerian-inhibiting substance. Curr. Top. Dev. Biol. **29:** 171–187.
5. PHOENIX, C.H., R.W. GOY, A.A. GERALL & W.C. YOUNG. 1959. Organizing action of prenatally administered testosterone propionate on the tissues mediating mating behavior in the female guinea pig. Endocrinology **65:** 369–382.
6. GOY, R.W. & B.S. MCEWEN. 1980. Sexual Differentiation of the Brain. MIT Press. Cambridge, MA.
7. MACLUSKY, N.J. & F. NAFTOLIN. 1981. Sexual differentiation of the central nervous system. Science **211:** 1294–1303.
8. ARNOLD, A.P. & R.A. GORSKI. 1984. Gonadal steroid induction of structural sex differences in the CNS. Annu. Rev. Neurosci. **7:** 413–442.
9. STURTEVANT, A.H. 1965. A History of Genetics. Harper & Row. New York.
10. CLINE, T.W. & B.J. MEYER. 1996. Vive la difference: males vs females in flies vs worms. Annu. Rev. Genet. **30:** 637–702.
11. WELSHONS, W.J. & L.B. RUSSELL. 1959. The Y chromosome as the bearer of male determining factors in the mouse. Proc. Natl. Acad. Sci. USA **45:** 560–566.
12. GOODFELLOW, P.N. & R. LOVELL-BADGE. 1993. *SRY* and sex determination in mammals. Annu. Rev. Genet. **27:** 71–92.
13. LYON, M.F. 1999. X-chromosome inactivation. Curr. Biol. **9:** R235–R237.
14. CARREL, L., A.A. COTTLE, K.C. GOGLIN & H.F. WILLARD. 1999. A first-generation X-inactivation profile of the human X chromosome. Proc. Natl. Acad. Sci. USA **96:** 14440–14444.
15. DELBRIDGE, M.L. & J.A. GRAVES. 1999. Mammalian Y chromosome evolution and the male-specific functions of Y chromosome-borne genes. Rev. Reprod. **4:** 101–109.
16. SKALETSKY, H., T. KURODA-KAWAGUCHI, P.J. MINX, *et al.* 2003. The male-specific region of the human Y chromosome is a mosaic of discrete sequence classes. Nature **423:** 825–837.
17. XU, J., P.S. BURGOYNE & A.P. ARNOLD. 2002. Sex differences in sex chromosome gene expression in mouse brain. Hum. Mol. Genet. **11:** 1409–1419.
18. MAXSON, S.C. 1996. Searching for candidate genes with effects on an agonistic behavior, offense, in mice. Behav. Genet. **26:** 471–476.
19. LEIGHTON, P.A., J.R. SAAM, R.S. INGRAM & S.M. TILGHMAN. 1996. Genomic imprinting in mice: its function and mechanism. Biol. Reprod. **54:** 273–278.
20. SKUSE, D.H., R.S. JAMES, D.V.M. BISHOP, *et al.* 1997. Evidence from Turner's syndrome of an imprinted x-linked locus affecting cognitive function. Nature **387:** 705–708.
21. NOTTEBOHM, F. & A.P. ARNOLD. 1976. Sexual dimorphism in vocal control areas of the song bird brain. Science **194:** 211–213.
22. GURNEY, M.E. & M. KONISHI. 1980. Hormone-induced sexual differentiation of brain and behavior in zebra finches. Science **208:** 1380–1382.
23. JACOBS, E.C., W. GRISHAM & A.P. ARNOLD. 1995. Lack of a synergistic effect between estradiol and dihydrotestosterone in the masculinization of the zebra finch song system. J. Neurobiol. **27:** 513–519.
24. GAHR, M. & R. METZDORF. 1999. The sexually dimorphic expression of androgen receptors in the song nucleus hyperstriatalis ventrale pars caudale of the zebra finch develops independently of gonadal steroids. J. Neurosci. **19:** 2628–2636.
25. ARNOLD, A.P. 1997. Sexual differentiation of the zebra finch song system: positive evidence, negative evidence, null hypotheses, and a paradigm shift. J. Neurobiol. **33:** 572–584.

26. DITTRICH, F., Y. FENG, R. METZDORF & M. GAHR. 1999. Estrogen-inducible, sex-specific expression of brain-derived neurotrophic factor mRNA in a forebrain song control nucleus of the juvenile zebra finch. Proc. Natl. Acad. Sci. USA **96:** 8241–8246.
27. HOLLOWAY, C.C. & D.F. CLAYTON. 2001. Estrogen synthesis in the male brain triggers development of the avian song control pathway in vitro. Nat. Neurosci. **4:** 170–175.
28. ARNOLD, A.P. 1996. Genetically triggered sexual differentiation of brain and behavior. Horm. Behav. **30:** 495–505.
29. WADE, J. & A.P. ARNOLD. 1996. Functional testicular tissue does not masculinize development of the zebra finch song system. Proc. Natl. Acad. Sci. USA **93:** 5264–5268.
30. ERICKSON, R.P. 1997. Does sex determination start at conception? BioEssays **19:** 1027–1032.
31. ARNOLD, A.P. 2002. Concepts of genetic and hormonal induction of vertebrate sexual differentiation in the twentieth century, with special reference to the brain. *In* Hormones, Brain, and Behavior. D.W. Pfaff, A.P. Arnold, A. Etgen, S. Fahrbach & R. Rubin, Eds.: 105–135. Academic Press. San Diego.
32. BURGOYNE, P.S. 1993. A Y-chromosomal effect on blastocyst cell number in mice. Dev. **117:** 342–345.
33. THORNHILL, A.R. & P.S. BURGOYNE. 1993. A paternally imprinted X chromosome retards the development of the early mouse embryo. Development **118:** 171–174.
34. RENFREE, M.B. & R.V. SHORT. 1988. Sex determination in marsupials: evidence for a marsupial-eutherian dichotomy. Phil. Trans. R. Soc. Lond. B **322:** 41–53.
35. PILGRIM, CH. & I. REISERT. 1992. Differences between male and female brains—developmental mechanisms and implications. Horm. Metab. Res. **24:** 353–359.
36. REISERT, I. & C. PILGRIM. 1991. Sexual differentiation of monoaminergic neurons—genetic or epigenetic. Trends Neurosci. **14:** 467–473.
37. AGATE, R.J., W. GRISHAM, J. WADE, *et al.* 2003. Neural not gonadal origin of brain sex differences in a gynandromorphic finch. Proc. Natl. Acad. Sci. USA **100:** 4873–4878.
38. HUGHES, R.L., A. PEARSE, D.W. COOPER, *et al.* 1993. The genetic basis of marsupial gonadogenesis and sexual phenytype. *In* Sex Chromosomes and Sex Determining Genes. K.C. Reed & J.A.M. Graves, Eds.: 17–48. Harwood Academic Publishers. Chur, Switzerland.
39. COOPER, D.W. 1993. The evolution of sex determination, sex chromosome dimorphism, and X-inactivation in therian mammals: a comparison of metatherians (marsupials) and eutherians ("placentals"). *In* Sex Chromosomes and Sex Determining Genes. K.C. Reed & J.A.M. Graves, Eds.: 183–200. Harwood Academic Publishers. Chur, Switzerland.
40. MAXSON, S.C. 1999. Sex differences in genetic mechanisms for mammalian brain and behavior. Biomed. Rev. **7:** 85–90.
41. SLUYTER, F., G.A. VAN OORTMERSSEN, A.J.H. DE RUITER & J.M. KOOLHAAS. 1996. Aggression in wild house mice: current state of affairs. Behav. Genet. **26:** 489–496.
42. JUTLEY, J.K. & A.D. STEWART. 1986. Genetic analysis of the Y-chromosome of the mouse: evidence for two loci affecting androgen metabolism. Genet. Res. **47:** 29–34.
43. TORDJMAN, S., P.L. ROUBERTOUX, M. CARLIER, *et al.* 1995. Linkage between brain serotonin concentration and the sex-specific part of the Y-chromosome in mice. Neurosci. Lett. **183:** 190–192.
44. GUILLOT, P.V., P.L. ROUBERTOUX, H. DEGRELLE, *et al.* 1993. Y chromosome and adult plasma testosterone levels in mice. Behav. Genet. **23:** 553.
45. SELMANOFF, M.K., B.D. GOLDMAN, S.C. MAXSON & B.E. GINSBURG. 1977. Correlated effects of the Y-chromosome of mice on developmental changes in testosterone levels and intermale aggression. Life Sci. **20:** 359–365.
46. LOVELL-BADGE, R. & E. ROBERTSON. 1990. XY female mice resulting from a heritable mutation in the primary testis-determining gene, Tdy. Development **109:** 635–646.
47. MAZEYRAT, S., N. SAUT, V. GRIGORIEV, *et al.* 2001. A Y-encoded subunit of the translation initiation factor Eif2 is essential for mouse spermatogenesis. Nat. Genet. **29:** 49–53.

48. MAHADEVAIAH, S.K., R. LOVELL-BADGE & P.S. BURGOYNE. 1993. Tdy-negative XY, XXY and XYY female mice: breeding data and synaptonemal complex analysis. J. Reprod. Fertil. **97:** 151–160.
49. DE VRIES, G.J., E.F. RISSMAN, R.B. SIMERLY, *et al.* 2002. A model system for study of sex chromosome effects on sexually dimorphic neural and behavioral traits. J. Neurosci. **22:** 9005–9014.
50. MARKHAM, J.A., H.A. JURGENS, C.J. AUGER, *et al.* 2003. Sex differences in mouse cortical thickness are independent of the complement of sex chromosomes. Neurosci. **116:** 71–75.
51. CARRUTH, L.L., I. REISERT & A.P. ARNOLD. 2002. Sex chromosome genes directly affect brain sexual differentiation. Nat. Neurosci. **5:** 933–934.
52. PARKER, K.L. & B.P. SCHIMMER. 1997. Steroidogenic factor 1: a key determinant of endocrine development and function. Endocr. Rev. **18:** 361–377.
53. GAHR, M. 2003. Male Japanese quails with female brains do not show male sexual behaviors. Proc. Natl. Acad. Sci. USA **100:** 7959–7964.

Puberty: A Finishing School for Male Social Behavior

CHERYL L. SISK, KALYNN M. SCHULZ, AND JULIA L. ZEHR

Neuroscience Program and Department of Psychology, Michigan State University, East Lansing, Michigan 48824, USA

Abstract: The classical view of steroid-dependent organization of brain and behavior holds that gonadal steroid hormones, acting during an early critical period of development, cause permanent structural changes in neural circuits that determine behavioral responses to hormones in adulthood. This classical view has been modified to incorporate evidence that organizational effects of steroids can occur outside of the established perinatal critical period and that multiple critical periods may exist during development. Experiments in this laboratory indicate that steroid-dependent organization of neural circuits underlying male social behaviors occurs during puberty. This work shows that adult-typical reproductive and flank marking behaviors cannot be activated by gonadal steroids in male Syrian hamsters prior to puberty, suggesting that developmentally timed processes during puberty render the nervous system responsive to activating effects of gonadal steroids in adulthood. Additional experiments demonstrate that the presence or absence of gonadal hormones during puberty is a major factor in the ability of steroids to activate reproductive and flank marking behavior in adult male hamsters and in androgen receptor expression within the neural circuit underlying these behaviors. Thus, gonadal hormones during puberty appear to exert long-lasting changes in neural circuits that are responsible for the programming of activational responses to steroids later in adulthood. A two-stage model for maturation of male social behaviors is proposed: a perinatal critical period for sexual differentiation of neural circuits, followed by the pubertal period, during which gonadal steroids further organize the circuits to enhance behavioral responsiveness to hormones in adulthood. Whether puberty is a critical period for the proposed second wave of steroid-dependent organization of behavioral circuits remains to be determined.

Keywords: puberty; organization; male social behavior; gonadal steroids

INTRODUCTION

The central thesis of this paper is that puberty is not only the time during which reproductive maturation occurs, but it is also a period of development of the nervous system that is dissociable from gonadal maturation. Pubertal maturation of the brain

Address for correspondence: Cheryl L. Sisk, Neuroscience Program, 108 Giltner Hall, Michigan State University, East Lansing, MI 48864. Voice: 517-355-5253; fax: 517-432-2744. sisk@msu.edu

Ann. N.Y. Acad. Sci. 1007: 189–198 (2003).
doi: 10.1196/annals.1286.019

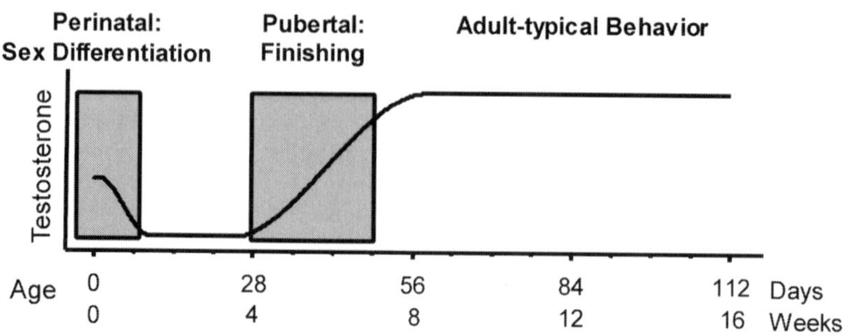

FIGURE 1. Two-stage model for the development of male social behavior. During the perinatal period, exposure to steroid hormones results in sexual differentiation. During the pubertal period, exposure to steroid hormones produces the final maturational changes necessary for adult-typical expression of social behavior.

and reproductive system normally occur around the same time in an individual, and these processes are interactive. Reproductive maturation is initiated through activation of the forebrain gonadotropin-releasing hormone (GnRH) neuronal system, and increased neurosecretory activity of GnRH neurons results in increased production of gonadal steroid hormones. Gonadal steroids, in turn, regulate physiological functions and facilitate the expression of many social behaviors. These actions of steroid hormones are typically described as activational effects. There is increasing evidence that steroid hormones also exert long-lasting organizational effects on neural circuits during puberty.[1,2] In this paper, we develop the idea that developmentally timed events, occurring during pubertal maturation of the brain, render neural circuits sensitive to steroid-dependent organizational change at this stage of development.

The concept of steroid-dependent organization of the nervous system is discussed first and the criteria historically used to establish that organizational effects have occurred are outlined. Next, we review experiments from this laboratory demonstrating that full hormonal activation of male social behaviors in adulthood is dependent in part on long-lasting structural modifications in behavioral circuits organized by steroid hormones during puberty. A two-stage model is proposed for the maturation of adult male social behaviors (FIG. 1). The model incorporates sexual differentiation of neural circuits during a perinatal critical period, followed by further steroid-dependent organization of these circuits during puberty that enhances behavioral responsiveness to hormones in adulthood.

ORGANIZATION OF THE BRAIN AND BEHAVIOR BY STEROID HORMONES

The concept of the organization of behavior and its underlying neural circuits originated with the demonstration that perinatal manipulation of gonadal steroids affected the propensity to display masculine or feminine sexual behavior in response to hormone treatment in adulthood.[3] The classical definition of organizational effects of steroid hormones includes (1) permanent or long-lasting effects of perinatal steroid hormone manipulation on behavior and structural features of underlying neural circuits; (2) the programming of behavioral responses to steroid hormones in adulthood; and (3) the existence of a perinatal critical period during which sensitivity to the organizational effects of steroid hormones is highest.

Several revisions to the organizational hypothesis have occurred over the past 40 years. Scott and colleagues laid the theoretical groundwork for the existence of multiple critical periods during development and suggested that organizational change in earlier critical periods may determine the capacity and direction of organizational change in successive critical periods.[4] Arnold and Breedlove[5] pointed out that steroid hormones can exert long-lasting structural changes in the nervous system well beyond the perinatal critical period. Finally, demonstrations that manipulations of gonadal steroids during puberty irreversibly alter the emergence of sex differences in nonreproductive adult social interactions indicated that puberty is a sensitive period for further steroid-dependent organization of behavioral circuits.[1] Data from this laboratory reviewed below support the idea that puberty is a sensitive period for hormonal organization of neural circuits underlying male reproductive and communicative behaviors.

ACTIVATION AND ORGANIZATION OF BEHAVIOR DURING PUBERTY

One of the first indications that organization of neural circuits underlying male reproductive behavior occurs during puberty came from observations that in a number of species doses of testosterone that reliably activate copulatory behavior in adult males do not activate behavior to the same extent in prepubertal males.[6–8] In a series of studies, we compared the activation of reproductive behavior in sexually naive prepubertal and adult male Syrian hamsters that were castrated and treated for one week with one of three doses of either testosterone, dihydrotestosterone, or estradiol benzoate via subcutaneous pellet implants.[8–10] Hormone treatment increased anogenital investigation of the female by both prepubertal and adult males, indicating

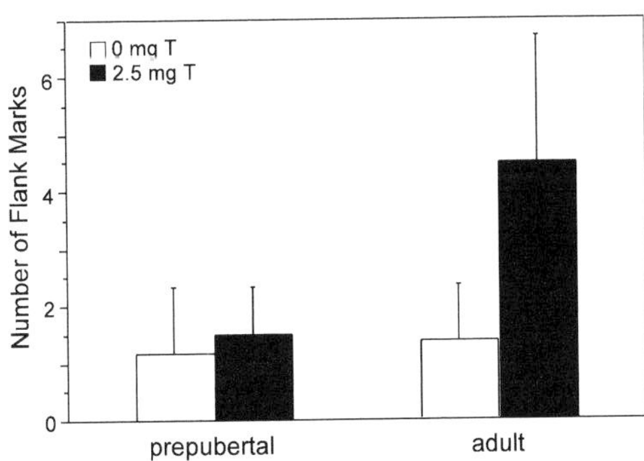

FIGURE 2. Number of mounts displayed by prepubertal and adult males during an interaction with an estrous female. All behavior tests occurred one week after castration and treatment with either TP (2.5 mg), DHT (0.5 mg), or EB (0.05 mg). Data are expressed as mean ± SEM.

similar activational effects of gonadal steroids on this component of reproductive behavior before and after puberty. In contrast, mounts (FIG. 2), intromissions, and ejaculations were activated by hormone treatment only in adults. These data suggest that developmental events occurring during puberty render the nervous system responsive to the activating effects of gonadal steroids on these components of reproductive behavior.

Another social behavior regulated by testosterone in Syrian hamsters is flank marking.[11,12] Males and females rub pigmented sebaceous glands located on their dorsal flank region against objects in the environment as an important form of communication about reproductive and social status.[13] Recent data from this laboratory suggest that testosterone does not facilitate flank marking during male social interactions until after pubertal development. Prepubertal and adult males were gonadectomized and treated with 0 or 2.5 mg of testosterone. After one week of treatment with testosterone, the flank marking behavior of prepubertal and adult males was observed during a social interaction with an unfamiliar male in a resident-intruder test. In adults, testosterone increased flank marking during the social interaction but, in juveniles, testosterone did not increase flank marking. These data suggest that, similar to neural circuits underlying reproductive behavior, circuits underlying flank marking are not responsive to the activating effects of testosterone until *after* pubertal maturation (FIG. 3).

The developmental processes during puberty that permit activating effects of steroid hormones on reproductive and flank marking behaviors in adulthood are still unknown. Recent work in this laboratory provides evidence that these processes include organizational change in neural circuits underlying behavior and, further, that gonadal hormones are the agents for organization. Two experiments investigated the effects of the presence of gonadal hormones during puberty on reproductive and flank marking behavior. In both studies, groups of male hamsters were gonadectomized either before or after puberty. Thus, the testes and gonadal hormones were not present during puberty in males castrated before puberty (NoTduringP), whereas gonadal hormones were present during puberty in males castrated afterward

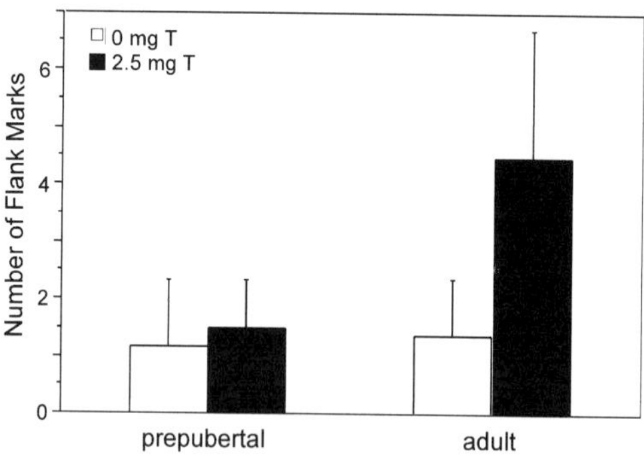

FIGURE 3. Number of flank marks displayed by prepubertal and adult males in their home cage during an interaction with an unfamiliar age- and weight-matched male intruder. All behavior tests occurred one week after castration and treatment with either T (2.5 mg) or vehicle (T, 0 mg). Data are expressed as mean ± SEM.

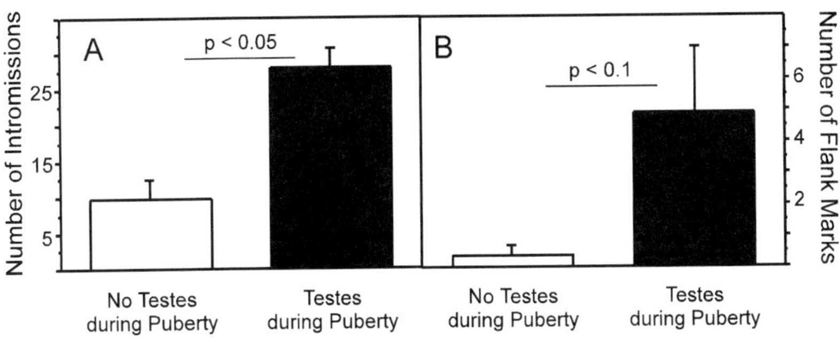

FIGURE 4. Number of intromissions during a reproductive test with a female (**A**) and number of flank marks during a resident-intruder test with an intact stimulus male (**B**) displayed by experimental males gonadectomized before (No Testes during Puberty) or after puberty (Testes during Puberty). Testosterone (2.5–3.0 mg) was administered 6 weeks after gonadectomy, and behavior tests occurred one week following the onset of testosterone treatment (7 weeks after gonadectomy). Each subject was tested in only one behavioral paradigm. Data are expressed as mean ± SEM.

(TduringP). Six weeks after prepubertal or postpubertal gonadectomy, when all males were chronologically adults, males were treated with testosterone and tested one week later either for reproductive behavior with a receptive female or for flank marking behavior during interactions with a male in a resident-intruder paradigm. NoTduringP males displayed fewer intromissions (FIG. 4A) and ejaculations than TduringP males, and these differences persisted even after 17 days of testosterone treatment. Similarly, NoTduringP males gonadectomized before puberty flank marked less frequently than TduringP males (FIG. 4B). Since behavioral differences between NoTduringP and TduringP males were present more than 7 weeks after gonadectomy, exposure to gonadal hormones during puberty appear to exert long-lasting changes in steroid-sensitive neural circuits underlying reproductive and flank marking behaviors. Furthermore, these changes induced by the presence of gonadal hormones during puberty alter the ability of testosterone to activate reproductive and flank marking behavior in adulthood. Thus, these outcomes of the presence of gonadal hormones during puberty fulfill two of the criteria for classical organizational effects: *long-lasting changes* that *program activational responses* to steroids in adulthood.

ACTIVATION AND ORGANIZATION OF BEHAVIORAL NEURAL CIRCUITS DURING PUBERTY

Pubertal development of sexual and flank marking behavior is paralleled by developmental changes within the neural circuits underlying social behaviors. Some differences in neural circuits before and after puberty are directly related to pubertal changes in circulating hormones, representing activational effects of steroid hormones on brain structure. For example, androgen and estrogen treatment of prepu-

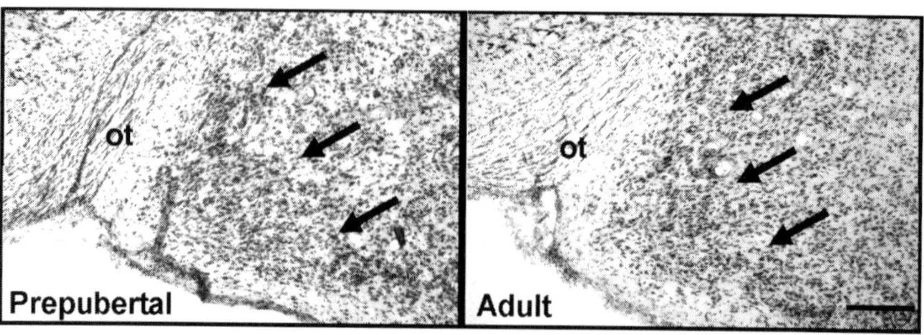

FIGURE 5. Photomicrograph of the anterior portion of the medial amygdala (MeA) in a prepubertal and adult male hamster. *Arrows* outline the outer boundary of the MeA. *Bar*, 200 µm. *Abbreviation*: ot, optic tract.

bertal male hamsters increases hypothalamic aromatase activity and progesterone receptor immunoreactivity, respectively, to levels comparable to those found in adults.[10,14] Therefore, in these respects prepubertal males can be made "adults" simply by experimentally increasing circulating steroids to adult levels.

Other experiments indicate that structural change in the amygdala occurs during puberty as the result of increased steroid secretion. The cross-sectional area of the posterodorsal portion of the medial amygdala (MePD) increases during puberty in male hamsters, and this increase in MePD area is reversible if adult males are housed in short photoperiods to induce gonadal regression and reduced testosterone secretion.[15] Experiments from other laboratories show that in adulthood, MePD size and dendritic branching are elaborated by testosterone and its estrogenic metabolites.[16,17] Thus, structural plasticity in the MePD appears to be related to circulating steroid levels during puberty and in adulthood.

In contrast to the MePD, the cross-sectional area of the medial amygdala (MeA) *decreases* during puberty in gonad-intact male hamsters (FIG. 5), and the MeA area does not revert back to the larger prepubertal size when males are exposed to short days to induce gonadal regression.[15] Whether the pubertal decrease in MeA area is dependent upon exposure to testosterone during puberty has not been determined. However, in adulthood, dendritic branching of MeA neurons is not influenced by circulating testosterone.[16] Collectively, these experiments suggest that pubertal development of the MeA involves regressive events that result in permanent structural organization that is not modifiable by testosterone in adulthood.

Androgen receptor (AR) expression within cell groups forming the forebrain neural circuit underlying male reproductive behavior is influenced by testosterone. Similar to behavioral activation by testosterone, AR regulation by testosterone differs in prepubertal and adult hamsters. However, unlike behavioral responses which are of less magnitude prior to puberty, the AR response is of *greater* magnitude in prepubertal males compared to adults. For example, the cells/unit area (density) of androgen receptor-immunoreactive (AR-ir) cells is higher in preoptic area nuclei of castrated, androgen-treated prepubertal males compared with similarly treated adults (FIG. 6).[8,9] Interestingly, as we found with behavioral activation, AR immunoreactivity in adulthood is influenced by whether gonadal hormones are present

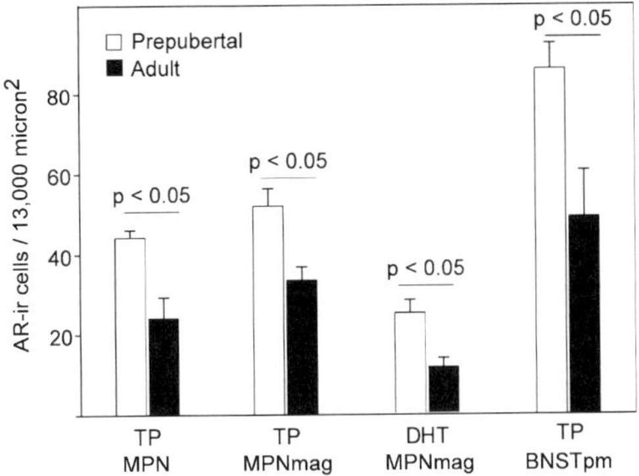

FIGURE 6. Androgen-receptor immunoreactivity (AR-ir cells/unit area) in brain regions controlling male sexual behavior after treatment of gonadectomized prepubertal and adult males with testosterone propionate (TP, 2.5 mg) or dihydrotestosterone (DHT, 0.5 mg) for one week prior to tissue collection. Data are expressed as mean ± SEM. *Abbreviations*: MPN, medial preoptic nucleus; MPNmag, magnocellular medial preoptic nucleus; BNSTpm, posterodorsal division of the bed nucleus of the stria terminalis.

during puberty. In an experiment similar in design to behavioral experiments described above, males were castrated either before (noTduringP) or after (TduringP) puberty, and several weeks later when all males were adults, a single injection of testosterone was administered 4 h prior to sacrifice to translocate AR to the nucleus for immunocytochemical visualization. The density of AR-ir cells in both preoptic area nuclei and bed nucleus of the stria terminalis (BNST) was *higher* in males gonadectomized before puberty (NoTduringP) when compared with males gonadectomized after puberty (TduringP) (FIG. 7).[18] These experiments suggest that prepubertal gonadectomy prevented a testosterone-dependent decrease in the number of AR-expressing cells in these brain areas, which caused AR expression to remain at prepubertal levels. These findings corroborate the observations on the MeA area in providing evidence that pubertal development of the nervous system involves steroid-dependent regressive events resulting in long-lasting structural and functional change in the forebrain neural circuits underlying male social behaviors.

CONCLUSIONS

The experiments substantiate the claim that prepubertal and adult males differ in more than just circulating gonadal steroid hormone levels, because adult levels of hormone administered to prepubertal males fail to elicit certain behavioral responses. These findings further suggest that the prepubertal brain is not merely an adult brain in limbo waiting for steroids to exert activational effects, but rather that the prepubertal brain requires additional development and maturation during puberty before full expression of adult-typical behavioral responses to hormones can occur.

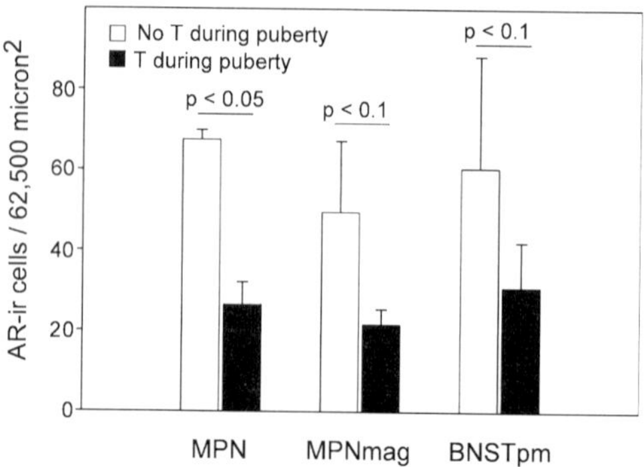

FIGURE 7. Androgen-receptor immunoreactivity (AR-ir cells/unit area) in brain regions controlling male sexual behavior in adult males gonadectomized before puberty (no T during puberty) and in adult males gonadectomized after puberty (T during puberty). All subjects received a subcutaneous injection of testosterone propionate (2.5 mg) 4 h prior to tissue collection. Data are expressed as mean ± SEM. *Abbreviations*: MPN, medial preoptic nucleus; MPNmag, magnocellular medial preoptic nucleus; BNSTpm, posterodorsal division of the bed nucleus of the stria terminalis.

They also provide evidence that pubertal maturation of the brain involves, at least in part, steroid-dependent organizational changes within forebrain behavioral circuits.

These observations have led us to propose a two-stage model for development of male social behavior (Fig. 1). The model holds that maturation of adult-typical behavioral responses to gonadal steroid hormones involves a perinatal critical period of steroid-dependent sexual differentiation of neural circuits underlying behavior, which determines whether male-typical or female-typical behavioral responses to gonadal steroids will occur in adulthood. A second period for steroid-dependent organizational change occurs during puberty when gonadal steroids further organize sexually differentiated neural circuits to enhance male-typical responses to steroid hormones in adulthood.

To date, our experiments provide evidence that effects of steroid hormones during puberty on adult behavior satisfy two of the criteria associated with the classical definition of organizational effects: *long-lasting* changes that *program activational responses* to hormones in adulthood. Arnold and Breedlove[5] effectively argued that steroid hormones can exert organizational effects on the nervous system outside of a critical period, and we contend that steroid hormones do organize neural circuits during puberty. However, Scott[4] made a compelling case for multiple critical periods during behavioral development and even argued that puberty is a likely candidate for a critical period because it is a time of rapid developmental change. While the proposed two-stage model incorporates puberty as a second developmental period during which steroids organize neural circuits and behavior, it does not *require* that puberty be a critical period for organizational change. That is, steroid hormones could theoretically further organize sexually differentiated neural circuits at any time following the initial perinatal critical period. Puberty may not be a critical period per se, but the second stage of organization may normally occur during puberty because that is when the reproductive neuroendocrine axis is reactivated. However, preliminary evidence from this laboratory suggests that puberty may indeed be a second critical period for steroid-dependent organizational change. First, treatment of prepubertal males with testosterone for up to two weeks (days 14–28 of age) still does not permit the activation of reproductive behavior prior to puberty. This finding suggests that neural circuits are not sensitive to potential organizing effects of testosterone prior to puberty. Second, up to 17 days of testosterone treatment administered to adult males that were castrated prior to puberty still does not permit adult-typical activation of reproductive behavior. This finding suggests that neural circuits are not sensitive to potential organizing effects of testosterone after puberty. Future work will include direct tests of the hypothesis that puberty is a critical period for steroid-dependent organization of behavior and focused investigation of the structural mechanisms by which steroids organize neural circuits during puberty, regardless of whether puberty is a critical period.

REFERENCES

1. PRIMUS, R. & C. KELLOGG. 1990. Gonadal hormones during puberty organize environment-related social interaction in the male rat. Horm. Behav. **24:** 311–323.
2. NUNEZ, J.L., J. SODHI & J.M. JURASKA. 2002. Ovarian hormones after postnatal day 20 reduce neuron number in the rat primary visual cortex. J. Neurobiol. **52:** 312–321.
3. PHOENIX, C., *et al.* 1959. Organizing action of prenatally administered testosterone propionate on the tissues mediating mating behavior in the female guinea pig. Endocrinology **65:** 369–382.
4. SCOTT, J.P., J.M. STEWART & V.J. DE GHETT. 1974. Critical periods in the organization of systems. Dev. Psychobiol. **7:** 489–513.
5. ARNOLD, A.P. & S.M. BREEDLOVE. 1985. Organizational and activational effects of sex steroids on brain and behavior: a reanalysis. Horm. Behav. **19:** 469–498.
6. LARSSON, K. 1967. Testicular hormone and developmental changes in mating behavior of the male rat. J. Comp. Physiol. Psychol. **63:** 223–230.
7. SISK, C.L. *et al.* 1992. Photoperiod modulates pubertal shifts in behavioral responsiveness to testosterone. J. Biol. Rhythms **7:** 329–339.
8. MEEK, L. *et al.* 1997. Actions of testosterone in prepubertal and postpubertal male hamsters: dissociation of effects on reproductive behavior and brain androgen receptor immunoreactivity. Horm. Behav. **31:** 75–88.
9. ROMEO, R.D. *et al.* 2001. Dihydrotestosterone activates sexual behavior in adult male hamsters but not in juveniles. Physiol. Behav. **73:** 579–584.
10. ROMEO, R.D. *et al.* 2002. Estradiol induces hypothalamic progesterone receptors but does not activate mating behavior in male hamsters (*Mesocricetus auratus*) before puberty. Behav. Neurosci. **116:** 198–205.
11. VANDENBERGH, J.G. 1971. The effects of gonadal hormones on the aggressive behaviour of adult golden hamsters (*Mesocricetus auratus*). Anim. Behav. **19:** 589–594.
12. ALBERS, H.E., A.C. HENNESSEY & D.C. WHITMAN. 1992. Vasopressin and the regulation of hamster social behavior. Ann. N.Y. Acad. Sci. **652:** 227–242.
13. JOHNSTON, R.E. & K. RASMUSSEN. 1984. Individual recognition of female hamsters by males: role of chemical cues and of the olfactory and vomeronasal systems. Physiol. Behav. **33:** 95–104.
14. ROMEO, R. *et al.* 1999. Androgenic regulation of hypothalamic aromatase activity in prepubertal and postpubertal male golden hamsters. Endocrinology **140:** 112–117.
15. ROMEO, R.D. & C.L. SISK. 2001. Pubertal and seasonal plasticity in the amygdala. Brain Res. **889:** 71–77.
16. GOMEZ, D.M. & S.W. NEWMAN. 1991. Medial nucleus of the amygdala in the adult Syrian hamster: a quantitative Golgi analysis of gonadal hormonal regulation of neuronal morphology. Anat. Rec. **231:** 498–509.

17. Cooke, B.M., G. Tabibnia & S.M. Breedlove. 1999. A brain sexual dimorphism controlled by adult circulating androgens. Proc. Natl. Acad. Sci. USA **96:** 7538–7540.
18. Romeo, R.D., S.L. Diedrich & C.L. Sisk. 2000. Effects of gonadal steroids during pubertal development on androgen and estrogen receptor-alpha immunoreactivity in the hypothalamus and amygdala. J. Neurobiol. **44:** 361–368.

The MPN mag

Introducing a Critical Area Mediating Pheromonal and Hormonal Regulation of Male Sexual Behavior

JENNIFER M. SWANN, JING WANG, AND ELIZABETH K. GOVEK

Department of Biological Sciences, Lehigh University, Bethlehem, Pennsylvania 18015, USA

ABSTRACT: Mating behavior in male hamsters is regulated by a chemosensory pathway that converges on the bed nucleus of the stria terminalis (BST) and the medial nucleus of the amygdala (Me). Both the BST and the Me project to the lateral part of the medial preoptic area. Lesion studies have identified a small group of large cells referred to as the magnocellular medial preoptic nucleus (MPN mag) whose integrity is required for normal mating behavior. Our data, summarized within, indicate that the MPN mag is a sexually differentiated nucleus in a large steroid-responsive network that relays pheromonal signals from the sensory systems to the motor areas to affect behavior.

KEYWORDS: medial nucleus of the amygdala; BST; MPN mag; Syrian hamster; sexual differentiation; stereology

A wide range of behaviors are differentially expressed in males and females including aggression,[1] reproductive behavior,[2] parenting,[3] spatial orientation,[4] and verbal abilities.[4] The mechanisms that underlie sexual differentiation of behavior in humans are poorly understood. However, research in other mammals suggests that the presence or absence of gonadal steroids during development regulates sex-specific expression of these behaviors in adulthood.[5] Female rodents treated with gonadal steroids at birth show male typical behavior in adulthood (masculinization), whereas males castrated after birth fail to show male typical behaviors in adulthood (demasculinization). Thus, neonatal exposure to gonadal steroids is critical for the expression of male typical behaviors in adulthood.

As behavior is regulated by the central nervous system (CNS) it follows that sex differences in behavior arise from sex differences in the organization or function of the CNS. Sex differences have been described for several neural parameters in a variety of species.[5] Sex differences in the size and volume of nuclei, first discovered in the song system of birds,[6] continue to be identified throughout the CNS.[7] Researchers have extended these findings to include drastic differences in cell number, neural chemistry, and connections in a variety of avian species.[8] Similar studies in

Address for correspondence: Jennifer M. Swann, Department of Biological Sciences, Lehigh University, Bethlehem, PA 18015. Voice: 610-758-5484; fax: 610-758-4004.
jms5@lehigh.edu

Ann. N.Y. Acad. Sci. 1007: 199–210 (2003). © 2003 New York Academy of Sciences.
doi: 10.1196/annals.1286.020

mammals have been less successful. Although sex differences in the volume of rodent hypothalamic nuclei were discovered within 2 years of the initial discovery in birds,[9] the functional significance of sex differences in neural number and chemistry in mammals is, at best, poorly understood.

The Syrian hamster offers a useful model for the study of neural regulation of sexually differentiated behaviors. These hamsters are thought to live alone in the wild and rely on chemical signals from conspecifics for the correct expression of social behaviors. Male mating behavior, in particular, is keenly dependent on the detection of pheromonal cues from the female.[10] This finding has enabled researchers to trace the pathway that regulates male sex behavior from the olfactory bulbs to the medial preoptic area. As described below, this highly conserved pathway converges on a small critical nucleus, the MPN mag. Gonadal steroids, present during development and in adulthood regulate both the structure and function of the pathway.

CHEMOSENSORY PATHWAYS PLAY CRITICAL ROLE IN MALE SEX BEHAVIOR IN THE HAMSTER

Hamsters are keenly dependent on chemosensory signals from females for the initiation of male copulatory behavior. These chemicals, which are released from several glands,[11] are detected by two distinct sensory systems in the hamster: the main and accessory olfactory systems.[12] The olfactory mucosa and the vomeronasal organ detect chemosensory signals and project to the main and accessory olfactory bulbs, respectively. The accessory olfactory system plays the greater role in the regulation of male mating behavior in the hamster.[13] Disruption of the input to the accessory olfactory bulbs immediately and permanently eliminates mating in approximately half of the male hamsters examined.[14] Disruption of main olfactory input has no effect on these measures. Simultaneous destruction of the receptors to each system or the main (MOB) and accessory olfactory bulbs (AOBs) immediately and permanently eliminates copulatory behavior in male hamsters,[14–16] Thus, these two systems are the only sensory systems required for the initiation of copulation.

In the hamster, as in other mammals, efferents from the main and accessory olfactory bulbs travel via separate routes to the amygdala and bed nucleus of the stria terminalis (BST; reviewed in Wood and Swann[17]). The accessory olfactory bulb projects to the medial nucleus of the amygdala (Me), the posteromedial cortical nucleus, and the posteromedial subdivision of the BST.[18,19] The main olfactory bulb sends projections to the anterior and posterior cortical nuclei.[20] The anterior cortical nucleus projects to the medial nucleus. Thus, Me is the first nucleus in the pathway to integrate the signals from both the MOB and AOB. Me maintains bidirectional connections with the BST.[21] Both the BST and Me project to the preoptic area.[22–24]

Both the Me and BST are readily partitioned into subdivisions based on bidirectional connections, concentration of steroid receptors, stimulation by pheromones and role in male reproduction (FIG. 1). In the hamster,[21] anterior Me (MeA) is bidirectionally connected to the posterior intermediate BST (BSTpi), and posterior Me (MeP) is bidirectionally connected to the posterior medial BST (BSTpm). Although all four areas contain receptors for androgen and estrogen receptor alpha (ERα), these receptors are more densely concentrated in the BSTpm and MeP.[25] Neurons in the BSTpm and MeP are stimulated by both sexually relevant pheromones that serve to initiate male sexual behavior[26,27] and ejaculation which may serve to terminate male sexual behavior.[28,29] Nonetheless, it is the MeA that plays the more critical role.[23] Destruction of the MeA eliminates both copulation and anogenital investigation in male hamsters. Destruction of the MeP only disrupts anogenital investigation.

ROLE OF THE MEDIAL PREOPTIC AREA: INTRODUCING THE MPN MAG

The medial preoptic area has been implicated in the regulation of male sexual behavior in every species examined to date including the hamster. Lesion studies in the

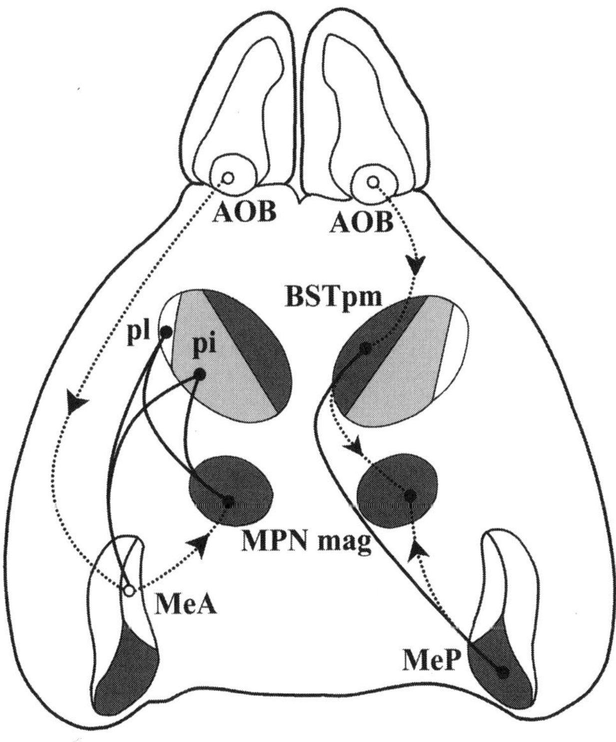

FIGURE 1. Schematic diagram of the connections between the accessory olfactory bulb, extended amygdala (BST and Me) and the MPN mag. *Dashed lines* indicate a unidirectional connection with projections in the direction indicated by the arrow. *Solid lines* indicate a bidirectional connection. *Shading* indicates the relative concentration of ERα-immunoreactive neurons: *black* shading indicates an area with high density of ERα-immunoreactive neurons, *gray* shading indicates an area with low density of ERα-immunoreactive neurons, *white* shading indicates an area with few ERα-immunoreactive neurons. AOB, accessory olfactory bulb; BST, bed nucleus of the stria terminalis; PM, posterior-medial BST; PI, posterior intermediate BST; PL, posterior lateral; MeA, anterior subdivision of the medial nucleus of the amygdala; cMePD, posterior subdivision of the medial nucleus of the amygdala; MPN mag, magnocellular subdivision of the medial preoptic nucleus.

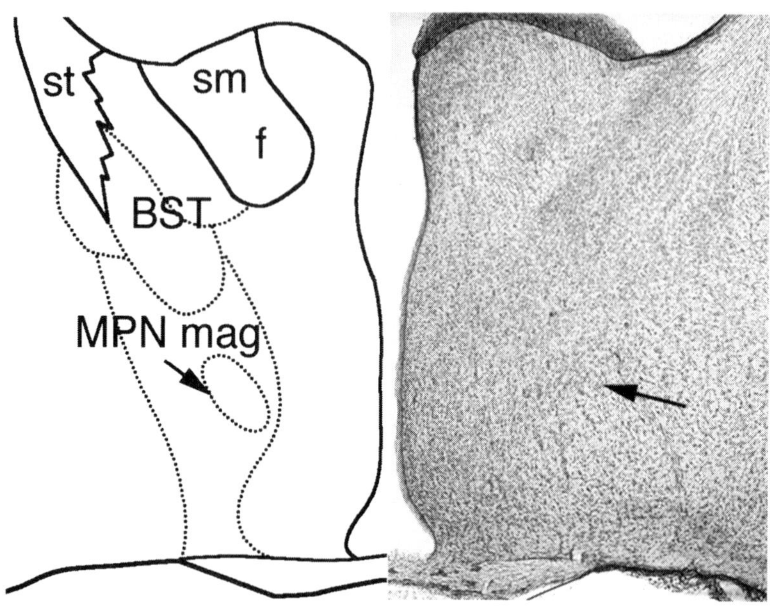

FIGURE 2. Schematic drawing (**A**) and photomicrograph (**B**) of a cresyl violet stained coronal section through the MPN mag. The MPN mag is indicted in both panels by an arrow. BST, bed nucleus of the stria terminalis; f, fornix; MPN mag, magnocellular subdivision of the medial preoptic nucleus; sm, stria medularis; st, stria terminalis.

male hamster have identified a small group of cells in the lateral aspect of the medial preoptic area that play a critical role.[30] This group has been named the magnocellular medial preoptic nucleus (MPN mag) because of the predominance of large cells[24] and is shown in FIGURE 2. Bilateral destruction of the MPN mag eliminates copulation in male hamsters but fails to disrupt anogenital investigation suggesting a more specific role for the MPN mag in the regulation of male mating behavior than that of the extended amygdala. Several studies utilizing anterograde tracers have suggested that the Me and BST are connected to the MPN mag.[22–24] Our laboratory recently has confirmed and extended these findings.[31]

We described the afferent connections of the MPN mag using the retrograde tract tracer cholera toxin-B (List Biologicals, CTB). Injections of CTB into the MPN mag labeled cells in both the MeA and MeP as well as the BSTpm and BSTpi. Thus, the MPN mag receives input from both circuits of the extended amygdala that process signals from the accessory olfactory system. We also found retrogradely labeled cells in the anterior and posterior cortical nuclei of the amygdala (ACo and PMCo, respectively), regions that receive direct input from the main olfactory bulbs. Taken together, our results suggest that the MPN mag integrates information from both the main and accessory olfactory systems to regulate male sexual behavior.

We also have used an anterograde tracer to identify the targets of the MPN mag.[31] Our results indicate that the MPN mag projects to the ACo and BSTpi, allowing the MPN mag to modify input from these areas. We found that the MPN mag does not project to the medial amygdala or the BSTpm, indicating that information relayed to the MPN mag from these areas is not directly affected by the MPN mag. Our findings are summarized in FIGURE 1.

The MPN mag sends projections to several brainstem nuclei implicated in the regulation of male mating behavior including the ventral tegmental area (VTA), the deep mesencephalic nuclei (DpMe), retrorubral field, and paragigantocellular nucleus (nPGi). Lesions of the dorsal tegmentum that include the DpMe eliminate sex behavior in adult male rats.[32] Lesions of the retrorubral field eliminate male mating behavior in adult gerbils.[33] The nPGi sends projections to the spinal nuclei that regulate ejaculation.[34] Projections between these brainstem nuclei and the MPN mag are unidirectional providing anatomical support for a role for the MPN mag in relaying chemosensory information to brainstem areas involved in reproduction.

THE MPN MAG IS PART OF A STEROID-RESPONSIVE NETWORK

In hamsters, as in most mammals, copulatory behavior is dependent on circulating gonadal steroids. Gonadectomy eliminates male mating behavior and systemic treatment with testosterone or its metabolites, DHT and estrogen, restores it.[35] Receptors for gonadal steroids have been localized to specific nuclear groups, and steroids are effective in restoring copulation when placed directly into these areas.[36–38] In light of these findings, it is interesting that the MPN mag maintains bidirectional connections with several neural groups that are immunopositive for the estrogen receptor alpha. As shown in FIGURE 3, most of these connections are bidirectional, suggesting that the MPN mag is part of a larger network of steroid-concentrating neurons. Interestingly, the steroid-concentrating neurons with unidirectional connections are found in the amygdala and BST. Both the BSTpm and the MePD project to the MPN mag, but neither area receives projections from it.[31] Both the BST and Me are sites for steroid action in the regulation of male sex behavior. Gonadal steroids placed in the BST or the Me stimulate mating behavior in castrated hamsters.[37] Moreover, an elegant study by Wood and Newman[39] indicates that the BST and Me integrate chemosensory and hormonal signals to regulate male mating behavior. This study utilized the fact that the pathways that process chemosensory information are highly conserved and do not cross the midline before reaching the MPOA. Hamsters were castrated and given a unilateral bulbectomy and an intracerebral steroid implant. The implant in the BST and Me restored sexual activity but only when the implant was placed on the unlesioned side. Thus, both hormonal and pheromonal input must arrive at the same neural groups to restore male sexual behavior. Finally, our research indicates that circulating gonadal steroids in the adult serve to maintain connections among the BST, Me, and MPN mag.[40] Exposure to pheromones found in female hamster vaginal secretions (FHVSs) induces copulatory behavior in male hamsters.[41] Exposure to FHVSs stimulates neurons in the BST, Me, and MPN mag in intact males.[26] The BST and Me show fos in castrated males exposed to FHVS but the MPN mag does not.[42] Pheromonal stimulation of the MPN mag is restored in castrates treated with testosterone. Because pheromonal signals are relayed to the MPN mag via the BST and Me, our results suggest that connections among the BST, Me, and MPN mag are disrupted in castrated males and that functional maintenance of connections among these nuclei are dependent on testosterone.

SEX DIFFERENCES IN NEURAL PARAMETERS CHARACTERIZE THE MATING BEHAVIOR PATHWAY

Male mating behavior is sexually dimorphic. Although female sexual behavior can be elicited from males in some species under the right hormonal conditions, male sexual behavior is predominately expressed by males. Sex differences in several neural parameters have been described in the vomeronasal pathway of several rodent species.[43] We have found a physiologic sex difference in the vomeronasal pathway. Exposure to FHVS stimulates the MPN mag in males but not in female hamsters. This sex difference is not the result of differential steroid milieu in the two sexes. Stimulation of the MPN mag is not induced in females treated with testosterone in adulthood.[42] Because several preoptic nuclei have been described as sexually dimorphic in other species,[9,44–47] we reasoned that the MPN mag of hamsters is also sexually dimorphic. To this end, we examined the number of neurons in the MPN mag of male and female hamsters using a stereologic approach. Our results show that adult male hamsters (60 days) have more neurons than females and that the neurons in the male are more densely packed than those in the female (FIG. 3).[48] We are currently measuring other neural parameters to determine if sex differences in density are caused by differences in glial cell number or neuropil. Note that the overall volume of the MPN mag is not different between the sexes. Because volume is the measure most often utilized in studies of sex difference in neural groups, our results stand as a cautionary tale to those that use this measure to infer a lack of sex differences within a neural area.

GONADAL STEROIDS ORGANIZE THE SEX DIFFERENCES IN BEHAVIOR AND BRAIN

Gonadal steroids play powerful and critical roles in the differentiation of male sexual behavior. In most mammals, it is the increase in circulating gonadal steroids, generated by the developing testis, that permanently masculinizes behavior. In a variety of rodents, including the hamster, postnatal treatment with testosterone or estrogen induces male sexual behavior in females (masculinization), whereas removal of gonadal steroids by postnatal castration eliminates male sexual behavior in males (demasculinization).[49] The window for masculinization is very narrow in the hamster.[50] Treatment with steroids is most effective on the first day of birth and gradually declines in effectiveness during the subsequent 3 days and has no effect from postnatal day 5 to adulthood.

We have found that sex differences in the number of neurons in the MPN mag arise between postnatal day 5 and 10 immediately after the critical period for the differentiation of the behavior. These findings suggest that the effect of steroids on cell number is delayed. Studies in two other models of sexual differentiation suggest a possible model. Neurons in the spinal nucleus of the bulbocavernosus (SNB) of rats are sexually differentiated such that males have more neurons than females.[51] Sexual differentiation of the SNB is regulated by the presence of testosterone during a critical period just before and after birth.[52] This nuclear group innervates muscles in the peritoneum[53] and steroids appear to regulate motor neuron number through actions on the muscle rather than the neurons.[54–57] Recently, Forger and coworkers

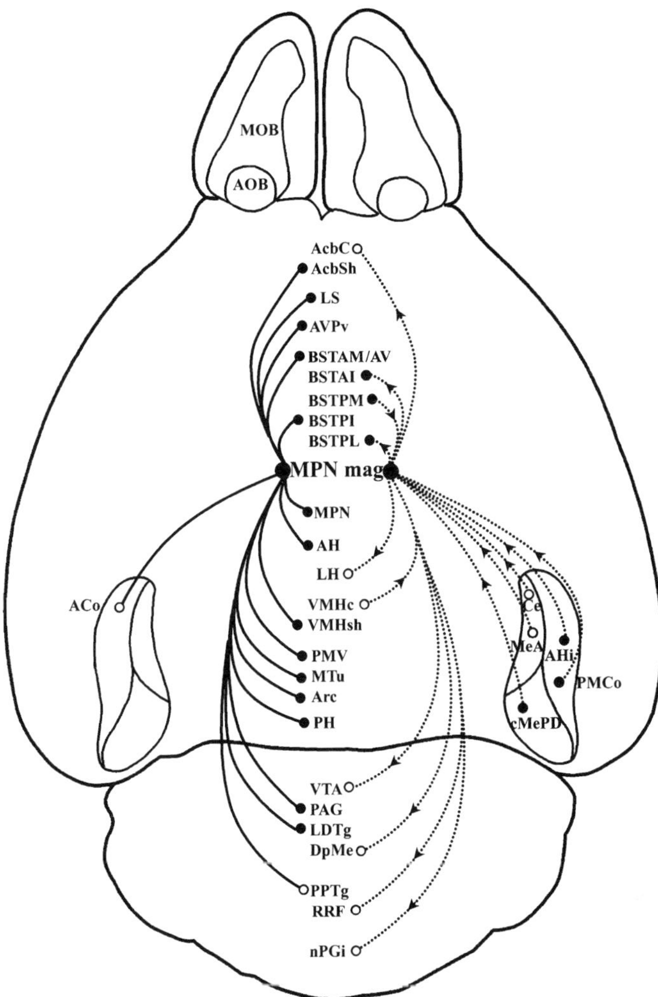

FIGURE 3. Schematic summary of the afferent and efferent connections of the MPN mag. Bidirectional connections are indicated with a solid line on the left, and unidirectional connections are indicated with dashed line on the right. The direction of the unidirectional connections is indicated with an arrowhead. Areas containing ERα immunoreactivity are indicated with a filled dot; those without ERα are indicated with an open dot. AOB, accessory olfactory bulb; AcbC, accumbens nucleus core; AcbSh, accumbens nucleus shell; ACo, anterior cortical nucleus of the amygdala; Ahi, anterior hippocampus; AOB, accessory olfactory bulb; ARC, arcuate nucleus; AVPv, anteroventral periventricular nucleus; BSTAI, anterior intermediate subdivision of the BST; BSTAL, anterior lateral subdivision of the BST; BSTAM, anterior medial subdivision of the BST; BSTAV, anterior ventral subdivision of the BST; BSTPI, posterior intermediate subdivision of the BST; BSTPL, posterior lateral subdivision of the BST; BSTPM, posterior medial subdivision of the BST; DpMe, deep mesencephalic nucleus; LH, lateral hypothalamus; LS, lateral septum; MeA, medial nucleus of

have produced evidence that sexual differentiation is mediated by a growth factor produced in the target muscle.[58] These researchers propose that steroids regulate neural survival by stimulating the production of growth factors in target areas that attract and support additional neurons in the male. This mechanism appears to underlie sexual differentiation in the rat CNS as well. Projections from the BST to the AVPv are strikingly dimorphic; this pathway is 10 times larger in males than in females.[59] Cocultures of explants from the BST and AVPv suggest that neurotrophic chemicals mediate the formation of this pathway.[60] Neurons in cultures of the BST taken from perinatal males will extend axons toward neurons in cultures of the AVPv taken from perinatal males when these two cultures are grown in close approximation. Moreover, whereas similar cultures from females do not show this growth, neurons in explants of the female BST will grow toward those in the male AVPv. Taken together, these results suggest that the cells in the AVPv release a growth factor that attracts the axons of the BST. We predict that a similar mechanism is at work during the development and sexual differentiation of the MPN mag. One potential problem with this hypothesis is the substantial distance between the MPN mag (in the preoptic area) and its target nuclei in the brainstem. We speculate that the efferents of the MPN mag are guided to their furthest targets by steroid-concentrating nuclei along the way.

IS THE MPN MAG ONLY FOUND IN THE HAMSTER?

Cellular groups analogous to the MPN mag may be present in the gerbil and the rat. Anatomically, the MPN mag is in the same location as the lateral sexually dimorphic area (lSDA) of the gerbil. The afferent connections of the lSDA are similar but not identical to those of the MPN mag.[61] The lSDA, like the MPN mag, receives projections from the MeA, VMH shell, PAG, and pedunculopontine tegmental nucleus (PPTg), which also project to the MPN mag. However, the lSDA does not receive projections from the BSTpm or VMH core. Instead, these areas project to a more medial nucleus, the mSDA. The efferents of the gerbil lSDA and mSDA are similar but not identical to those of the MPN mag in the caudal hypothalamus and brainstem.[62] For example, the lSDA fails to project to the PMV, a target of the MPN mag. Conversely, the mSDA projects to both anterior and posterior Me but the MPN mag does not. Because both the mSDA and lSDA play a role in the regulation of male sexual behavior in the gerbil,[63] the hamster MPN mag may be an interesting anatomical combination of these nuclei.

The analogous area in the rat has been labeled the "preoptic BST,"[64] the "ventral and magnocellular" BST,[65]the BSTpi,[66] and the "vBST-MPOA."[67] The vBST-

---

the amygdala, anterior; cMePD, caudal portion of the medial nucleus of the amygdala, posterodorsal; MOB, main olfactory bulb; MPN, medial preoptic nucleus; MPN mag, magnocellular medial preoptic nucleus; Mtu, medial tuberal nucleus; nPGi, paragigantocellular nucleus; PAG, periaqueductal gray; PH, posterior hypothalamus; PMCo, posterior medial cortical nucleus of the amygdala; PMV, ventral premamillary nucleus; PPTg, pedunculopontine tegmental nucleus; RRF, retrorubral field; VMHc, ventral medial nucleus of the hypothalamus, core; VMHsh, ventral medial nucleus of the hypothalamus, shell.

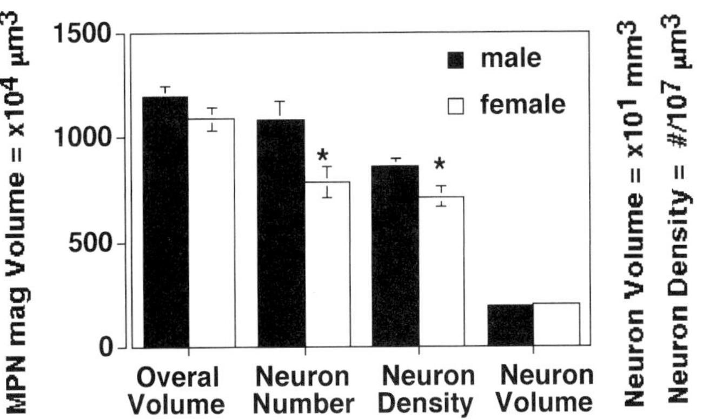

FIGURE 4. Sex differences in stereologic parameters of the MPN mag. The average number of neurons per MPN mag is indicated on the left axis. (N = 10 for all groups.)

MPOA projects to areas in the brainstem that include those of the hamster MPN mag. Moreover, the vBST-MPOA, like the MPN mag, fails to project to any subdivision of the Me. These findings have been confirmed and extended by Murphy and Hoffman who found that cells that label positively for steroid receptors in this region project to the PAG.[68] Projections from these neurons terminate in close proximity to neurons projecting to the nucleus paragigantocellularis, suggesting that the preoptic neurons are part of a circuit that regulates male sexual behavior. Clearly, more studies are warranted to determine the role of this more lateral cell group in the regulation of male sexual behavior in the rat.

In conclusion, the MPN mag offers an exciting new anatomical model for the study of the role of steroids in the differentiation and maintenance of male sexual behavior. Comparison with studies in the gerbil points out interesting species differences. The location of brain areas playing similar critical roles in rats and mice has not been described. We urge researchers in these models to look in more lateral parts of the MPOA for analogous areas that will extend our understanding of this complicated brain region.

REFERENCES

1. Archer, J. 2000. Sex differences in aggression between heterosexual partners: a meta-analytic review. Psychol. Bull. **126:** 651–680.
2. Breedlove, S. 1993. Sexual differentiation of the brain and behavior. *In* Behvioral Endocrinology. J. Becker, S. Breedlove & D. Crews, Eds.: 39–70. MIT. Cambridge, MA.
3. Lonstein, J.S. & G.J. De Vries. 2000. Sex differences in the parental behavior of rodents. Neurosci. Biobehav. Rev. **24:** 669–686.
4. Neave, N., M. Menaged & D.R. Weightman. 1999. Sex differences in cognition: the role of testosterone and sexual orientation. Brain Cogn. **41:** 245–262.
5. Cooke, B. *et al.* 1998. Sexual differentiation of the vertebrate brain: principles and mechanisms. Front. Neuroendocrinol. **19:** 323–362.

6. Nottebohm, F. & A.P. Arnold. 1976. Sexual dimorphism in vocal control areas of the songbird brain. Science **194:** 211–213.
7. Madeira, M.D. & A.R. Lieberman. 1995. Sexual dimorphism in the mammalian limbic system. Prog. Neurobiol. **45:** 275–333.
8. Ball, G.F. & S.A. MacDougall-Shackleton. 2001. Sex differences in songbirds 25 years later: what have we learned and where do we go? Microsc. Res. Tech. **54:** 327–334.
9. Gorski, R.A. *et al.* 1978. Evidence for a morphological sex difference within the medial preoptic area of the rat brain. Brain Res. **148:** 333–346.
10. Johnston, R.E. 1998. Pheromones, the vomeronasal system, and communication. From hormonal responses to individual recognition. Ann. N.Y. Acad. Sci. **855:** 333–348.
11. Johnston, R.E. 1990. Chemical communication in golden hamsters: from behavior to molecules and neural mechanisms. *In* Contemporary Issues in Comparative Psychology. D.A. Dewsbury, Ed.: 381–409. Sinauer. Sunderland, MA.
12. Meredith, M. 1991. Sensory processing in the main and accessory olfactory systems: comparisons and contrasts. Steroid Biochem. Mol. Biol. **39:** 610–614.
13. Meredith, M. 1986. Vomeronasal organ removal before sexual experience impairs male hamster mating behavior. Physiol. Behav. **36:** 737–743.
14. Winans, S.S. & J.B. Powers. 1977. Olfactory and vomeronasal differentiation of male hamsters: histological and behavioral analyses. Brain Res. **126:** 325–344.
15. Murphy, M.R. & G.E. Schneider. 1970. Olfactory bulb removal eliminates mating behavior in the male golden hamster. Science **167:** 302–304.
16. Lisk, R.D., J. Zeiss & L.A. Ciaccio. 1972. The influence of olfaction on sexual behavior in the male golden hamster (*Mesocricetus auratus*). J. Exp. Zool. **181:** 69–78.
17. Wood, R.I. & J.M. Swann. 1999. Neuronal integration of chemosensory and hormonal signals in the control of male sexual behavior. *In* Reproduction in Context. K. Wallen & J. Schneider, Eds.: 423–444. MIT Press. Cambridge, MA.
18. Scalia, F. & S.S. Winans. 1975. The differential projections of the olfactory bulb and accessory olfactory bulb in mammals. J. Comp. Neurol. **161:** 31–56.
19. Davis, B.J. *et al.* 1978. Efferents and centrifugal afferents of the main and accessory olfactory bulbs in the hamster. Brain Res. Bull. **3:** 59–72.
20. Kevetter, G.A. & S.S. Winans. 1981. Connections of the corticomedial amygdala in the golden hamster. II. Efferents of the "olfactory amygdala." J. Comp. Neurol. **197:** 99–111.
21. Coolen, L.M. & R.I. Wood. 1998. Bidirectional connections of the medial amygdaloid nucleus in the Syrian hamster brain: simultaneous anterograde and retrograde tract tracing. J. Comp. Neurol. **399:** 189–209.
22. Gomez, D.M. & S.W. Newman. 1992. Differential projections of the anterior and posterior regions of the medial amygdaloid nucleus in the Syrian hamster. J. Comp. Neurol. **317:** 195–218.
23. Lehman, M.N., S.S. Winans & J.B. Powers. 1980. Medial nucleus of the amygdala mediates chemosensory control of male hamster sexual behavior. Science **210:** 557–560.
24. Maragos, W.F. *et al.* 1989. Neurons of origin and fiber trajectory of amygdalofugal projections to the medial preoptic area in Syrian hamsters. J. Comp. Neurol. **280:** 59–71.
25. Wood, R.I. & S.W. Newman. 1995. Androgen and estrogen receptors coexist within individual neurons in the brain of the Syrian hamster. Neuroendocrinology **62:** 487–497.
26. Fiber, J.M., P. Adames & J.M. Swann. 1993. Pheromones induce c-*fos* in limbic areas regulating male hamster mating behavior. Neuroreport **4:** 871–874.
27. Kollack-Walker, S. & S. Newman. 1997. Mating-induced expression of c-fos in the male Syrian hamster brain: role of experience, pheromones, and ejaculations. J. Neurobiol. **32:** 481–501.
28. Coolen, L.M. *et al.* 1997. Demonstration of ejaculation-induced neural activity in the male rat brain using 5-HT1A agonist 8-OH-DPAT. Physiol. Behav. **62:** 881–891.
29. Parfitt, D.B. & S.W. Newman. 1998. Fos-immunoreactivity within the extended amygdala is correlated with the onset of sexual satiety. Horm. Behav. **34:** 17–29.

30. Powers, J.B., S.W. Newman & M.L. Bergondy. 1987. MPOA and BNST lesions in male Syrian hamsters: differential effects on copulatory and chemoinvestigatory behaviors. Behav. Brain Res. **23:** 181–195.
31. Wang, J. & J.M. Swann. 2001. Connections of the magnocellular medial preoptic nucleus. Abstr. Soc. Neurosci. **27**.
32. Brackett, N.L. & D.A. Edwards. 1984. Medial preoptic connections with the midbrain tegmentum are essential for male sexual behavior. Physiol. Behav. **32:** 79–84.
33. Finn, P.D. & P. Yahr. 1994. Projections of the sexually dimorphic area of the gerbil hypothalamus to the retrorubral field is essential for male sexual behavior: role of A8 and other cells. Behav. Neurosci. **108:** 362–378.
34. Murphy, A.Z. *et al.* 1999. The organization of preoptic-medullary circuits in the male rat: evidence for interconnectivity of neural structures involved in reproductive behavior, antinociception and cardiovascular regulation. Neuroscience **91:** 1103–1116.
35. Powers, J.B., M.L. Bergondy & J.A. Matochik. 1985. Male hamster sociosexual behaviors: effects of testosterone and its metabolites. Physiol. Behav. **35:** 607–616.
36. Wood, R.I. *et al.* 1992. Androgen and estrogen concentrating neurons in chemosensory pathways of the male Syrian hamster brain. Brain Res. **596:** 89–98.
37. Wood, R. & S. Newman. 1995. The medial amygdaloid nucleus and medial preoptic area mediate steroidal control of sexual behavior in the male Syrian hamster. Horm. Behav. **29:** 338–353.
38. Wood, R.I. & S.J. Williams. 2001. Steroidal control of male hamster sexual behavior in Me and MPOA: effects of androgen dose and tamoxifen. Physiol. Behav. **72:** 727–733.
39. Wood, R.I. & S.W. Newman. 1995. Integration of chemosensory and hormonal cues is essential for mating in the male Syrian hamster. J. Neurosci. **15:** 7261–7269.
40. Swann, J.M. & S.W. Newman. 1992. Testosterone regulates substance P within neurons of the medial nucleus of the amygdala, the bed nucleus of the stria terminalis and the medial preoptic area of the male golden hamster. Brain Res. **590:** 18–28.
41. Murphy, M.R. 1973. Effects of female hamster vaginal discharge on the behavior of male hamsters. Behav. Biol. **9:** 367–375.
42. Fiber, J.M. & J.M. Swann. 1996. Testosterone differentially influences sex-specific pheromone-stimulated fos expression in limbic regions of Syrian hamsters. Horm. Behav. **30:** 455–473.
43. Guillamon, A. & S. Segovia. 1997. Sex differences in the vomeronasal system. Brain Res. Bull. **44:** 377–382.
44. Raisman, G. & P.M. Field. 1973. Sexual dimorphism in the neuropil of the preoptic area of the rat and its dependence on neonatal androgen. Brain Res. **54:** 1–29.
45. Shapiro, L.E. *et al.* 1991. Comparative neuroanatomy of the sexually dimorphic hypothalamus in monogamous and polygamous voles. Brain Res. **541:** 232–240.
46. Yahr, P. *et al.* 1994. Sexually dimorphic cell groups in the medial preoptic area that are essential for male sex behavior and the neural pathways needed for their effects. Psychoneuroendocrinology **19:** 463–470.
47. Davis, E.C., J.E. Shryne & R.A. Gorski. 1996. Structural sexual dimorphisms in the anteroventral periventricular nucleus of the rat hypothalamus are sensitive to gonadal steroids perinatally, but develop peripubertally. Neuroendocrinology **63:** 142–148.
48. Govek, E.K., J. Wang & J.M. Swann. 2003. Sex differences in the magnocellular subdivision of the medial preoptic nucleus in Syrian hamsters. Neuroscience **116:** 593–598.
49. Breedlove, S.M., B.M. Cooke & C.L. Jordan. 1999. The orthodox view of brain sexual differentiation. Brain Behav. Evol. **54:** 8–14.
50. Coniglio, L.P. & L.G. Clemens. 1976. Period of maximal susceptibility to behavioral modification by testosterone in the golden hamster. Horm. Behav. **7:** 267–282.
51. Breedlove, S.M. & A.P. Arnold. 1980. Hormone accumulation in a sexually dimorphic motor nucleus of the rat spinal cord. Science **210:** 564–566.
52. Breedlove, S.M. & A.P. Arnold. 1983. Hormonal control of a developing neuromuscular system. II. Sensitive periods for the androgen-induced masculinization of the rat spinal nucleus of the bulbocavernosus. J. Neurosci. **3:** 424–432.

53. McKenna, K.E. & I. Nadelhaft. 1986. The organization of the pudendal nerve in the male and female rat. J. Comp. Neurol. **248:** 532–549.
54. Fishman, R.B. & S.M. Breedlove. 1988. Neonatal androgen maintains sexually dimorphic muscles in the absence of innervation. Muscle Nerve **11:** 553–560.
55. Fishman, R.B. *et al.* 1990. Evidence for androgen receptors in sexually dimorphic perineal muscles of neonatal male rats. Absence of androgen accumulation by the perineal motoneurons. J. Neurobiol. **21:** 694–704.
56. Freeman, L.M., N.V. Watson & S.M. Breedlove. 1996. Androgen spares androgen-insensitive motoneurons from apoptosis in the spinal nucleus of the bulbocavernosus in rats. Horm. Behav. **30:** 424–433.
57. Jordan, C.L. *et al.* 1997. Ontogeny of androgen receptor immunoreactivity in lumbar motoneurons and in the sexually dimorphic levator ani muscle of male rats. J. Comp. Neurol. **379:** 88–98.
58. Xu, J. *et al.* 2001. Blockade of endogenous neurotrophic factors prevents the androgenic rescue of rat spinal motoneurons. J. Neurosci. **21:** 4366–4372.
59. Hutton, L., G. Gu & R. Simerly. 1998. Development of a sexually dimorphic projection from the bed nuclei of the stria terminalis to the anteroventral periventricular nucleus in the rat. J. Neurosci. **18:** 3003–3013.
60. Ibanez, M.A., G. Gu & R.B. Simerly. 2001. Target-dependent sexual differentiation of a limbic-hypothalamic neural pathway. J. Neurosci. **21:** 5652–5659.
61. De Vries, G., C. Gonzales & P. Yahr. 1988. Afferent connections of the sexually dimorphic area of the hypothalamus of male and female gerbils. J. Comp. Neurol. **271:** 91–105.
62. Finn, P.D., G.J. De Vries & P. Yahr. 1993. Efferent projections of the sexually dimorphic area of the gerbil hypothalamus: anterograde identification and retrograde verification in males and females. J. Comp. Neurol. **338:** 491–521.
63. Yahr, P. & J. Gregory. 1993. The medial and lateral cell groups of the sexually dimorphic area of the gerbil hypothalamus are essential for male sex behavior and act via separate pathways. Brain Res. **631:** 287–296.
64. Moga, M.M., C.B. Saper & T.S. Gray. 1989. Bed nucleus of the stria terminalis: cytoarchitecture, immunohistochemistry, and projection to the parabrachial nucleus in the rat. J. Comp. Neurol. **283:** 315–332.
65. Ju, G., L.W. Swanson & R.B. Simerly. 1989. Studies on the cellular architecture of the bed nuclei of the stria terminalis in the rat. II. Chemoarchitecture. J. Comp. Neurol. **280:** 603–621.
66. Alheid, G.F. *et al.* 1998. The neuronal organization of the supracapsular part of the stria terminalis in the rat: the dorsal component of the extended amygdala. Neuroscience **84:** 967–996.
67. Numan, M. & T.P. Sheehan. 1997. Neuroanatomical circuitry for mammalian maternal behavior. Ann. N.Y. Acad. Sci. **807:** 101–125.
68. Murphy, A.Z. & G.E. Hoffman. 2001. Distribution of gonadal steroid receptor-containing neurons in the preoptic-periaqueductal gray-brainstem pathway: a potential circuit for the initiation of male sexual behavior. J. Comp. Neurol. **438:** 191–212.

The Activation of Birdsong by Testosterone

Multiple Sites of Action and Role of Ascending Catecholamine Projections

GREGORY F. BALL,[a] CHRISTINA B. CASTELINO,[a] DONNA L. MANEY,[a] DIDIER APPELTANTS,[b] AND JACQUES BALTHAZART[b]

[a]*Department of Psychological and Brain Sciences, Johns Hopkins University, Baltimore, Maryland 21218, USA*

[b]*Center for Cellular and Molecular Neurobiology, Research Group in Behavioral Neuroendocrinology, University of Liège, B-4020 Liège, Belgium*

ABSTRACT: Birdsong is a species-typical stereotypic vocalization produced in the context of reproduction and aggression. Among temperate-zone songbirds, it is produced primarily by males, and its frequency and quality are enhanced by the presence of the gonadal steroid hormone testosterone in the plasma. In the brain, the effects of testosterone on song behavior involve both estrogenic and androgenic metabolites of testosterone that are locally produced and act via their cognate receptors. Androgen, and in some cases estrogen, receptors are present in many specialized forebrain song control nuclei. Testosterone can regulate catecholamine steady-state levels and turnover in these song control regions. Tracing studies combined with immunocytochemistry for tyrosine hydroxylase (a marker of catecholamine synthesis) reveal several catecholamine cell groups that project to forebrain song control nuclei. These brain areas also express the mRNA for either androgen receptors or estrogen receptor alpha, and androgens enhance the expression of tyrosine hydroxylase. Dopaminergic cell groups that project to song nuclei express the protein product of the immediate early gene *fos* in association with the production of territorial song. Thus, testosterone may be acting on song behavior via these ascending catecholamine cell groups. Chemical lesioning studies suggest that noradrenergic projections to the song system are involved in the latency to produce song and the ability to discriminate conspecific from heterospecific song. The song control circuit may thus be modulated in significant ways via the androgen regulation of forebrain catecholamine systems.

KEYWORDS: estradiol; norepinephrine; song learning; seasonal reproduction; zebra finch; European starling

Address for correspondence: Gregory F. Ball, Department of Psychological and Brain Sciences, Johns Hopkins University, 3400 N. Charles Street, Baltimore, MD 21218. Voice: +1 410-516-7910; fax: +1 410-516-6008.
gball@jhu.edu

Ann. N.Y. Acad. Sci. 1007: 211–231 (2003).
doi: 10.1196/annals.1286.021

BEHAVIORAL NEUROENDOCRINOLOGY AND THE STUDY OF HORMONAL REGULATION OF BIRDSONG

A key observation that forms the foundation for behavioral neuroendocrinology is that the presence or absence of a hormone greatly influences the probability and intensity of a behavioral response.[1] Among the first attempts to link an important social behavior with the action of sex steroid hormones were studies of sexual behavior.[1] Initial studies in this tradition utilized techniques that removed or restored the source of the hormone in question to causally link the presence of the hormone with the behavioral response (e.g., Ref. 2). Related studies measured hormone concentrations in the plasma to assess whether variation in the hormone correlated with behavioral changes (e.g., Ref. 2). The next important advance was to identify neural sites(s) where hormones act to facilitate behavior (e.g., Refs. 3–5). This era of the behavioral neuroendocrinology research program led to the identification of a few brain nuclei that clearly play key roles in the facilitation of certain behaviors (e.g., the ventrolateral ventromedial nucleus of the hypothalamus (VMN) and the lordotic response in female rodents, or the preoptic area and male sexual response in many species; see Refs. 6–8). It is now clear that these key sites of hormone action are part of much more complex neural circuits that involve sensory inputs of various sorts—connections to the appropriate motor outputs, as well as ascending inputs from brainstem modulatory circuits. Hormone–brain–behavior interrelationships need to be understood in this broader context. Hormones can potentially exert their behavioral effects by acting directly on the sensory inputs or motor outputs or via ascending modulatory transmitter systems (e.g., Ref. 9).

One of the challenges of the systems approach to the study of neuroendocrinology and behavior therefore is to characterize functionally the neural circuits that regulate the behavioral system of interest. For example, the importance of the preoptic region in relation to male sexual response and the VMN for female-typical lordosis has long been known.[10,11] Current studies on the neuroendocrine control of male sexual behavior carried out by Hull and colleagues analyze how inputs from the medial amygdala to the preoptic region are important for dopamine action in this area in relation to male sexual response.[12] Work on the lordosis circuit by Calizo and Flanagan-Cato[13] has identified specific neurons within the VMN that exhibit changes in spine density regulated by estrogens that also project to the periacqueductal central gray (PAG) that in turn project to spinal areas responsible for activating back muscles involved in the lordotic reflex. Thus, in these well-known research paradigms in behavioral neuroendocrinology, brain areas initially discovered as playing a key role in certain behaviors are being placed in the broader context of the entire circuit that regulates the behavior of interest.

The study of the hormonal control of birdsong is a particularly good example of how a neuroendocrine research strategy has developed based on decades of research. Song is a male reproductive behavior that functions primarily for territorial defense and mate attraction.[14] It is controlled by a clearly defined neural circuit that is an example of a neural specialization unique in several respects to members of the songbird suborder (suborder passeres or oscines of the order passeriformes[15,16]). This circuit is also clearly regulated by gonadal sex steroid hormones as one might expect of a behavior so closely tied to reproduction.[17,18] What is unusual to some degree is that the specialized forebrain brain nuclei that control song also express in many cases androgen receptors (AR) as well as estrogen receptors α (ERα).[19–23] Investigation of this specialized steroid-sensitive forebrain circuit has provided neuroendocrinologists with a unique opportunity to study hormone-induced neuroplasticity both in adulthood and during ontogeny.[24] Most research has focused on characterizing the action of steroids within these forebrain nuclei and on related chemical neuroanatomical studies of the phenotype of cells expressing steroid receptors, as well as investigation of steroid metabolizing enzymes in and around these nuclei. Recently, it has become clear that even a complex multisynaptic circuit such as the song control system receives projections from and is modulated by brain systems that may coordinate song with other behaviors.[17] In this paper, we review studies linking testosterone (T) and the activation of song behavior. We will focus on how T may be acting at multiple sites both within the song system *per se* and outside of it to regulate this behavior. We will stress the role of T in relation to ascending catecholamine inputs in this behavioral regulation.

SINGING AND THE SONG CONTROL SYSTEM AS MODELS IN NEUROBIOLOGY— A LEARNED COMPLEX BEHAVIOR CONTROLLED BY STEROIDS AND ASSOCIATED WITH EXTENSIVE PLASTICITY

Songbirds are notable because they learn and produce vocalizations called songs. Song behavior refers to complex vocalizations used in the context of mate attraction and territorial defense. Unlike most calls, songs are learned; they develop abnormally if a young male is reared without hearing the sounds of adults. Song learning displays a striking number of analogies with the acquisition of human speech.[25] Avian vocal development therefore provides one of the few tractable animal models for studying the behavioral and neural bases of vocal plasticity.[16]

Song learning and production are also modulated by steroid hormones and controlled by a discrete network of brain nuclei that ultimately control the activity of the syrinx. Some of these nuclei display an unusual degree of plasticity for homeothermic vertebrates and seasonally recruit high numbers of new neurons in response to changes in the endocrine environment (e.g., Ref. 26). Therefore, singing and the underlying neural circuitry that supports this behavior represent a useful model to analyze the behavioral, anatomical, endocrine, and neural bases of a complex behavior. It is especially interesting because this is one of the few examples where a reproductive behavior regulated by gonadal steroids involves specialized brain nuclei in the pallium that mediate a complex learned behavior.[24] Thus, in this system, questions relevant to cognitive neuroscience and affective neuroscience are united.

BRIEF OVERVIEW OF THE ANATOMY OF THE SONG CONTROL SYSTEM

Songbirds have evolved, in association with their unusual vocal abilities, a suite of neural specializations that include an interconnected circuit of telencephalic, diencephalic, mesencephalic, and myencephalic nuclei that regulate the learning, production, and perception of song.[15,27,28]

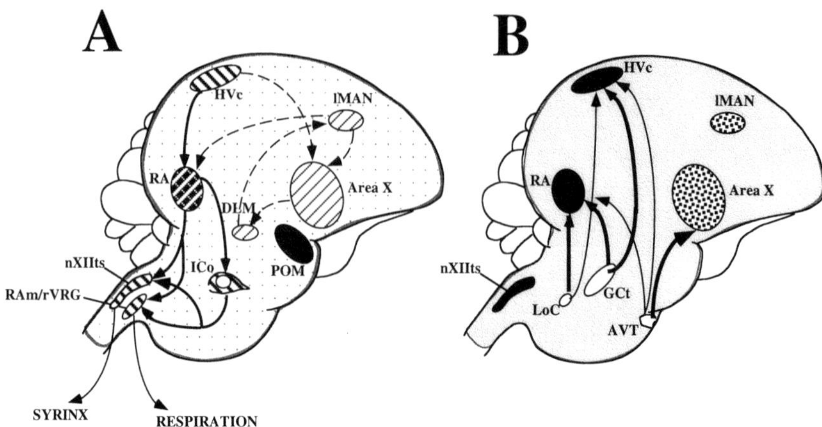

FIGURE 1. Panel A: A generalized view of the songbird vocal control system. Several of these telencephalic nuclei including HVC, RA, and lMAN represent neural specializations for vocal learning that were only observed in songbird species. One forebrain pathway, HVC to RA to nXIIts, is involved in song production. Another pathway HVC to X to lMAN to RA is involved in song learning during ontogeny and song maintenance in adulthood. The POM, a key area in the control of male sexual behaviors, is also illustrated. See text for more detail. **Panel B:** A diagrammatic representation of catecholamine cell groups that have been described which project to the forebrain song control nuclei. The LoC projection is noradrenergic in nature while GCt and AVT are primarily dopaminergic. The thickness of the lines corresponds to the number of cells that project to these areas.

A generalized model song circuit has been described based primarily on studies of zebra finches and canaries, as well as a selection of other wild species, mainly from the temperate zone, such as European starlings (*Sturnus vulgaris*). This circuit can be divided into two main parts: a caudal motor pathway and an anterior forebrain pathway (see FIG. 1A).

The caudal pathway originates in HVC (originally misnamed as hyperstriatum ventrale, pars caudale and now known simply as its abbreviation, see Ref. 29). HVC is a key part of the song system involved in the learning, production, and perception of song.[15,30,31] HVC projects to the nucleus robustus archistriatalis (RA) that in turn projects to nucleus intercollicularis (ICo), in particular, the dorsomedial portion of this complex (DM). Both RA and DM project to several medullary components of this circuit, including the tracheosyringeal part of the nucleus of the XIIth cranial nerve (nXIIts) that innervates the vocal production organ the syrinx, as well as to nucleus retroambigualis (RAm) and the rostral ventral respiratory group of neurons (rVRG) that coordinate respiratory activity with song production (see FIG. 1A). This caudal pathway (HVC→RA→ICo→nXIIts) is involved in the motor production of song. HVC also receives projections from two additional nuclei, the thalamic nucleus uvaeformis (Uva) and the neostriatal nucleus interfacialis (Nif), which also play a key role in the control of vocalization and should be considered as part of the motor pathway of the oscine song system.[15]

The second major pathway, the anterior forebrain pathway, also includes HVC and RA, and these nuclei are connected here but by an indirect route. HVC projects to area X, a part of the parolfactory lobe (homologue to parts of the corpus striatum in mammals), then to the medial part of the dorsolateral thalamic nucleus (DLM), which in turn projects to the lateral part of the magnocellular nucleus of the anterior neostriatum (lMAN), and finally back to RA (HVC→X→DLM→lMAN→RA; see FIG. 1A). lMAN also projects to area X.

Thus, there are two circuits that can transfer information from HVC to RA. The caudal pathway, described above, is clearly essential for song production based on lesion studies,[32,33] immediate early gene induction,[34,35] and electrophysiological recordings.[36] The indirect anterior forebrain pathway, in contrast, plays a key role in song learning (see Ref. 37 for a review) and in the maintenance of stereotypic adult song,[38] but lesions to nuclei within this pathway do not block adult song production.[39–41]

THE LINK BETWEEN SONG BEHAVIOR AND TESTOSTERONE

Song is a reproductive behavior, and its occurrence is therefore generally correlated positively with the onset of breeding behavior.[14,42] In temperate-zone bird species, long photoperiods that occur in the spring stimulate the recrudescence of the reproductive system.[43,44] One consequence of this vernal recrudescence is a marked increase in circulating gonadal steroid hormones that is thought to be a prerequisite for the observed increase in a suite of courtship behaviors.[43,45] In songbirds, castration combined (or not) with T replacement clearly indicates that song behavior is enhanced by T of gonadal origin.[46,47] However, although song is a good example of a T-enhanced behavior, the correlation is far from perfect. Song sparrows (*Melospiza melodia*) breeding in Washington state, USA stay on territory all year round and will sing in response to a challenging playback in the spring when plasma T concentrations are high, as well as in the fall when they are low.[48] European starlings exhibit female-directed song in the spring but will also sing in a more nonspecific manner in the fall and winter.[49,50] Castration and hormone replacement studies indicate that only the female-directed song characteristic of the spring is clearly dependent on T of gonadal origin.[51,52]

EFFECTS OF TESTOSTERONE BEFORE AND AFTER AROMATIZATION INTO 17β-ESTRADIOL

Many of the behavioral effects of T are mediated at the cellular level by the interaction of T metabolites, in particular 17β-estradiol (E2) and 5α-dihydrotestosterone (5α-DHT), with specific receptors, ER and AR, respectively. The receptors, when occupied by their specific ligand, act as transcription factors and modulate gene expression, which in turn result in a host of neurochemical changes (yet to be identified) that lead to behavioral as well as morphological changes. These general principles apply broadly in vertebrates including songbirds (for references reviewing the avian literature in particular, see Refs. 18, 53–59).

Most studies of steroid-specificity in relation to male reproductive behaviors in songbirds have focused on zebra finches (e.g., Ref. 60). Castration markedly decreases or totally suppresses all measures of reproductive behavior that were considered including singing; treatments that provided a combination of androgenic and estrogenic stimulation (T, androstenedione, E2 + 5α-DHT) restored these behaviors to normal levels typical of sexually active males. Other treatments providing pure androgenic stimulation were ineffective as also was the case for the low dose of E2 that had been selected for study.[60] These data therefore indicated that in zebra finches, singing and the associated courtship behaviors are activated synergistically by estrogens and androgens. This role of estrogens was subsequently confirmed in another study demonstrating that the behavioral effects of an aromatizable androgen such as androstenedione are markedly reduced by a simultaneous treatment with the aromatase inhibitor 1,4,6-androstatriene-3,17-dione (ATD).[61]

The synergistic action of estrogens and androgens on the activation of reproductive behaviors in songbirds may be a general feature of this taxa. This is indicated by the fact that in red-winged blackbirds (*Agelaius phoeniceus*) the frequencies of singing and of three common vocalizations (chucks, checks, and ips) that had been markedly decreased by castration were restored by treatments that provided both androgenic and estrogenic metabolites (e.g., T, androstenedione, E2 + 5α-DHT), but not by nonaromatizable androgens or estrogens alone.[62] The role of aromatase inhibitors has not been investigated exhaustively in relation to male song. However, treating female canaries with exogenous T induces male-like song patterns, but the simultaneous administration of the aromatase inhibitor fadrozole results in songs lacking a stable song structure characteristic of fall male song (produced in the presence of low T) and a low syllable repetition pattern more characteristic of female song than male song.[63] These data are consistent with the idea that estrogenic metabolites of T are important for the activation of some aspects of male-typical song in canaries.

DISTRIBUTION OF ANDROGEN AND ESTROGEN RECEPTORS IN THE SONG CONTROL SYSTEM

Both estrogenic and androgenic stimulation are thus required for the optimal activation of singing behavior. One of the first questions asked by behavioral endocrinologists was where T might be acting in the songbird brain.[19] Initial autoradiographic studies utilizing [^{3}H] T revealed uptake in several of the forebrain song control nuclei.[19] The presence of AR in the telencephalon represents another neural specialization that distinguishes songbirds from other vertebrates.[64,65] In this section we will review briefly what is known about the distribution of AR and ER in the song control system.

Androgen Receptors

In general, the distribution of AR in birds is restricted to the septal-preoptic area and to various nuclei in the hypothalamus and in the midbrain (for review, Refs. 45, 66, and 67), as is commonly observed in all vertebrate classes.[68–70] In addition to the receptors present in all avian (and vertebrate) species, songbirds possess androgen-

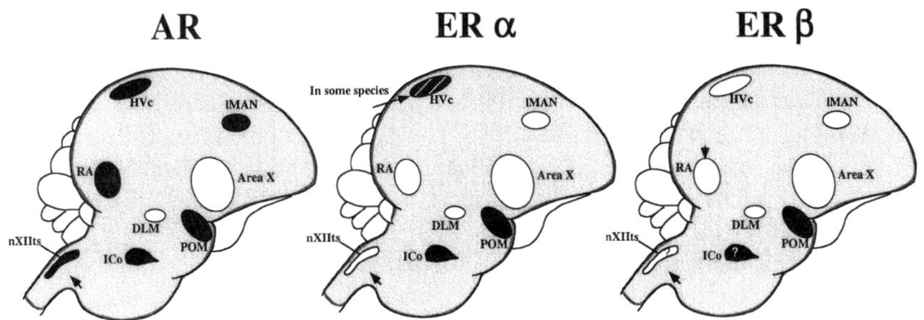

FIGURE 2. A diagrammatic representation of the distribution of androgen receptors (AR), estrogen receptor α (ERα), and estrogen receptor β (ERβ) in song control nuclei. *Dark shading* means that the receptor is expressed in the brain area. In the case of ERα in HVC, there is species diversity in this expression. See text for more details.

sensitive brain areas that make up the song control system.[19,30,71–73] HVC, RA, and MAN contain AR based on both autoradiographic[19,74–76] (for review, Refs. 66 and 67) and binding assay[77] methods. Additional autoradiographic studies utilizing the nonaromatizable androgen [^{3}H]dihydrotestosterone as a ligand[78–80] have confirmed that these telencephalic binding sites, identified by testosterone autoradiography, are specific for androgens. The presence of AR in these nuclei has also been confirmed by immunocytochemistry.[20,81,82] In addition, the androgen receptor has been cloned and sequenced in canaries[83,84] and starlings,[22] and probes based on this information have been used to localize the AR mRNA in the canary[23,85,86] and starling brain[22,87]). These *in situ* hybridization studies have largely confirmed the AR distribution identified by *in vivo* autoradiography or immunocytochemistry.

A concordant pattern of distribution for AR has generally been described by these three independent experimental approaches in the preoptic area–hypothalamus–limbic system, in the mesencephalic ICo of songbirds and non-songbirds, and in the song control system of songbirds (see FIG. 2).

Specifically, three song control nuclei—HVC, RA, and MAN—accumulate radioactive T (e.g., Refs. 19, 30, 72, 75, and 76) or 5α-dihydrotestosterone[78–80,88] in autoradiographic studies, and they contain AR-ir cells (e.g., Refs. 20, 81, and 82). Weakly labeled AR-ir cells were also observed in a position adjacent to the canary RA, in a "hook-like" structure that runs laterally and then ventrally.[20] This area has been previously identified in zebra finches as a region receiving projections from the lateral MAN[89] and labeled by the high density of α_2 adrenergic receptors in starlings.[66,90] This area should thus be considered as part of the song system. Several medullary nuclei that receive inputs from RA, such as the nucleus hypoglossus pars tracheosyringealis (syringeal motonucleus or nXIIts), the nucleus retroambigualis (RAm), and the rostroventral respiratory group (rVRG),[28,91,92] are also defined by the presence of AR.[93] In contrast, to our knowledge, no report has mentioned the presence of AR in these nuclei in non-songbirds,[94] with one exception—the Anna's hummingbirds (*Calypte anna*), a species that belongs to another bird family where song learning has been identified.[94]

Estrogen Receptors of the Alpha Subtype

The distribution of ER has been investigated in a few avian species, including songbirds, by the same methods used in the case of AR (*in vivo* autoradiography, *in vitro* binding, immunocytochemistry, and, in a few cases, *in situ* hybridization). In the late 1990s, a new ER was cloned in mammals[95–97] and later identified in avian species.[22,98,99] This second ER was called estrogen receptor beta (ERβ) to distinguish it from the previously described receptor that was then renamed ERα. We first review work that was performed before the second receptor was known—that is, work involving the first-identified form of receptor (ERα). The distribution of ERβ will be considered subsequently.

Similar to what has been observed for AR, ER binding sites appear to be restricted to the hypothalamic and limbic structures and to the mesencephalic intercollicular nucleus in non-songbirds and songbirds (e.g., Refs. 100–103), but additional binding sites are found in telencephalic song nuclei of oscines (e.g., Refs. 104 and 105).

Immunocytochemistry has also been used to analyze the distribution of ERα in zebra finches and canaries first[106] and then in many avian species ($n = 26$) belonging to a large number of avian orders—namely, anseriformes, galliformes, columbiformes, psittaciformes, apodiformes, and passeriformes (17 species).[21] These data confirm that the distribution of ERα immunoreactive cells in the diencephalic and limbic structures is very similar across all species that have been studied. All songbirds, however, also display significant numbers of ERα-expressing cells in three structures of the nonlimbic forebrain: the caudal neostriatum including, in some species, HVC, the dorsorostral area surrounding RA, and an area in the rostral forebrain, dorsal to the lamina hyperstriatica and rostral to the nucleus MAN (see FIG. 2). A fourth forebrain area, the hyperstriatum accessorium, also contains many ERα-immunoreactive cells in songbirds, but a few positive cells are also found in this location in budgerigars.[21]

ERα was also cloned in zebra finches and canaries, and the distribution of the corresponding mRNA was analyzed in the brain of these species by *in situ* hybridization. These studies confirmed, with a few exceptions, results previously established by autoradiographic and immunocytochemical methods (e.g., presence of ERα in the neo- and archistriatal areas adjacent to HVC and RA; see Ref. 107). One noticeable difference between canaries and zebra finches should be highlighted here, however: ERα mRNA and protein are present within HVC in canaries, but in zebra finches they are located in the surrounding neostriatum but not in HVC proper.[23,84,85]

Estrogen Receptors of the Beta Subtype

The identification of a second type of ER (see above) raised new issues about the action of estrogens.[95,108] It is possible, for example, that effects of estrogen on singing behavior in species that do not express ERα in HVC (e.g., the zebra finch or starling) are mediated, at least in part, through the binding of the steroid to ERβ present in this nucleus. Following the cloning and sequencing of ERβ in Japanese quail[98] and then in European starlings,[22] a specific riboprobe was used to analyze the neuroanatomical distribution of the mRNA in the starling brain, with a special focus on the brain areas containing the song control nuclei.[22] ERβ mRNA was not expressed at detectable levels in any forebrain song control nucleus. A low level of expression was observed in the caudomedial neostriatum close to, but not within, HVC in a pattern distinct from ERα. As was observed in a non-songbird species, the Japanese quail,[98] a high level of expression was observed in starlings in the medial preoptic nucleus (POM), an area implicated in the mediation of sexual behavior and in the nucleus taeniae, the avian homologue of parts of the mammalian amygdala.[109] These data therefore provide no evidence that ERβ mediates the control of singing in the telencephalic song control nuclei.

STEROID MODULATION OF CATECHOLAMINERGIC ACTIVITY AND CONTROL OF SINGING

The presence of sex steroid receptors in various nuclei in the song control system is consistent with the idea that T and its metabolites regulate song behavior by acting directly on steroid-expressing cells in these nuclei.[30] However, several lines of evidence indicate that steroid hormones may also regulate song behavior indirectly by modulating the activity of ascending inputs from catecholaminergic nuclei that project to the song control nuclei. This notion is supported by anatomical, neuroendocrine, and pharmacological data reviewed below.

Anatomy of Catecholaminergic Cell Groups in Songbirds and Their Projections to the Song Control Nuclei

A prominent catecholaminergic innervation of the song control system has been demonstrated in several songbird species, most notably zebra finches, by the presence of fibers immunoreactive for the catecholamine-synthesizing enzymes tyrosine hydroxylase (TH)[110,111] and/or dopamine β-hydroxylase.[112] Similarly, immunocytochemical studies of TH in male canaries have found that the boundaries of HVC and RA can be defined in a manner in agreement with Nissl-defined boundaries—by the presence of a higher density of fibers immunoreactive for TH compared to the surrounding neostriatum.[113]

High concentrations of NE and DA have accordingly been measured in the song control nuclei of zebra finches.[114–116] Autoradiographic studies have revealed binding sites for [^{3}H] RX821002, a ligand specific for α_2- adrenergic receptors, to be enriched in forebrain song control nuclei of this species.[117] In European starlings, high densities of noradrenergic receptors of the α_2 and β1/β2 subtypes are also present in several song control nuclei (HVC, RA, and area X)[90,118,119] (see FIG. 3), and high densities of dopamine D1 receptors have been described in area X of the lobus parolfactorius in the same species.[120] In these cases, boundaries of these song control nuclei can be defined based on the high receptor densities compared to the surrounding brain area that are consistent with Nissl-defined boundaries.

Further understanding of the relationships between steroids, catecholamines, and song learning/production was until recently limited by the lack of precise knowledge concerning the anatomical organization of CAergic projections to the song control nuclei. The origins of the catecholaminergic innervation of the song control nuclei have been investigated to some extent by tract-tracing in canaries. HVC receives dopaminergic inputs mainly from the mesencephalic central gray (GCt; group A11 in the nomenclature of Dahlström and Fuxe;[121] see Ref. 122 for a review of this no-

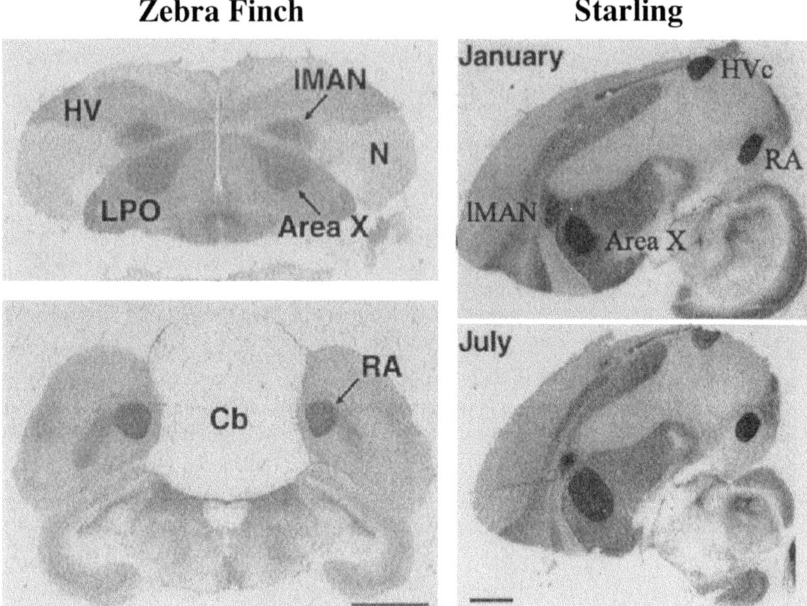

FIGURE 3. Autoradiograms illustrating the distribution of α_2 adrenergic receptors based on the binding of the α_2 specific ligand [^{3}H] RX 821002. Two sections in the transverse plane from a male zebra finch are illustrated, and two sections in the sagittal plan from a male European starlings collected at two different months of the year are also illustrated. Note the high densities of these receptors in the song control nuclei HVC, RA, X, and lMAN in both species. Data were modified from Refs. 117 and 119. See text for more details.

menclature use in birds) and to a lesser extent from the AVT (group A10) and noradrenergic inputs from the complex of the locus coeruleus (Loc; group A6).[123] Similarly, dopaminergic inputs to RA come mostly from the A11 (mesencephalic central gray) and A10 (AVT) cell groups, and noradrenergic inputs come from the locus coeruleus and subcoeruleus (A6)[124] (see FIG. 1B). In contrast, area X, a key nucleus of the rostral forebrain pathway controlling song learning but not song production, seems to receive catecholamine (CA) inputs exclusively from AVT.[125] These data thus suggest that different populations of CA cell groups could control the motor and anterior forebrain pathways (see FIG. 1B).

Sex Differences and Effects of T on the CAergic Innervation of Song Control Nuclei

The prominent catecholaminergic innervation of some song control nuclei is sexually dimorphic in the songbirds species that have been investigated. For example, the high density of TH-immunoreactive fibers that is observed in the HVC and RA of male canaries is not present in females, who sing less than males. In females, these nuclei either have the same density of immunoreactive fibers as the surrounding neo-

and archistriatum, respectively, or in other subjects they are identified by the nearly complete absence of immunoreactivity.[113] The volume of HVC based on relative densities of α_2-adrenergic receptors is also larger in male than in female starlings similar to sex differences based Nissl-defined critiera.[90,118] In zebra finches, the pattern of α_2-adrenergic receptor densities reveal even more dramatic sex differences in three nuclei; HVC, area X, and lMAN exhibit high densities in males with no obvious ligand binding in these areas in females.[117]

Some of these sex differences originate at least in part through a differential activation by steroids in adult males and females as indicated by the fact that catecholaminergic activity in several song control nuclei is clearly modulated by steroids. In zebra finches, androgens and their metabolites have been found to regulate NE and DA baseline levels and turnover in forebrain song control nuclei.[114,115] There are also pronounced seasonal changes in the density of α_2-adrenergic receptors in HVC and RA of starlings, suggesting steroid regulation of this receptor subtype.[119]

Given that the density of immunoreactive catecholaminergic fibers innervating telencephalic song nuclei in canaries is higher in males than in females, we recently hypothesized that some of these sex differences were directly controlled by T. Therefore, we investigated the effects of a treatment with exogenous T on song production, on the volume of song control nuclei, and on the catecholaminergic innervation of these nuclei in female canaries, as assessed by immunocytochemical visualization of TH. As expected, T induced male-like singing in all females and increased the volume of HVC and RA by about 80%. T also significantly increased the fractional area covered by TH-immunoreactive structures (fibers and varicosities) in most telencephalic song control nuclei (HVC, the lateral and medial parts of the magnocellular nucleus of the anterior neostriatum, the nucleus interfacialis, and to a lesser extent RA). In contrast, T did not affect the catecholaminergic innervation of the telencephalic areas adjacent to HVC and RA.[126]

Together, these data demonstrate that, in parallel to its effects on song behavior and on the morphology of the song control system, T also regulates the catecholaminergic innervation of most telencephalic song control nuclei in canaries.This effect of T provides one way to explain the mechanistic basis of sex differences in catecholaminergic innervation of these nuclei, given that plasma T concentrations are substantially higher in males than in females (e.g., Ref. 127).

Presence of Steroid Receptors in Catecholaminergic Cell Groups

Chemical neuroanatomical studies have identified one potential way that sex steroid hormones could regulate these catecholaminergic inputs. *In situ* hybridization was used to analyze the distribution of AR and ER in the brainstem[87] of male canaries. Significant concentrations of AR mRNA were found in several catecholaminergic nuclei including the locus coeruleus, the substantia nigra, and the AVT (homologous to the ventral tegmental area). Dense ERα mRNA labeling overlapping with TH immunoreactivity was also detected in the locus coeruleus and the AVT.[87]

We do not know at present whether these receptors are truly co-localized in catecholaminergic neurons or simply coexist in the same general area. However, studies in mammalian species demonstrate that ERα are specifically expressed in a significant percentage of dopaminergic neurons at the level of the infundibular hypothalamus (e.g., arcuate nucleus) and in the zona incerta,[128–130] as well as in similar brainstem catecholamine cell groups.[131,132] The presence of ER and AR within these cell groups is thus consistent with the possibility that sex steroid hormones may affect song production by modulating the catecholaminergic system at the site of synthesis by acting both as androgens or as estrogens (see below).

This steroid modulation of catecholaminergic inputs represents one way that steroids may influence song production.[37,58,60] Indeed, functional interactions between steroids and catecholamines have been reported in many vertebrate species, and catecholamines are involved in the control of a variety of steroid-regulated reproductive behaviors.[133–137] It is therefore reasonable to hypothesize that steroid hormones may influence song control nuclei and singing activity at least in part by a direct action at the level of catecholaminergic structures. This notion has not been extensively tested to date, but it is nevertheless already supported by a number of experimental studies that will be reviewed in the remainder of this paper.

DOPAMINE AND SONG CONTROL—DOPAMINERGIC CELL GROUPS EXPRESS THE IMMEDIATE EARLY GENE FOS IN ASSOCIATION WITH TERRITORIAL SONG

In birds as in mammals, dopamine (DA) is implicated in the control of a wide diversity of physiological and behavioral responses. The anatomically complex nature of the dopaminergic innervation of the song system has made it difficult to assess the specific effects of this transmitter on song learning and production. Most of the data on this topic collected to date are therefore essentially correlational in nature.

One way to assess the potential involvement of a brain area in a behavior of interest is to establish whether engaging in the behavior is associated with immediate early gene expression in the brain area of interest.[138] This approach has been particularly successful in relation to the study of neural circuits regulating song production and perception.[139,140] In order to establish the potential involvement of dopamine expressing areas in the control of song behavior, the expression of the protein product of the immediate early gene c-fos was studied in song sparrows experiencing a territorial challenge.[141] Free-living male song sparrows were subjected to simulated territorial intrusion (STI), which stimulates territorial singing. Control birds received an "intrusion" consisting of an empty cage together with a recording of heterospecific song. The resulting fos-like immunoreactivity (FLI) was quantified in two dopaminergic regions of the brainstem that project to the song system: the AVT and the midbrain central gray (GCt). Males subjected to STI exhibited more FLI in both of these regions than did control males. In addition, FLI in both nuclei was correlated positively with the number of songs sung in response to STI. These results suggest a role for AVT and GCt, and thus possibly catecholamines, in the regulation of territorial song in songbirds.[141]

NOREPINEPHRINE AND SONG CONTROL

Because of the complex anatomical organization of NA innervation of the song system, producing lesions that specifically affect noradrenergic afferents to the song control nuclei is difficult with the technologies currently available. A specific noradrenergic drug, DSP4, specifically affects central noradrenergic pathways while leaving the peripheral system relatively intact. In addition, DSP4 preferentially depletes the telencephalic innervation by norepinephrine (NE) and has only a modest impact on the diencephalon. This drug has therefore been used in a number of experiments to test the effects of noradrenergic denervation of the telencephalon on song learning, expression, and detection.

Effects of Noradrenergic Lesions on Song Behavior in Zebra Finches and Female Responses to Song in Canaries

In zebra finches, systemic injections of DSP4 decrease male courtship behavior including female-directed singing.[134,135] This effect appears to result from attention deficits rather than from impairments of the motor aspects of song because in DSP4-treated birds the latency to initiate singing was increased; once song began, however, it was quite normal.

In female canaries, the pharmacological depletion of central norepinephrine levels obtained by injection of DSP4 decreases the incidence of copulation solicitation displays that are produced in response to the playback of sexually stimulating male songs.[142] This effect of DSP4 was observed in conditions where the sexually stimulating songs were partly masked by nonstimulating wild-canary songs or heterospecific songs, but not when the songs were masked by simpler signals such as white noise. These data therefore suggest that central noradrenergic inputs (presumably to the song system) modulate sexual responsiveness of female canaries by affecting the ability of the birds to attend to species-specific auditory signals, in particular, sexually stimulating male songs.

Noradrenergic Lesions Modify Immediate Early Gene Expression in the Song System

Immediate early genes such as *zenk* are expressed in the avian song system in a motor-driven fashion in that such expression is even observed in deafened birds when they sing.[34] In male zebra finches, this immediate early gene expression induced by song is context dependent.[143] Males singing songs directed at females exhibit very low induction of the immediate early gene *zenk* in area X, whereas *zenk* induction is high in males that sing the same amount of song but produce song either in isolation or in the presence of other males.[143] Similar findings have been reported about electrophysiological activity; multiunit activity in area X is much lower when the birds engage in directed song than when they sing in social isolation.[144,145] These findings suggest that this anterior forebrain circuit may modulate song output in adulthood, but may not be directly responsible for the motor output.

We administered the noradrenergic neurotoxin DSP4 to male zebra finches prior to singing either directed or undirected song and found that those who sang song directed at females had high levels of zenk protein expression characteristic of males singing undirected song.[146] These data implicate the noradrenergic system in regulating social context effects on song system activity.

CONCLUSIONS

The avian song control system has emerged as a valuable model system for the study of at least some aspects of a complex human cognitive ability, namely, language.[25] This interest has driven much research on this system. Once it was established that certain forebrain song nuclei are essential for song production, most recent research relevant to the neurobiology of song has focused on studying the well-defined song circuit as it relates to song learning and perception (e.g., Refs. 147 and 148). However, song behavior is produced in a variety of contexts that have very different functional consequences for the individual producing the song (e.g., in the context of mate attraction versus aggression[14]). The hormone, testosterone, is a powerful regulator of song production that helps ensure that song is produced in a contextually appropriate way. Because several nuclei in the song circuit itself are a direct target of T, it was appealing to hypothesize that hormonal effects on song were mediated exclusively or primarily within the song circuit itself.[30] However, the effects of the social and environmental contexts on a neural circuit often involve more general modulatory systems such as the catecholamines. We have reviewed much of the current evidence supporting a role for catecholamine systems as a key site of action of T on song production and perception in the context of reproduction and aggression. Further studies investigating the connectivity and chemical neuroanatomy of defined cell types, as well as perhaps utilizing precise immunolesioning strategies (e.g., Ref. 149) to assess function, are now needed to confirm the importance of this system in relation to song behavior. Such a research strategy is essential for the next generation of studies of hormone-modulated neural circuits.

ACKNOWLEDGMENTS

We thank Dr. Lauren V. Riters and Ms. Jennifer Sartor for discussion about many issues considered in this review. Research from our laboratories described in the review was supported by grants from the National Institute of Neurological Diseases and Stroke (NS 35467) to G.F.B.; grants from the National Science Foundation (DBN 9804129), and the National Insitutes of Health (T32 MH15330-24) to D.L.M. and grants from the Belgian Fonds de la Recherche Fondamentale Collective (2.4555.01), the French Community of Belgium (ARC 99/04-241), and the University of Liège (Fonds Spéciaux pour la Recherche) to J.B.

REFERENCES

1. Becker, J.B. & S.M. Breedlove. 2002. Introduction to behavioral endocrinology. *In* Behavioral Endocrinology. J.B. Becker, S.M. Breedlove, D. Crews & M.M. McCarthy, Eds.: 3–38. MIT Press. Cambridge, MA.
2. Silver, R. 1978. The parental behavior of ring doves. Am. Scientist **66:** 209–215.
3. Barfield, R.J. 1969. Activation of copulatory behavior by androgen implanted into the preoptic area of the male fowl. Horm. Behav. **1:** 37–52.
4. Lisk, R.D. 1962. Diencephalic placement of estradiol and sexual receptivity in the female rat. Am. J. Physiol. **203:** 493–496.

5. Lisk, R.D. 1967. Neural localization for androgen activation of copulatory behavior in the male rat. Endocrinology **80:** 754–761.
6. Hull, E.M., R.L. Meisel & B.D. Sachs. 2002. Male sexual behavior. *In* Hormones, Brain, and Behavior. Vol. 2. D.W. Pfaff, A.P. Arnold, A.M. Etgen, *et al.*, Eds.: 1–137. Academic Press. San Diego, CA.
7. Blaustein, J.D. & M.S. Erskine. 2002. Feminine sexual behavior: cellular integration of hormonal and afferent information in the rodent brain. *In* Hormones, Brain, and Behavior. Vol. 1. D.W. Pfaff, A.P. Arnold, A.M. Etgen, *et al.*, Eds.: 139–214. Academic Press. San Diego, CA.
8. Pfaff, D.W., S. Ogawa, K. Kia, *et al.* 2002. Genetic mechansims in neural and hormonal controls over female reproductive behaviors. *In* Hormones, Brain, and Behavior. Vol. 3. D.W. Pfaff, A.P. Arnold, A.M. Etgen, *et al.*, Eds.: 441–510. Academic Press. San Diego, CA.
9. Etgen, A.M. 2002. Estrogen regulation of neurotransmitter and growth factor signaling in the brain. *In* Hormones, Brain, and Behavior. D.W. Pfaff, A.P. Arnold, A.M. Etgen, *et al.*, Eds. Vol. 3: 381–440. Academic Press. San Diego.
10. Larsson, K. & L. Heimer. 1964. Mating behaviour of male rats after lesions in the preoptic area. Nature **202:** 413–414.
11. Heimer, L. & K. Larsson. 1966. Impairment of mating behavior in male rats following lesions in the preoptic-anterior hypothalamic continuum. Brain Res. **3:** 248–263.
12. Dominguez, J., J.V. Riolo, Z.J. Xu & E.M. Hull. 2001. Regulation by the medial amygdala of copulation and medial preoptic dopamine release. J. Neurosci. **21:** 349–355.
13. Calizo, L.H. & L.M. Flanagan-Cato. 2002. Estrogen-induced dendritic spine elimination on female rat ventromedial hypothalamic neurons that project to the periaqueductal gray. J. Comp. Neurol. **447:** 234–248.
14. Catchpole, C.K. & P.J.B. Slater. 1995. Bird Song: Biological Themes and Variations. 1st edit. Cambridge University Press. New York.
15. Brenowitz, E.A. 1997. Comparative approaches to the avian song system. J.Neurobiol. **33:** 517–531.
16. Ball, G.F. & S.H. Hulse. 1998. Bird song. Am. Psychol. **53:** 37–58.
17. Ball, G.F., L.V. Riters & J. Balthazart. 2002. Neuroendocrinology of song behavior and avian brain plasticity: multiple sites of action of sex steroid hormones. Front. Neuroendocrinol. **23:** 137–178
18. Schlinger, B.A. & E.A. Brenowitz. 2002. Neural and hormonal control of birdsong. *In* Hormones, Brain, and Behavior. Vol. 2. D.W. Pfaff, A.P. Arnold, A.M. Etgen, *et al.*, Eds.: 799–839. Academic Press. San Diego.
19. Arnold, A.P., F. Nottebohm & D.W. Pfaff. 1976. Hormone concentrating cells in vocal control areas of the brain of the zebra finch (*Poephila guttata*). J. Comp. Neurol. **165:** 487–512.
20. Balthazart, J., A. Foidart, E.M. Wilson & G.F. Ball. 1992. Immunocytochemical localization of androgen receptors in the male songbird and quail brain. J. Comp. Neurol. **317:** 407–420.
21. Gahr, M., H.-R. Güttinger & D.E. Kroodsma. 1993. Estrogen receptors in the avian brain: Survey reveals general distribution and forebrain areas unique to songbirds. J. Comp. Neurol. **327:** 112–122.
22. Bernard, D.J., G.E. Bentley, J. Balthazart, *et al.* 1999. Androgen receptor, estrogen receptor alpha, and estrogen receptor beta show distinct patterns of expression in forebrain song control nuclei of European starlings. Endocrinology **140:** 4633–4643.
23. Metzdorf, R., M. Gahr & L. Fusani. 1999. Distribution of aromatase, estrogen receptor, and androgen receptor mRNA in the forebrain of songbirds and nonsongbirds. J. Comp. Neurol. **407:** 115–129.
24. Arnold, A.P. 1990. The passerine bird song system as a model in neuroendocrine research. J. Exp. Zool. **4:** 22–30.
25. Doupe, A.J. & P.K. Kuhl. 1999. Birdsong and human speech: common themes and mechanisms. Annu. Rev. Neurosci. **22:** 567–631.
26. Alvarez-Borda, B. & F. Nottebohm. 2002. Gonads and singing play separate, additive roles in new neuron recruitment in adult canary brain. J. Neurosci. **22:** 8684–8690.

27. Margoliash, D. 1997. Functional organization of forebrain pathways for song production and perception. J. Neurobiol. **33:** 671–693.
28. Wild, J.M. 1997. Neural pathways for the control of birdsong production. J.Neurobiol. **33:** 653–670.
29. Brenowitz, E.A., D. Margoliash & K.W. Nordeen. 1997. An introduction to birdsong and the avian song system. J. Neurobiol. **33:** 495–500.
30. Nottebohm, F. 1980. Brain pathways for vocal learning in birds: a review of the first 10 years. *In* Progress in Psychobiology and Physiological Psychology. Vol. 9. J.M. Sprague & A.N. Epstein, Eds.: 85–214. Academic Press. New York.
31. Nottebohm, F. 1993. The search for neural mechanisms that define the sensitive period for song learning in birds. Neth. J. Zool. **43:** 193–234.
32. Nottebohm, F., T.M. Stokes & C.M. Leonard. 1976. Central control of song in the canary, Serinus canarius. J. Comp. Neurol. **165:** 457–486.
33. Simpson, H.B. & D.S. Vicario. 1990. Brain pathways for learned and unlearned vocalizations differ in zebra finches. J. Neurosci. **10:** 1541–1556.
34. Jarvis, E.D. & F. Nottebohm. 1997. Motor-driven gene expression. Proc. Natl. Acad. Sci. USA **94:** 4097–4102.
35. Kimpo, R.R. & A.J. Doupe. 1997. FOS is induced by singing in distinct neuronal populations in a motor network. Neuron **18:** 315–325.
36. Yu, A.C. & D. Margoliash. 1996. Temporal hierarchical control of singing in birds. Science **273:** 1871–1875.
37. Bottjer, S.W. & F. Johnson. 1997. Circuits, hormones, and learning: vocal behavior in songbirds. J. Neurobiol. **33:** 602–618.
38. Benton, S., D.A. Nelson, P. Marler & T.J. DeVoogd. 1998. Anterior forebrain pathway is needed for stable song expression in adult male white-crowned sparrows (*Zonotrichia leucophrys*). Behav. Brain Res. **96:** 135–150.
39. Bottjer, S.W., E.A. Miesner & A.P. Arnold. 1984. Forebrain lesions disrupt development but not maintenance of song in passerine birds. Science **224:** 901–903.
40. Scharff, C. & F. Nottebohm. 1991. A comparative study of the behavioral deficits following lesions of various parts of the zebra finch song system: implications for vocal learning. J. Neurosci. **11:** 2896–2913.
41. Sohrabji, F., E.J. Nordeen & K.W. Nordeen. 1990. Selective impairment of song learning following lesions of a forebrain nucleus in juvenile zebra finches. Behav. Neural Biol. **53:** 51–63.
42. Ball, G.F. 1999. Neuroendocrine basis of seasonal changes in vocal behavior among songbirds. *In* The Design of Animal Communication. M. Hauser & M. Konishi, Eds.: 213–253. MIT Press. Cambridge, MA.
43. Wingfield, J.C. & D.S. Farner. 1993. Endocrinology of reproduction in wild species. *In* Avian Biology. Vol. 9. D.S. Farner, J. King & K.C. Parkes, Eds: 163–327. Vol. 9. Academic Press. New York.
44. Dawson, A., V.M. King, G.E. Bentley & G.F. Ball. 2001. Photoperiodic control of seasonality in birds. J. Biol. Rhythms **16:** 365–380.
45. Balthazart, J. 1983. Hormonal correlates of behavior. *In* Avian Biology. Vol. 7. D.S. Farner, J. R. King, K. C. Parkes, Eds.: 221–365. Academic Press. New York.
46. Pröve, E. 1974. Der Einfluss von Kastration und Testosteronsubstitution auf das Verhalten manlicher Zebrafinken. J. Ornithol. **115:** 338–347.
47. Arnold, A.P. 1975. The effects of castration and androgen replacement on song courtship, and aggression in zebra finches. J. Exp. Zool. **191:** 309–326.
48. Wingfield, J.C. & T.P. Hahn. 1994. Testosterone and territorial behaviour in sedentary and migratory sparrows. Anim. Behav. **47:** 77–89.
49. Eens, M. 1997. Understanding the complex song of the European starling: an integrated ethological approach. Adv. Study Anim. Behav. **26:** 355–434.
50. Riters, L.V., M. Eens, R. Pinxten, *et al.* 2000. Seasonal changes in courtship song and the medial preoptic area in male European starlings (*Sturnus vulgaris*). Horm. Behav. **38:** 250–261.
51. De Ridder, E., R. Pinxten & M. Eens. 2000. Experimental evidence of a testosterone-induced shift from paternal to mating behaviour in a facultatively polygynous songbird. Behav. Ecol. Sociobiol. **49:** 24–30.

52. Pinxten, R., E. De Ridder, J. Balthazart & M. Eens. 2002. Context-dependent effects of castration and testosterone treatment on song in male European starlings. Horm. Behav. **42:** 307–318.
53. Adkins-Regan, E. 1981. Hormone specificity, androgen metabolism, and social behavior. Am. Zool. **21:** 257–271.
54. Adkins-Regan, E. 1983. Sex steroids and the differentiation and activation of avian reproductive behaviour. *In* Hormones and Behaviour in Higher Vertebrates. J. Balthazart & R. Gilles, Eds.: 219–228. Springer-Verlag. Berlin.
55. Balthazart, J. 1989. Steroid metabolism and the activation of social behavior. *In* J. Balthazart, Ed.: 105–159. Advances in Comparative and Environmental Physiology, 1st edit. Vol. 3. Springer Verlag. Berlin.
56. Hutchison, J.B. 1987. A role for brain metabolism in the behavioural action of androgen. *In* C. Christiansen & B.J. Riis, Eds.: 429–436. Highlights on Endocrinology Bogtrykkeri. Copenhagen.
57. Balthazart, J., O. Tlemçani & G.F. Ball. 1996. Do sex differences in the brain explain sex differences in the hormonal induction of reproductive behavior? What 25 years of research on the Japanese quail tells us. Horm. Behav. **30:** 627–661.
58. Schlinger, B.A. 1997. Sex steroids and their actions on the birdsong system. J.Neurobiol. **33:** 619–631.
59. Ball, G.F. & J. Balthazart. 2002. Neuroendocrine mechanisms regulating reproductve cycles and reproductive behavior in birds. *In* Hormones, Brain, and Behavior. Vol. 2. D. W. Pfaff, A.P. Arnold, A.M. Etgen, *et al.*, Eds.: 649–798. Academic Press. San Diego.
60. Harding, C.F., K. Sheridan & M.J. Walters. 1983. Hormonal specificity and activation of sexual behavior in male zebra finches. Horm. Behav. **17:** 111–133.
61. Walters, M.J. & C.F. Harding. 1988. The effects of an aromatization inhibitor on the reproductive behavior of male zebra finches. Horm. Behav. **22:** 207–218.
62. Harding, C.F., M.J. Walters, D. Collado & K. Sheridan. 1988. Hormonal specificity and activation of social behavior in male red-winged blackbirds. Horm. Behav. **22:** 402–418.
63. Fusani, L., R. Metzdorf, J.B. Hutchison & M. Gahr. 2003. Aromatase inhibition affects testosterone-induced masculinization of song and the neural song system in female canaries. J. Neurobiol. **54:** 370–379.
64. Kelley, D.B. & D.W. Pfaff. 1978. Generalizations from comparative studies on neuroanatomical and endocrine mechanisms of sexual behaviour. *In* Biological Determinants of Sexual Behaviour. J.B. Hutchison, Ed.: 225–254. John Wiley & Sons. Chichester.
65. Morrell, J.I. & D.W. Pfaff. 1978. A neuroendocrine approach to brain function: localization of sex steroid concentrating cells in vertebrate brains. Am. Zool. **18:** 447–460.
66. Ball, G.F. 1990. Chemical neuroanatomical studies of the steroid-sensitive songbird vocal control system: a comparative approach. *In* Hormones, Brain, and Behaviour in Vertebrates. Vol. 8: Sexual Differentiation, Neuroanatomical Aspects, Neurotransmitters, and Neuropeptides. J. Balthazart, Ed.: 148–167. Karger. Basel.
67. Brenowitz, E.A. 1991. Evolution of the vocal control system in the avian brain. Semin. Neurosci. **3:** 399–407.
68. Morrell, J.I., D.B. Kelley & D.W. Pfaff. 1975. Sex steroid binding in the brain of vertebrates. *In* Brain-Endocrine Interactions II. K.M. Knigge, D.E. Scott, H. Kobayashi, *et al.*, Eds.: 230–256. Karger. Basel.
69. Pfaff, D.W. 1976. The neuroanatomy of sex hormone receptors in the vertebrate brain. *In* Neuroendocrine Regulation of Fertility. T.C. Anand Kumar, Ed.: 30–45. Karger. Basel.
70. Stumpf, W.E. & M. Sar. 1978. Anatomical distribution of estrogen, androgen, progestin, corticoid and thyroid hormone target sites in the brain of mammals: phylogeny and ontogeny. Am. Zool. **18:** 435–445.
71. Konishi, M. 1985. Birdsong: from behavior to neuron. Annu. Rev. Neurosci. **8:** 125–170.
72. Nottebohm, F. & A.P. Arnold. 1976. Sexual dimorphism in the vocal control areas in the song bird brain. Science **194:** 211–213.

73. Nottebohm, F., A. Alvarez-Buylla, J. Cynx, *et al.* 1990. Song learning in birds: the relation between perception and production. Philos. Trans. R. Soc. Lond. [Biol.] **329:** 115–124.
74. Gahr, M. 1990. Localization of androgen receptors and estrogen receptors in the same cells of the songbird brain. Proc. Natl. Acad. Sci. USA **87:** 9445–9448.
75. Lücke, J. & E. Haase. 1980. Autoradiographische Untersuchungen am Gehirn von Bergfinken (*Fringilla montifringilla* L.) nach injektion von 3H-Testosteron. J. Hirnforsch. **21:** 369–380.
76. Zigmond, R.E., F. Nottebohm & D.W. Pfaff. 1973. Androgen-concentrating cells in the midbrain of a songbird. Science **179:** 1005–1007.
77. Harding, C.F., M.J. Walters & B. Parsons. 1984. Androgen receptor levels in hypothalamic and vocal control nuclei in the male zebra finch. Brain Res. **306:** 333–339.
78. Arnold, A.P. & A. Saltiel. 1979. Sexual difference in pattern of hormone accumulation in the brain of a song bird. Science **205:** 702–705.
79. Nordeen, E.J., K.W. Nordeen & A.P. Arnold. 1987. Sexual differentiation of androgen accumulation within the zebra finch brain through selective cell loss and addition. J. Comp. Neurol. **259:** 393–399.
80. Sohrabji, F., K.W. Nordeen & E.J. Nordeen. 1989. Projections of androgen-accumulating neurons in a nucleus controlling avian song. Brain Res. **488:** 253–259.
81. Smith, G.T., E.A. Brenowitz & G.S. Prins. 1996. Use of PG-21 immunocytochemistry to detect androgen receptors in the songbird brain. J. Histochem. Cytochem. **44:** 1075–1080.
82. Soma, K.K., V.N. Hartman, J.C. Wingfield & E.A. Brenowitz. 1999. Seasonal changes in androgen receptor immunoreactivity in the song nucleus HVc of a wild bird. J. Comp. Neurol. **409:** 224–236.
83. Nastiuk, K.L. & D.F. Clayton. 1994. Seasonal and tissue-specific regulation of canary androgen receptor messenger ribonucleic acid. Endocrinology **134:** 640–649.
84. Gahr, M. & R. Metzdorf. 1997. Distribution and dynamics in the expression of androgen and estrogen receptors in vocal control systems of songbirds. Brain Res. Bull. **44:** 509–517.
85. Fusani, L., T. Van't Hof, J.B. Hutchison & M. Gahr. 2000. Seasonal expression of androgen receptors, estrogen receptors, and aromatase in the canary brain in relation to circulating androgens and estrogens. J. Neurobiol. **43:** 254–268.
86. Nastiuk, K.L. & D.F. Clayton. 1995. The canary androgen receptor mRNA is localized in the song control nuclei of the brain and is rapidly regulated by testosterone. J. Neurobiol. **26:** 213–224.
87. Maney, D.L., D.J. Bernard & G.F. Ball. 2001. Gonadal steroid receptor mRNA in catecholaminergic nuclei of the canary brainstem. Neurosci. Lett. **311:** 189–192.
88. Nordeen, K.W., E.J. Nordeen & A.P. Arnold. 1986. Estrogen establishes sex differences in androgen accumulation in zebra finch brain. J. Neurosci. **6:** 734–738.
89. Bottjer, S.W., K.A. Halsema, S.A. Brown & E.A. Miesner. 1989. Axonal connections of a forebrain nucleus involved with vocal learning in zebra finches. J. Comp. Neurol. **279:** 312–326.
90. Ball, G.F. 1994. Neurochemical specializations associated with vocal learning and production in songbirds and budgerigars. Brain Behav. Evol. **44:** 234–246.
91. Reinke, H. & J.M. Wild. 1998. Identification and connections of inspiratory premotor neurons in songbirds and budgerigar. J. Comp. Neurol. **391:** 147–163.
92. Wild, J.M., D.F. Li & C. Eagleton. 1997. Projections of the dorsomedial nucleus of the intercollicular complex (DM) in relation to respiratory-vocal nuclei in the brainstem of pigeon (*Columba livia*) and zebra finch (*Taeniopygia guttata*). J. Comp. Neurol. **377:** 392–413.
93. Gahr, M. & J.M. Wild. 1997. Localization of androgen receptor mRNA-containing cells in avian respiratory-vocal nuclei: an *in situ* hybridization study. J. Neurobiol. **33:** 865–876.
94. Gahr, M. 2000. Neural song control system of hummingbirds: comparison to swifts, vocal learning (songbirds) and nonlearning (suboscines) passerines, and vocal learning (budgerigars) and nonlearning (dove, owl, gull, quail, chicken) nonpasserines. J. Comp. Neurol. **426:** 182–196.

95. KUIPER, G.G.J.M., E. ENMARK, M. PELTO-HUIKKO, *et al.* 1996. Cloning of a novel estrogen receptor expressed in rat prostate and ovary. Proc. Natl. Acad. Sci. USA **93:** 5925–5930.
96. MOSSELMAN, S., J. POLMAN & R. DIJKEMA. 1996. ER beta: identification and characterization of a novel human estrogen receptor. FEBS Lett. **392:** 49–53.
97. TREMBLAY, G.B., A. TREMBLAY, N.G. COPELAND, *et al.* 1997. Cloning, chromosomal localization, and functional analysis of the murine estrogen receptor beta. Mol. Endocrinol. **11:** 353–365.
98. FOIDART, A., B. LAKAYE, T. GRISAR, *et al.* 1999. Estrogen receptor-beta in quail: cloning, tissue expression and neuroanatomical distribution. J. Neurobiol. **40:** 327–342.
99. BALL, G.F., D.J. BERNARD, A. FOIDART, *et al.* 1999. Steroid sensitive sites in the avian brain: does the distribution of the estrogen receptor alpha and beta types provide insight into their function? Brain Behav. Evol. **54:** 28–40.
100. KIM, Y.S., W.E. STUMPF, M. SAR & M.C. MARTINEZ-VARGAS. 1978. Estrogen and androgen target cells in the brain of fishes, reptiles, and birds: phylogeny and ontogeny. Am. Zool. **18:** 425–433.
101. MARTINEZ-VARGAS, M.C., W.E. STUMPF & M. SAR. 1975. Estrogen localization in the dove brain. Phylogenetic considerations and implications for nomenclature. *In* Anatomical Neuroendocrinology. W.E. Stumpf & P.P. Grant, Eds.: 166–175. Karger. Basel.
102. MARTINEZ-VARGAS, M.C., W.E. STUMPF & M. SAR. 1976. Anatomical distribution of estrogen target cells in the avian CNS: a comparison with the mammalian CNS. J. Comp. Neurol. **167:** 83–104.
103. WATSON, J.T. & E. ADKINS-REGAN. 1989. Neuroanatomical localization of sex steroid-concentrating cells in the Japanese quail (*Coturnix japonica*): autoradiography with [^{3}H]-testosterone, [^{3}H]-estradiol, and [^{3}H]-dihydrotestosterone. Neuroendocrinology **49:** 51–64.
104. BRENOWITZ, E.A. & A.P. ARNOLD. 1989. Accumulation of estrogen in a vocal control brain region of a duetting song bird. Brain Res. **480:** 119–125.
105. NORDEEN, K.W., E.J. NORDEEN & A.P. ARNOLD. 1987. Estrogen accumulation in zebra finch song control nuclei: implications for sexual differentiation and adult activation of song behavior. J. Neurobiol. **18:** 569–582.
106. GAHR, M., G. FLÜGGE & H.R. GÜTTINGER. 1987. Immunocytochemical localization of estrogen binding neurons in the songbird brain. Brain Res. **402:** 173–177.
107. JACOBS, E.C., A.P. ARNOLD & A.T. CAMPAGNONI. 1996. Zebra finch estrogen receptor cDNA: cloning and mRNA expression. J. Steroid Biochem. Mol. Biol. **59:** 135–145.
108. KUIPER, G.G.J.M., P.J. SHUGHRUE, I. MERCHENTHALER & J.-A. GUSTAFFSON. 1998. The estrogen receptor b subtype: a novel mediator of estrogen action in neuroendocrine systems. Front. Neuroendocrinol. **19:** 253–286.
109. THOMPSON, R.R., J.L. GOODSON, M.G. RUSCIO & E. ADKINS-REGAN. 1998. Role of the archistriatal nucleus taeniae in the sexual behavior of male Japanese quail (*Coturnix japonica*): a comparison of function with the medial nucleus of the amygdala in mammals. Brain Behav. Evol. **51:** 215–229.
110. BOTTJER, S.W. 1993. The distribution of tyrosine hydroxylase immunoreactivity in the brains of male and female zebra finches. J. Neurobiol. **24:** 51–69.
111. SOHA, J.A., T. SHIMIZU & A.J. DOUPE. 1996. Development of the catecholaminergic innervation of the song system of the male zebra finch. J. Neurobiol. **29:** 473–489.
112. MELLO, C.V., R. PINAUD & S. RIBEIRO. 1998. Noradrenergic system of the zebra finch brain: immunocytochemical study of dopamine-beta-hydroxylase. J. Comp. Neurol. **400:** 207–228.
113. APPELTANTS, D., G.F. BALL & J. BALTHAZART. 2001. The distribution of tyrosine hydroxylase in the canary brain: demonstration of a specific and sexually dimorphic catecholaminergic innervation of the telencephalic song control nuclei. Cell Tissue Res. **304:** 237–259.
114. BARCLAY, S.R. & C.F. HARDING. 1988. Androstenedione modulation of monoamine levels and turnover in hypothalamic and vocal control nuclei in the male zebra finch: steroid effects on brain monoamines. Brain Res. **459:** 333–343.

115. BARCLAY, S.R. & C.F. HARDING. 1990. Differential modulation of monoamine levels and turnover rates by estrogen and/or androgen in hypothalamic and vocal control nuclei of male zebra finches. Brain Res. **523:** 251–262.
116. SAKAGUCHI, H. & N. SAITO. 1989. The acetylcholine and catecholamine contents in song control nuclei of zebra finch during song ontogeny. Dev. Brain Res. **47:** 313–317.
117. RITERS, L.V. & G.F. BALL. 2002. Sex differences in the densities of alpha2-adrenergic receptors in the song control system, but not the medial preoptic nucleus in zebra finches. J. Chem. Neuroanat. **23:** 269–277.
118. BALL, G.F., J.M. CASTO & D.J. BERNARD. 1994. Sex differences in the volume of avian song control nuclei: comparative studies and the issue of brain nucleus delineation. Psychoneuroendocrinology **19:** 485–504.
119. RITERS, L.V., M. EENS, R. PINXTEN & G.F. BALL. 2002. Seasonal changes in the densities of alpha2-noradrenergic receptors are inversely related to changes in testosterone and the volumes of song control nuclei in male European starlings. J. Comp. Neurol. **444:** 63–74.
120. CASTO, J.M. & G.F. BALL. 1994. Characterization and localization of D1 dopamine receptors in the sexually dimorphic vocal control nucleus, area X, and the basal ganglia of European starlings. J.Neurobiol. **25:** 767–780.
121. DAHLSTRÖM, A. & K. FUXE. 1964. Evidence for the existence of monoamine-containing neurons in the central nervous system. I. Demonstration of monoamines in the cell bodies of brain stem neurones. Acta Physiol. Scand. **62:** 1–55.
122. REINER, A., E.J. KARLE, K.D. ANDERSON & L. MEDINA. 1994. Catecholaminergic perikarya and fibers in the avian nervous system. *In* Phylogeny and Development of Catecholamine Systems in the CNS of Vertebrates. W.J.A.J. Smeets & A. Reiner, Eds.: 135–181. Cambridge University Press. Cambridge, UK.
123. APPELTANTS, D., P. ABSIL, J. BALTHAZART & G.F. BALL. 2000. Identification of the origin of catecholaminergic inputs to HVc in canaries by retrograde tract tracing combined with tyrosine hydroxylase immunocytochemistry. J. Chem. Neuroanat. **18:** 117–133.
124. APPELTANTS, D., G.F. BALL & J. BALTHAZART. 2002. The origin of catecholaminergic inputs to the song control nucleus RA in canaries. Neuroreport **13:** 649–653.
125. LEWIS, J.W., S.M. RYAN, A.P. ARNOLD & L.L. BUTCHER. 1981. Evidence for catecholamine projection to area X in the zebra finch. J. Comp. Neurol. **196:** 347–354.
126. APPELTANTS, D., G.F. BALL & J. BALTHAZART. 2003. Song activation by testosterone is associated with increased catecholaminergic innervation of the song control system in female canaries. Neuroscience **121:** 801–814.
127. NOTTEBOHM, F. 1980. Testosterone triggers growth of brain vocal control nuclei in adult female canaries. Brain Res. **189:** 429–436.
128. GRANT, L.D. & W.E. STUMPF. 1975. Hormone uptake sites in CNS biogenic amines systems. *In* Anatomical Neuroendocrinology. W.E. Stumpf, L.D. Grant, Eds.: 445–463. Karger. Basel.
129. SAR, M. 1984. Estradiol is concentrated in tyrosine hydroxylase-containing neurons of the hypothalamus. Science **223:** 938–940.
130. BATAILLER, M., D. BLACHE, J. THIBAULT & Y. TILLET. 1992. Immunohistochemical colocalization of tyrosine hydroxylase and estradiol receptors in the sheep arcuate nucleus. Neurosci. Lett. **146:** 125–130.
131. KRITZER, M.F. 1997. Selective colocalization of immunoreactivity for intracellular gonadal steroid hormone receptors and tyrosine hydroxylase in the ventral tegmental area, substantia nigra, and retrorubral fields in the rat. J. Comp. Neurol. **379:** 247–260.
132. HERITAGE, A.S., W.E. STUMPF, M. SAR & L.D. GRANT. 1980. Brainstem catecholaminergic neurons are target sites for sex steroid hormones. Science **207:** 1377–1379.
133. BALTHAZART, J. & G.F. BALL. 1989. Effects of the noradrenergic neurotoxin DSP-4 on luteinizing hormone levels, catecholamine concentrations, alpha2-adrenergic receptor binding, and aromatase activity in the brain of the Japanese quail. Brain Res. **492:** 163–175.
134. BARCLAY, S.R., C.F. HARDING & S.A. WATERMAN. 1991. Correlations between catecholamine levels and sexual behavior in male zebra finches. Pharmacol. Biochem. Behav. **41:** 195–201.

135. Barclay, S.R., C.F. Harding & S.A. Waterman. 1996. Central DSP-4 treatment decreases norepinephrine levels and courtship behavior in male zebra finches. Pharmacol. Biochem. Behav. **53:** 213–220.
136. Blaustein, J.D. & D.H. Olster. 1989. Gonadal steroid hormone receptors and social behaviors. *In* Advances in Comparative and Environmental Physiology. Vol. 33. J. Balthazart, Ed.: 31–104. Springer Verlag. Berlin.
137. Blaustein, J.D., M.J. Tetel & J.M. Meredith. 1995. Neurobiological regulation of hormonal response by progestin and estrogen receptors. *In* Neurobiological Effects of Sex Steroid Hormones. P.E. Micevych, R.P.J. Hammer, Eds.: 324–349. Cambridge University Press. Cambridge, UK.
138. Curran, T. & J.I. Morgan. 1995. Fos: an immediate-early transcription factor in neurons. J. Neurobiol. **26:** 403–412.
139. Ball, G.F. & T.Q. Gentner. 1998. They're playing our song: gene expression and birdsong perception. Neuron **21:** 271–274.
140. Mello, C.V. 2002. Mapping vocal communication pathways in birds with inducible gene expression. J. Comp. Physiol. A **188:** 943–959.
141. Maney, D.L. & G.F. Ball. 2003. Territorial behavior induces fos-like immunoreactivity in catecholaminergic brain nuclei in free-living song sparrows. J. Neurobiol. **56:** 163–170.
142. Appeltants, D., C. Del Negro & J. Balthazart. 2002. Noradrenergic control of auditory information processing in female canaries. Behav. Brain Res. **133:** 221–235.
143. Jarvis, E.D., C. Scharff, M.R. Grossman, *et al.* 1998. For whom the bird sings: context-dependent gene expression. Neuron **21:** 775–788.
144. Hessler, N.A. & A.J. Doupe. 1999. Social context modulates singing-related neural activity in the songbird forebrain. Nat. Neurosci. **2:** 209–211.
145. Hessler, N.A. & A.J. Doupe. 1999. Singing-related neural activity in a dorsal forebrain-basal ganglia circuit of adult zebra finches. J. Neurosci. **19:** 10461–10481.
146. Castelino, C.B. & G.F. Ball. 2002. Noradrenergic regulation of context-dependent zenk expression related to song production in male zebra finches. Society for Neuroscience. Washington, DC. Abstr. **680.9**.
147. Brenowitz, E.A. 2002. Birdsong: integrating physics, physiology, and behavior. J. Comp. Physiol. **188:** 827–828.
148. Margoliash, D. 2002. Evaluating theories of bird song learning: implications for future directions. J. Comp. Physiol. **188:** 851–866.
149. Baxter, M.G. 2001. Effects of selective immunotoxic lesions on learning and memory. Methods Mol. Biol. **166:** 249–265.

Gonadectomy Affects Hormonal and Behavioral Responses to Repetitive Nociceptive Stimulation in Male Rats

ANNA MARIA ALOISI, ILARIA CECCARELLI, AND PAOLO FIORENZANI

Department of Physiology, University of Siena, Via Aldo Moro, 53100 Siena, Italy

ABSTRACT: Sex differences have been observed repeatedly in chronic pain syndromes in both humans and animals, with females showing a higher incidence; it is likely that the gonadal hormones are responsible for these differences. To examine the role of male gonadal hormones on repetitive nociceptive stimulation, we studied male rats, half of them gonadectomized (GDX) and half left intact (INT). Starting from the third week after gonadectomy, they were subjected to the formalin test once a week for 3 weeks (50 μl formalin 5% injected s.c. in the dorsum of the hind paw: right, left, and right). Formalin-induced licking, flexing, and jerking of the injected paw were recorded and analyzed for each of the three trials. Analysis of variance showed significant differences between GDX and INT animals depending on the trial considered: Trial 1: the GDX and INT groups showed a similar amount of licking, flexing, and paw-jerk; Trials 2 and 3: these responses showed a sort of adaptation in INT animals, not present in the GDX ones, resulting in lower levels of pain responses in INT than GDX. Corticosterone was higher in GDX animals than in INT animals. Testosterone plasma levels were drastically decreased by gonadectomy, whereas estradiol was increased. These data indicate that male gonadal hormones play a key role in inhibiting the behavioral responses to repeated nociceptive stimulation. This suggests that the lower incidence of chronic pain syndromes in males could be caused by the presence of these hormones.

KEYWORDS: pain; androgens; estrogens; behavior; formalin test; male rats

INTRODUCTION

Many studies of the involvement of gonadal hormones in chronic pain syndromes suggest that estrogens have a pronociceptive role, which could explain, at least in part, the higher incidence of chronic pain syndromes in women.[1] However, not enough information is available about the effect of androgens in pain, although most of the studies performed indicate that androgens are helpful in women suffering chronic pain.[2] In male rats, testosterone was found to play a protective role in adjuvant-induced arthritis.[3]

Address for correspondence: Anna Maria Aloisi, Department of Physiology, University of Siena, Via Aldo Moro, 53100 Siena, Italy. Voice: 39-05-7723-4103; fax: 39-05-7723-4037. aloisi@unisi.it

Ann. N.Y. Acad. Sci. 1007: 232–237 (2003). © 2003 New York Academy of Sciences. doi: 10.1196/annals.1286.022

Like estrogen receptors, androgen receptors are present in tissues associated with reproduction, in skeletal muscle and in the central nervous system (CNS).[4] In the brain, there is a high concentration of these receptors in the hypothalamus and in parts of the limbic forebrain thought to regulate homeostasis, reproduction, emotional behavior, and pain.

The aim of this experiment was to test the hypothesis that gonadectomy modifies the behavioral and hormonal changes that can accompany the repetition of a painful stimulus. The formalin test is a well-known method to induce acute persistent pain.[5] The occurrence in the injected animals of different behavioral responses (licking, flexing, jerking of the injected paw) makes the formalin test one of the best methods to study acute pain. In this experiment, the formalin or sham injection was administered up to three times, with a week between each treatment. Plasma levels of corticosterone, estradiol, and testosterone were determined in blood collected from deeply anesthetized animals at the end of the final test to evaluate the effects of gonadectomy and of repeated sham/formalin treatment on the hypothalamic-pituitary-adrenal and hypothalamic-pituitary-gonadal axes.

METHODS

Sixty-six adult male Wistar rats (Harlan Italia, Milan, Italy), 10 weeks of age, weighing 220–240 g at the beginning of the experiment, were used. Animals were kept on an inverted 12-h-light/12-h-dark cycle with lights on at 19:00. Food and water were available *ad libitum*. In all experiments, attention was paid to the ethical guidelines for investigation of experimental pain in conscious animals issued by the ad hoc Committee of the International Association for the Study of Pain.[6] Particular efforts were made to minimize animal suffering and to reduce the number of animals used.

Gonadectomy was performed as previously described.[7] Behavioral testing was conducted 3 weeks after surgery. Both intact (INT) and gonadectomized (GDX) animals were randomly assigned to four experimental groups, depending on whether they received formalin (F = one injection of formalin) or sham (S = one sham injection) treatment on Days 1, 8, and 15: Group FFF: Days 1, 8, 15: formalin treatment ($n = 6$ INT, $n = 6$ GDX); Group SFF: Day 1: sham treatment; Days 8, 15: formalin treatment ($n = 6$ INT, $n = 6$ GDX); Group SSF: Days 1, 8: sham treatment; Day 15: formalin treatment ($n = 6$ INT, $n = 6$ GDX); Group SSS: Days 1, 8, 15: sham treatment ($n = 5$ INT, $n = 5$ GDX). On Day 22, the animals' spontaneous behavior was observed in an open-field apparatus (Final Open Field). In addition to the four experimental groups, one group was added as controls: the controls (CRL, $n = 5$; INT, $n = 5$ GDX) always remained in their home cage and were subjected only to the Final Open-Field test (Day 22).

The open-field apparatus was used to conduct the formalin test (60 min) and the Final Open-Field test (15 min). It consisted of a transparent square-floor cage (50 × 50 × 30-high cm). Each animal's behavior was video-recorded and subsequently analyzed by an observer who was unaware of the treatment group of each animal. Immediately before being placed in the open-field apparatus, each animal was sham injected (S, only a prick in the dorsum of the hind paw) or formalin injected (F; 5% formalin, 50 μl into the dorsum of the hind paw). The first week, the injection (F or

S) was done in the right hind paw, the second week in the left, and the third week again in the right hind paw. The formalin-evoked responses were licking (time spent licking the foot), flexing (time spent with the leg held off the floor, flexed, close to the body), and paw-jerk (number of phasic flexions of the leg). Immediately after the end of the Final Open-Field test, the animals were deeply anesthetized to collect blood from the abdominal aorta. Blood was collected in EDTA, centrifuged, and frozen. Corticosterone, estradiol, and testosterone plasma levels were determined as previously described.[7] All data were assessed by ANOVA followed by Fisher's protected least significant difference post hoc test as appropriate. The criterion for statistical significance was $P < 0.05$.

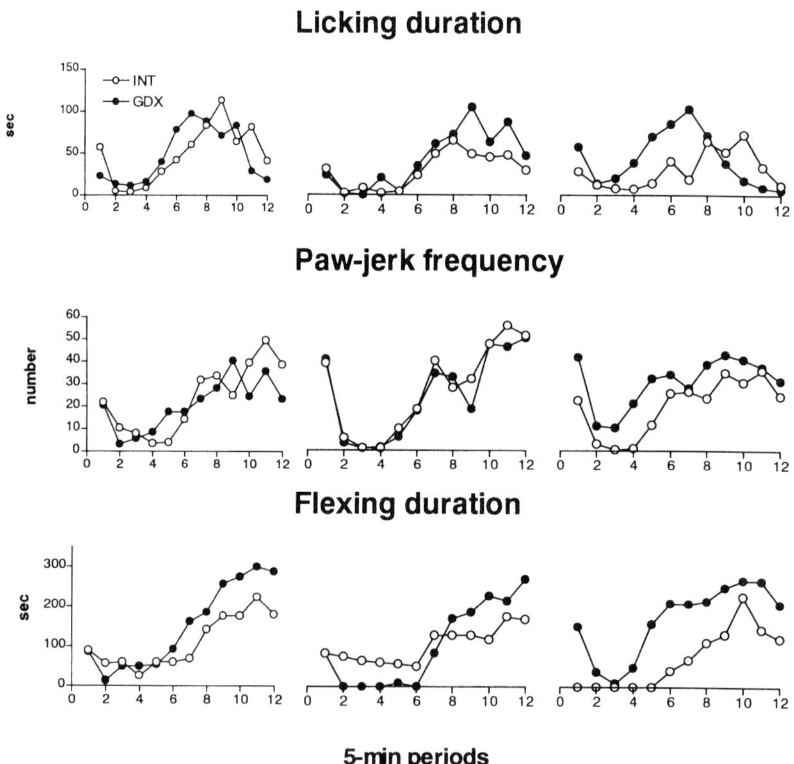

FIGURE 1. Formalin test: licking duration (seconds), paw-jerk frequency (number), and flexing duration (seconds). Behavior was scored for a 1-h period after formalin injection (50 μl, 5%) in animals belonging to Group FFF, receiving formalin in each trial. The time after formalin injection (in 5-min periods) is indicated on the abscissa. Indications of significance for single time points and standard errors were not included to maintain the clarity of the graph. (*closed symbols*) Gonadectomized animals; (*open symbols*) intact animals.

RESULTS

Formalin Test

Sham-treated animals spent most of their time exploring the environment; the locomotor/exploratory activity decreased progressively from the beginning to the end of the test. In formalin-treated animals, the formalin-induced licking, flexing, and jerking of the injected paw were recorded in all groups and were mostly directed toward the injected foot.

To compare the formalin-induced responses in the same animal during the three experimental sessions, we applied ANOVA to licking duration, flexing duration, and jerking frequency in Group FFF, treated with formalin three times. The main factors were gonadectomy (2 levels: INT, GDX), trial (3 levels: Trials 1, 2, 3), and Time (12 levels: 12 5-min periods, repeated).

Licking: Repetition of the test had a significantly different effect on licking in the intact and gonadectomized animals, as revealed by ANOVA: Gonadectomy × Trial × Time ($P < 0.02$). As shown in FIGURE 1, no differences were found between INT and GDX animals during Trial 1, whereas licking duration was lower in INT than GDX in Trials 2 and 3 (both $P < 0.04$). In fact, licking duration decreased from the first to the third trials in INT but not in GDX.

Flexing: ANOVA applied to flexing duration values showed no significance for any of the factors considered.

Jerking: ANOVA applied to jerking frequencies revealed a significant interaction Trial × Time ($P < 0.02$). During Trial 3, paw-jerk frequency remained high in GDX animals but was lower than during Trial 1 in INT.

Final Open-Field Test

ANOVA was applied with the factors gonadectomy and group (five levels: CRL, SSS, SSF, SFF, and FFF) to the spontaneous behaviors (data not shown). Inner and outer crossing frequencies did not differ among groups. ANOVA applied to rearing frequency showed a significant effect of gonadectomy ($P<0.02$), because of the higher levels of rearing in INT than GDX. There were no significant effects on self-grooming duration.

Neuroendocrine Assay

ANOVA applied to corticosterone plasma levels revealed a significant effect of gonadectomy ($P < 0.001$), because of the higher levels in GDX than in INT. ANOVA applied to testosterone and estradiol plasma levels revealed a significant effect of the factor gonadectomy ($P < 0.001$, for both). Testosterone was lower and estradiol was higher in GDX than INT (TABLE 1).

DISCUSSION

To study the effects of circulating androgens on the responses to repeated acute short-lasting nociceptive stimulation, we subjected intact and gonadectomized male rats to the formalin test one, two, or three times. Formalin pain-induced behavioral

TABLE 1. Corticosterone, estradiol, and testosterone plasma levels determined in all groups at the end of the experimental tests.

Groups	Surgery	Corticosterone (μg/100 mL)	Testosterone (ng/mL)	Estradiol (pg/mL)
CRL	INT	18.8 ± 6.2	2.9 ± 0.9	36.7 ± 5.2
	GDX	17.3 ± 3.3	0.6 ± 0.2	85.0 ± 5.5
SSS	INT	11.9 ± 2.7	2.2 ± 1.0	32.3 ± 3.0
	GDX	21.1 ± 3.9	0.6 ± 0.3	75.3 ± 9.8
SSF	INT	14.8 ± 2.6	2.0 ± 0.6	48.5 ± 11.0
	GDX	21.6 ± 3.4	0.6 ± 0.2	65.9 ± 11.0
SFF	INT	11.8 ± 1.2	4.4 ± 0.9	68.5 ± 6.0
	GDX	23.8 ± 4.3	0.4 ± 0.1	66.0 ± 10.0
FFF	INT	13.7 ± 1.9	1.3 ± 0.5	45.5 ± 8.0
	GDX	24.7 ± 5.1	0.5 ± 0.1	86.3 ± 3.0

responses indicative of pain depending on the number of times the animals were exposed to the noxious stimulus: whereas in intact animals the responses decreased from the first to the third formalin test; in gonadectomized animals no differences were found among trials. The presence of circulating androgens seemed to help the animals to "habituate" to the nociceptive stimulus, whereas this "ability" was lost in gonadectomized animals.

Because pain-related behaviors decreased in intact animals, we must infer the presence of an inhibitory, rather than excitatory, modulation by repetition of the noxious stimulus. This agrees with numerous behavioral, electrophysiological, and neuronal data showing the inhibitory effects of descending fibers on peripheral afferent and/or spinal nociceptive second-order neurons during the development of peripheral inflammation.[8–10] The progressive decrease of nociceptive responses in intact rats can be explained by increased sensitivity to opioids; indeed, as recently summarized by Ren *et al.*,[11] the descending inhibitory pathways would become more active in response to inflammation and the whole descending system would be maximally activated by the persistent afferent barrage. The fact that there was no decrease of the formalin-induced responses in gonadectomized animals suggests that androgens play a key role in these processes. Our results generally agree with those of other studies indicating the important role played by normal levels of androgens in decreasing the reactivity of the CNS during both physiological and aversive events.[12–14]

Interestingly, in gonadectomized animals there are not only lower testosterone levels, but also higher estradiol levels (probably to be ascribed to the common increase in fat mass—the substrate of peripheral aromatization—after gonadectomy); this condition could per se be pronociceptive considering estrogen as part in the higher incidence of chronic painful syndromes in females.

In conclusion, these findings strongly support our hypothesis that male gonadal hormones acting at central levels decrease the "ability" of the CNS to retain information, including information related to nociceptive input.

REFERENCES

1. BERKLEY, K.J. 1997. Sex differences in pain. Behav. Brain Sci. **20:** 371–380.
2. KAERGAARD, A. *et al.* 2000. Association between plasma testosterone and work-related neck and shoulder disorders among female workers. Scand. J. Work Environ. Health **26:** 292–298.
3. HARBUZ, M.S. *et al.* 1995. A protective role for testosterone in adjuvant-induced arthritis. Br. J. Rheumatol. **34:** 1117–1122.
4. MANOLAGAS, S.C. & S. KOUSTENI. 2001. Perspective: nonreproductive sites of action of reproductive hormones. Endocrinology **142:** 2200–2204.
5. ALOISI, A.M., M.E. ALBONETTI & G. CARLI. 1996. Formalin-induced changes in adrenocorticotropic hormone and corticosterone plasma levels and hippocampal choline acetyltransferase activity in male and female rats. Neuroscience **74:** 1019–1024.
6. ZIMMERMANN, M. 1983. Ethical guidelines for investigations of experimental pain in conscious animals. Pain **16:** 109–110.
7. ALOISI, A.M. & I. CECCARELLI. 2000. Role of gonadal hormones in formalin-induced pain responses of male rats: modulation by estradiol and naloxone administration. Neuroscience **95:** 559–566.
8. DANZIGER, N. *et al.* 1999. Alteration of descending modulation of nociception during the course of monoarthritis in the rat. J. Neurosci. **19:** 2394–2400.
9. GOGAS, K.R., J.D. LEVINE & A.I. BASBAUM. 1996. Differential contribution of descending controls to the antinociceptive actions of kappa and mu opioids: an analysis of formalin-evoked C-fos expression. J. Pharmacol. Exp. Ther. **276:** 801–809.
10. GOZARIU, M. *et al.* 1997. Temporal summation of C-fiber afferent inputs: competition between facilitatory and inhibitory effects on C-fiber reflex in the rat. J. Neurophysiol. **78:** 3165–3179.
11. REN, K., M. ZHUO & W.D. WILLIS. 2000. Multiplicity and plasticity of descending modulation of nociception: implications for persistent pain. *In* Proceedings of the 9th World Congress on Pain, Progress in Pain Research and Management, M. Devor, M.C. Rowbotham & Z. Wiesenfeld-Hallin, Eds.: 387–400. IASP Press. Seattle.
12. HADID, R. *et al.* 1995. Repeated endotoxin treatment decreases immune and hypothalamo-pituitary-adrenal axis responses: effects of orchidectomy and testosterone therapy. Neuroendocrinology **62:** 348–355.
13. HANDA, R.J. *et al.* 1994. Androgen regulation of adrenocorticotropin and corticosterone secretion in the male rat following novelty and foot shock stressors. Physiol. Behav. **55:** 117–124.
14. VIAU, V., L. SORIANO & M.F. DALLMAN. 2001. Androgens alter corticotropin releasing hormone and arginine vasopressin mRNA within forebrain sites known to regulate activity in the hypothalamic-pituitary-adrenal axis. J. Neuroendocrinol. **13:** 442–452.

Progestin Receptors

Neuronal Integrators of Hormonal and Environmental Stimulation

JEFFREY D. BLAUSTEIN

Center for Neuroendocrine Studies, University of Massachusetts, Amherst, Massachusetts 01003-9271, USA

ABSTRACT: Although it originally was believed that neuronal steroid hormone receptors require binding to cognate ligand for activation, more recent evidence suggests that the receptors can be activated indirectly by other compounds, such as neurotransmitters and growth factors, acting through their own membrane receptors and specific intracellular signaling pathways. For example, as is the case with facilitation of sexual behavior by progesterone, facilitation of sexual behavior by D_1/D_5 dopamine receptor agonists is blocked by disruption of progestin receptors. Therefore, some dopamine agonists facilitate sexual behavior at least in part by a progestin receptor–dependent mechanism, as does progesterone. This "ligand-independent activation" of neuronal progestin receptors is not limited to dopamine agonists; a variety of other compounds, as well as mating stimulation, facilitate sexual receptivity by a progestin receptor–dependent process. Steroid hormone receptors also can be regulated by afferent input in another way. Various neurotransmitters upregulate or downregulate steroid hormone receptors in some neurons. This, in turn, presumably confers greater or decreased sensitivity to the particular factors that can activate the particular steroid receptor in those particular neurons. Therefore, steroid hormones are but one class of factors that can regulate and activate steroid hormone receptors. Some additional factors that activate steroid hormone receptors have been identified, as have some factors that can regulate concentrations of receptors. Relatively little is known at this time about the range of neurotransmitters, humoral factors, and intracellular signaling pathways that are involved.

KEYWORDS: progestin receptor; estrogen receptor; progesterone; estradiol; neural integration; hypothalamus; forebrain; sexual behavior; reproductive behavior; steroid hormones; ligand-independent activation

INTRODUCTION

Ovarian hormones have many effects in the brain which result in changes in behaviors and reproductive physiology.[1–3] A model that often is used to study the cellular mechanisms of ovarian hormones in the brain is the regulation of feminine

Address for correspondence: Jeffrey D. Blaustein, Center for Neuroendocrine Studies, 135 Hicks Way, University of Massachusetts, Amherst, MA 01003-9271, USA. Voice: 413-545-1524; fax: 413-545-0769.

blaustein@cns.umass.edu

Ann. N.Y. Acad. Sci. 1007: 238–250 (2003). © 2003 New York Academy of Sciences. doi: 10.1196/annals.1286.023

sexual behavior by estradiol and progesterone. In this article, the role of neuronal progestin receptors in mediating the effects of progesterone on sexual behavior is discussed. Also, the influences of afferent input conveyed from the social environment via changes in neurotransmitter pathways on steroid hormone receptors are elaborated. We suggest that there is the potential for a great deal of regulation of progestin receptor–dependent processes in specific neurons by particular neurotransmitter pathways that convey environmental regulation of steroid hormone receptors.

Although the cellular processes of hormone action in the brain have been most extensively studied in rats, there is much commonality in the hormonal regulation of feminine sexual behavior in a variety of other rodent species, including guinea pigs, hamsters, and mice. During the estrous cycle,[4–8] the sequential secretion of estradiol and progesterone from the ovaries induces a period of sexual behavior around the time of ovulation. Ovariectomy eliminates the expression of feminine sexual behaviors by terminating the cyclic release of ovarian hormones.[4,9,10] Although ovariectomized rats, guinea pigs, and mice may respond to estradiol alone, sequential treatment with estradiol and progesterone is more effective,[9–11] and it makes the onset and termination of heat more predictable.[4,9,10] After heat terminates, the animals become transiently refractory to the effect of progesterone on sexual receptivity.[1,2,12–14] Because estradiol and progesterone have very predictable influences on feminine sexual behavior, the hormonal regulation of feminine sexual behavior provides a physiologically relevant model with which to investigate the cellular processes by which estradiol, progesterone, and other factors act on the brain to influence behavior and by which other afferent factors may influence neuronal function and behavior through these processes.

There is general agreement that steroid hormones act through steroid hormone receptors functioning as transcriptional regulators, as well as by other mechanisms. Steroid hormones diffuse freely into and out of all cells, but, in target cells containing receptors for the particular hormone, the hormones bind with high affinity to unoccupied receptors. Ligand binding to the receptor results in a conformational change, activation, and dimerization. Once bound to the chromatin, the hormone–receptor complex causes changes in gene expression,[15] leading to alterations in protein synthesis and consequently to changes in cellular function. Although some experiments suggested that the receptors are entirely or primarily nuclear proteins,[16,17] others suggested the presence of receptors in both cytoplasmic and nuclear locations, particularly in the brain.[18] However, the site of action of the receptors acting as transcriptional regulators is the cell nucleus, where they bind in concert with steroid receptor coregulators,[19,20] to steroid response elements on particular genes.

NEURAL PROGESTIN RECEPTORS AND BEHAVIOR

The dependence of progesterone-facilitated sexual behavior on progestin receptors in guinea pigs, rats, and mice has been shown by the use of progesterone antagonists,[21] antisense oligonucleotides to progestin receptor mRNA,[22–24] and progestin receptor gene disruption in mice.[25] Generally, when progestin receptor levels are elevated, animals respond to progesterone with the expression of sexual behavior, and when they are reduced, either by interference with the receptor, by lack of estradiol, or by down-regulation by progesterone itself, animals are hyposensitive or unresponsive to progesterone.[1,2] Although there are numerous differences in the expression of sexual behaviors in different rodent species, rats, guinea pigs, and mice each require activation of neuronal progestin receptors for progesterone-facilitated sexual behavior.

LIGAND-INDEPENDENT ACTIVATION OF PROGESTIN RECEPTORS

Although it had been assumed that binding of receptors to their cognate ligands—the steroid hormones—was necessary for activation of the transcription factor receptors, it was shown more recently[26,27] that the COUP receptor, progestin receptor and estrogen receptor could each be activated *in vitro* by activation of D_1 dopamine receptors. The process by which dopamine or other compounds *indirectly* activate steroid hormone receptors through intracellular signaling pathways is referred to as *ligand-independent activation.*

A good deal of evidence now supports the idea that both progestin receptors and estrogen receptors can undergo ligand-independent activation. Most of this work, done *in vitro* and with peripheral tissues, has focused on activation of estrogen receptors by growth factors, such as epidermal growth factor[28] and insulin-like growth factor.[29] However, ligand-independent activation seems to be a common mechanism by which steroid hormone receptors are activated. Additional factors that can activate estrogen receptors and/or progestin receptors in various tissues by ligand-independent activation as well include GnRH,[30,31] D_1/D_5 dopaminergic agonists,[27] phorbol esters,[32] and cAMP,[29] MAP kinase,[33] and cyclins[34] (for review see Cenni and Picard[35]).

Despite the wealth of information concerning ligand-independent activation of steroid hormone receptors in nonneural tissues, relatively little work has been done on the idea that *neural* steroid hormone receptors can be activated by afferent influences. What is known is summarized here. Intracerebroventricular infusion of a D_1/D_5-specific dopamine receptor agonist substitutes for progesterone in facilitating sexual behavior in estradiol-primed rats.[36] As with progesterone activation of sexual behavior, progesterone antagonists, antisense oligonucleotides directed at the progestin receptor mRNA[22–24,37] or progestin receptor gene disruptions in mice[25] block this facilitation, supporting the idea that ligand-independent activation of progestin receptors mediates dopamine-facilitated feminine sexual behavior.

Ligand-independent activation of neuronal progestin receptors is not limited to activation by dopamine though. In fact, facilitation of sexual receptivity by a progestin receptor–dependent process has been observed for GnRH,[38,39] prostaglandin E2,[38] and nitric oxide.[40] Furthermore, stimulation of cAMP[38] and cGMP[41] each facilitate the expression of sexual behavior by a progestin receptor–dependent mechanism, implicating protein kinase A and protein kinase G in ligand-independent activation. Although the idea that many drugs that facilitate sexual behavior do so by influencing a common second messenger system was first proposed by Whalen and Lauber for cGMP[42] and by Beyer and Gonzalez-Mariscal for cAMP in 1986,[43] more recent data suggest that progestin receptors may be a component of a final common signaling pathway.

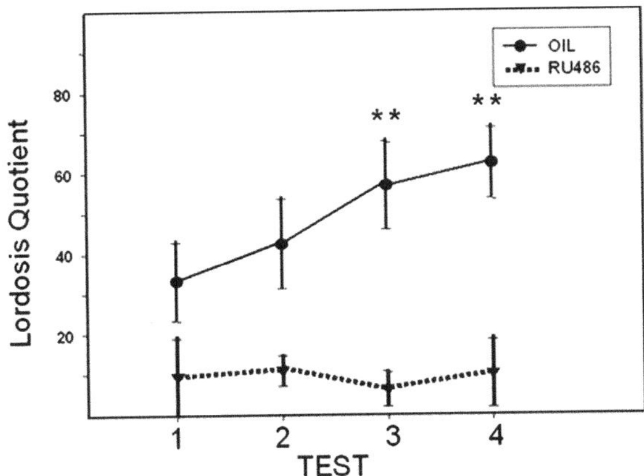

FIGURE 1. Effects of the progesterone antagonist RU486 or oil vehicle on sexual behavior of estradiol-primed female rats in response to repeated testing with a male rat. Each test is based on 15 min of mating with a male rat followed by 15 min without the male. Although rats were given vaginocervical stimulation with a plastic probe 15 min before the start of testing in this experiment, the additional stimulation is not essential for the enhancement of sexual behavior by mating. Data redrawn from Auger *et al.*[45]

Ligand-independent activation by afferent input appears to have an important role in the regulation of feminine sexual behavior by afferent input derived from mating stimulation in rats. When estradiol-treated, ovariectomized rats are repeatedly exposed to males, for example, for 15 min at a time followed by 15 min away for the male,[44] their lordosis increases over the course of a few hours, a response that is not dependent on the ovaries or adrenal glands.[45] Treatment with a progestin antagonist just before exposure to the males completely blocks this response (FIG. 1), although it does not block the rapid lordosis response to manual palpation *at the time of* vaginocervical stimulation.[45] This suggests that ligand-independent activation of progestin receptors is involved in the process by which environmental stimulation (i.e., mating stimulation) enhances subsequent sexual behavior. Most importantly, these results also suggest that neuronal progestin receptors can undergo ligand-independent activation *in vivo* by a *physiologically relevant stimulus* in addition to pharmacologically by a D_1/D_5 dopamine agonist.

Ligand-independent activation of progestin receptors also is involved in the regulation of ovulation during the rat and mouse estrous cycle. Blockade of progestin receptors or inhibition of progestin receptor synthesis in the anteroventral periventricular area blocks some of the effects of estradiol on GnRH regulation. This is believed to be caused by inhibition of activation of progestin receptors, which occurs as a neuronal consequence of estradiol action (see Levine *et al.*[46] for review).

In a study of a vaginocervical stimulation–induced neuronal response that is apparently mediated by ligand-independent activation of progestin receptors, we found that injection of a progesterone antagonist an hour before vaginocervical stimulation with a plastic probe inhibits stimulation-induced Fos expression (a protein marker for a neuronal response to the stimulation) in the rostral medial preoptic

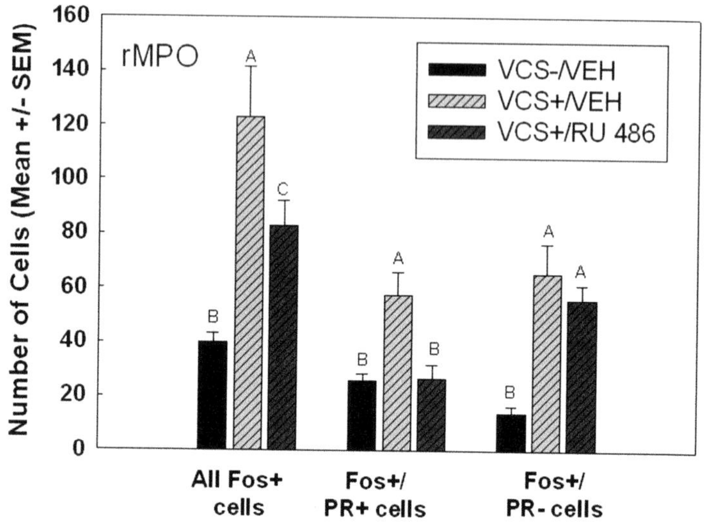

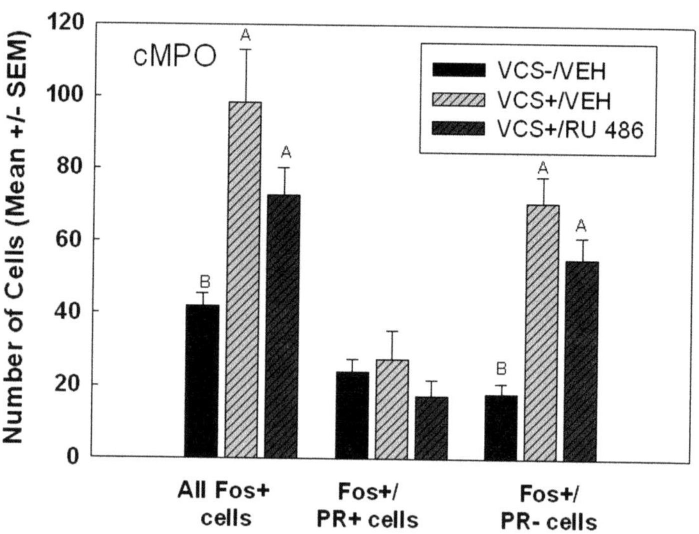

FIGURE 2. Number of cells expressing Fos-ir (all Fos+ cells), Fos-ir, and PR-ir (Fos+/PR+ cells) or Fos+ without PR-ir (Fos+/PR– cells) in the rostral medial preoptic area (rMPO) or caudal medial preoptic area (cMPO) after control stimulation (VCS–) preceded by vehicle (VCS–/VEH), vaginocervical stimulation preceded by vehicle (VCS+/VEH) or vaginocervical stimulation preceded by RU486 (VCS+/RU486). Bars with different letters over them denote statistically significant differences between groups. Data redrawn from Blaustein and Greco.[47]

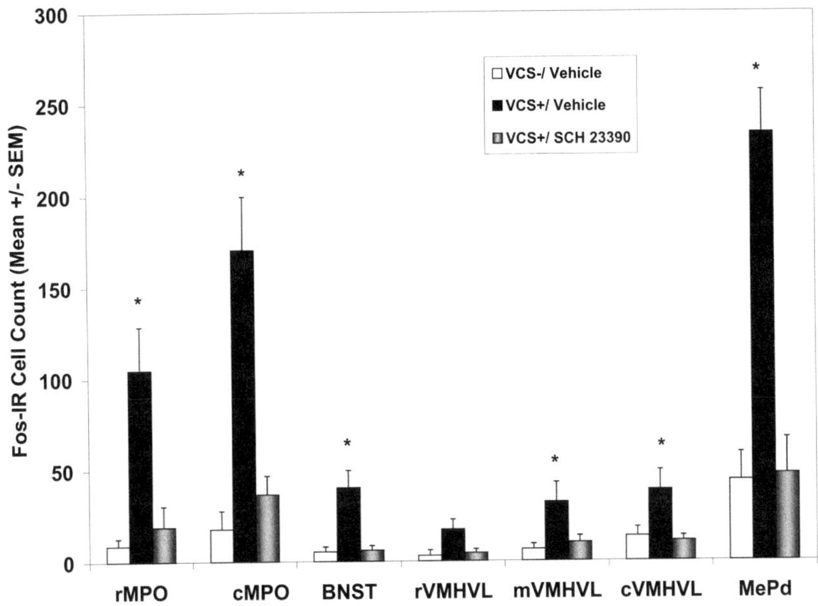

FIGURE 3. Numbers of Fos-ir cells (mean ± SEM) in forebrain areas after control stimulation (VCS–) or vaginocervical stimulation (VCS+) preceded by an injection of either saline or SCH 23390. Asterisks above bars indicate statistically significant difference between VCS + and other groups. rMPO, cMPO, rostral, caudal medial preoptic area; BNST, bed nucleus of stria terminalis; rVMHVL, mVMHVL, cVMHVL, rostral, mid, and caudal ventrolateral aspect of ventromedial hypothalamus; MePd, posterodorsal medial amygdala. Data redrawn from Quysner and Blaustein.[55]

area, bed nucleus of stria terminalis, and parts of the ventromedial hypothalamus, but not other areas studied.[45,47] Many of the neurons that responded with Fos expression coexpress progestin receptors.[48] In the rostral medial preoptic area, a progestin antagonist specifically blocked Fos expression in progestin receptor–containing cells, not in progestin receptor–negative cells (FIG. 2).[47] In contrast, in the caudal medial preoptic area, vaginocervical stimulation induced Fos expression only in progestin receptor–negative neurons, and the progestin antagonist was without effect. These results are consistent with the idea that, although Fos can be induced by mating stimulation in both neurons expressing and neurons not expressing progestin receptors, in those containing progestin receptors, the response to afferent input is *gated* by the progestin receptor. Furthermore, although not necessarily the *only* site involved, the data show that the rostral medial preoptic area is likely to be *one* of the sites at which genital stimulation can activate progestin receptors by the ligand-independent mechanism.

Consistent with the hypothesis that dopamine is one of the critical factors that is released in response to mating-related stimulation, resulting in ligand-independent activation of progestin receptors, mating-related stimuli induce the release of dopamine,[49–52] as well as norepinephrine,[53,54] in the forebrain under a variety of circumstances. These neurotransmitters then act on their receptors in specific neurons, which activate intracellular second messendger signaling pathways. Vaginocervical stimulation-induced Fos is completely blocked by a D_1/D_5 dopamine receptor antagonist in all forebrain areas studied (FIG. 3),[55] suggesting that dopamine is released in response to the vaginocervical stimulation which then stimulates D_1/D_5 dopamine receptors, which, in turn, induce a neuronal response (Fos expression). Preliminary immunocytochemical data suggest that D_5 dopamine receptors are coexpressed with progestin receptors in the ventromedial hypothalamus (J. C. Turcotte and J. D. Blaustein, unpublished material), suggesting a neuronal substrate by which dopaminergic neurotransmission might activate progestin receptors in some neurons.

Recent evidence suggests the importance of the phosphatase-1 inhibitor, DARPP-32,[56] in the process by which sexual behavior is induced by either progesterone or ligand-independent activation.[57] Activation of D_1/D_5 dopamine receptors induces an increase in the level of intracellular cAMP, which, in turn, induces phosphorylation on the Thr_{32} residue of DARPP-32, an inhibitor of protein phosphatase-1. Behavioral response to both progesterone and a D_1 dopamine receptor agonist, but not to serotonin, is blocked in DARPP-32 knockout mice, suggesting that DARPP-32 may be involved in phosphorylation and dephosphorylation of progestin receptors.[57] Because of this finding and the fact that vaginocervical stimulation induces the phosphorylation of DARPP-32 in some forebrain neurons, including progestin receptor–rich areas,[58] we suggested that one mechanism by which vaginocervical stimulation influences progestin receptor–dependent neuronal and behavioral changes is by activation of the DARPP-32 pathway. This, in turn, may lead to increased phosphorylation of progestin receptors or its coactivators resulting in activation of progestin receptors. Although much of the evidence is consistent with mating stimulation activating progestin receptors and facilitating sexual receptivity *via* a dopaminergic pathway, note that DARPP-32 can be phosphorylated by a variety of other neurotransmitters that act through either a protein kinase A or protein kinase G pathway, as well as by other intracellular signaling pathways.[56]

Steroid receptors can be activated by circulating hormones, so why might receptors in some neurons also be activated by afferent neurotransmitter input? We speculate that the teleological raison d'être for ligand-independent activation of neuronal steroid hormone receptors is to enable nonhormonal factors (i.e., afferent stimulation in the form of neurotransmitter release) to *fine-tune* and, perhaps in some, cases *turn on* the expression of neuronal and behavioral responses. This is best seen in the example of mating stimulation enhancing sexual receptivity over the course of a few hours described earlier. Although purely speculative, the purpose of this may be to synchronize the onset of receptive behavior in the female with the presence of adequate stimulation by male rats. In other words, if a female rat emerges from her burrow before she is fully receptive,[59] her initial interactions with male rats may hasten the onset of full sexual receptivity earlier than the progesterone would have done so. Although relatively little is known about the mechanisms of reflex ovulation, perhaps mating-induced, ligand-independent activation of progestin receptors provides a mechanism by which males can induce reflex ovulation by a neuronal pathway similar to that proposed for spontaneous ovulation.[46]

The duration of the period of sexual receptivity is the result of a complex interplay between factors that enhance and those that inhibit the further display. Interest-

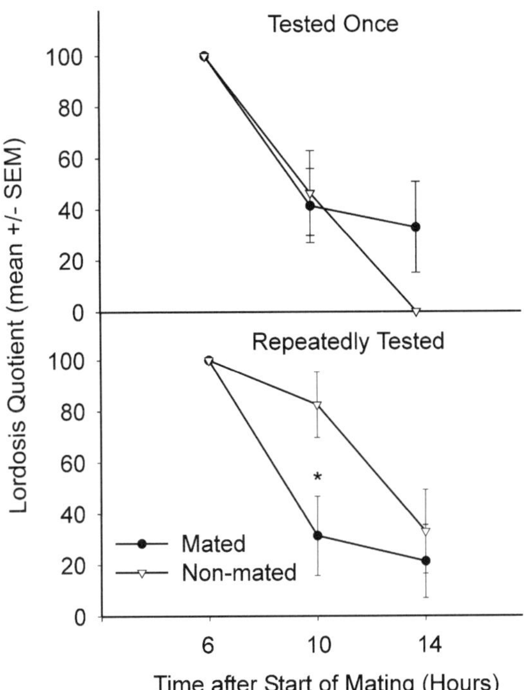

FIGURE 4. Lordosis quotients of female rats that had not been mated previously and those that received mounts and intromissions resulting in two ejaculations and were then tested 6, 10, and 14 h later (*top*). Lordosis quotients of female rats that had not been mated previously and those that received mounts and intromissions resulting in two ejaculations and then were tested at either 6, 10, or 14 h later (*bottom*). Contrast between the nonmated controls demonstrates that the testing at 6 and 10 h prolonged the duration of sexual receptivity. Prior mating exposure shortened heat duration only in the animals that were tested repeatedly, not in the animals tested only once. Data redrawn from reference Bennett *et al.*[60]

ingly, while mating stimulation in which intromissions were allowed abbreviated the period of sexual receptivity, mating stimulation in which intromissions were prevented somewhat delayed heat termination.[60] That is, although some aspects of mating stimulation shorten heat duration, others lengthen it (FIG. 4), and, as discussed earlier, some induce it. Some of this microregulation of sexual receptivity by the interactions of the female with a male might well involve acute regulation of activated progestin receptors by these stimuli from the social environment in concert with activation caused by hormonal changes. There is also one report of another signaling pathway involving epidermal growth factor activating neuronal estrogen receptors resulting in the expression of lordosis.[61] The possible contribution of ligand-independent activation of estrogen receptors also must be considered.

We also have suggested that a similar process could be involved in the induction or maintenance of maternal behavior by stimulation from pups, that is, the process

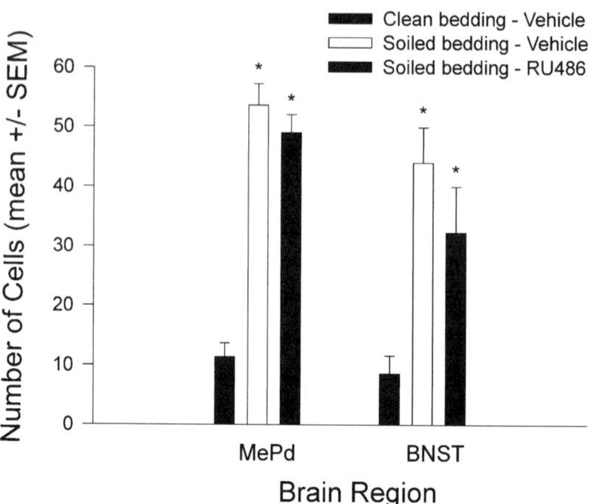

FIGURE 5. Mean number (±SEM) of Fos-immunoreactive cells in the posterodorsal medial amygdala (MePd) and bed nucleus of stria terminalis (BNST) after treatment with vehicle and exposure to clean bedding (Clean bedding - Vehicle), treatment with vehicle and exposure to male-soiled bedding (Soiled bedding - Vehicle), or treatment with RU486 and exposure to male-soiled bedding (Soiled bedding - RU486). *Significant difference from females treated with vehicle and exposure to clean bedding. Data redrawn from Bennett *et al.*[65]

by which rat pups induce maternal behavior in the absence of the typical hormonal changes associated with the onset of maternal behavior postpartum and also maintain maternal behavior in the absence of high estradiol levels. Perhaps one or more of the sensory stimuli associated with the pups results in the activation of estrogen receptors in critical neurons involved in the onset or maintenance of maternal behavior.[62]

AFFERENT REGULATION OF RECEPTOR CONCENTRATION

Not *all* influences of afferent input on steroid hormone-sensitive processes can be attributed to ligand-independent activation. Mating-induced enhancement of sexual behavior is also dependent on an accessory olfactory pathway.[44,63,64] However, unlike the case with vaginocervical stimulation, neurons in which Fos is induced after exposure to male-soiled bedding do not contain estradiol-induced progestin receptors.[65] Furthermore, unlike the case with vaginocervical stimulation-induced Fos expression, which is blocked by progesterone antagonists,[45] odor-induced Fos expression is not (FIG. 5).[65] Thus, the evidence suggests that, unlike vaginocervical stimulation, the effects of this particular olfactory pathway on sexual receptivity do not involve ligand-independent activation of progestin receptors.

The fact that odors do not seem to activate progestin receptors in the same way as genital stimulation does not imply that odors do not influence steroid receptors. First of all, although estrogen-induced progestin receptors were not coexpressed with Fos after exposure to odors from bedding soiled by male rats, ERα is coexpressed, leaving open the possibility that ligand-independent activation of ERα is involved. Furthermore, a second mode of interaction of afferent input with steroid hormone receptors is the regulation of steroid hormone receptor concentrations by neurotransmitters.[2] In fact, olfactory bulbectomy, which increases sensitivity to estradiol, increases the *concentration* of estrogen receptors in the medial amygdala.[66] An increase in receptor levels would be expected to alter *sensitivity* or *responsiveness* of particular neurons to estradiol or to other factors that can activate estrogen receptors. That is, a greater concentration of receptors in a particular neuron would increase the probability of activation by a particular ligand or other factor. Note that regulation of the concentrations of neuronal progestin, estrogen, and glucocorticoid receptors by an array of neurotransmitters and social environmental factors has been described (for review, see Blaustein and Erskine[2]).

SUMMARY

In summary, there are at least two modes of regulation of neuronal steroid hormone receptors by afferent input. Neurotransmitters and perhaps humoral factors as well can activate steroid hormone receptors independently of cognate hormone by ligand-independent activation. Ligand-independent activation of neuronal progestin receptors with consequent neuronal and behavioral changes can be induced not only by pharmacological means, but also by elements of the social environment as well. In addition, some neurotransmitters can, under some circumstances, regulate the concentrations of particular steroid hormone receptors in populations of neurons. This regulation of the concentration of receptors would be expected to alter the sensitivity of particular neurons to factors (including steroid hormones as well as neurotransmitters and other factors conveying input from the social environment) that can activate the receptors. Besides demonstrating novel mechanisms by which the social environment influences neuronal function and behavior, these modes of regulation of steroid receptors are relevant to other work in neuroendocrinology. It is possible that in some experiments in which the effects of neurotransmitters on progesterone-influenced neuronal and behavioral responses are assessed, the drugs may be inducing ligand-independent activation of progestin receptors with consequent progestin receptor–dependent changes in behavior and physiology. Alternatively, in other cases, drugs may influence the sensitivity of particular neurons to a particular steroid hormone by up- or down-regulation of steroid hormone receptors. A comprehensive understanding of the neuronal processes involved in the regulation of feminine sexual behavior requires an understanding of the identity of the afferent factors that influence these processes, as well as the cellular mechanisms by which this occurs.

ACKNOWLEDGMENTS

The work from the authors' laboratory discussed in this article was supported by Senior Scientist Award MH 01312 and research grants NS 19327 and MH 56187, all from the National Institutes of Health.

REFERENCES

1. Blaustein, J.D. & D.H. Olster. 1989. Gonadal steroid hormone receptors and social behaviors. *In* Advances in Comparative & Endrocrine Physiololgy, Vol. 3, Molecular and Cellular Basis of Social Behavior in Vertebrates. J. Balthazart, Ed.: 31–104. Springer-Verlag. Berlin.
2. Blaustein, J.D. & M.S. Erskine. 2002. Feminine sexual behavior: cellular integration of hormonal and afferent information in the rodent forebrain. *In* Hormones, Brain and Behavior. D.W. Pfaff, Ed.: 139–214. Academic Press. New York.
3. Pfaff, D.W., S. Schwartz-Giblin, M.M. McCarthy, *et al.* 1994. Cellular and molecular mechanisms of female reproductive behaviors. *In* The Physiology of Reproduction. 2nd ed. E. Knobil & J.D. Neill, Eds.: 107–220. Raven Press Ltd. New York.
4. Boling, J.L. & R.J. Blandau. 1939. The estrogen-progesterone induction of mating responses in the spayed female rat. Endocrinology **25:** 359–364.
5. Powers, J.B. 1970. Hormonal control of sexual receptivity during the estrous cycle of the rat. Physiol. Behav. **5:** 831–835.
6. Dempsey, E.W., R. Hertz & W.C. Young. 1936. The experimental induction of oestrus (sexual receptivity) in the normal and ovariectomized guinea pig. Am. J. Physiol. **116:** 201–209.
7. Collins, V.J., J.I. Boling, E.W. Dempsey, *et al.* 1938. Quantitative studies of experimentally induced sexual receptivity in the spayed guinea pig. Endocrinology **23:** 188–196.
8. Joslyn, W.D., H.H. Feder & R.W. Goy. 1971. Estrogen conditioning and progesterone facilitation of lordosis in guinea pigs. Physiol. Behav. **7:** 477–482.
9. Ring, J.R. 1944. The estrogen-progesterone induction of sexual receptivity in the spayed female mouse. Endocrinology **34:** 269–275.
10. Young, W.C. 1969. Psychobiology of sexual behavior in the guinea pig. *In* Advances in the Study of Behavior. D.S. Lehrman, R.A. Hinde & E. Shaw, Eds.: 1–110. Academic Press. New York.
11. Whalen, R.E. 1974. Estrogen-progesterone induction of mating in female rats. Horm. Behav. **5:** 157–162.
12. Morin, L.P. 1977. Progesterone: inhibition of rodent sexual behavior. Physiol. Behav. **18:** 701–715.
13. Feder, H.H. & B.L. Marrone. 1977. Progesterone: its role in the central nervous system as a facilitator and inhibitor of sexual behavior and gonadotropin release. Ann. N.Y. Acad. Sci. **286:** 331–354.
14. Edwards, D.A. 1970. Induction of estrus in female mice: estrogen-progesterone interactions. Horm. Behav. **1:** 299–304.
15. Tsai, M.J. & B.W. O'Malley. 1994. Molecular mechanisms of action of steroid/thyroid receptor superfamily members. Annu. Rev. Biochem. **63:** 451–486.
16. King, W.J. & G.L. Greene. 1984. Monoclonal antibodies localize oestrogen receptor in the nuclei of target cells. Nature **307:** 745–747.
17. Welshons, W.V., M.E. Lieberman & J. Gorski. 1984. Nuclear localization of unoccupied oestrogen receptors. Nature **307:** 747–749.
18. Blaustein, J.D. 1994. Estrogen receptors in neurons: new subcellular locations and functional implications. Endocr. J. **2:** 249–258.
19. Tetel, M.J. 2000. Nuclear receptor coactivators in neuroendocrine function. J. Neuroendocrinol. **12:** 927–932.
20. McKenna, N.J., R.B. Lanz & B.W. O'Malley. 1999. Nuclear receptor coregulators: cellular and molecular biology. Endocr. Rev. **20:** 321–344.
21. Brown, T.J. & J.D. Blaustein. 1984. Inhibition of sexual behavior in female guinea pigs by a progestin receptor antagonist. Brain Res. **301:** 343–349.
22. Pollio, G., P. Xue, M. Zanisi, *et al.* 1993. Antisense oligonucleotide blocks progesterone-induced lordosis behavior in ovariectomized rats. Mol. Brain Res. **19:** 135–139.
23. Ogawa, S., U.E. Olazabal, I.S. Parhar, *et al.* 1994. Effects of intrahypothalamic administration of antisense DNA for progesterone receptor mrna on reproductive behavior and progesterone receptor immunoreactivity in female rat. J. Neurosci. **14:** 1766–1774.

24. MANI, S.K., J.D. BLAUSTEIN, J.M. ALLEN, *et al.* 1994. Inhibition of rat sexual behavior by antisense oligonucleotides to the progesterone receptor. Endocrinology **135:** 1409–1414.
25. MANI, S.K., J.M.C. ALLEN, J.P. LYDON, *et al.* 1996. Dopamine requires the unoccupied progesterone receptor to induce sexual behavior in mice. Mol. Endocrinol. **10:** 1728–1737.
26. POWER, R.F., J.P. LYDON, O.M. CONNEELY, *et al.* 1991. Dopamine activation of an orphan of the steroid receptor superfamily. Science **252:** 1546–1548.
27. POWER, R.F., S.K. MANI, J. CODINA, *et al.* 1991. Dopaminergic and ligand-independent activation of steroid hormone receptors. Science **254:** 1636–1639.
28. IGNAR-TROWBRIDGE, D.M., K.G. NELSON, M.C. BIDWELL, *et al.* 1992. Coupling of dual signaling pathways: epidermal growth factor action involves the estrogen receptor. Proc. Natl. Acad. Sci. USA **89:** 4658–4662.
29. ARONICA, S.M. & B.S. KATZENELLENBOGEN. 1993. Stimulation of estrogen receptor-mediated transcription and alteration in the phosphorylation state of the rat uterine estrogen receptor by estrogen, cyclic adenosine monophosphate, and insulin- like growth factor-1. Mol. Endocrinol. **7:** 743–752.
30. DEMAY, F., M. DE MONTI, C. TIFFOCHE, *et al.* 2001. Steroid-independent activation of ER by GnRH in gonadotrope pituitary cells. Endocrinology **142:** 3340–3347.
31. WARING, D.W. & J.L. TURGEON. 1992. A pathway for luteinizing hormone releasing-hormone self-potentiation—cross-talk with the progesterone receptor. Endocrinology **130:** 3275–3282.
32. JOEL, P.B., A.M. TRAISH & D.A. LANNIGAN. 1995. Estradiol and phorbol ester cause phosphorylation of serine 118 in the human estrogen receptor. Mol. Endocrinol. **9:** 1041–1052.
33. KATO, S., H. ENDOH, Y. MASUHIRO, *et al.* 1995. Activation of the estrogen receptor through phosphorylation by mitogen-activated protein kinase. Science **270:** 1491–1494.
34. TROWBRIDGE, J.M., I. ROGATSKY & M.J. GARABEDIAN. 1997. Regulation of estrogen receptor transcriptional enhancement by the cyclin A Cdk2 complex. Proc. Natl. Acad. Sci. USA **94:** 10132–10137.
35. CENNI, B. & D. PICARD. 1999. Ligand-independent activation of steroid receptors: new roles for old players. Trends Endocrinol. Metab. **10:** 41–46.
36. MANI, S.K., J.M.C. ALLEN, J.H. CLARK, *et al.* 1994. Convergent pathways for steroid hormone- and neurotransmitter-induced rat sexual behavior. Science **265:** 1246–1249.
37. APOSTOLAKIS, E.M., J. GARAI, C. FOX, *et al.* 1996. Dopaminergic regulation of progesterone receptors: brain D5 dopamine receptors mediate induction of lordosis by D1-like agonists in rats. J. Neurosci. **16:** 4823–4834.
38. BEYER, C., O. GONZALEZ-FLORES & G. GONZALEZ-MARISCAL. 1997. Progesterone receptor participates in the stimulatory effect of LHRH, prostaglandin E_2, and cyclic AMP on lordosis and proceptive behaviours in rats. J. Neuroendocrinol. **9:** 609–614.
39. MANI, S.K., J.M.C. ALLEN, J.H. CLARK, *et al.* 1995. Progesterone receptor involvement in the LHRH-facilitated sexual behavior of female rats. Abstracts of the 77th Annual Meeting of the Endocrine Society **77:** P1–440.
40. MANI, S.K., J.M.C. ALLEN, V. RETTORI, *et al.* 1994. Nitric oxide mediates sexual behavior in female rats. Proc. Natl. Acad. Sci. USA **91:** 6468–6472.
41. CHU, H.P., J.C. MORALES & A.M. ETGEN. 1999. Cyclic GMP may potentiate lordosis behaviour by progesterone receptor activation. J. Neuroendocrinol. **11:** 107–113.
42. WHALEN, R.E. & A.H. LAUBER. 1986. Progesterone substitutes: cGMP mediation. Neurosci. Biobehav. Rev. **10:** 47–53.
43. BEYER, C. & G. GONZALEZ-MARISCAL. 1986. Elevation in hypothalamic cyclic AMP as a common factor in the facilitation of lordosis in rodents: a working hypothesis. Ann. N.Y. Acad. Sci. **474:** 270–281.
44. RAJENDREN, G., C.A. DUDLEY & R.L. MOSS. 1990. Role of the vomeronasal organ in the male-induced enhancement of sexual receptivity in female rats. Neuroendocrinology **52s:** 368–372.
45. AUGER, A.P., C.A. MOFFATT & J.D. BLAUSTEIN. 1997. Progesterone-independent activation of rat brain progestin receptors by reproductive stimuli. Endocrinology **138:** 511–514.

46. LEVINE, J.E., P.E. CHAPPELL, J.S. SCHNEIDER, *et al.* 2001. Progesterone receptors as neuroendocrine integrators. Front. Neuroendocrinol. **22:** 69–106.
47. BLAUSTEIN, J.D. & B. GRECO. 2002. A progestin antagonist blocks vaginocervical stimulation-induced Fos expression in neurones containing progestin receptors in the rostral medial preoptic area. J. Neuroendocrinol. **14:** 109–115.
48. AUGER, A.P., C.A. MOFFATT & J.D. BLAUSTEIN. 1996. Reproductively-relevant stimuli induce Fos-immunoreactivity within progestin receptor-containing neurons in localized regions of female rat forebrain. J. Neuroendocrinol. **8:** 831–838.
49. VATHY, I. & A.M. ETGEN. 1989. Hormonal activation of female sexual behavior is accompanied by hypothalamic norepinephrine release. J. Neuroendocrinol. **1:** 383–388.
50. MERMELSTEIN, P.G. & J.B. BECKER. 1995. Increased extracellular dopamine in the nucleus accumbens and striatum of the female rat during paced copulatory behavior. Behav. Neurosci. **109:** 354–365.
51. KOHLERT, J.G., R.K. ROWE & R.L. MEISEL. 1997. Intromissive stimulation from the male increases extracellular dopamine release from fluoro-gold-identified neurons within the midbrain of female hamsters. Horm. Behav. **32:** 143–154.
52. MATUSZEWICH, L., D.S. LORRAIN & E.M. HULL. 2000. Dopamine release in the medial preoptic area of female rats in response to hormonal manipulation and sexual activity. Behav. Neurosci. **114:** 772–782.
53. VATHY, I. & A.M. ETGEN. 1988. Ovarian steroids and hypothalamic norepinephrine release: studies using in vivo brain microdialysis. Life Sci. **43:** 1493–1499.
54. ETGEN, A.M. & J.C. MORALES. 2002. Somatosensory stimuli evoke norepinephrine release in the anterior ventromedial hypothalamus of sexually receptive female rats. J. Neuroendocrinol. **14:** 213–218.
55. QUYSNER, A. & J.D. BLAUSTEIN. 2001. A dopamine antagonist blocks vaginocervical stimulation-induced neuronal responses in the rat forebrain. Brain Res. **921:** 173–182.
56. GREENGARD, P., P.B. ALLEN & A.C. NAIRN. 1999. Beyond the dopamine receptor: the DARPP-32/protein phosphatase-1 cascade. Neuron **23:** 435–447.
57. MANI, S.K., A.A. FIENBERG, J.P. O'CALLAGHAN, *et al.* 2000. Requirement for DARPP-32 in progesterone-facilitated sexual receptivity in female rats and mice. Science **287:** 1053–1056.
58. MEREDITH, J.M., C.A. MOFFATT, A.P. AUGER, *et al.* 1998. Mating-related stimulation induces phosphorylation of dopamine- and cyclic AMP-regulated phosphoprotein-32 in progestin receptor-containing areas in the female rat brain. J. Neurosci. **18:** 10189–10195.
59. CALHOUN, J.B. 1962. The Ecology and Sociology of the Norway Rat. PHS Publication no. 1008. US Government Printing Office. Washington, DC.
60. BENNETT, A.L., M.E. BLASBERG & J.D. BLAUSTEIN. 2002. Mating stimulation required for mating-induced estrous abbreviation in female rats: effects of repeated testing. Horm. Behav. **42:** 206–211.
61. APOSTOLAKIS, E.M., J. GERAI, J.E. LOHMANN, *et al.* 2000. Epidermal growth factor activates reproductive behavior independent of ovarian steroids in female rodents. Mol. Endocrinol. **14:** 1086–1098.
62. LONSTEIN, J.S., B. GRECO, G. DE VRIES, *et al.* 2000. Maternal behavior stimulates c-fos activity within estrogen receptor alpha-containing neurons in lactating rats. Neuroendocrinology **72:** 91–101.
63. RAJENDREN, G. & R.L. MOSS. 1993. The role of the medial nucleus of amygdala in the mating-induced enhancement of lordosis in female rats—the interaction with luteinizing hormone-releasing hormone neuronal system. Brain Res. **617:** 81–86.
64. RAJENDREN, G., C.A. DUDLEY & R.L. MOSS. 1991. Role of the ventromedial nucleus of hypothalamus in the male-induced enhancement of lordosis in female rats. Physiol. Behav. **50:** 705–710.
65. BENNETT, A.L., B. GRECO, M.E. BLASBERG, *et al.* 2002. Response to male odours in progestin receptor- and oestrogen receptor-containing cells in female rat brain. J. Neuroendocrinol. **14:** 442–449.
66. MCGINNIS, M.Y., A.R. LUMIA & B.S. MCEWEN. 1985. Increased estrogen receptor binding in amygdala correlates with facilitation of feminine sexual behavior induced by olfactory bulbectomy. Brain Res. **334:** 19–25.

The Aromatase Knockout (ArKO) Mouse Provides New Evidence That Estrogens Are Required for the Development of the Female Brain

J. BAKKER,[a] S. HONDA,[b] N. HARADA,[b] AND J. BALTHAZART[a]

[a]*Center for Cellular and Molecular Neurobiology, Research Group in Behavioral Neuroendocrinology, University of Liège, B-4020 Liège, Belgium*

[b]*Division of Molecular Genetics, Fujita Health University, Toyoake, Aichi, Japan*

ABSTRACT: The classic view of sexual differentiation is that the male brain develops under the influence of testicular secretions, whereas the female brain develops in the absence of any hormonal stimulation. However, several studies have suggested a possible role of estradiol in female neural development, although they did not provide unequivocal evidence that estradiol is indispensable for the development of the female brain and behavior. As a result, the hypothesis subsequently languished because of the lack of a suitable animal model to test estrogen's possible contribution to female differentiation. The recent introduction of the aromatase knockout (ArKO) mouse, which is deficient in aromatase activity because of a targeted mutation in the CYP19 gene and therefore cannot aromatize androgen to estrogen, has provided a new opportunity to reopen the debate of whether estradiol contributes to the development of the female brain. Female ArKO mice showed reduced levels of lordosis behavior after adult treatment with estradiol and progesterone, suggesting that estradiol is required for the development of the neural mechanisms controlling this behavior in female mice. The neural systems affected may include the olfactory systems in that ArKO females also showed impairments in olfactory investigation of odors from conspecifics. Thus, the classic view of sexual differentiation, that is, the female brain develops in the absence of any hormonal secretion, needs to be re-examined.

KEYWORDS: estradiol; aromatase; female differentiation; sexual behavior; olfaction

INTRODUCTION

The classic view of sexual differentiation of the brain in mammalian species is that testosterone secreted by the testes causes masculinization ("increase in male-typical characteristics") and defeminization ("decrease in female-typical character-

Address for correspondence: J. Bakker, Center for Cellular and Molecular Neurobiology, Research Group in Behavioral Neuroendocrinology, University of Liège, B-4020 Liège, Belgium. Voice: 32-4-366-5978; fax: 32-4-366-5971.
jbakker@ulg.ac.be

Ann. N.Y. Acad. Sci. 1007: 251–262 (2003). © 2003 New York Academy of Sciences.
doi: 10.1196/annals.1286.024

istics") of the brain and behavior, whereas the ovaries are functionally inactive during early development. According to this view, the female state is considered to be the "default" within mammals, meaning that only the absence of testosterone is required for complete feminine development ("passive feminization"). This concept is based on some early studies that showed that female guinea pigs treated *in utero* with testosterone propionate displayed elevated levels of male-typical sexual behaviors in adulthood, whereas male rats castrated on the day of birth showed female-typical sexual behaviors when treated with ovarian hormones in adulthood.[1–3] However, a possible role of estrogens in the differentiation of the female brain was suggested by Toran-Allerand[4] who found that estradiol promotes neurite outgrowth from fetal hypothalamic explants of both sexes. This hypothesis was further supported by several behavioral studies that showed that perinatal exposure to low levels of estrogens facilitates the capacity to display female sexual behavior in adulthood.[5–7] However, these studies did not provide unequivocal evidence that estradiol is required for the development of the female brain. For example, Döhler and co-workers[6] found that neonatal treatment of female rats with tamoxifen, an estrogen receptor antagonist, decreases their later capacity to show female sexual behavior, whereas concurrent neonatal administration of a low dose of estradiol prevents this effect. However, tamoxifen can exert estrogen-like agonist actions in the brain.[8] Therefore, the observed reduction in female sexual behavior induced by administering tamoxifen neonatally to female rats[6] actually may have resulted from a partial defeminization of the brain by the estradiol-like actions of tamoxifen acting on neural estrogen receptors. Thus, the hypothesis subsequently languished because of the lack of a suitable animal model in which to test estrogen's possible contribution to the development of the female brain.

The introduction of the aromatase knockout (ArKO) mouse,[9–11] which is deficient in aromatase activity because of a targeted mutation in the CYP19 gene, has provided a new model in which to study the role of estradiol in the female-typical differentiation of brain and behavior. Unlike estrogen receptor knockout mouse models, the ArKO mouse has functional estrogen receptors. Thus, by administering estradiol to adult ArKO mice one can assess the consequences of the absence of estradiol biosynthesis and cellular action earlier in life. This makes the ArKO mouse an ideal model in which to ask whether estradiol is required for the development of the female brain. We will show here some recent results obtained in female ArKO mice which suggest that estradiol is indeed required for the development of the neural mechanisms regulating female sexual behavior.[12]

ESTRADIOL IS NEEDED FOR THE DEVELOPMENT OF FEMALE SEXUAL BEHAVIOR

Beach[13] proposed to divide female sexual behavior into three components: (1) attractivity, (2) proceptivity, and (3) receptivity. Attractivity has been defined as the stimulus value of the female for a male conspecific; proceptivity has been defined as the extent to which the female initiates copulation and thus reflects her underlying motivational state, whereas receptivity has been defined as the responsiveness of the female to copulation and is mostly characterized by the display of species-specific mating postures. Female rodents display the lordosis posture characterized by an

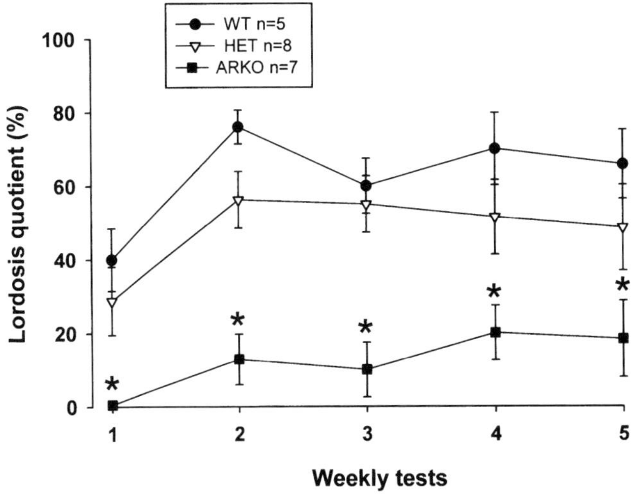

FIGURE 1. Lordosis quotients displayed in tests with an intact male by wild-type (WT), heterozygous (HET), and homozygous ArKO female mice. All subjects were treated with estradiol and progesterone in adulthood. $^{*}P < 0.05$ compared with WT and HET females. (Data are taken from Bakker *et al.*[12])

arching of the back, in response to mounting stimulation from the male. This behavior is only observed when female rodents are in estrus, that is, when preovulatory follicles are present in their ovaries, thereby ensuring fertilization and pregnancy. However, lordosis behavior can be induced by treating female rodents with estrogens and progesterone, thereby mimicking their estrous cycle.

To determine whether estradiol is also required for the development of female sexual behavior as has been suggested by Döhler *et al.*[6] and Toran-Allerand,[14] among others, we tested ovariectomized female ArKO mice for their lordosis behavior after treatment with estradiol and progesterone in adulthood. We found that the display of lordosis in response to mounts from a stimulus male was severely impaired in ArKO females[12] (FIG. 1). The same hormone treatment was, however, effective, in inducing lordosis behavior in wild-type (WT) and heterozygous (HET) females. Although ArKO females are possibly exposed to increased testosterone levels during ontogeny,[9] it seems unlikely that the deficit in lordosis observed in ArKO females resulted somehow from a defeminizing action of testosterone exposure during early development. After ovariectomy in adulthood and treatment with either testosterone or estradiol, female mice typically show high (male-typical) levels of mounting and even intromission-like behavior in tests with an estrous female (e.g., Wersinger *et al.*[15]), perhaps caused by fetal exposure to high levels of testosterone derived from the placenta. ArKO females that received testosterone + estradiol showed significantly lower levels of male-typical sexual behavior (mounts and intromission-like movements) in tests with an estrous female[12] (FIG. 2) than either WT or HET controls. Such an outcome would not have occurred had ArKO females been exposed perinatally to high levels of testosterone capable of masculinizing their co-

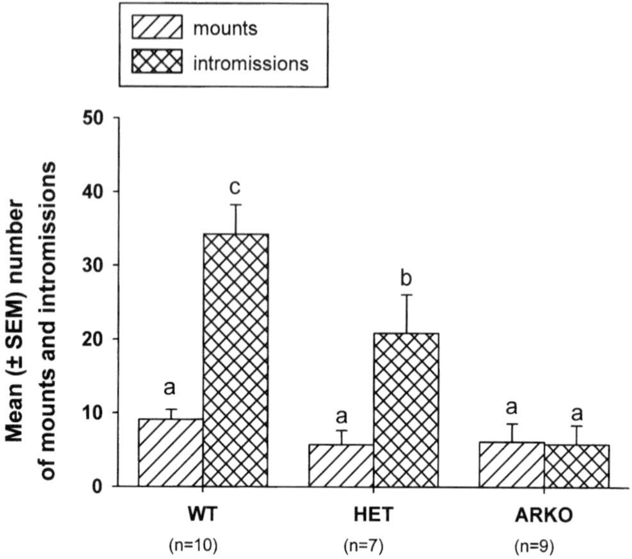

FIGURE 2. Mean number of mounts and intromission-like responses displayed in tests with an estrous female by wild-type (WT), heterozygous (HET), and homozygous ArKO female mice. Females were treated with testosterone and estradiol. Means with different letters above them are significantly different from each other by post hoc comparisons. (Data are taken from Bakker *et al.*[12])

ital capacity. Thus, it seems most likely that the reduction in lordosis behavior of ArKO females resulted from a perinatal deprivation of estradiol that disrupted the normal development of the neural mechanisms controlling the expression of lordosis behavior in adulthood.

NEURAL SYSTEMS INVOLVED IN FEMALE SEXUAL BEHAVIOR

If estradiol is indeed required for the development of the female brain as has been suggested by recent results obtained in ArKO females,[12] where in the brain does it act? In other words, which neural mechanisms regulate female sexual behavior and therefore depend on estrogenic stimulation during development? Historically, studies of female sexual behavior have concentrated on the neural and hormonal control of lordosis behavior in the female rat (for detailed description, see Pfaff *et al.*[16]). In brief, male mounting stimulates pressure receptors on the flanks, posterior rump, tail base, and perineum of the female. Axons from these receptors form a sensory nerve that projects to the dorsal root of the ganglion of the spinal cord. Then, the signal is transmitted to the reticular formation in the brainstem and the midbrain central gray area. When the female is in estrus, that is, when estrogen concentrations are high, several brain regions including the ventromedial nucleus of the hypothalamus

(VMN) and the medial preoptic area (POA), activate via the midbrain central gray, medullary reticular formation, and medial geniculate body, the spinal motoneurons innervating the back muscles critical to the display of lordosis. Thus, the VMN plays a critical role in integrating hormonal and sensory information necessary for the display of lordosis in female rodents. Accordingly, lesions of the VMN, or destruction of its afferent and efferent fibers, typically reduce the frequency of lordosis in female rats (reviewed in Emery and Moss[17]), whereas implants of estradiol into the VMN induce lordosis behavior in ovariectomized female rats.[18]

In contrast with the neural control of lordosis behavior, very few studies have concentrated on other aspects of female sexual behavior, including proceptivity (i.e., sexual motivation) and sexual partner preference. Nevertheless, the ability to seek out and identify potential mates is as critical to female sexual behavior as is the capacity to display the lordosis reflex when mounted by a male. Rodent species use primarily odors to identify individuals of their own species and accordingly release to their environment a wide variety of volatile and nonvolatile odors via skin glands, urine, and feces. These socially relevant odors are also known as pheromones, which have been defined as "substances which are secreted to the outside by an individual and received by a second individual, in which they release a specific reaction such as a behavior, developmental process or physiological change, for example, hormone release to their mutual benefit."[19,20] In female mice, olfactory cues have been shown to facilitate the display of lordosis behavior. Bilateral removal of the olfactory bulbs severely attenuated lordosis behavior in ovariectomized female mice which were treated with estradiol and progesterone.[21] Likewise, peripherally induced anosmia by intranasal application of zinc sulfate solution attenuated lordosis behavior in hormone-primed female mice, although not to the same extent as olfactory bulbectomy.[22] These findings suggest that the neural mechanisms regulating female sexual behavior may include the olfactory systems.

Two olfactory systems have evolved in vertebrates that differ considerably in their anatomy and function. The first of these, the main olfactory system, is used to detect a wide variety of volatile odorants derived from food prey and potential predators, among many sources.[23] Volatile odors initially are detected by olfactory sensory neurons in the main olfactory epithelium whose axons project to specific clusters of glomeruli in the main olfactory bulb (MOB), resulting in a spatial map of activation. The mitral and tufted relay neurons of the MOB, in turn, transmit signals onto the olfactory cortical structures, including the olfactory tubercle, anterior olfactory nucleus, piriform, and entorhinal cortex.[24–26] A second accessory olfactory system evolved in vertebrates to detect and process a subset of nonvolatile pheromones that influence a variety of reproductive and aggressive behaviors in mammalian species.[27] Sensory neurons in the vomeronasal organ (VNO), a cigar-shaped organ located at the base of the nasal septum, detect nonvolatile pheromones which gain access to the VNO via a pumping mechanism.[28] The sensory neurons located in the apical zone of the VNO send their axons to the glomerular layer of the rostral accessory olfactory bulb (AOB), whereas sensory neurons in the basal zone of the VNO send their axons to the caudal AOB.[29] Neuronal tracing studies have shown that mitral cells in the AOB project exclusively to the anterior and posterior amygdala which, in turn, conveys inputs to hypothalamic regions including the bed nucleus of the stria terminalis (BNST), medial POA, and the VMN.[25,30,31] As described before, the VMN is part of the neural circuitry regulating lordosis behavior[16] and thus may play a critical role in integrating hormonal and sensory (somatosensory and chemosensory) information necessary for the display of female sexual behavior.

ESTRADIOL IS NEEDED FOR OLFACTORY INVESTIGATION

The reduction in lordosis behavior previously observed in female ArKO mice[12] may reflect deficits in (1) the neural circuitry regulating the lordosis reflex and/or (2) the neural mechanisms regulating sexual motivation and sexual partner preference. Note that the impairment in lordosis behavior observed in ArKO females tended to decrease toward the end of the test, possibly as a result of repeated mounting and stimulation of the flanks and back of the female.[12] Thus, female ArKO mice seem to be capable of showing the lordosis reflex; however, they show it significantly less, suggesting that the reduction in lordosis behavior actually may reflect deficits in sexual motivation and/or sexual partner preference. It is possible that ArKO females simply did not recognize the stud male as being male on the basis of his body odors and as a result did not become sexually receptive. Therefore, we tested here whether olfactory investigation of odors was affected in female ArKO mice.

Ovariectomized, testosterone-treated ArKO females spent significantly less time than WT females investigating both volatile and nonvolatile odors from male and estrous female conspecifics in a Y-maze[12] (FIG. 3A and B). However, ArKO females did not seem to differ much from HET females in olfactory investigation.[12] The behavioral differences between ArKO and WT females could have reflected differences in activation of olfactory investigation by estradiol, because testosterone treatment presumably generated higher levels of estradiol biosynthesis in WT females than in ArKO females. Therefore, to distinguish between activational and organizational effects of estradiol on olfactory investigation, the same ovariectomized female subjects were tested again for odor preferences after receiving estradiol treatment for several weeks in adulthood. The impairment in olfactory investigation of volatile odors by ArKO females persisted after estradiol treatment, suggesting that the normal, female-typical differentiation of the main olfactory system to detect volatile body odors may depend on the presence of estradiol at some point during development (FIG. 3C). In contrast, estradiol-treated ArKO females spent as much time as WT females investigating nonvolatile odors present in bedding soiled bygonadally intact males and estrous females (FIG. 3D). This finding suggests that the accessory olfactory system may be functional in ArKO females provided that they are treated with estradiol in adulthood. This conclusion was corroborated by Lau *et al.*[32] In their study, nonvolatile odors derived from gonadally intact males induced neuronal Fos immunoreactivity (ir), which is commonly used as a marker of neuronal activation, in sensory neurons located throughout the accessory olfactory system, that is, in the apical and basal zones of the VNO, the granular layer of the AOB, the anterior and posterior medial amygdala, the BNST, and the medial POA of ovariectomized, estradiol-treated ArKO females. However, the number of Fos-ir neurons was significantly reduced in the apical and basal zones of the VNO and in the anterior amygdala and BNST in ArKO females compared with WT controls. Taken together, these results point to a slight reduction in the responsiveness of the accessory olfactory system to odors in ArKO females.

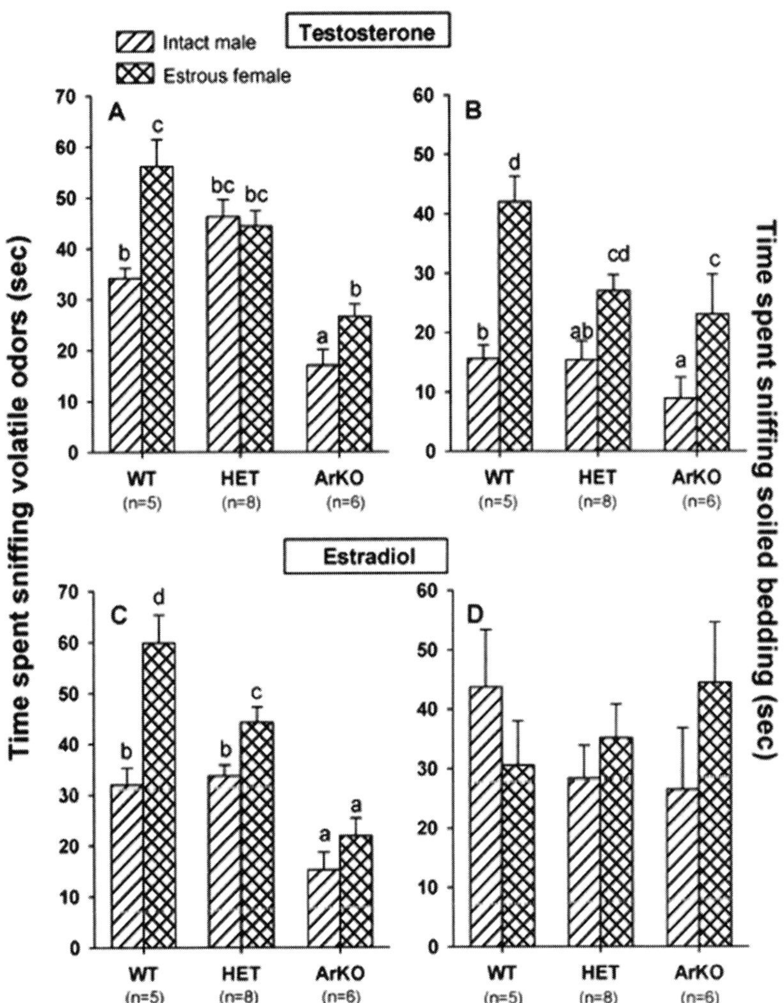

FIGURE 3. Mean amount of time that wild-type (WT), heterozygous (HET), and homozygous ArKO female mice spent investigating volatile and nonvolatile odors when given a choice between intact male and estrous female odor stimuli in a Y-maze. First, females were tested while treated with testosterone (**A** and **B**). Then, the same subjects were retested for odor preferences while receiving estradiol (**C** and **D**). Panels **A** and **C** show the results when females were given a choice between volatile odor stimuli. Panels **B** and **D** show the results when females were given a choice between nonvolatile odor stimuli (soiled bedding). Means with different letters above them are significantly different from each other by post hoc comparisons. (Redrawn from data published in Bakker *et al.*[12])

DISCUSSION

The introduction of the ArKO mouse has provided a new opportunity to reopen the debate of whether estradiol contributes to the development of the female brain. Recent results obtained in female ArKO mice have provided new evidence that estradiol is indeed required for the development of the neural mechanisms controlling female sexual behavior.[12] These neural mechanisms may include the olfactory systems in that female ArKO mice also showed some impairments in olfactory investigation of odors from conspecifics. Thus, it is possible that ArKO females fail to recognize the stimulus male on the basis of his body odors and as a result do not become sexually receptive. However, the observation[12] that ArKO females, when ovariectomized and treated with testosterone, showed a significant preference to approach volatile and nonvolatile odors from estrous females as opposed to males implies that these females are capable of discriminating between male and female odors even though they showed no significant preference for one over the other when tested with estradiol. Therefore, the impairments in olfactory investigation of odors by ArKO females may be caused by a reduction in the sensitivity of their olfactory systems (both main and accessory) to detect odors. Future studies should address these questions and determine whether the impairment of olfactory function observed in mice treated with estrogens persist when they are in addition treated with progesterone. In summary, these results suggest that estrogens are required for the development of the main and accessory olfactory system and, in this way, may regulate female sexual behavior.

POSSIBLE SOURCES OF ESTRADIOL IN THE FEMALE BRAIN

If female neural development requires estrogenic stimulation, what might be its source? At least two possible sources of estradiol come to mind. First, estradiol may be taken up directly from the circulation. However, basal estrogen secretion by the embryonic rodent ovary is undetectable before postnatal day 5,[33,34] implying that any estrogens during the fetal period either must come from external sources (e.g., the mother) or be synthesized locally from androgenic precursor. Much evidence suggests that any estradiol produced by the mother or male siblings developing in close proximity will not be available for action in the fetal female brain because it will be bound with high affinity to α-fetoprotein (AFP), which circulates in high concentrations in the fetal blood.[35–37] Thus, AFP is thought to protect the developing female rodent brain from excessive exposure to estrogens and thus from becoming masculinized and defeminized.[37] Therefore, a more likely source of estradiol in the female brain during perinatal development involves the localized, neural aromatization of testosterone which can freely enter the brain, because in mice it is not bound by plasma proteins. Beyer *et al.*[38] and Hutchison *et al.*[39] reported that aromatase activity, measured in hypothalamic homogenates, is higher in male than female mice on embryonic day 17 and on the day of birth. Because prenatal testosterone levels are thought to be higher in males than females, possibly as early as embryonic day 14,[40] it can be assumed that neural estradiol biosynthesis will be higher in males as well. However, aromatase activities are still quite substantial in the female hypothalamus at these early ages, suggesting that estradiol derived from neural aromatization of testosterone is available to affect female neural development. Another possibility is that estradiol is synthesized *de novo* from cholesterol in the brain without any gonadal or adrenal contribution, as has been suggested in songbirds (reviewed in Schlinger *et al.*[41]). Holloway and Clayton[42] showed that brain slices from male zebra finches that are cultured *in vitro* synthesize more estradiol *de novo* than those of female zebra finches, suggesting that neurosteroidogenesis can occur in the developing zebra finch brain. It is not unreasonable to expect complete synthesis of estradiol in the mouse brain because all five enzymes required to catalyze reactions that lead from cholesterol to estradiol have been detected.[43]

An obvious question raised by the proposition that the development of both the male and female brain normally requires estrogens is how estradiol can have these biphasic effects on neural differentiation and thus elicit quite different developmental patterns in the two sexes. There are two possible answers to this question. First, quantitative differences in local estradiol concentrations may be one mechanism by which a male or female brain develops.[6] Thus, in the genetic female, perinatal exposure of the developing brain to low "priming" concentrations of estradiol, derived from local aromatization of testosterone, may elicit neuronal growth and differentiation in a female-specific manner. The higher levels of testosterone and of aromatase activity available perinatally in the male brain may produce higher neural concentrations of estradiol and thereby induce a male-typical profile of brain sexual differentiation. Second, the critical period for female neural development may occur later than that for male neural development. Different critical periods also have been suggested for masculinization (primarily prenatally) and defeminization (primarily postnatally) of the brain in male mammals.[44–48] Work by the group of Denenberg[49–52] demonstrated that the sexually dimorphic corpus callosum, which is larger in male than female rats, has different developmental periods in the two sexes. The testosterone-dependent organization of the male-like corpus callosum seems to occur prenatally, whereas the estradiol-dependent organization of the female-like corpus callosum extends much later into postnatal life (sometime between postnatal days 25 and 70).

In conclusion, recent results obtained in estradiol-deficient ArKO mice suggest that estradiol *is* required during development for the expression of female sexual behavior in adult female mice. Thus, the classic view of sexual differentiation, that is, the female brain develops in the absence of any hormonal secretion needs to be reexamined. Future studies should focus on the neural mechanisms regulating female sexual behavior and on the identification of those mechanisms on which estrogens may act to induce female-typical differentiation. For example, the main and accessory olfactory system may be important for female sexual behavior in that female ArKO mice also showed impairments in olfactory investigation of odors from conspecifics. In addition, special attention should be paid to the neural systems regulating sexual motivation because the decrease in lordosis behavior and olfactory investigation may reflect a pervasive reduction in feminine sexual motivation among ArKO females.

ACKNOWLEDGMENTS

This work was supported by grants from the French Community of Belgium (ARC 99/04-241) and National Institutes of Health (MH-50388).

REFERENCES

1. PHOENIX, C.H., R.W. GOY, A.A. GERALL & W.C. YOUNG. 1959. Organizational action of prenatally administered testosterone propionate on the tissues mediating mating behavior in the female guinea pig. Endocrinology **65:** 369–382.
2. FEDER, H.H. & R.E. WHALEN. 1965. Feminine behavior in neonatally castrated and estrogen-treated male rats. Science **147:** 306–307.
3. GRADY, K.L., C.H. PHOENIX & W.C. YOUNG. 1965. Role of the developing rat testis in differentiation of the neural tissues mediating mating behavior. J. Comp. Physiol. Psychol. **59:** 176–182.
4. TORAN-ALLERAND, C.D. 1976. Sex steroids and the development of the newborn mouse hypothalamus and preoptic area in vivo: implications for sexual differentiation. Brain Res. **106:** 407–412.
5. GERALL, A.A., J.L. DUNLAP & S.E. HENDRICKS. 1973. Effect of ovarian secretions on female behavioral potentiality in the rat. J. Comp. Physiol. Psychol. **82:** 449–465.
6. DÖHLER, K.D., J.L. HANCKE, S.S. SRIVASTAVA, *et al.* 1984. Participation of estrogens in female sexual differentiation of the brain: neuroanatomical, neuroendocrine, and behavioral evidence. *In* Progress in Brain Research. Vol. 61. Sex Differences in the Brain: The Relation between Structure and Function. G.J. de Vries, J.P.C. de Bruin, H.B.M. Uylings & M.A. Corner, Eds.: 99–117. Elsevier Science Publishers. Amsterdam.
7. BAUM, M.J. & S.A. TOBET. 1986. Effect of prenatal exposure to aromatase inhibitor, testosterone, or antiandrogen on the development of feminine sexual behavior in ferrets of both sexes. Physiol. Behav. **37:** 111–118.
8. MATHEWS, G.A., E.W. BRENOWITZ & A.P. ARNOLD. 1988. Paradoxical hypermasculinization of the zebra finch song system by an antiestrogen. Horm. Behav. **22:** 540–551.
9. FISHER, C.R., K.H. GRAVES, A.F. PARLOW & E.R. SIMPSON. 1998. Characterization of mice deficient in aromatase (ArKO) because of targeted disruption of the Cyp19 gene. Proc. Natl. Acad. Sci. USA **95:** 6965–6970.
10. HONDA, S., N. HARADA, S. ITO, *et al.* 1998. Disruption of sexual behavior in male aromatase-deficient mice lacking exons 1 and 2 of the Cyp19 gene. Biochem. Biophys. Res. Commun. **252:** 445–449.
11. TODA, K., T. OKADA, K. TAKEDA, *et al.* 2001. Oestrogen at the neonatal stage is critical for the reproductive ability of male mice as revealed by supplementation with 17β-oestradiol. J. Endocrinol. **170:** 99–111.
12. BAKKER, J., S. HONDA, N. HARADA & J. BALTHAZART. 2002. The aromatase knockout mouse provides new evidence that estradiol is required during development in the female for the expression of socio-sexual behaviors in adulthood. J. Neurosci. **22:** 9104–9112.
13. BEACH, F.A. 1976. Sexual attractivity, proceptivity, and receptivity in female mammals. Horm. Behav. **7:** 105–138.
14. TORAN-ALLERAND, C.D. 1984. On the genesis of sexual differentiation of the central nervous system: morphogenetic consequences of steroidal exposure and possible role of a-fetoprotein. *In* Progress in Brain Research. Vol. 61. Sex Differences in the Brain: The Relation between Structure and Function. G.J. de Vries, J.P.C. de Bruin, H.B.M. Uylings, M.A. Corner, Eds.: 63–98. Elsevier Science Publishers. Amsterdam.
15. WERSINGER, S.R., K. SANNEN, C. VILLALBA, *et al.* 1997. Masculine sexual behavior is disrupted in male and female mice lacking a functional estrogen receptor α. Horm. Behav. **32:** 176–183.
16. PFAFF, D.W., S. SCHWARTZ-GIBLIN, M.M. MCCARTHY & L.-M. KOW. 1994. Cellular and molecular mechanisms of female reproductive behaviors. *In* The Physiology of Reproduction. Vol. 2. E. Knobil & J. Neill, Eds.: 107–220. Raven Press. New York.
17. EMERY, D.E. & R.L. MOSS. 1984. Lesions confined to the ventromedial hypothalamus decrease the frequency of coital contacts in female rats. Horm. Behav. **18:** 313–329.
18. RUBIN, B.S. & R.J. BARFIELD. 1980. Priming of estrous responsiveness by implants of 17 beta-oestradiol in the ventromedial hypothalamic nucleus of female rats. Endocrinology **106:** 504–509.

19. KARLSON, P. & M. LUSCHER. 1959. "Phermones": a new term for a class of biologically active substances. Nature **183:** 55–56.
20. Meredith, M. 2001. Human vomeronasal organ function. Chem. Sens. **24:** 433–445.
21. THOMPSON, M.L. & D.A. EDWARDS. 1972. Olfactory bulb ablation and hormonally induced mating in spayed female mice. Physiol. Behav. **8:** 1141–1146.
22. EDWARDS, D.A. & K.G. BURGE. 1973. Olfactory control of the sexual behavior of male and female mice. Phsyiol. Behav. **11:** 867–872.
23. FIRESTEIN, S. 2001. How the olfactory system makes sense of scents. Nature **413:** 211–218.
24. SCOTT, J.W. 1986. The olfactory bulb and central pathways. Experientia **42:** 223–232.
25. PRICE, J.L. 1987. *In* Neurobiology of Taste and Smell. T.E. Finger & W.L. Sliver, Eds.: 179–203. Wiley. New York.
26. SHIPLEY, M.T. & M. ENNIS. 1996. Functional organization of the olfactory system. J. Neurobiol. **30:** 123–176.
27. KEVERNE, E.B. 1999. The vomeronasal organ. Science **286:** 716–720.
28. MEREDITH, M. & R.J. O'CONNELL. 1979. Efferent control of stimulus access to the hamster vomeronasal organ. J. Physiol. (Lond.) **286:** 301–316.
29. HALPERN, M., L.S. SHAPIRO & C. JIA. 1995. Differential localisation of G proteins in the opossum vomeronasal system. Brain Res. **677:** 157–161.
30. SCALIA, F. & S.S. WINANS. 1975. The differential projections of the olfactory bulb and accessory olfactory bulb in mammals. J. Comp. Neurol. **161:** 31–55.
31. KEVETTER, G.A. & S.S. WINANS. 1981. Connections of the corticomedial amygdala in the golden hamster. I. Efferents of the "vomeronasal amygdala." J. Comp. Neurol. **197:** 81–98.
32. LAU, Y.E., J.A. CHERRY, M.J. BAUM & S.K. MANI. 2003. Induction of Fos in the accessory olfactory system by male odors persists in female mice with a null mutation of the aromatase (Cyp19) gene. Brain Res. Bull. **60:** 143–150.
33. WENIGER, J.P. 1993. Estrogen production by fetal rat gonads. J. Steroid Biochem. Mol. Biol. **44:** 459–462.
34. WENIGER, J.P., A. ZEIS & J. CHOURAQUI. 1993. Estrogen production by fetal and infantile rat ovaries. Reprod. Nutr. Dev. **33:** 129–136.
35. RAYNAUD, P. 1971. Influence of rat estradiol binding plasma protein (EBP) on uterotrophic activity. Steroids **21:** 249–258.
36. LIEBERBURG, I. & B.S. MCEWEN. 1975. Estradiol-17b: a metabolite of testosterone recovered in cell nuclei from limbic areas of neonatal rat brains. Brain Res. **85:** 165–170.
37. MCEWEN, B.S., L. PLAPINGER, C. CHAPTAL, *et al.* 1975. The role of fetoneonatal estrogen binding proteins in the association of estrogen with neonatal brain cell nuclear receptors. Brain Res. **96:** 400–407.
38. BEYER, C., A. WOZNIAK & J.B. HUTCHISON. 1993. Sex-specific aromatization of testosterone in mouse hypothalamic neurons. Neuroendocrinology **58:** 673–681.
39. HUTCHISON, J.B., C. BEYER, R.E. HUTCHISON & A. WOZNIAK. 1995. Sexual dimorphism in the developmental regulation of brain aromatase. J. Steroid. Biochem. Mol. Biol. **53:** 307–313.
40. POINTIS, G., M.T. LATREILLE & L. CEDARD. 1980. Gonado-pituitary relationships in the fetal mouse at various times during sexual differentiation. J. Endocrinol. **86:** 483–488.
41. SCHLINGER, B.A., K.K. SOMA & S.E. LONDON. 2001. Neurosteroids and brain sexual differentiation. TINS **24:** 429–431.
42. HOLLOWAY, C.C. & D.E. CLAYTON. 2001. Estrogen synthesis in the male brain triggers development of the avian song control pathway in vitro. Nat. Neurosci. **4:** 170–175.
43. COMPAGNONE, N.A. & S.H. MELLON. 2000. Neurosteroids: biosynthesis and function of these novel neuromodulators. Front. Neuroendocrinol. **21:** 1–56.
44. GOY, R.W. 1970. Experimental control of psychosexuality. Philos. Trans. R. Soc. Lond. B Biol. Sci. **259:** 149–162.
45. VREEBURG, J.T.M., P.D.M. VAN DER VAART & P. VAN DER SCHOOT. 1977. Prevention of central defeminization but not masculinization in male rats by inhibition of oestrogen biosynthesis. J. Endocrinol. **74:** 375–382.

46. BAUM, M.J. 1979. Differentiation of coital behavior in mammals: a comparative analysis. Neurosci. Biobehav. Rev. **3:** 265–284.
47. DAVIS, P.G., C.V. CHAPTEL & B.S. MCEWEN. 1979. Independence of differentiation of masculine and feminine sexual behavior in rats. Horm. Behav. **12:** 12–19.
48. BAKKER, J., T. BRAND, J. VAN OPHEMERT & A.K. SLOB. 1993. Hormonal regulation of adult partner preference behavior in neonatally ATD-treated male rats. Behav. Neurosci. **107:** 480–487.
49. FITCH, R.H., A.S. BERREBI, P.E. COWELL, *et al.* 1990. Corpus callosum: effects of neonatal hormones on sexual dimorphism in the rat. Brain Res. **515:** 111–116.
50. MACK, C.M., R.H. FITCH, P.E. COWELL, *et al.* 1993. Ovarian estrogen acts to feminize the female rat's corpus callosum. Dev. Brain Res. **71:** 115–119.
51. MACK, C.M., R.F. MCGIVERN, L.H. HYDE & V.H. DENENBERG. 1996. Absence of postnatal testosterone fails to demasculinize the male rat's corpus callosum. Dev. Brain Res. **95:** 252–255.
52. BIMONTE, H.A., C.M. MACK, A.J. STAVNEZER & V.H. DENENBERG. 2000. Ovarian hormones can organize the rat corpus callosum in adulthood. Dev. Brain Res. **21:** 637–645.

Aromatase (Estrogen Synthase) Activity in the Dorsal Horn of the Spinal Cord: Functional Implications

HENRY C. EVRARD[a] AND JACQUES BALTHAZART

Center for Cellular and Molecular Neurobiology, Research Group in Behavioral Neuroendocrinology, University of Liège, Liège, Belgium

ABSTRACT: The presence of aromatase (estrogen synthase) in neurons in the dorsal horn of the spinal cord in Japanese quail suggests that estrogens produced locally from androgens could control spinal sensory processes including nociception. We used the hot water nociceptive test (54°C) to appraise the long-term effect of an inhibition of aromatization on the foot withdrawal latency in male quail. Four weeks after the ablation of their main source of testosterone (testes), castrated males displayed a significantly higher foot withdrawal latency than gonadally intact males. A prolonged treatment with subcutaneous capsules filled with testosterone or 17 beta-estradiol restored the baseline latency within 2 weeks. The effect of testosterone in castrated quail was almost completely blocked by systemic injections of Vorozole™, a nonsteroidal aromatase inhibitor or tamoxifen, an estrogen receptor antagonist (one injection per day for 10 days). Taken together, these data demonstrate for the first time to our knowledge an effect of estrogens formed by aromatization of androgens on nociception. Because aromatase-immunoreactive neurons and aromatase activity are present in the dorsal horns of the spinal cord, this control of pain thresholds is presumably mediated, at least in part, by estrogens produced at the spinal level that act locally via slow, presumably genomic, mechanisms mediated by the activation of spinal nuclear estrogen receptors.

KEYWORDS: spinal cord; nociception; reproduction; estrogen receptor; Japanese quail

INTRODUCTION

The enzyme aromatase catalyzes the conversion of androgens (e.g., testosterone, T) into estrogens (e.g., 17 beta-estradiol, E2). This enzyme has been known for many years to be present in the limbic system (preoptic area, bed nucleus striae terminalis, amygdala), but it is also expressed in most sensory nuclei of the hindbrain and in the sensory (dorsal) horn of the spinal cord in male and female Japanese quail and in

Address for correspondence: Henry C. Evrard, Center for Cellular and Molecular Neurobiology, Research Group in Behavioral Neuroendocrinology, University of Liège, 17 Place Delcour, B-4020 Liège, Belgium. Voice: 1-617-353-6813; fax: 1-617-358-2754.
henry.evrard@ulg.ac.be
[a]Present address: Department of Biology, Boston University, 5 Cummington Street, Boston MA 02215.

Ann. N.Y. Acad. Sci. 1007: 263–271 (2003).
doi: 10.1196/annals.1286.025

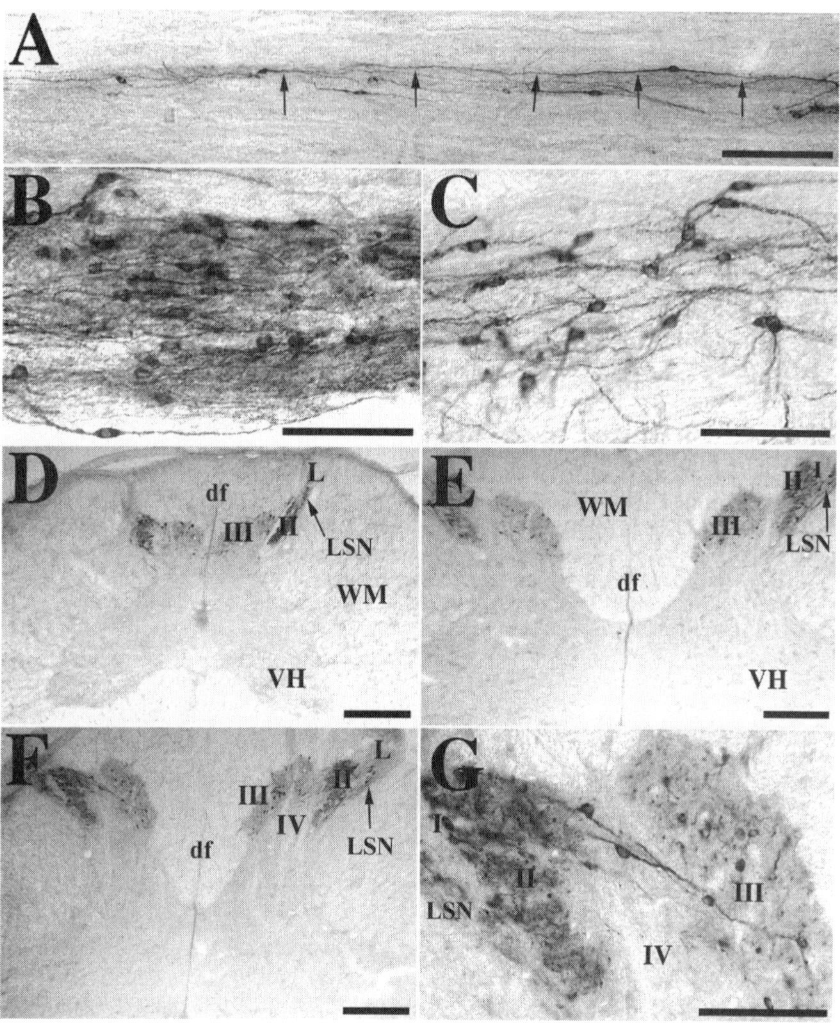

FIGURE 1. Photomicrographs illustrating the distribution of aromatase-immunoreactive (ARO-ir) neurons in 40-μm-thick sections of quail spinal cord (for methods, see Evrard *et al.*[1]). Panels **A**, **B**, and **C** represent longitudinal sections through laminae I, II, and III, respectively. In **A** to **C**, *arrows* point to relatively long ARO-ir processes orientated parallel to the rostro-caudal axis; *arrowheads* point to short ARO-ir processes without predominant orientation. Panels **D–G** represent transversal sections at the cervical (**D**), brachiothoracic (**E**), and lumbar (**F**, **G**). **G** is a higher magnification of **F**. *Legends*: I to X, laminae I to X; cc, central canal; df, dorsal funiculus; IZ, intermediary zone; L, tract of Lissauer; LSN, lateral spinal nucleus; VH, ventral horn; WM, white matter. Bars = 100 μm (**A**, **B**); 200 μm (**D–H**).

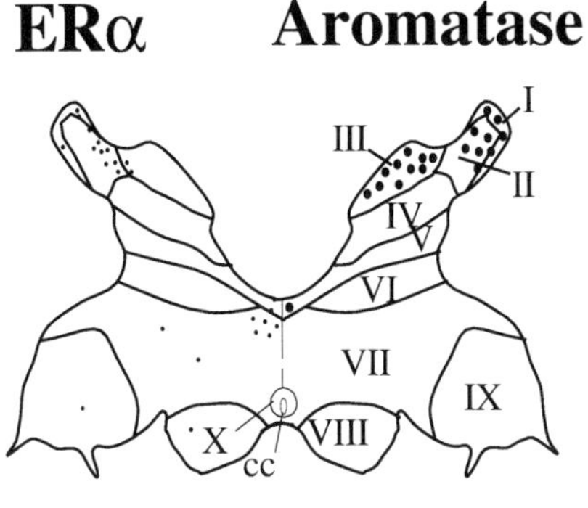

FIGURE 2. Schematic drawing illustrating the distribution of estrogen receptors of the alpha subtype (ERα: left, *small dots*) and aromatase (right, *large dots*) as detected by immunocytochemistry in the spinal cord of Japanese quail.[1,5] The number of symbols has been adjusted to provide a qualitative estimate of the number of immunoreactive cells. The section illustrated here was collected at the brachial level, but similar distributions are observed throughout the rostrocaudal extent of the spinal cord. cc, central canal; I to X, laminae I to X. Bar = 1 mm.

rats.[1–4] In adult male and female Japanese quail, aromatase-immunoreactive neurons are present in the spinal dorsal horn from the upper cervical segment to the lower caudal area. These immunoreactive nerve cells are mostly located in laminae I, II, and III, with additional sparse cells being present in the medial part of lamina V and, at the cervical level exclusively, in lamina X around the central canal (see FIG. 1). A variety of tests confirms the specificity of this immunocytochemical signal, and the morphology of the labeled cells clearly indicates their neuronal nature. Furthermore, radioenzyme assays based on the measurement of tritiated water release confirm the presence of substantial levels of aromatase activity throughout the rostrocaudal extent of the spinal cord.[1] Interestingly, the mechanisms that control this enzymatic activity are different from what has been described in the limbic system. Contrary to what is observed in the brain, the spinal aromatase activity and the number of aromatase-immunoreactive cells in five representative segments of the spinal cord are not different in sexually mature males or females and are not influenced in males by castration associated or not with a treatment with testosterone.

These data demonstrated, for the first time to our knowledge, the presence of a local estrogen production in the spinal cord of an amniote vertebrate. Interestingly, in rats and quail, the dorsal horns of the spinal cord also contain nuclear estrogen receptors of the alpha subtype[5,6] (see FIG. 2). In rats, experimental studies had established that the activation of estrogen receptors in the dorsal horn modulates nociceptive thresholds through relatively slow, presumably genomic, mechanisms.[7,8] In addition, androgens themselves had been shown to exert a significant control over pain-related mechanisms (nociception) in males,[9,10] but data were not available to determine whether this control was, at least partly, mediated through aromatization.

The recent anatomical data collected in quail, demonstrating a production of estrogens in the sensory fields of dorsal horns where estrogen receptors also had been identified in several avian and mammalian species, suggested an implication of aromatase in the modulation of sensory and, in particular, nociceptive processes. The demonstration of this notion, however, required some additional investigation.

ASSESSMENT OF PAIN THRESHOLDS IN QUAIL

After the discovery of aromatase in the spinal cord of male quail, we initiated a research program to assess the effects of spinal aromatization on nociception. We shall review here studies currently completed demonstrating that T and E2 have similar effects on the responsiveness of male quail to an aversive stimulus and that a chronic inhibition of estrogen production or action results in a long-lasting inhibition of the effect of T on nociception. A first step in this research required the establishment and validation of methods that could reliably assess pain thresholds in quail. Preliminary studies revealed indeed that tests classically used in rats and mice are not necessarily valid in birds. Quail, for example, never learned to avoid a hot plate, making the hot plate test inadequate for this species. In one set of studies,[11] we evaluated the efficacy of two nociceptive tests, the hot water and the foot pressure tests, and one non-nociceptive test (Semmes–Weinstein test) in assessing skin sensitivity in conscious Japanese quail. All stimuli elicited a reflex-like, strongly reproducible response. Responses in the hot water test and foot pressure test were identified as

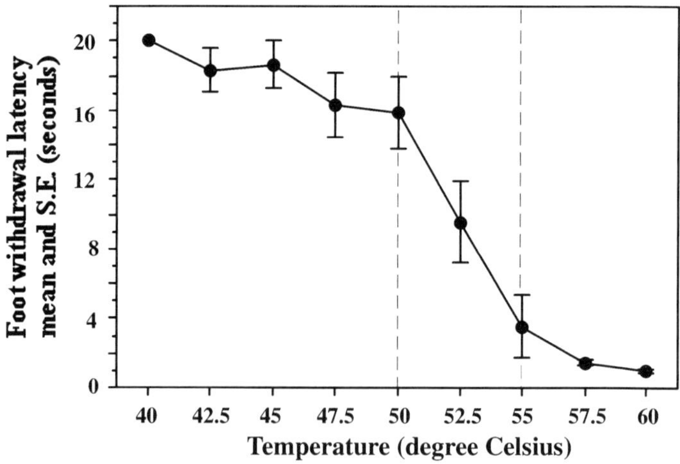

FIGURE 3. Effect of the water bath temperature (from 40 to 60°C ± 0.3°C) on the mean latency (in seconds) of foot withdrawal in the Hot Water Nociceptive Test. A rapid decrease in latency is observed from temperatures ranging between 50 and 55°C. Redrawn from data in Evrard and Balthazart.[11]

typical nocifensive flight-fight behavior. In untreated birds, these responses occurred at temperatures and forces described previously as noxious. In the Semmes–Weinstein test, two responses were observed: a slight ruffling of the cloacal gland feathers due to the stimulation of the cloacal gland, and a brief extension of the limbs due to the stimulation of the ilium or pectoral apterium. These reactions occurred at intensities recognized as innocuous. Morphine significantly altered the response latency and threshold in the hot water and the foot pressure tests but had no effect in the Semmes–Weinstein test. However, the Semmes–Weinstein test response threshold was significantly increased by local application of xylocaine (Astra Pharmaceuticals SA, Brussels). Taken together, the pattern of the responses, the intensities, and the effects of morphine and xylocaine allowed to us to distinguish between nociceptive and non-nociceptive tests. They also demonstrate the efficacy of these tests to evaluate skin sensitivity in quail and to assess its modulation by chemical factors that affect somatosensory processes. The hot water test was finally found to be the easiest, most sensitive, and most reliable method to assess skin sensitivity to noxious stimuli in quail. Birds were found to react to this test in a very reproducible manner (see small error bars in FIG. 3), and their response (latency to foot withdrawal) was clearly related to the temperature of the water bath (FIG. 3). This test therefore was selected for further studies.

EFFECTS OF SEX STEROIDS ON FOOT WITHDRAWAL LATENCY IN THE HOT WATER TEST

The effects of sex steroids on the sensitivity to an acute noxious stimulus were assessed in male quail by the hot water test in which a foot of the bird is immerged in a 54°C water bath and the experimenter records the latency of foot withdrawal in seconds.[11] The maximum duration of immersion was arbitrarily set at 20 s (cutoff), and a latency of 20 s was assigned for all experiments during which birds did not remove their foot from the water within the cutoff time. Previous work had shown that intact males (i.e., noncastrated, sexually mature males exposed to a long-day photoperiod and having a high plasma concentration of T) display a mean foot withdrawal latency in the hot water test that was equal to approximately 4.00 s (see FIG. 3; see baseline in the following text and in FIG. 4).[11] In our set of experiments, male quail that had been castrated 2 weeks before the beginning of the experiment were implanted subcutaneously with two 20-mm-long Silastic™capsules (1.57-mm inner diameter, 2.41-mm outer diameter; Degania Silicone, Israel) that were empty (CX, $n = 6$) or filled with crystalline T (CX+T, $n = 8$; T-1500; Sigma-Aldrich, USA) or crystalline E2 (CX+E2, $n = 8$; E-4260, Sigma-Aldrich, USA). Two weeks after implantation, the foot withdrawal latency was measured in each bird with the hot water test at 54°C. CX birds displayed a markedly longer latency than intact subjects (FIG. 4A). E2 and T similarly restored the withdrawal latency to the baseline level typical of intact males (FIG. 4A). Accordingly, a Kruskal–Wallis nonparametric analysis of variance revealed the presence of significant differences between the summed ranked latencies of the different groups (KW = 9.950, df = 2, $P = 0.0069$). Post hoc multiple comparisons between groups based on the Kruskal–Wallis analysis showed that CX+E2 and CX+T latencies were not significantly different but significantly smaller than in CX birds (see the symbols in FIG. 4A).

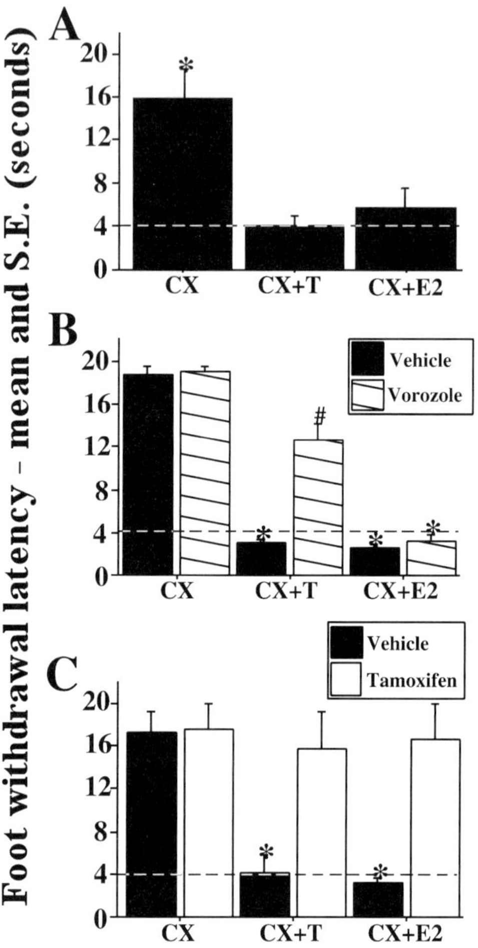

FIGURE 4. Histograms illustrating the mean foot withdrawal latencies measured with the hot water test at 54°C in male quail that were either castrated (CX) or castrated and treated with testosterone (CX+T) or 17 alpha-estradiol (CX+E2) subcutaneous implants. (**A**) Effects of castration and hormonal replacement with T or E2. (**B**) Half of the subjects in each of the three groups received a daily intraperitoneal injection of Vorozole for 10 days *(hatched bars)*, whereas the other half received vehicle injections *(black bars)*. (**C**) Half of the subjects in each of the three groups received a daily intraperitoneal injection of tamoxifen for 10 days *(empty bars)*, whereas the other half received vehicle injections *(black bars)*. The horizontal dashed line represents the baseline latency previously measured in similar conditions in intact, noncastrated male quail.[11] The symbols above the bars summarize the results of multiple comparisons by nonparametric post hoc tests; $^{*}P < 0.05$ compared with all other groups except those also labeled by an asterisk; $^{\#}P < 0.05$ compared with all groups.

INHIBITION OF ESTROGEN ACTION AND FOOT WITHDRAWAL LATENCY IN THE HOT WATER TEST

During a 10-day period beginning 2 weeks later, half of the birds in each group (randomly selected) received a daily intraperitoneal injection of a nonsteroidal aromatase inhibitor, Vorozole™ (3 mg/kg, R083842; Janssen Pharmaceutica, Belgium), whereas the other birds were injected daily with the vehicle (these treatments resulted in six subgroups). All birds were then submitted to the hot water test 1 day after the last injection. Injections were discontinued, and birds were tested again 2 weeks and 4 weeks after the last injection to follow the vanishing of the effect of vorozole. Twenty-four hours after the last injection, Vorozole™ significantly increased the latency in CX+T birds but had no effect in the CX+E2 and CX groups (FIG. 4B; results of a Kruskal–Wallis test with the six subgroups considered as six independent samples: KW = 16.42, df = 5, $P = 0.0057$; see symbols in FIG. 3B for results of multiple post hoc comparisons). The effect of Vorozole™ had totally disappeared 2 and 4 weeks after the last injection (results not shown here). After about 30 days when behavioral effects of Vorozole™ had disappeared, a similar procedure was used to test the effects of the estrogen receptor antagonist, tamoxifen (4 mg/kg; T-6292; Sigma-Aldrich, USA). One-half of the birds in each group (CX, T, or E2) were again selected randomly and injected daily for 10 days with the antagonist, whereas the other birds received control injections. The foot withdrawal latency then was measured 24 h after the last injection as well as 2 and 4 weeks later. The 10-day treatment with tamoxifen completely blocked the effects of both E2 and T on mean foot withdrawal latency (FIG. 4C; results of a Kruskal-Wallis test with the six subgroups considered as six independent samples: KW = 11.907, df = 5, $P = 0.0181$; see symbols in FIG. 4C for results of multiple comparisons). The effect of tamoxifen vanished in CX+T birds after 2 weeks. In contrast, after 2 weeks, CX+E2 birds retained a latency higher than the baseline (14.433 ± 5.57 s, $P = 0.081$) and only reached the baseline 4 weeks after the end of the injections (results not shown here).

DISCUSSION

The studies described above show that aromatization of T into E2 controls nociception and possibly other sensory modalities. Based on the time-course of the observed changes in foot withdrawal latencies, it appears that this control reflects long-term effects of E2 on nociception probably mediated by the activation of nuclear estrogen receptors. Accordingly, a repeated chronic treatment with either vorozole or tamoxifen disrupted these effects of E2 that subsequently required a relatively long period to recover from these pharmacological treatments. Previous immunocytochemical data in quail suggest that these effects could depend partly on the spinal aromatization of androgens and on the activation of nuclear estrogens receptors found in the vicinity of aromatase-immunoreactive neurons in the dorsal horns.[1,6] The long-lasting effects of castration and hormonal replacements in quail are consistent with the increase of nocifensive behaviors in the late phase of the formalin test observed previously in castrated male rats bearing T implants[9] and with the hyperalgesia in ovariectomized female rats bearing E2 implants and submitted to the hot plate test.[12] However, reverse effects of T and E2 (increase in tail withdrawal and jump latency or threshold after a treatment with T or E2 in gonadectomized male and female rats) also have been observed in male and female rats,[13–15] suggesting a certain plasticity of the steroidal control of sensitivity. The factors controlling the direction of the effect (pro- or antinociceptive) of T and E2 remain to be determined. Interestingly, in male house sparrows T administration increased, whereas a treatment with flutamide and ATD decreased the foot withdrawal latency in the hot water test (M. Hau, O. Dominguez, and H.C. Evrard, unpublished data). Previous studies have demonstrated that androgens exert a substantial influence over pain-related mechanisms in male rats and humans.[10,12,13] The current study provides the first evidence to our knowledge for a role of aromatase in this control. As observed for the effect of T on the activation of copulatory behavior in the preoptic area in male, T aromatization in the spinal cord could play a critical role for the action of T on nociception and sensory processes in general. However, in male rats, both castration and flutamide (an androgen receptor antagonist) treatment induced antinociception in the late phase of formalin tests[9] indicating that T also could modulate nociception by a direct action as an androgen. In the current experiments, the mean latency in CX+E2 birds was still higher than the baseline 2 weeks after the last injection of tamoxifen, whereas mean latency in CX+T had returned to the baseline level. This difference in the long-term effect of tamoxifen between CX+E2 and CX+T birds may account for an additional effect androgens *per se* on nociception in CX+T birds. The mechanisms through which spinal aromatase and estrogens influence pain should be clarified in future studies. From a functional perspective, the slow effect of estrogens on pain thresholds could play a significant role in the control of sensory processes during reproduction.

ACKNOWLEDGMENTS

This work was supported by the National Institute of Mental Health (NIMH50388), the Belgian Fonds de la Recherche Fondamentale Collective (2.4555.01), and the government of the French Community of Belgium (ARC99/04-241).

REFERENCES

1. Evrard, H., M. Baillien, A. Foidart, *et al.* 2000. Localization and controls of aromatase in the quail spinal cord. J. Comp. Neurol. **423:** 552–564.
2. Evrard, H.C. & J. Balthazart. 2001. Localization of estrogen-synthase (aromatase) in the rat spinal cord. Abstr. Soc. Neurosci. **1:** 260.
3. Evrard, H.C. & J. Balthazart. 2000. Localization of estrogen-synthase and estrogen receptor immunoreactive cells in the descending nucleus of the trigeminal nerve in Japanese quail. Eur. J. Neurosci. **12:** 147.
4. Evrard, H.C., N. Harada & J. Balthazart. 2003. Immunocytochemical localization of aromatase in sensory and integrating nuclei of the hindbrain in Japanese quail (*Coturnix japonica*). J. Comp. Neurol. In press.
5. Amandusson, A., O. Hermanson & A. Blomqvist. 1995. Estrogen receptor-like immunoreactivity in the medullary and spinal dorsal horn of the female rat. Neurosci. Lett. **196:** 25–28.
6. Evrard, H.C. & J. Balthazart. 2002. Localization of estrogen receptors in the sensory and motor areas of the spinal cord in Japanese quail (*Coturnix japonica*). J. Neuroendocrinol. **14:** 894–903.

7. ALOISI, A.M. 2000. Sensory effects of gonadal hormones. *In* Sex, Gender, and Pain. R.B. Fillingim, Ed.: 7–24. IASP Press. Seattle.
8. LIU, N.J. & A.R. GINTZLER. 2000. Prolonged ovarian sex steroid treatment of male rats produces antinociception: identification of sex-based divergent analgesic mechanisms. Pain **85:** 273–281.
9. NAYEBI, A.R. & A. AHMADIANI. 1999. Involvement of the spinal serotonergic system in analgesia produced by castration. Pharmacol. Biochem. Behav. **64:** 467–471.
10. KLIMEK, A. 1999. Use of testosterone in the treatment of cluster headache. Eur. Neurol. **24:** 53–56.
11. EVRARD, H.C. & J. BALTHAZART. 2002. The assessment of nociceptive and non- nociceptive skin sensitivity in the Japanese quail (*Coturnix japonica*). J. Neurosci. Methods **116:** 135–146.
12. RATKA, A. & J.W. SIMPKINS. 1991. Effects of estradiol and progesterone in the sensitivity to pain and on morphine-induced antinociception in female rats. Horm. Behav. **25:** 217–228.
13. FORMAN, L.J., V. TINGLE, S. ESTILOW, *et al.* 1989. The response to analgesia testing is affected by gonadal steroids in the rat. Life Sci. **45:** 447–454.
14. FRYE, C.A. & A.M. SELIGA. 2001. Testosterone increases analgesia, anxiolysis, and cognitive performance of male rats. Cogn. Affect. Behav. Neurosci. **1:** 371–381.
15. DAWSON-BASOA, M.B. & A.R. GINTZLER. 1993. 17-Beta-estradiol and progesterone modulate an intrinsic opioid analgesic system. Brain Res. **601:** 241–245.

Sex Steroids and Human Behavior: Prenatal Androgen Exposure and Sex-Typical Play Behavior in Children

MELISSA HINES

Department of Psychology, City University, Northampton Square, London, EC1V 0HB, United Kingdom

ABSTRACT: Gonadal hormones, particularly androgens, direct certain aspects of brain development and exert permanent influences on sex-typical behavior in nonhuman mammals. Androgens also influence human behavioral development, with the most convincing evidence coming from studies of sex-typical play. Girls exposed to unusually high levels of androgens prenatally, because they have the genetic disorder, congenital adrenal hyperplasia (CAH), show increased preferences for toys and activities usually preferred by boys, and for male playmates, and decreased preferences for toys and activities usually preferred by girls. Normal variability in androgen prenatally also has been related to subsequent sex-typed play behavior in girls, and nonhuman primates have been observed to show sex-typed preferences for human toys. These findings suggest that androgen during early development influences childhood play behavior in humans at least in part by altering brain development.

KEYWORDS: androgen; behavior; human; play; sex differences; gender; hormones

Gonadal steroids, particularly androgens, have dramatic influences on the development of the mammalian brain. During critical periods of prenatal or neonatal life, they direct basic developmental processes, including the death versus survival of neurons, the anatomical connections among cells in different neural regions, and the specification of neurochemicals that are used for cell to cell communication. As a consequence of these influences on neural development, levels of androgens during early life influence sex-typical behavior across the lifespan (see reviews, see Refs. 1–4).

HORMONES AND SEXUAL DIFFERENTIATION IN NONHUMAN MAMMALS

The effects of gonadal steroids on brain development and behavior have been established in experimental research on a variety of mammals, ranging from rodents to

Address for correspondence: Melissa Hines, Department of Psychology, City University, Northhampton Square, London, EC1V 0HB, U.K. Voice: 20-7040-8351; fax: 20-7040-8947. m.hines@city.ac.uk

Ann. N.Y. Acad. Sci. 1007: 272–282 (2003). © 2003 New York Academy of Sciences. doi: 10.1196/annals.1286.026

nonhuman primates. For instance, XX rats treated with a single injection of androgen on the day of birth show increased capacity for male sexual behavior and decreased capacity for female sexual behavior in adulthood. They also show increased male typical behavior and decreased female typical behavior for other characteristics that show sex differences, even if they do not relate directly to reproduction. To give one example, female rats treated shortly after birth with androgen show increased rough-and-tumble play, a behavior that is normally seen more often in juvenile males than females, as well as the alterations in sexual behavior described above. Similar effects on both juvenile play behavior and adult sexual behavior are seen in the female offspring of pregnant rhesus monkeys who were treated with testosterone during pregnancy.

The difference in the timing of the effects of androgen on behavior for rhesus monkeys (prenatal) versus rats (early postnatal) occurs because rats are born at an earlier developmental stage than rhesus monkeys. The times when hormone manipulations are effective correspond to the times when testosterone is elevated in developing males of the species compared with developing females. For rats, this is roughly from days 17 to 19 of a 22-day gestation and for the first 10 days postnatally. In humans, testosterone is elevated prenatally from approximately week 8 to week 24 of gestation, and postnatally from about the first to the sixth month of life.[5] Thus, these times are potential critical periods for hormonal influences on human brain development and behavior.

In addition to differences among species in the overall critical period for hormonal influences on behavior, there are different subperiods within the overall critical period for each species during which particular behavioral characteristics are maximally sensitive to hormonal influences. For example, in rats, the critical period for hormonal influences on the female-typical sexual behavior, lordosis, occurs earlier than that for hormonal influences on the male-typical sexual behavior, mounting.[6] Similarly, in rhesus monkeys, the critical period for hormonal influences on maternal grooming by offspring occurs earlier than that for hormonal influences on juvenile play.[7]

HORMONES AND HUMAN SEXUAL DIFFERENTIATION

In studies of rodents and nonhuman primates, hormones are manipulated during early development, and the effects of these manipulations on sex-related behaviors then are determined. True experiments of this kind are not possible in human beings, because it is generally unethical to alter hormone levels during early life for these experimental purposes. Instead, information on the role of hormones in human development has come from other sources, including so-called experiments of nature, where people have developed in unusual hormone environments for other reasons, for instance, because of genetic disorders. A second approach to understanding the role of hormones in human development has been to relate normal variability in the early hormone environment to subsequent behavior. Data from both of these approaches, as well as additional research involving nonhuman primates, are described in the next sections of this article.

Hormones and Sexual Differentiation of the External Genitalia

Genetic female animals treated with androgens during early life resemble males not only behaviorally, but also physically. This occurs because androgens direct development of the external genitalia, as well as of the brain. Whether they are XX or XY, animals begin life with identical primordial genitalia. These primordia develop as penis and scrotum in the presence of high levels of androgens, and as clitoris and labia in the presence of low levels of androgens. Evidence that androgens direct development of the human external genitalia in a manner similar to that documented experimentally in other mammals has come from individuals with genetic disorders that cause hormonal abnormalities beginning before birth, including congenital adrenal hyperplasia (CAH) and androgen insensitivity syndrome (AIS).

CAH is caused by deficiency in an enzyme, usually 21 hydroxylase, that is needed to produce cortisol. Because of the enzymatic deficiency, precursors to cortisol are shunted into the androgen pathway, resulting in elevated levels of androgens in females with the disorder, beginning prenatally. Human XX infants with CAH are typically born with varying degrees of genital virilization, ranging from minor labial fusion and clitoral enlargement in some girls to complete fusion and enlargement of the phallus to resemble a penis in others. This genital virilization demonstrates that androgen promotes male-typical development of the external genitalia in humans as it does in other species.

Individuals with the disorder AIS have defective androgen receptors, impairing the ability of their cells to respond to testosterone and other androgens. The disorder can be partial or complete. XY infants with the complete form of AIS are born with external genitalia that resemble those of females, and, in fact, are not usually identified at birth as XY or as suffering from any disorder. Their feminine appearance is so convincing that the condition typically is not detected until they fail to menstruate at the time of normal puberty. Individuals with partial AIS are often born with ambiguous genitalia, similar to those of girls with CAH. Both the complete feminization in individuals with complete AIS and the ambiguous genitalia in those with partial AIS further document the important role of androgen in development of the external genitalia in humans.

Hormones and Human Behavior

Hormonal influences on human behavior are more difficult to establish conclusively than are hormonal influences on the external genitalia. This is partly because behavioral sex differences generally are more subtle than physical sex differences, partly because they are harder to measure reliably and partly because behavioral outcomes are influenced by the social environment as well as by physical factors, making it difficult to attribute behavioral differences in individuals with disorders such as CAH directly to hormones. As is discussed in more detail below, the physical consequences of CAH themselves have even been suggested to explain behavioral differences between women with and without CAH.

Androgen and Childhood Play

The best evidence that androgens influence human behavioral development has come from studies of childhood play behaviors that show sex differences, such as toy choices and activity and playmate preferences. Sex differences in play begin early in life. By 12 months of age, boys and girls prefer different toys, and these sex differences continue through childhood. Boys gravitate towards vehicles, like toy cars, trucks and airplanes, or weapons, like guns and swords, whereas girls prefer dolls and doll clothes, dress-up toys and cosmetics, and tea sets. Like other mammals, boys also spend more time than girls do in rough-and-tumble play, including play fighting and wrestling. In addition, boys and girls differ in their playmate choices. Boys generally play with boys and girls generally play with girls (see Hines[4] for a more detailed review of these sex differences in the play behavior of children, and for additional primary references).

In the 1960s, girls exposed prenatally to high levels of androgenic hormones were reported to be "tomboys," preferring boys' toys and activities, boys as playmates, and rough, active utdoor play.[8,9] Interviews with androgen-exposed girls and their mothers suggested that the girls showed unusually high levels of these behaviors. Mothers also indicated that they would use the word "tomboy" to describe their daughters. "Tomboyish" behavior was reported in girls exposed to high levels of androgen prenatally because of CAH, as well as in girls whose pregnant mothers had been prescribed synthetic progestins that stimulated androgen receptors. Thus, evidence from a genetic disorder, as well as from an external source of hormone exposure, provided convergent evidence, suggesting a hormonal influence on this aspect of human psychological development.

Additional evidence of increased male-typical play behavior in girls with CAH has come from several subsequent studies using questionnaires and interviews to assess sex-typed interests and activities, as well as direct observation of girls with CAH. One study videotaped children in a playroom containing toys typically preferred by girls (e.g., dolls, doll clothes, a tea set), toys typically preferred by boys (e.g., a car, a truck, a helicopter), and toys that boys and girls typically enjoy equally (e.g., books, board games, a puzzle).[10] Unaffected siblings and first cousins of the children with CAH served as controls in the study, and they showed the expected sex differences in time spent with each type of toy. However, compared with the control girls, girls with CAH spent more time with "masculine" toys, less time with "feminine" toys, and a similar amount of time with "neutral" toys.

Similar findings of increased male-typical interests have been reported based on analyses of the drawings of girls with CAH in Japan,[11] and differences between girls with CAH and other girls are seen whether children are observed playing with a parent or on their own.[12,13] In addition, findings of increased male-typical play behavior or interests have been reported for girls with CAH in a variety of countries, including the United States, Great Britain, Canada, the Netherlands, Sweden, Germany, and Japan, in comparison with same-sex relatives and with matched controls, with concurrent and retrospective assessments, and with interviews, questionnaires, and direct observation of behavior (for review, see Hines[4]).

Early reports of masculinized play in girls exposed to androgens prenatally were viewed by some with skepticism, partly because experimenters often knew the medical status (CAH vs. control) of individual children, or because control groups were lacking or poorly matched.[14–16] However, subsequent studies have produced similar findings without these problems. Thus, the masculinized play behavior seen in androgenized girls could be evidence of gonadal hormone influences on the developing brain similar to those documented in nonhuman mammals.

ALTERNATIVE PERSPECTIVES ON THE CAUSES OF SEX-TYPED PLAY

It also has been suggested that the altered play behavior seen in girls with CAH can be explained by alterations in their external genitalia (e.g., Quadagno *et al.*[16]). From this perspective, girls with CAH show increased male-typical play behavior, because they are born with masculine-appearing genitalia. For instance, this physical masculinization could cause their parents or the girls themselves to view them as less feminine or cause their parents to treat them differently because of their genital abnormalities at birth. It also has been suggested that the illness aspects of CAH, particularly salt-losing crises and hospitalizations during infancy for these crises and for genital surgery, could increase male-typical behavior in girls with the disorder independent of androgen exposure.[17]

Nonhormonal perspectives on gender development emphasize social and cognitive processes that influence sex-typical behavior. For instance, from the social learning perspective, girls and boys learn to choose different toys and activities, because they are taught to do so (e.g., through reward and punishment).[18,19] In support of this perspective, parents, peers, and teachers are more likely to reward children for sex-appropriate play than for cross-sex play, and discourage or even punish play that is viewed as sex-inappropriate.[20–22] From the cognitive perspective, each child's gender identity (i.e., awareness of being a boy or a girl) leads him or her to value and engage in activities associated with that identity, thus promoting what society views as sex-appropriate behavior.[23,24] In support of this perspective, children do prefer items or activities that they have been told are for children of their own sex,[25] and they preferentially model item and activity preferences that they have seen displayed by others of their own sex.[26]

From these social/cognitive perspectives, male-typical behavior in girls with CAH could be caused by parents reinforcing girls with CAH differently or could result from reduced female gender identification in girls with CAH. Parents say that they do not treat their daughters with CAH differently from how they would treat other girls.[10,27] However, parents have been observed treating their healthy sons and daughters differently, despite saying that they do not do so,[20] raising the possibility that they treat their daughters with CAH differently without being aware of it. Detailed information on parental treatment of girls with CAH has not been published, and it might be impossible to completely rule out the possibility that at some stage of development girls with CAH are treated differently from other girls. Similarly, it is hard to rule out the possibility that girls with CAH do not identify as strongly with the female gender as do other girls. However, other empirical approaches to this question suggest that hormones influence sex-typical toy preferences independent of these social and cognitive mechanisms. These approaches have linked normal variability in the prenatal hormone environment to sex-typical toy preferences in healthy girls[28] and have documented sex-typical toy preferences in nonhuman primates.[29]

Prenatal Hormonal Variability and Childhood Sex-Typed Behavior

The relationship of normal variability in hormones during prenatal development to postnatal behavior was studied in a sample of 679 children.[28] These girls and boys were participants in a longitudinal, population study of children born in a geographically defined area (Avon, England) during a specified time period (April 1, 1991 to December 21, 1992). All pregnant women in the area were notified about the study, and approximately 90% participated, totaling 13,998 pregnancies and 14,138 offspring.

When the children in the study were 3½ years old, sex-typed behavior was assessed using the Pre-School Activities Inventory (PSAI), a standardized questionnaire that is completed by a parent, usually the mother, to indicate the child's sex-typed toy, playmate, and activity preferences. Six groups of children were selected based on PSAI scores for further study: highly feminine girls ($n = 118$), highly masculine girls ($n = 113$), highly feminine boys ($n = 112$), highly masculine boys ($n = 128$), a random sample of girls ($n = 106$), and a random sample of boys ($n = 102$). Testosterone and sex hormone binding globulin (SHBG) then were measured in samples of maternal blood that had been obtained during the pregnancies that produced these 679 children. The blood samples had been taken during routine medical visits, and the mean time of sampling was gestational week 16 (standard deviation, 8 weeks). As mentioned above, testosterone levels are elevated in developing male fetuses from approximately week 8 to 24 of gestation, peaking at approximately week 16. Thus, the timing of the samples was centered on the time when testosterone is elevated in developing males, a putative critical period for hormonal influences on human development.

Testosterone related positively and linearly to gestational age, and negatively and linearly to maternal age, in women carrying both male and female fetuses. Because of these relationships, analyses relating prenatal testosterone to postnatal behavior were conducted using gestational age and maternal age as covariates. These analyses revealed that testosterone related in the predicted direction to sex-typical play behavior in girls; women with higher levels of testosterone during pregnancy had daughters with higher levels of male-typical play behavior than those with lower levels of testosterone during pregnancy. Maternal testosterone during pregnancy did not relate to sex-typed behavior in male offspring. There also was no relationship between SHBG and sex-typed behavior in either sex, and the ratio of testosterone to SHBG showed the same relationship to sex-typed behavior as testosterone alone. These data suggest that normal variability in testosterone prenatally relates to sex-typed behavior in girls in the general population. Because these girls all had normal appearing genitalia at birth, and were as healthy as girls in general, the relationship between androgen and behavior cannot be attributed to illness or to genital ambiguity.

What causes the association between maternal testosterone levels during pregnancy and sex-typical play behavior in female offspring? One possibility is that testosterone from the maternal system has passed through the placenta to influence the female fetus. The daughters of women with medical conditions causing elevated androgen during pregnancy, and the daughters of women prescribed androgenic hormones during pregnancy, sometimes can be born with virilized genitalia,[8,30,31] indicating that androgens can pass from the mother to the fetus. Hormones do not appear to pass in appreciable amounts in the other direction (i.e., from the fetus to the mother). If they did, women pregnant with male fetuses (who have high levels of testosterone) would be expected to have higher levels of testosterone than women carrying female fetuses (who have low levels of testosterone), and this generally has not been found to be the case.[28] The movement of testosterone from the mother to the fetus, but not from the fetus to the mother, may explain the lack of a relationship between maternal testosterone and sex-typed behavior in male offspring. Boys already have high levels of testosterone during prenatal development, causing any testosterone that they might receive from the maternal circulation to have no additional impact.

A second possible explanation of the relationship between maternal testosterone during pregnancy and the sex-typical behavior of daughters, but not sons, relates to genetic factors. Individual differences in levels of testosterone are determined partly by genetic factors, with heritability estimates ranging from 40 to 60%,[32,33] and this genetic connection is clearer in females than in males.[32] Thus, mothers with high testosterone may have daughters with high testosterone because of the influence of genetic factors that show closer relationships in mothers and daughters than in mothers and sons. The available information does not allow determination of whether the relationship between maternal testosterone and the behavior of daughters is caused by shared genetic factors or by testosterone passing from the maternal circulation to the fetal circulation. Either way, however, the linkage between the maternal hormone environment and the postnatal behavior of daughters suggests that normal variability in the prenatal hormone environment contributes to normal variability in sex-typed behavior among girls.

Sex-Typical Toy Preferences in Nonhuman Primates

In another study,[29] colonies of vervet monkeys were provided with toys typically preferred by boys (a toy police car and a ball), toys typically preferred by girls (a rag doll and a cooking pot), and toys preferred equally by boys and girls (a picture book and a stuffed dog). Videotapes were made of the animals interacting with the toys. Subsequently, researchers who did not know which animals were male and which were female recorded the amount of time that male and female vervets spent in contact with each type of toy. Results indicated that male animals spent more time than females did contacting the toys usually preferred by boys, female animals spent more time than males did contacting the toys usually preferred by girls, and male and female animals spent similar amounts of time contacting the toys that both girls and boys enjoy. These results suggest that nonhuman primates show similar preferences for sex-typed toys to those seen in human children. The vervet monkeys had no prior experience with any of the toys used in the study and had no cultural expectations about which toys were for males versus females. Therefore, the differences between male and female vervets in toy contact cannot be attributed to social/cognitive mechanisms.

SUMMARY, CAVEATS, AND CONCLUSIONS

Prenatal levels of androgen appear to influence the development of children's sex-typical play behavior. This conclusion is suggested by studies of children who were exposed to abnormal levels of hormones beginning before birth, by research relating normal variability in prenatal hormones to postnatal behavior, and by the observation of sex-typed toy preferences in nonhuman primates. Therefore, hormones appear to influence at least some aspects of human brain development and behavior in a manner similar to that seen in other species.

Nevertheless, hormones cannot be assumed to exert similar influences to those seen for childhood play on all human behaviors that show sex differences. In fact, sexual orientation and core gender identity (or the basic sense of self as male or female) appear to be less susceptible to influences of prenatal hormones than is childhood play. For instance, females with CAH are more likely than other females to be lesbian or bisexual and to suffer from gender dysphoria.[34–37] However, these effects occur more rarely, or are less drastic, than those on play behavior.[35,37] Most women with CAH are heterosexual as adults and the vast majority have a female core gender identity, despite their prenatal androgen exposure and despite alterations in their childhood play interests (for review, see Hines[4]).

In addition, not all of the specific hormonal influences that have been described in other mammals, even for play behavior, can be assumed to be directly relevant to human development. An example comes from research on prenatal stress. In rodents, stress during pregnancy influences sexual differentiation of both male and female offspring, and the effects involve many of the same behaviors, including sexual behavior and rough-and-tumble play, as are influenced by manipulations of androgen.[38–41] In general, prenatal stress reduces male-typical behavior and increases female-typical behavior in male offspring and has the opposite effects (reduced female-typical characteristics and increased male-typical characteristics) in female offspring. These effects are thought to occur because stress alters the timing of the prenatal androgen surge in developing male rodents[40] and increases levels of androgens in pregnant female rodents and their fetuses.[42,43]

Stress during prenatal life does not appear to have the same influences on sex-related development in humans as have been observed in rodents. Although one early report suggested that mothers of homosexual men recalled more prenatal stress than mothers of heterosexual men,[44] subsequent studies have not found similar results.[45–47] Fewer studies are available relating prenatal stress to sexual differentiation in females than in males, but for females also prenatal stress appears to exert minimal, or no, influence on sexual-related behavior.[45,48] For instance, the longitudinal, population-based study of over 14,000 pregnancies in Avon, England found no relationship between prenatal stress and sex-typed play behavior in boys, and only small relationships in girls.[48]

Why might the effects of prenatal stress differ for rodents versus humans? Stress has been found to alter androgen levels in adult humans,[49–51] but no data are available on fetal androgen responses to stress. The reduced influence of prenatal stress on sexual differentiation in humans also may occur because adrenal androgen production in response to stress is less dramatic in humans than in rodents[52] (cited in Bailey *et al.*[45]). In addition, the prenatal critical period for hormonal influences on sexual differentiation is much longer in humans (approximately 16 weeks) than in rats (approximately 2–3 days). This longer period may allow the male fetus to compensate for stress-related hormone perturbations, for example, via feedback mechanisms that adjust testicular androgen production[53,54] and thus prevent disruption of sexual differentiation.

Finally, although hormones, particularly androgens, influence the development of children's interest in sex-typed toys and activities, hormones are not the only important factors. For instance, in the longitudinal population study of children from Avon, England, many factors in addition to maternal testosterone during pregnancy were found to relate to individual differences in sex-typical behavior as assessed with the PSAI.[48,55] In both boys and girls, these factors included the presence of older brothers or sisters in the home, maternal education, and the degree to which the parents conformed to traditional gender roles. Older brothers were associated with more male-typical behavior, and older sisters with more female-typical behavior, in both boys and girls. In addition, more educated mothers had children who were less sex-typed and parents who conformed to traditional gender roles had children who were more sex-typed. Nevertheless, the relationship between prenatal testosterone and postnatal behavior persisted when these other factors were controlled.[28] Thus, the prenatal hormone environment appears to be one of several factors that contribute to variability from one child to the next in sex-typed play behavior in childhood.

ACKNOWLEDGMENTS

This work has been supported by the United States Public Health Service (HD 24542) and by the Wellcome Trust, UK.

REFERENCES

1. Arnold, A.P. & R.A. Gorski. 1984. Gonadal steroid induction of structural sex differences in the central nervous system. Annu. Rev. Neurosci. **7:** 413–442.
2. De Vries, G.J. & R.B. Simerly. 2002. Anatomy, development, and function of sexually dimorphic neural circuits in the mammalian brain. *In* Hormones, Brain and Behavior. D.W. Pfaff, A.P. Arnold, A.M. Etgen, S.E. Fahrbach & R.T. Rubin, Eds.: 137–191. Academic Press. San Diego.
3. Goy, R.W. & B.S. McEwen. 1980. Sexual Differentiation of the Brain. MIT Press. Cambridge, MA.
4. Hines, M. 2004. Brain Gender. Oxford University Press. New York.
5. Smail, P.J., F.I. Reyes, J.S.D. Winter & C. Faiman. 1981. The fetal hormone environment and its effect on the morphogenesis of the genital system. *In* Pediatric Andrology. S.J. Kogan & E.S.E. Hafez, Eds: 9–20. Martinus Nijhoff. The Hague.
6. Christensen, L.W. & R.A. Gorski. 1978. Independent masculinization of neuroendocrine systems by intracerebral implants of testosterone or estradiol in the neonatal female rat. Brain Res. **146:** 325–340.
7. Goy, R.W., F.B. Bercovitch & M.C. McBrair. 1988. Behavioral masculinization is independent of genital masculinization in prenatally androgenized female rhesus macaques. Horm. Behav. **22:** 552–571.
8. Ehrhardt, A.A. & J. Money. 1967. Progestin-induced hermaphroditism: IQ and psychosexual identity in a study of ten girls. J. Sex Res. **3:** 83–100.
9. Ehrhardt, A.A., R. Epstein & J. Money. 1968. Fetal androgens and female gender identity in the early-treated adrenogenital syndrome. Johns Hopkins Med. J. **122:** 165–167.
10. Berenbaum, S.A. & M. Hines. 1992. Early androgens are related to childhood sex-typed toy preferences. Psychol. Sci. **3:** 203–206.
11. Iijima, M., O. Ariska, F. Minamoto & Y. Arai. 2001. Sex differences in children's free drawings: a study on girls with congenital adrenal hyperplasia. Horm. Behav. **40:** 99–104.
12. Nordenstrom, A., A. Servin, G. Bohlin, *et al.* 2002. Sex-typed play behavior correlates with the degree of prenatal androgen exposure as assessed by CYP21 genotypes in girls with congenital adrenal hyperplasia. J. Clin. Endocrinol. Metab. **87:** 5119–5124.
13. Pasterski, V.L. 2002. Development of gender role behaviour in children: prenatal hormones and parental socialisation. Ph.D. thesis. City University. London.
14. Fausto-Sterling, A. 1992. Myths of Gender. Basic Books. New York.

15. HINES, M. 1982. Prenatal gonadal hormones and sex differences in human behavior. Psychol. Bull. **92:** 56–80.
16. QUADAGNO, D.M., R. BRISCOE & J.S. QUADAGNO. 1977. Effects of perinatal gonadal hormones on selected nonsexual behavior patterns: a critical assessment of the nonhuman and human literature. Psychol. Bull. **84:** 62–80.
17. SLIJPER, F.M.E. 1984. Androgens and gender role behaviour in girls with congenital adrenal hyperplasia (CAH). *In* Progress in Brain Research. G.J. De Vries, J.P.C. De Bruin, H.B.M. Uylings & M.A. Corner, Eds.: 417–422. Elsevier. Amsterdam.
18. BANDURA, A. 1977. Social learning theory. Prentice Hall. Englewood Cliffs, NJ.
19. MISCHEL, W. 1966. A social learning view of sex differences in behavior. *In* The Development of Sex Differences. E.E. Maccoby, Ed.: 56–81. Stanford University Press. Stanford, CA.
20. FAGOT, B.I. 1978. The influence of sex of child on parental reactions to toddler children. Child Dev. **49:** 459–465.
21. FAGOT, B.I. & R. HAGAN. 1991. Observations of parent reactions to sex-stereotyped behaviors: age and sex effects. Child Dev. **62:** 617–628.
22. LANGLOIS, J.H. & A.C. DOWNS. 1980. Mothers, fathers and peers as socialization agents of sex-typed play behaviors in young children. Child Dev. **51:** 1237–1247.
23. BUSSEY, K. & A. BANDURA. 1984. Influence of gender constancy and social power on sex-linked modeling. J. Pers. Soc. Psychol. **47:** 1292–1302.
24. KOHLBERG, L. 1966. A cognitive-developmental analysis of children's sex-role concepts and attitudes. *In* The Development of Sex Differences. E.E. Maccoby, Ed.: 82–173. Stanford University Press. Stanford, CA.
25. MASTERS, J.C., M.E. FORD, R. AREND, *et al.* 1979. Modeling and labelling as integrated determinants of children's sex-typed imitative behavior. Child Dev. **50:** 364–371.
26. PERRY, D.G. & K. BUSSEY. 1979. The social learning theory of sex difference: imitation is alive and well. J. Pers. Soc. Psychol. **37:** 1699–1712.
27. EHRHARDT, A.A. & S.W. BAKER. 1974. Fetal androgens, human central nervous system differentiation, and behavior sex differences. *In* Sex Differences in Behavior. R.C. Friedman, R.M. Richart & R.L. van de Wiele, Eds.: 33–52. Wiley. New York.
28. HINES, M., S. GOLOMBOK, J. RUST, *et al.* 2002. Testosterone during pregnancy and childhood gender role behavior: a longitudinal population study. Child Dev. **73:** 1678–1687.
29. ALEXANDER, G.M. & M. HINES. 2002. Sex differences in response to children's toys in nonhuman primates (Cercopithecus aethiops sabaeus). Evol. Hum. Behav. **23:** 467–479.
30. BARBIERI, R.L. 1999. Endocrine disorders in pregnancy. *In* Reproductive Endocrinology: Physiology, Pathophysiology and Clinical Management. S.S.C. Yen, R.B. Jaffe & R.L. Barbieri, Eds.: 785–812. W.B. Saunders. Philadelphia.
31. WILKINS, L. 1960. Masculinization of female fetus due to use of orally given progestins. J. Am. Med. Assoc. **172:** 1028–1032.
32. HARRIS, J.A., P.A. VERNON & D.I. BOOMSMA. 1998. The heritability if testosterone: a study of Dutch adolescent twins and their parents. Behav. Genet. **28:** 165–171.
33. SLUYTER, F., J.M. KEIJSER, D.I. BOOMSMA, *et al.*. 2000. Genetics of testosterone and the aggression-hostility-anger (AHA) syndrome: a study of middle aged male twins. Twin Res. **3:** 266–276.
34. DITTMANN, R.W., M.E. KAPPES & M.H. KAPPES. 1992. Sexual behavior in adolescent and adult females with congenital adrenal hyperplasia. Psychoneuroendocrinology **17:** 153–170.
35. HINES, M., C. BROOK & G.S. CONWAY. 2004. Androgen and psychosexual development: core gender identity, sexual orientation and recalled childhood gender role behavior in women and men with congenital adrenal hyperplasia (CAH). J. Sex Res. In press.
36. MONEY, J., M. SCHWARTZ & V. LEWIS. 1984. Adult erotosexual status and fetal hormonal masculinization and demasculinization: 46 XX congenital virilizing adrenal hyperplasia and 46 XY androgen-insensitivity syndrome compared. Psychoneuroendocrinology **9:** 405–414.
37. ZUCKER, K.J., S.J. BRADLEY, G. OLIVER, *et al.* 1996. Psychosexual development of women with congenital adrenal hyperplasia. Horm. Behav. **30:** 300–318.

38. HERRENKOHL, L.R. 1979. Prenatal stress reduces fertility and fecundity in female offspring. Science **206:** 1097–1099.
39. SACHSER, N. & S. KAISER. 1996. Prenatal social stress masculinizes the females behaviour in guinea pigs. Physiol. Behav. **60:** 589–594.
40. WARD, I.L. 1984. The prenatal stress syndrome: current status. Psychoneuroendocrinology **9:** 3–11.
41. WARD, I.L. & K.E. STEHM. 1991. Prenatal stress feminizes juvenile play patterns in male rats. Physiol. Behav. **50:** 601–605.
42. BECKHARDT, S. & I.L. WARD. 1983. Reproductive functioning in the prenatally stressed female rat. Dev. Psychobiol. **16:** 111–118.
43. VOM SAAL, F.S., D.M. QUADAGNO, M.D. EVEN, *et al.* 1990. Paradoxical effects of maternal stress in fetal steroids and postnatal reproductive traits in female mice from different intrauterine positions. Biol. Reprod. **43:** 761.
44. DORNER, G., B. SCHENK, B. SCHMIEDEL & L. AHRENS. 1983. Stressful events in prenatal life of bi-and homosexual men. Exp. Clin. Endocrinol. **81:** 83–87.
45. BAILEY, J.M., L. WILLERMAN & C. PARKS. 1991. A test of the maternal stress theory of human male homosexuality. Arch. Sex. Behav. **20:** 277–293.
46. ELLIS, L., M.A. AMES, W. PECKHAM & D. BURKE. 1988. Sexual orientation of human offspring may be altered by severe maternal stress during pregnancy. J. Sex Res. **25:** 152–157.
47. SCHMIDT, G. & U. CLEMENT. 1990. Does peace prevent homosexuality? Arch. Sex. Behav. **19:** 183–187.
48. HINES, M., K. JOHNSTON, S. GOLOMBOK, *et al.* 2002. Prenatal stress and gender role behavior in girls and boys: a longitudinal, population study. Horm. Behav. **42:** 126–134.
49. NAKASHIMA, A., K. KOSHIYAMA, T. UOZUMI, *et al.* 1975. Effects of general anaesthesia and severity of surgical stress on serum LH and testosterone in males. Acta Endocrinol. (Copenh.) **78:** 258–269.
50. LINDH, A., K. CARLSTROM, J. EKLUND & N. WILKING. 1992. Serum steroids and prolactin during and after major surgical trauma. Acta Anaesthesiol. Scand. **36:** 119–124.
51. KLIBANSKI, A., I.Z. BEITINS, R. BADGER, *et al.* 1981. Reproductive function during fasting in men. J. Clin. Endocrinol. Metabol. **53:** 258–263.
52. SACHAR, E.J. 1980. Hormonal changes in stress and mental illness. *In* Neuroendocrinology. D.T. Krieger & J.C. Hughes, Eds.: 177–183. H.P. Publishing. New York.
53. BROWN-GRANT, K., G. FINK, F. GREIG & M.A.F. MURRAY. 1975. Altered sexual development in male rats after oestrogen administration during the neonatal period. J. Reprod. Fertil. **44:** 25–42.
54. PANG, S., L.S. LEVINE, D.M. CHOW, *et al.* 1979. Serum androgen concentrations in neonates and young infants with congenital adrenal hyperplasia due to 21-hydroxylase deficiency. Clin. Endocrinol. **11:** 575–584.
55. RUST, J., S. GOLOMBOK, M. HINES, *et al.* 2000. The role of brothers and sisters in the gender development of preschool children. J. Exp. Child Psychol. **77:** 292–303.

Estradiol Modulation of Astrocytes and the Establishment of Sex Differences in the Brain

M.M. McCARTHY, B.J. TODD, AND S.K. AMATEA

Department of Physiology and Program in Neuroscience, University of Maryland, Baltimore, School of Medicine, Baltimore, Maryland 21201, USA

ABSTRACT: The role of steroid hormones as a conduit for reciprocal glial–neuronal communication is an emerging but relatively unexplored concept. Research in our laboratory has discovered that the relationship between astrocytic and neuronal morphology during development is distinct for different brain regions and provides a fundamental basis for region-specific sexual differentiation. The functional significance of estradiol-induced differentiation of astrocytes and the cross-talk of these cells with neurons includes permanent changes in synaptic patterning and control of adult reproductive behaviors. The cellular mechanisms as currently understood for each region are discussed and unanswered questions as well as other areas for future research are reviewed.

KEYWORDS: preoptic area; development; arcuate nucleus; reproductive behavior

INTRODUCTION

Astrocytes, a subtype of glia found throughout the brain, including the hypothalamus and preoptic area (POA), compose up to 10–20% of the neuropil.[6] Many of these cells are considered protoplasmic astrocytes because of the pronounced morphological plasticity that they show in response to extracellular stimuli, including steroid hormones, neurotransmitters, injury, and osmotic stress. Changes in astrocyte morphology can occur as rapidly as 10 min or can span several hours to days. Having a relatively restricted radius of 50 µm, they have an impact on the local environment by communicating with neighboring astrocytes, endothelial cells, and neurons. Involvement of astrocytes in synaptic functioning is in part evident by preferential coverage at synapses as compared with other portions of the neuron.[6] Additional evidence is the presence of neurotransmitter receptors on astrocytes,[56] which when activated can increase intracellular calcium concentrations.[7] Moreover, glial cells release transmitters of their own in response to elevated intracellular calcium.[4,54] These and other observations provide support for the concept that glial cells play a crucial role in regulating synaptic transmission. This regulation may be indirect, via uptake or release of critical neurochemicals, a direct physical effect in which astrocytic process retract from or ensheath synapses, or some combination of the two. The degree of ensheathment can be altered by endogenous[5,32] or

Address for correspondence: Margaret M. McCarthy, Ph.D., Department of Physiology, 655 W. Baltimore Street, Baltimore, MD 21201. Voice: 410-706-2655; fax: 410-706-8341. mmccarth@umaryland.edu

Ann. N.Y. Acad. Sci. 1007: 283–297 (2003). © 2003 New York Academy of Sciences.
doi: 10.1196/annals.1286.027

exogenous[19] stimuli. The gonadal steroid hormone, estradiol, is a potent regulator of glial ensheathment of synapses in some brain areas, most notably the arcuate nucleus.[18,19,21,39] Glial ensheathment of synapses also is related to modulation of neurotransmission indirectly as proximity influences the ability of astrocytic processes to uptake or release neurochemicals.

ESTRADIOL MEDIATES SEXUAL DIFFERENTIATION OF THE RODENT BRAIN

The establishment of sex differences in the brain occurs during a restricted perinatal sensitive period and is consequent to dimorphic gonadal steroid hormone exposure in males versus females. The conversion of testicular testosterone to estradiol by neurons of the perinatal brain is an obligatory step in the establishment of a male phenotype for numerous sexually dimorphic brain traits in rodents.[62] Sex differences in the brain occur on multiple levels, from the molecular to global, but two fundamental characteristics amenable to investigation are differences in the size or volume of distinct structures, including nuclei, and the synaptic patterning present in a particular region. The latter refers to the density of axosomatic versus axodendritic spinous synapses, which have been shown to vary drastically between males and females in the arcuate nucleus[33] and are less well documented in the POA.[58] Volumetric sex differences, such as the larger sexually dimorphic nucleus (SDN) in males and the larger anteroventral periventricular nucleus (AVPv) in females, are the result of greater naturally occurring cell death in one sex over the other.[62] Beyond a role for estradiol, the signal cascades regulating this differential cell death remain entirely unknown. Likewise, beyond a role for estradiol, the cellular mechanisms regulating sexually dimorphic synaptic patterning also remain elusive. We review here the role of estradiol in cross-talk between the neurons and astrocytes of the arcuate nucleus and POA and present evidence that this relationship is critical to the establishment of sex differences in synaptic patterning but may play little role in controlling cell death and hence volumetric sex differences.

ASTROCYTES ARE SEXUALLY DIFFERENTIATED BY ESTRADIOL EARLY IN DEVELOPMENT IN THE ARCUATE NUCLEUS AND PREOPTIC AREA

Protoplasmic astrocytes of the developing arcuate nucleus and POA can be visualized with immunocytochemistry for glial fibrillary acidic protein (GFAP) as early as the first day of life, a trait not found in some other sexually dimorphic brain regions, such as the ventromedial hypothalamus.[2,39] GFAP is a structural protein found throughout the numerous processes of astrocytes and allows for morphometric analysis of these complex cells. Using region-specific strategies for assessing astrocyte morphology, we have determined the same endpoint for the arcuate nucleus and POA, which is that astrocytes in males are more complex than those in females, having more, longer, and more frequently branching process. In females, astrocytes of these two brain regions remain relatively bipolar, having shorter primary processes with infrequent branching. In both regions, the conversion of testosterone to estradi-

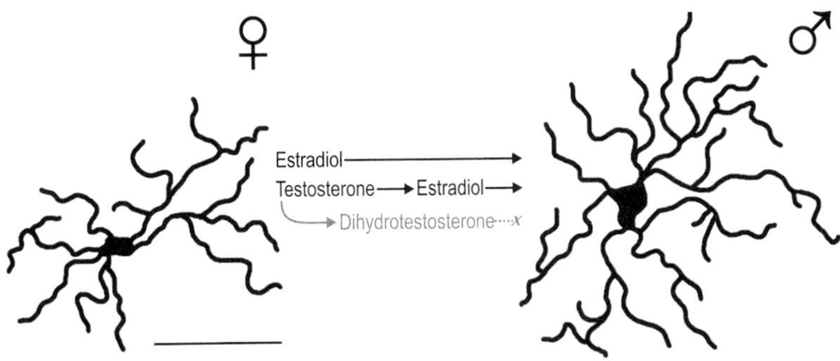

FIGURE 1. GFAP reveals sexually dimorphic astrocytes in the arcuate nucleus and preoptic area as early as the day of birth. Representative tracings of two perinatal POA astrocytes. Immunocytochemical detection of GFAP reveals dimorphic astrocytes in the arcuate and POA on the first day of life with those of the female (*left*) exhibiting less complex morphology compared with those of the male (*right*). Exposure to either estradiol or testosterone, but not the non-aromatizable steroid, dihydrotestosterone, masculinizes the morphology of the female astrocyte, suggesting that this steroid hormone mediates the naturally occurring sex difference (scale bar = 25 μM).

ol is a requisite for establishing dimorphic astrocyte morphology[36] (see FIG. 1). There is evidence to support the concept of a direct action of estradiol on astrocytes. Several studies[24,25,59,51,63] have demonstrated immunoreactivity or mRNA for both the alpha and beta forms of the estrogen receptor in cultured astrocytes from many brain regions including hypothalamus. To date, however, there is no evidence to suggest that either form of the estrogen receptor is present in astrocytes *in vivo*.[40] Thus, whereas there exists the potential for a direct effect of estradiol on the astrocytes, evidence for estrogen receptors in these cells remains lacking. Neurons of both the arcuate nucleus and POA, on the other hand, express high levels of estradiol receptors[11] Astrocytes within the arcuate nucleus and POA are sexually dimorphic as early as postnatal day 0 (PN0) , and this dimorphism is apparent through days 2, 5, 10, and 15 of life and continues into adulthood.[41] Astrocytes throughout the brain increase their expression of GFAP with age, but in the arcuate the magnitude of the sex difference does not change from that observed at PN0, indicating that once initial differentiation occurs, male rats maintain increased astrocyte differentiation throughout life. The ontogeny of sexually dimorphic astrocytes in the POA has been less well established than in the arcuate nucleus. As in the arcuate nucleus, the morphology of astrocytes in this area is sexually dimorphic as early as PN0,[2] and this sex difference is also apparent on PN3. As with the arcuate nucleus, perinatal exposure to estradiol or testosterone masculinizes the female brain, rendering astrocytes indistinguishable from those of males on PN3. The similarities between the POA and arcuate nucleus end here, because there is a striking divergence in the relationship between astrocytic and neuronal morphology in these two sexually dimorphic brain regions.

ESTRADIOL AFFECTS ASTROCYTE MORPHOLOGY AND NEURONAL DENDRITIC SPINE DENSITY THROUGH DIFFERENT PATHWAYS IN THE ARCUATE NUCLEUS AND PREOPTIC AREA

Although estradiol increases the complexity of astrocytes in both the arcuate nucleus and POA, it has opposite effects on neuronal dendritic spine density, decreasing dendritic spines in the arcuate nucleus while simultaneously increasing them in the POA. Thus, there is not a simple unitary mechanism by which estradiol mediates differentiation of the male brain. It is striking that the same hormone, estradiol, can have the same effect on one cell type, astrocytes, but the exact opposite on another, neurons, in brain regions separated by only a few millimeters. These two regions serve to highlight the simultaneous convergent and divergent effects of estradiol but are merely representative. Evidence suggests there are also distinct estradiol-mediated mechanisms at play in the ventromedial nucleus of the hypothalamus and the hippocampus, and likely other brain regions which have not yet been examined. Nonetheless, for purposes of review and speculation, we focus on the two regions best characterized as this point in time.

Arcuate Nucleus

In the arcuate nucleus, neuronally derived GABA mediates estradiol's effects on astrocyte morphology (see FIG. 2A). Estradiol increases the level of hypothalamic glutamic acid decarboxylase (GAD), the rate-limiting enzyme involved in the synthesis of GABA.[37] Levels of GABA and mRNA for GAD are higher in the arcuate nucleus of neonatal males compared with females,[8,9] corresponding with the critical period for steroid-mediated astrocyte differentiation. Manipulating this system in the neonatal male or masculinized female by knocking down GAD levels with antisense oligodeoxynucleotides results in blockade of steroid-induced astrocyte differentiation. Moreover, administration of the $GABA_A$ receptor agonist, muscimol, to neonatal females results in a male-like astrocytic phenotype; astrocytes are more complex, with increased stellation and greater mean process length than control females[42] (see FIG. 2B). This effect of GABA is also apparent *in vitro*, in which the $GABA_A$ receptor antagonist bicuculline blocks astrocyte differentiation in mixed astrocyte-neuronal cultures.[34,35] $GABA_A$ receptors are present on astrocytes in other regions of the brain[16,57] and are presumably present on arcuate astrocytes as well.

In mature mammalian neurons, GABA acts primarily as an inhibitory neurotransmitter, binding its ionotropic receptor to open a chloride channel, resulting in chloride influx and consequent membrane hyperpolarization. In neonatal astrocytes, however, the reversal potential for chloride is more positive than in mature neurons. $GABA_A$ receptor activation therefore causes chloride efflux sufficient to depolarize the cell membrane[17] and open voltage-gated calcium channels, leading to a calcium transient.[16,45,46] This effect can be blocked by nimodipine,[17] indicating that the L-type calcium channel is involved in $GABA_A$ receptor–mediated depolarization of astrocytes.

The assembly and disassembly of astrocytic intermediate filaments are modulated by the phosphorylation status of GFAP. There is increasing evidence that GFAP is phosphorylated by cAMP-dependent and calcium-dependent protein kinases.[30,47] Although there is as yet no evidence linking $GABA_A$ receptor activation to GFAP phosphorylation, increased intracellular calcium concentrations resulting from

$GABA_A$ receptor activation may stimulate these second messenger pathways, resulting in astrocyte process extension and branching. This may provide the molecular mechanism underpinning the physical relationship between astrocyte complexity and estradiol action on neurons to increase GABA synthesis and release.

Gonadal steroid-mediated increases in astrocyte complexity in the arcuate nucleus occur coincident with a reduction in both dendritic spine density[40] and axos-

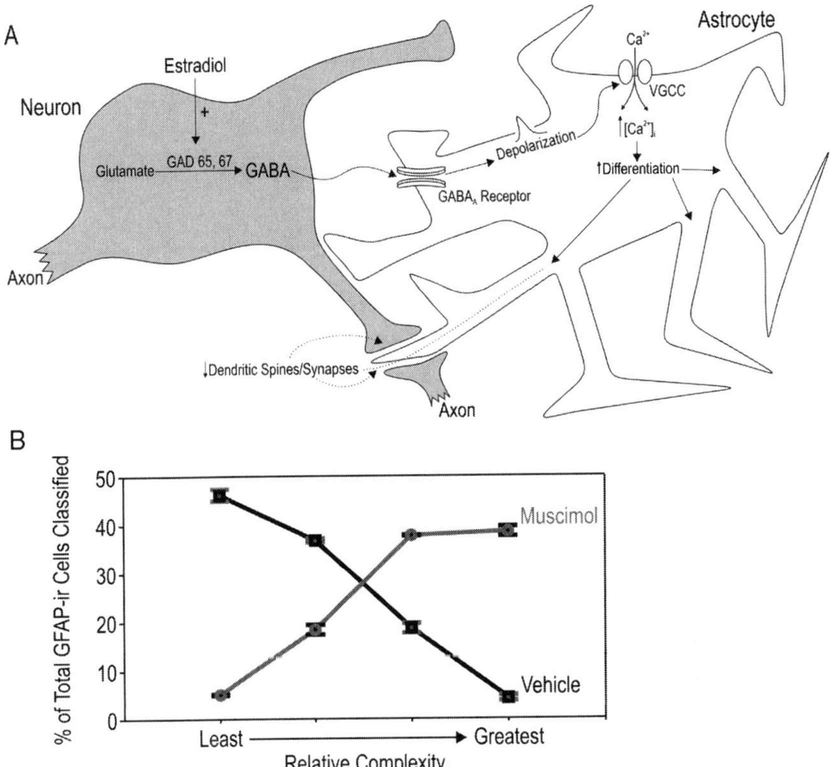

FIGURE 2. GABA as a messenger of estradiol-induced differentiation in the developing arcuate nucleus. (**A**) Schematic representation of gamma-amino butyric acid (GABA) as a messenger of differentiation from neurons to astrocytes in the developing arcuate. Estradiol increases the synthesis of neuronal GABA by up-regulating the expression of its synthetic enzyme, GAD. GABA diffuses from the neuron and binds to $GABA_A$ receptors of nearby astrocytes. Activation of these receptors generates a local depolarization sufficient to activate voltage gated calcium channels (VGCCs), causing a transient influx of calcium (Ca^{2+}). Although brief, this increase in internal Ca^{2+} may trigger any of several Ca^{2+}-dependent second messenger systems, including those responsible for the polymerization of glial fibrillary acidic protein (GFAP) and the subsequent differentiation of the astrocyte. (**B**) Perinatal females treated with the $GABA_A$ receptor agonist, muscimol, displayed within 48 h a drastic increase in the frequency of highly differentiated astrocytes in the arcuate compared with vehicle-treated females. These data implicate GABA, a purely neuronal factor, as the mediator of hormonally directed astrocyte differentiation in the arcuate nucleus (redrawn from original data presented in Mong, Nunez, and McCarthy, 2002, J. Neuroendo. **14:** 1–16).

pinous synapses.[43] The specific mechanisms by which gonadal steroids influence synaptic patterning are unknown, but astrocytes are recognized to play a crucial role in synaptogenesis. Indeed, in the adult female arcuate nucleus, astrocytes are responsive to the endogenous hormone changes across the estrous cycle and play an integral part in the synaptic remodeling that occurs in this region.[5,20,53] This remodeling is important to the function of the GnRH "surge generator." When circulating estrogens are high, astrocytic surface area increases, such that astrocyte processes ensheath arcuate neurons. This prevents inhibitory synaptic input, which provides a permissive environment for the preovulatory LH surge. Evidence is mounting that a similar physical mechanism is occurring in the male neonatal arcuate nucleus, resulting in the above-mentioned reduction in dendritic spine density and synapse formation compared with the female. However, in this instance, the estradiol-induced changes in astrocyte morphology, and hence neuronal morphology, are permanent as opposed to plastic like those in the adult female. A question that arises is how such a permanency can be maintained. Recent findings regarding synaptic plasticity in the hippocampus may provide a clue. The Eph family of receptor tyrosine kinases are activated by ligands that are themselves membrane bound and can reverse signal to their host cell, allowing for bidirectional signaling. In the case of the EphA receptor, which localizes to the region of dendritic spine synapses, the principle ligand, ephrin A3, is anchored in the membranes of immediately adjacent astrocytes. Activation of the EphA receptor by ephrin A3 results in spine retraction.[44] If there is a high level of EphA receptor activation by ephrin ligands anchored in the membranes of arcuate astrocytes, a permanent suppression of dendritic spines could be established, resulting in the sexually dimorphic patterning observed in adults.[33] This possibility remains to be investigated.

Preoptic Area

Like the arcuate, the astrocytes of the neonatal POA respond to gonadal steroids with increases in process number and branching.[2] Unlike the arcuate nucleus though, markers of dendritic spine density show that in this region, high levels of gonadal steroids in the brain are associated with increased dendritic spines.[1] This observation suggests a distinct mode of cross-talk between astrocytes and neurons in this more rostral region of the brain. Our laboratory has begun to elucidate the mechanisms by which astrocytes and neurons interact in the POA (see FIG. 3A). Prostaglandin-E_2 (PGE_2), but not other prostanoids, mimics the effect of estradiol on markers of spine density *in vivo* and *in vitro*. Indomethacin, an inhibitor of the prostanoid synthesis enzyme cyclooxygenase-2 (COX-2) blocks the action of estradiol on neurons. The actions of both estradiol and PGE_2 are attenuated by AMPA-kainate, but not NMDA receptor antagonists. These observations suggest a model in which the actions of estradiol, PGE_2, and glutamate are in series. Specifically, we propose that estradiol increases PGE_2 in neurons which then diffuses to act on local astrocytes causing release of glutamate which then acts back on the neurons to induce dendritic spines.

Experiments addressing the exact site of action of estrogen and PGE_2 in the neuron/astrocyte/neuron signaling pathway are still in progress. Once again, the issue of estrogen receptor location is relevant. In addition, it is uncertain whether COX-2 is present in the neurons, the astrocytes, or both.[29,52] Although we have not yet verified it in our system, evidence suggests that astrocytes are responsive to PGE_2,[14,26] and release glutamate after PGE_2 stimulation,[4,60] which in our model acts on neuronal AMPA-kainate receptors. Notably, this mechanism by which PGE_2 mediates the action of estradiol is region specific, because in the hippocampus, also an estrogen sensitive area of the brain, PGE_2 does not increase markers of neuronal spine density.[1] Finally, we have investigated whether PGE_2, presumably of neuronal origin, is the mediator of the sex differences in astrocyte morphology observed in the POA. The answer seems to be, partly, as treatment with exogenous PGE_2 increased the length of primary processes of POA astrocytes to only half the level induced by estradiol. Moreover, the effect of estradiol was reduced by approximately half when combined with the PGE_2 synthesis inhibitor, indomethacin (see FIG. 3B). Although it is possible that these partial effects are caused by dosage or access of the drugs, this seems

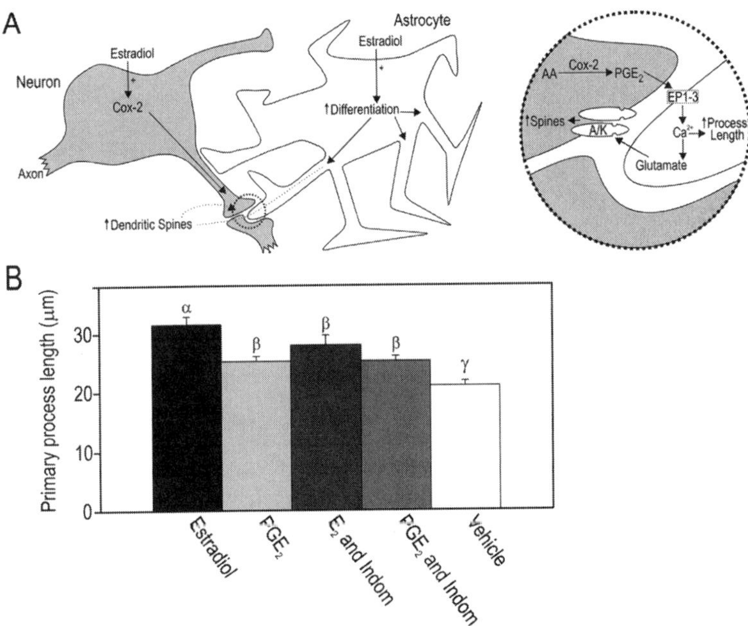

FIGURE 3. PGE_2 as a messenger of estradiol-induced differentiation in the developing preoptic area. (**A**) Schematic representation of reciprocal communication between neighboring astrocytes and neurons in the developing POA. Estradiol initiates the cascade, binding neuronal receptors and up-regulating proteins, such as the dendritic spine enriched COX-2, needed to specifically synthesize and release neuronal PGE_2. Neighboring astrocytes respond to diffusible PGE_2 by releasing glutamate, which back-communicates to activate neuronal non-NMDA ionotropic glutamate receptors, a process that has been implicated in dendritic spine modification. AA, arachidonic acid; EP, prostaglandin receptor subtypes 1–3; A/K, AMPA/kainate glutamate receptor. (**B**) Female preoptic area astrocytes exposed to 2 μg PGE_2 for 48 h beginning on the first day of life exhibited longer primary processes than those of vehicle-treated females, although to only half the length induced by estradiol. Importantly, coadministration of the COX-2 inhibitor indomethacin (subcutaneous injections of 25 μg) partially attenuated estradiol's effect on primary process length. These data suggest that multiple mechanisms, including one involving PGE_2, lie downstream of estradiol-mediated differentiation of preoptic astrocyte morphology (dissimilar letters denote significant differences, one-way ANOVA; Student-Neuman-Keuls post hoc analysis with significance at $\alpha < 0.5$, $P < 0.01$).

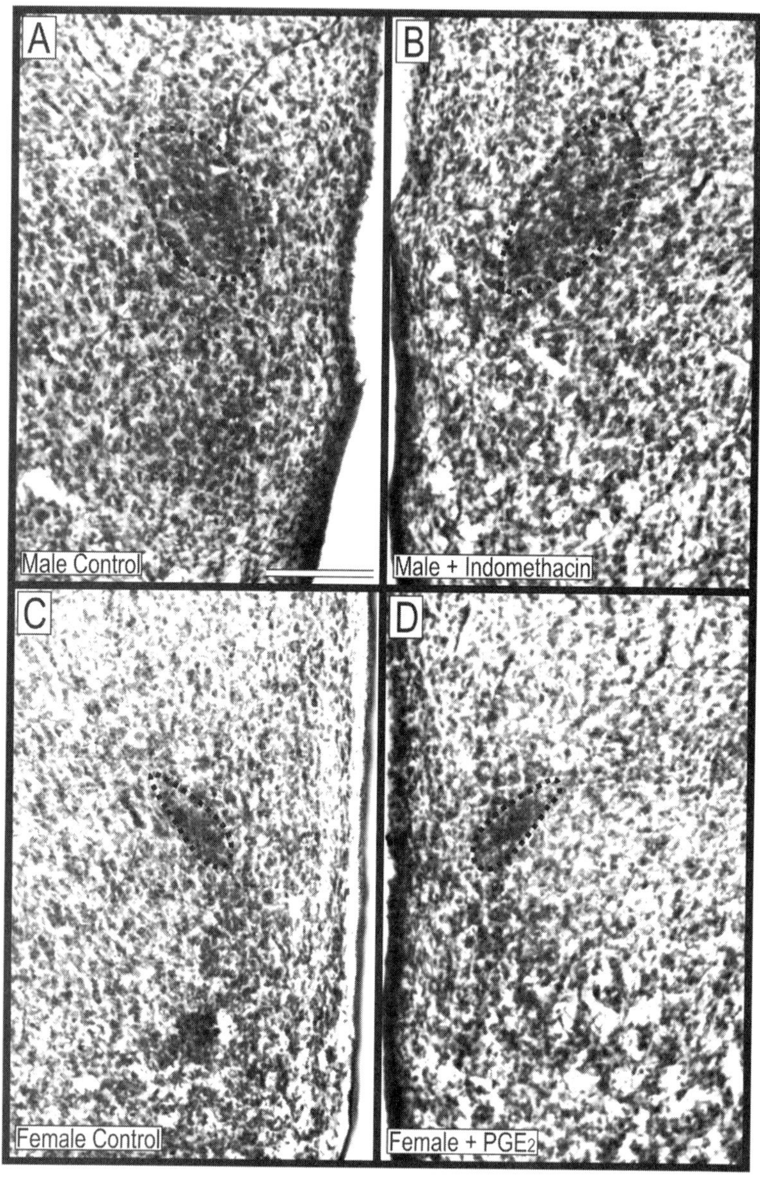

FIGURE 4. PGE_2-mediated estrogen action on the POA has no effect on the volume of the sexually dimorphic nucleus. (**A–D**) Representative photomicrographs of thionin-stained coronal brain sections collected at PN17 of the POA incorporating the SDN (outlined in each) from control males (**A**), indomethacin-treated males (**B**, 25 μg s.c., twice daily beginning on PN0 and ending on PN1), control females (**C**), and PGE_2-treated females (**D**, 2 μg bilateral i.c.v., twice daily beginning on PN0 and ending on PN1) (scale bar = 1 mm).

unlikely given the magnitude of the behavioral effects observed (see below). Thus, there appears to be more than one mechanism mediating astrocyte complexity in the POA and a direct action of estradiol on the astrocytes themselves cannot be ruled out.

FUNCTIONAL SIGNIFICANCE OF CHANGES IN ASTROCYTE MORPHOLOGY IN THE POA APPEARS SPECIFIC TO SYNAPTIC PATTERNING

Estrogens play a well-known role in modulating apoptotic pathways in many regions of the brain (reviewed in Wise[65]) and are crucial in establishing the sex difference in the volume of the SDN of the POA.[3,10,22] Data presented thus far speak only to the influence of this putative model on synaptic patterning, that is, neuronal spine density and synapse formation. We also have investigated the role of the prostaglandin-mediated estradiol signaling in development of the SDN (see FIG. 4). We used an identical paradigm to that which caused an up-regulation of dendritic spine markers in females and blocked estradiol's induction of spines in males. Animals were killed on PN17 and the SDN volume was calculated. Although we observed the predictable sex difference in volume, the SDN volume of PGE_2-treated females was not different from that of control females. There were also no differences between indomethacin-treated males and control males. Estrogens affect cell survival, and therefore nucleus volume by up-regulating antiapoptotic proteins such as bcl-2.[12,55]

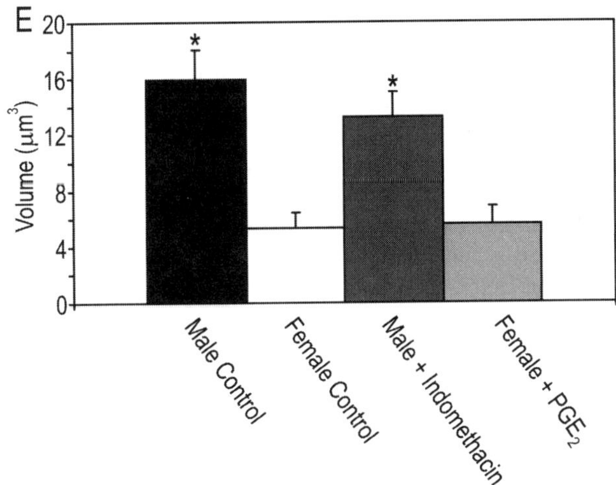

FIGURE 4E. Quantification of SDN volumes of each of the four groups displayed in the panels beside. Volumes were collected bilaterally under a Nikon ×4 objective from a minimum of six animals per group using the computer-integrated microscopic Neurolucida system. There was a significant difference in the SDN volume between males and females; however, there were no differences in SDN volume between treatment and control groups (*significantly different from female groups; one-way ANOVA; Student-Neuman-Keuls post hoc; $P < 0.001$). Therefore, we conclude that PGE_2 mediation of estradiol actions in the developing POA affects synaptic patterning but not cell survival.

Although we did not perform cell counts *per se*, there has been a reliable correlation between neuron number and volume of the SDN in numerous past studies (this is not the case for some song control nuclei in birds in which cell density and nuclear volume are not always concordant). This leads us to the speculation that, because PGE_2 had no effect on SDN volume in female POA, PGE_2-mediated estrogen action on the POA may be restricted to synaptic patterning rather than cell survival. This finding is particularly interesting in lieu of the profound effects of early treatment with PGE_2 or indomethacin on adult male sexual behavior.

BEHAVIORAL IMPLICATIONS OF CHANGES IN ASTROCYTE AND NEURONAL MORPHOLOGY IN THE NEONATAL POA FOR MALE SEXUAL BEHAVIOR

The POA is an essential brain area for expression of male sexual behavior by the adult.[38] Therefore, after establishing that estradiol exerts an organizational effect on POA neurons and astrocytes through a PGE_2–glutamate-mediated pathway, we next determined if the effects of neonatal estradiol on adult sexual behavior could be mimicked by treatment of neonatal females with exogenous PGE_2. Toward this end, neonatal PGE_2- and vehicle-treated controls were raised to adulthood, gonadectomized, and implanted with testosterone secreting capsules before being tested in a standard male sexual behavior paradigm using hormonally primed stimulus females. Three tests of 20 minutes duration at 1-week intervals revealed that males were unaffected by PGE_2 treatment, as would be expected. In contrast, females treated with PGE_2 exhibited a marked induction of male sexual behavior as evidenced by a decreased latency to mount and increased frequency of mounts and intromission-like behavior toward stimulus females. The behavior of PGE_2-treated females was significantly different from vehicle-treated females, which showed very little male sexual behavior and was indistinguishable from that of male littermates treated with either PGE_2 or vehicle (see FIG. 5). These behavioral observations strongly implicate an early establishment of sexually dimorphic patterning and changes in astrocyte morphology as major determinants of adult sexual behavior; to our knowledge, they constitute one of the first demonstrations of an association between early changes in brain morphology and adult behavior. Future experiments will examine the effects of treatment with the COX-2 inhibitor, indomethacin, as well as determine if changes in synaptic patterning observed in the first few days of life persist into adulthood.

ARE THERE BEHAVIORAL IMPLICATIONS OF CHANGES IN ASTROCYTE AND NEURONAL MORPHOLOGY IN THE NEONATAL POA FOR FEMALE REPRODUCTIVE BEHAVIORS?

Having established a positive correlation between neonatal neuronal morphology and male sexual behavior in the adult, we now have a unique opportunity to investigate if this morphology also correlates negatively with other sexually dimorphic behaviors. In other words, will a masculinized POA preclude the expression of female behaviors such as lordosis and maternal behavior? The POA is a key structure regulating the initiation and maintenance of maternal behavior.[48,50] Lesions in this

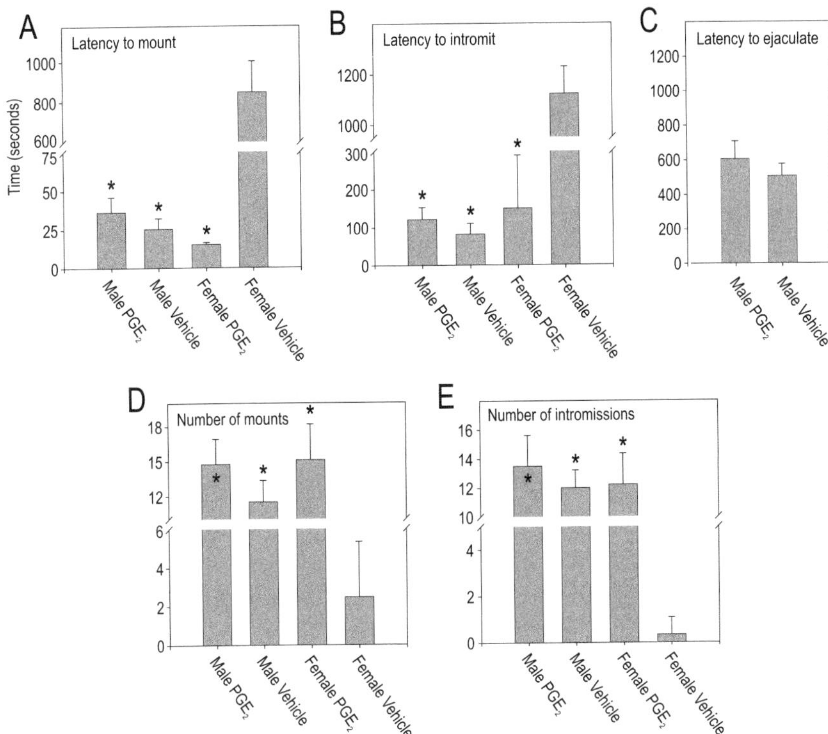

FIGURE 5. Early exposure to PGE_2 masculinizes the sex behavior of female rodents. Neonatal males and females were treated with PGE_2 (2 μg bilateral i.c.v., twice daily beginning on PN0 and ending on PN1) and raised to adulthood for behavioral testing. Around PN40, males and females were gonadectomized and implanted with a testosterone secreting silastic capsule. Three weeks later, they were observed for male sexual behavior with a sexually receptive female during a 20-min trial. Testing was repeated at weekly intervals for two more weeks. PGE_2-treated females exhibited marked masculinized sexual behaviors. The latency to both mount (**A**) and display intromission-like behaviors (**B**) decreased significantly to levels no different than those displayed by control males. The frequency of each also became male typic in PGE_2-treated females (**D**, **E**). Males were unaffected by PGE_2 treatment (*significantly different from vehicle-treated females; repeated measures ANOVA; Student-Neuman-Keuls post hoc analysis with significance at $\alpha < 0.5$, $P < 0.01$).

region[27,64] and lesions of projections between this and other regions such as the substantia nigra,[49] amygdala,[15] and ventral tegmental area[51] prevent proper maternal retrieval and grooming of pups. Moreover, Fos immunoreactivity is up-regulated in this region coincident with maternal behavior[31] Several circulating factors converge to act on the POA and modulate its effect on behavior. Estrogen implants in the POA stimulate maternal behavior in virgin female rats.[13] As with lordosis behavior, maternal behavior in the adult rat is influenced by the perinatal hormone environment. Because PGE_2 mediates the effects of estradiol in the developing POA, it is possible that it is also involved in the organizational effects of steroids in establishing brain connections for these female behaviors as well, and this will be the focus of future studies.

SUMMARY AND PERSPECTIVES

The importance of astrocytes to the establishment and maintenance of synapses is becoming increasingly evident. The closer we look, the more we find regarding the multitude of functions these cells serve. Of late, there has been a suggestion that their role may even go beyond the structural; that astrocytes *themselves* may be the source of memory formation and play an integral role in signaling associated with variance in behavior.[28] Comparative analyses between simple to complex organisms indicate that the glia-to-neuron ratio increases by a factor of 10 from nematodes to rodents and by 10 again from rodents to primates.[23] Rapid neuronal signaling is just as effective in the brain of a rat as in that of a primate, but what varies is the ability for complex thoughts and behaviors. These facts, and observations of plasticity exhibited by astrocytes in animals raised in enriched versus deprived environments, have led to the speculation that astrocytes themselves may be an important source of encoding information essential for behavioral variation.[28]

We have discussed here that astrocytes are also a heretofore unknown target of steroid hormone-mediated sexual differentiation, and we present evidence that this differentiation is likely indirect, requiring the steroid-addressed neuron as an essential partner. Astrocytes then communicate back to neurons, using regionally specific messengers, to alter the pattern of synapses, and ultimately functioning in the adult brain.

REFERENCES

1. Amateau, S.K. & M.M. McCarthy. 2002. A novel mechanism of dendritic spine plasticity involving estradiol induction of prostaglandin-E2. J. Neurosci. **22:** 8586–8596.
2. Amateau, S.K. & M.M. McCarthy. 2002. Sexual differentiation of astrocyte morphology in the developing rat preoptic area. J. Neuroendocrinol. **14:** 904–910.
3. Arai, Y., Y. Sekine & S. Murakami. 1996. Estrogen and apoptosis in the developing sexually dimorphic preoptic area in female rats. Neurosci. Res. **25:** 403–407.
4. Bezzi, P., G. Carmignoto, L. Pasti, *et al.* 1998. Prostaglandins stimulate calcium-dependent glutamate release in astrocytes. Nature **391:** 281–285.
5. Cashion, A.B., M.J. Smith & P.M. Wise. 2003. The morphometry of astrocytes in the rostral preoptic area exhibits a diurnal rhythm on proestrus: relationship to the luteinizing hormone surge and effects of age. Endocrinology **144**: 274–280.
6. Chao, T.I., M. Rickmann & J.R. Wolf. 2002. The synapse-astrocyte boundary: an anatomical basis for an integrative role of glia in synaptic transmission. *In* A. Volterra, P.J. Magistretti & P.G. Haydon, Eds.: 3–23. The Tripartite Synapse. Glia in Synaptic Transmission. Oxford University Press. New York.
7. Cornell-Bell, A.H. & S.M. Finkbeiner. 1991. Ca^{2+} waves in astrocytes. Cell Calcium **12:** 185–204.
8. Davis, A.M., D.R. Grattan, M. Selmanoff & M.M. McCarthy. 1996. Sex differences in glutamic acid decarboxylase mRNA in neonatal rat brain: implications for sexual differentiation. Horm. Behav. **30:** 538–552.
9. Davis, A.M., S.C. Ward, M. Selmanoff, *et al.* 1999. Developmental sex differences in amino acid neurotransmitter levels in hypothalamic and limbic areas of rat brain. Neuroscience **90:** 1471–1482.

10. DOHLER, K.D., S.S. SRIVASTAVA, J.E. SHRYNE, *et al.* 1984. Differentiation of the sexually dimorphic nucleus in the preoptic area of the rat brain is inhibited by postnatal treatment with an estrogen antagonist. Neuroendocrinology **38:** 297–301.
11. DONCARLOS, L.L. 1996. Developmental profile and regulation of estrogen receptor ER. mRNA expression in the preoptic area of prenatal rats. Dev. Brain Res. **20:** 224–233.
12. DUBAL, D.B., P.J. SHUGHRUE, M.E. WILSON, *et al.* 1999. Estradiol modulates bcl-2 in cerebral ischemia: a potential role for estrogen receptors. J. Neurosci. **19:** 6385–6393.
13. FAHRBACH, S.E. & D.W. PFAFF. 1986. Effect of preoptic region implants of dilute estradiol on the maternal behavior of ovariectomized, nulliparous rats. Horm. Behav. **20:** 354–363.
14. FIEBICH, B.L., S. SCHLEICHER, O. SPLEISS, *et al.* 2001. Mechanisms of prostaglandin E2-induced interleukin-6 release in astrocytes: possible involvement of EP4-like receptors, p38 mitogen-activated protein kinase and protein kinase C. J. Neurochem. **79:** 950–958.
15. FLEMING, A.S., M. MICELI & D. MORETTO. 1983. Lesions of the medial preoptic area prevent the facilitation of maternal behavior produced by amygdala lesions. Physiol. Behav. **31:** 503–510.
16. FRASER, D.D., S. DUFFY, K.J. ANGELIDES, *et al.* 1995. GABAA/benzodiazepine receptors in acutely isolated hippocampal astrocytes. J. Neurosci. **15:** 2720–2732.
17. GANDOLFO, P., E. LOUISET, C. PATTE, *et al.* 2001. The triakontatetraneuropeptide TTN increases $[CA^{2+}]i$ in rat astrocytes through activation of peripheral-type benzodiazepine receptors. Glia **35:** 90–100.
18. GARCIA-SEGURA, L.M., B. CANAS, A. PARDUCZ, *et al.* 1995. Estradiol promotion of changes in the morphology of astroglia growing in culture depends on the expression of polysialic acid of neural membranes. Glia **13:** 209–216.
19. GARCIA-SEGURA, L.M., J.A. CHOWEN, A. PARDUCZ & F. NAFTOLIN. 1994. Gonadal hormones as promoters of structural synaptic plasticity: cellular mechanisms. Prog. Neurobiol. **44:** 279–307.
20. GARCIA-SEGURA, L.M., M. DUENAS, S. BUSIGUINA, *et al.* 1995. Gonadal hormone regulation of neuronal-glial interactions in the developing neuroendocrine hypothalamus. J. Steroid Biochem. Mol. Biol. **53:** 293–298.
21. GARCIA-SEGURA, L.M., I. TORRES-ALEMAN & F. NAFTOLIN. 1989. Astrocytic shape and glial fibrillary acidic protein immunoreactivity are modified by estradiol in primary rat hypothalamic cultures. Brain Res. Dev. Brain Res. **47:** 298–302.
22. HANDA, R.J., P. CORBIER, J.E. SHRYNE, *et al.* 1985. Differential effects of the perinatal steroid environment on three sexually dimorphic parameters of the rat brain. Biol. Reprod. **32:** 855–864.
23. HAYDON, P.G. 2001. Glia: listening and talking to the synapse. Nat. Rev. Neurosci. **2:** 185–193.
24. HOSLI, E., K. JURASIN, W. RUHL, *et al.* 2001. Colocalization of androgen, estrogen and cholinergic receptors on cultured astrocytes of rat central nervous system. Int. J. Dev. Neurosci. **19:** 11–19.
25. HOSLI, E., W. RUHL & L. HOSLI. 2000. Histochemical and electrophysiological evidence for estrogen receptors on cultured astrocytes: colocalization with cholinergic receptors. Int. J. Dev. Neurosci. **18:** 101–111.
26. ITO, S., K. SUGAMA, N. INAGAKI, *et al.* 1992. Type-1 and type-2 astrocytes are distinct targets for prostaglandins D2, E2, and F2 alpha. Glia **6:** 67–74.
27. JACOBSON, C.D., J. TERKEL, R.A. GORSKI & C.H. SAWYER. 1980. Effects of small medial preoptic area lesions on maternal behavior: retrieving and nest building in the rat. Brain Res. **194:** 471–478.
28. JONES, T.A. & W.T. GREENOUGH. 2002. Behavioral experience-dependent plasticity of glial-neuronal interactions. *In* The Tripartite Synapse. A. Volterra, P.J. Magistretti & P.G. Haydon, Eds.: 248–265. Oxford University Press. New York.
29. KAUFMANN, W.E., P.F. WORLEY, J. PEGG, *et al.* 1996. COX-2, a synaptically induced enzyme, is expressed by excitatory neurons at postsynaptic sites in rat cerebral cortex. Proc. Natl. Acad. Sci. USA **93:** 2317–2321.
30. LEAL, R.B., C.A. GONCALVES & R. RODNIGHT. 1997. Calcium-dependent phosphorylation of glial fibrillary acidic protein (GFAP) in the rat hippocampus: a comparison of

the kinase/phosphatase balance in immature and mature slices using tryptic phosphopeptide mapping. Brain Res. Dev. Brain Res. **104:** 1–10.

31. LONSTEIN, J.S., D.A. SIMMONS, J.M. SWANN & J.M. STERN. 1998. Forebrain expression of c-fos due to active maternal behaviour in lactating rats. Neuroscience **82:** 267–281.
32. LUQUIN, S., F. NAFTOLIN & L.M. GARCIA-SEGURA. 1993. Natural fluctuation and gonadal hormone regulation of astrocyte immunoreactivity in dentate gyrus. J. Neurobiol. **24:** 913–924.
33. MATSUMOTO, A. & Y. ARAI. 1980. Sexual dimorphism in "wiring pattern" in the hypothalamic arcuate nucleus and its modification by neonatal hormonal environment. Brain Res. **19:** 238–242.
34. MATSUTANI, S. & N. YAMAMOTO. 1997. Neuronal regulation of astrocyte morphology in vitro is mediated by GABAergic signaling. Glia **20:** 1–9.
35. MATSUTANI, S. & N. YAMAMOTO. 1998. GABAergic neuron-to-astrocyte signaling regulates dendritic branching in coculture. J. Neurobiol. **37:** 251–264.
36. MCCARTHY, M.M., S.K. AMATEAU & J.A. MONG. 2002. Steroid modulation of astrocytes in the neonatal brain: implications for adult reproductive function. Biol. Reprod. **67:** 691–698.
37. MCCARTHY, M.M., L.C. KAUFMAN, P.J. BROOKS, *et al.* 1995. Estrogen modulation of mRNA levels for the two forms of glutamic acid decarboxylase (GAD) in female rat brain. J. Comp. Neurol. **360:** 685–697.
38. MEISEL, R.L. & B.D. SACHS. 1994. The physiology of male sexual behavior. *In* Physiology of Reproduction. Vol. 2. E. Knobil & J.D. Neill, Eds.: 3–106. Raven Press. New York.
39. MONG, J.A., E. GLASER & M.M. MCCARTHY. 1999. Gonadal steroids promote glial differentiation and alter neuronal morphology in the developing hypothalamus in a regionally specific manner. J. Neurosci. **19:** 1464–1472.
40. MONG, J.A. & M.M. MCCARTHY. 1999. Steroid-induced developmental plasticity in hypothalamic astrocytes: implications for synaptic patterning. J. Neurobiol. **40:** 602–619.
41. MONG, J.A. & M.M. MCCARTHY. 2002. Ontogeny of sexually dimorphic astrocytes in the neonatal rat arcuate. Brain Res. Dev. Brain Res. **139:** 151–158.
42. MONG, J.A., J.L. NUNEZ & M.M. MCCARTHY. 2002. GABA mediates steroid-induced astrocyte differentiation in the neonatal rat hypothalamus. J. Neuroendocrinol. **14:** 45–55.
43. MONG, J.A., R.C. ROBERTS, J.J. KELLY & M.M. MCCARTHY. 2001. Gonadal steroids reduce the density of axospinous synapses in the developing rat arcuate nucleus: an electron microscopy analysis. J. Comp. Neurol. **432:** 259–267.
44. MURAI, K.K., L.N. NGUYEN, F. IRIE, *et al.* 2003. Control of hippocampal dendritic spine morphology through ephrin-A3/EphA4 signaling. Nat. Neurosci. **6:** 153–160.
45. NILSSON, M., P.S. ERIKSSON, L. RONNBACK & E. HANSSON. 1993. GABA induces Ca^{2+} transients in astrocytes. Neuroscience **54:** 605–614.
46. NILSSON, M., E. HANSSON & L. RONNBACK. 1992. Agonist-evoked Ca^{2+} transients in primary astroglial cultures—modulatory effects of valproic acid. Glia **5:** 201–209.
47. NOETZEL, M.J. 1990. Phosphorylation of the glial fibrillary acidic protein. J. Neurosci. Res. **27:** 184–192.
48. NUMAN, M. 1974. Medial preoptic area and maternal behavior in the female rat. J. Comp. Physiol. Psychol. **87:** 746–759.
49. NUMAN, M. & D.S. NAGLE. 1983. Preoptic area and substantia nigra interact in the control of maternal behavior in the rat. Behav. Neurosci. **97:** 120–139.
50. NUMAN, M., J.S. ROSENBLATT & B.R. KOMISARUK. 1977. Medial preoptic area and onset of maternal behavior in the rat. J. Comp. Physiol. Psychol. **91:** 146–164.
51. NUMAN, M. & H.G. SMITH. 1984. Maternal behavior in rats: evidence for the involvement of preoptic projections to the ventral tegmental area. Behav. Neurosci. **98:** 712–727.
52. O'BANION, M.K., J.C. MILLER, J.W. CHANG, *et al.* 1996. Interleukin-1 beta induces prostaglandin G/H synthase-2 cyclooxygenase-2. in primary murine astrocyte cultures. J. Neurochem. **66:** 2532–2540.

53. OLMOS, G., F. NAFTOLIN, J. PEREZ, *et al.* 1989. Synaptic remodeling in the rat arcuate nucleus during the estrous cycle. Neuroscience **32:** 663–667.
54. PASTI, L., A. VOLTERRA, T. POZZAN & G. CARMIGNOTO. 1997. Intracellular calcium oscillations in astrocytes: a highly plastic, bidirectional form of communication between neurons and astrocytes in situ. J. Neurosci. **17:** 7817–7830.
55. PATRONE, C., S. ANDERSSON, L. KORHONEN & D. LINDHOLM. 1999. Estrogen receptor-dependent regulation of sensory neuron survival in developing dorsal root ganglion. Proc. Natl. Acad. Sci. USA **96:** 10905–10910.
56. PORTER, J.T. & K.D. MCCARTHY. 1997. Astrocytic neurotransmitter receptors in situ and in vivo. Prog. Neurobiol. **51:** 439–455.
57. POULTER, M.O. & L.A. BROWN. 1999. Transient expression of GABAA receptor subunit mRNAs in the cellular processes of cultured cortical neurons and glia. Brain Res. Mol. Brain Res. **69:** 44–52.
58. RAISMAN, G. & P.M. FIELD. 1973. Sexual dimorphism in the neuropil of the preoptic area of the rat and its dependence on neonatal androgen. Brain Res. **54:** 1–29.
59. SANTAGATI, S., R.C. MELCANGI, F. CELOTTI, *et al.* 1994. Estrogen receptor is expressed in different types of glial cells in culture. J. Neurochem. **63:** 2058–2064.
60. SANZGIRI, R.P., A. ARAQUE & P.G. HAYDON. 1999. Prostaglandin E2 stimulates glutamate receptor-dependent astrocyte neuromodulation in cultured hippocampal cells. J. Neurobiol. **41:** 221–229.
61. SAVASKAN, E., G. OLIVIERI, F. MEIER, *et al.* 2001. Hippocampal estrogen beta-receptor immunoreactivity is increased in Alzheimer's disease. Brain Res. **908:** 113–119.
62. SIMERLY, R.B. 2002. Wired for reproduction: organization and development of sexually dimorphic circuits in the mammalian forebrain. Annu. Rev. Neurosci. **25:** 507–536.
63. SU, J.D., J. QIU, Y.P. ZHONG, *et al.* 2001. Expression of estrogen receptor ER-alpha and -beta immunoreactivity in hippocampal cell cultures with special attention to GABAergic neurons. J. Neurosci. Res. **65:** 396–402.
64. TERKEL, J., R.S. BRIDGES & C.H. SAWYER. 1979. Effects of transecting lateral neural connections of the medial preoptic area on maternal behavior in the rat: nest building, pup retrieval and prolactin secretion. Brain Res. **169:** 369–380.
65. WISE, P.M. 2002. Estrogens and neuroprotection. Trends Endocrinol. Metab. **13:** 229–230.

Aromatase Expression by Reactive Astroglia Is Neuroprotective

IÑIGO AZCOITIA,[a] AMANDA SIERRA,[b] SERGIO VEIGA,[b] AND LUIS M. GARCIA-SEGURA[b]

[a]*Departamento de Biología Celular, Facultad de Biología, Universidad Complutense, E-28040 Madrid, Spain*

[b]*Instituto Cajal, C.S.I.C., E-28002 Madrid, Spain*

Abstract: The enzyme aromatase catalyzes the conversion of testosterone and other C19 steroids to estradiol. Under normal circumstances, the expression of aromatase in the central nervous system of mammals is restricted to neurons. However, the expression of the enzyme is induced in astrocytes *in vitro* by stressful stimuli. Furthermore, different types of brain injury induce *in vivo* the expression of aromatase in reactive astrocytes. The expression of aromatase by reactive astrocytes is neuroprotective, because the pharmacological inhibition of the enzyme in the brain exacerbates neuronal death after different forms of mild neurodegenerative stimuli that do not significantly affect neuronal survival under control conditions. These findings indicate that the induction of aromatase in reactive astrocytes, and the consecutive increase in the local production of estradiol in the brain at injured sites, may be an endogenous neural response to reduce the extent of neurodegenerative damage.

Keywords: steroidogenesis; aromatase; aromatase knockout mice; fadrozole; sex steroids; estradiol; androgens; glia; astroglia; astrocytes; neuroprotection; neurodegeneration; hippocampus; inferior olivary nucleus

INTRODUCTION

Sex steroids have a widespread collection of effects in the central nervous system (CNS). During brain development, sex hormones regulate cell death, neuronal migration, neurogenesis, axonal guidance, and synaptogenesis.[1,2] In the adult brain, sex steroids control synaptic efficacy by the modulation of postsynaptic currents,[3] the number of synapses[4] and dendritic spines,[5] and the expression of neurotransmitter receptors.[6] Adult neurogenesis is also influenced by sex hormones,[7,8] and neuroprotective effects have been demonstrated in different experimental animal models of neurodegenerative diseases[9] and are supported by some epidemiological studies.[10–17] Furthermore, the ability of steroids in the control of axonal growth during

Address for correspondence: Dr. I. Azcoitia, Departamento de Biología Celular, Facultad de Biología, Universidad Complutense, E-28040 Madrid, Spain. Voice: 34-913944861; fax: 34-913944981.
azcoitia@bio.ucm.es

**Ann. N.Y. Acad. Sci. 1007: 298–305 (2003). © 2003 New York Academy of Sciences.
doi: 10.1196/annals.1286.028**

development is reactivated in adulthood, improving axonal outgrowth after nerve crushing[18] and activating remyelination.[19]

In addition to neurons, sex steroids affect glial cells. Glia are a target as well as a source of steroids in the central and peripheral nervous system. Sex steroids affect the morphology and gene expression of astroglia *in vitro* and *in vivo*[20–22] and exert physiological effects on astrocytes during the estrous cycle.[23] Effects of sex steroids on glia are not restricted to astrocytes. The expression of myelin proteins in oligodendrocytes[24] and Schwann cells[25] is regulated by sex steroids and the phagocytic activity and rate of superoxide release by microglia depends on the presence of these hormones.[26]

Sex steroids may affect glia by classic nuclear receptor–mediated mechanisms, because estrogen receptors (ERs), androgen receptors (ARs), and progesterone receptors (PRs) have been identified in mixed astrocyte-oligodendrocyte CNS primary cultures and in peripheral nervous system glial cultures.[27,28] ER expression also has been found in cultures of rat microglía.[26,29] *In vivo* detection of receptors is more difficult, and some of them appear to be absent in peripheral nervous sytem.[30] In CNS, these receptors have been described in radial glia derived cells,[31] astrocytes,[32,33] and oligodendrocytes.[34] Furthermore, after injury, ER expression increases in astrocytes,[35] and AR are overexpressed in astrocytes, oligodendrocytes, and microglía.[35,36]

Sex steroids also may affect glia by non-classic mechanisms of action. For instance, $GABA_A$ channel conductance in Schwann cells is enhanced by direct binding of progesterone derivatives, with the result of increased transcription of the myelin protein PMP22. In this paradigm, the $GABA_A$ antagonist bicuculline and not the PR inhibitor RU486, down-regulates PMP22 transcription, confirming the nonclassic pathway of activation.[25] Sex steroids may also affect glia by regulating the levels of growth factors[37,38] and growth factor receptors.[38–40] Furthermore, steroids are able to interfere with signal cascades of growth factors in glial cells.[41]

GLIA ARE A SOURCE OF STEROIDS

In addition to circulating steroids produced by peripheral organs, neural cells are exposed to locally produced steroids. Steroidogenesis in the CNS is a process in which different types of cells, neurons and glia, act in coordination, transferring intermediate metabolites between them.[42] The brain synthesizes steroids from cholesterol, especially within glia, by a series of reactions catalyzed by P-450 and non P-450 enzymes.[43] The first and rate-limiting step of steroid biosynthesis is the steroidogenic acute regulatory protein (StAR) that mediates the transfer of cholesterol from outer to inner mitochondrial membrane. Then, the enzyme $P\text{-}450_{SCC}$ (cholesterol side-chain cleavage) converts cholesterol to pregnenolone. From pregnenolone, several steroids can be synthesized within central and peripheral nervous system.[43,44] King *et al.*[45] have recently identified by immunocytochemical methods the presence of StAR in neurons and astrocytes in several brain areas. Moreover, these authors have established that the levels of StAR mRNA in cultured astrocytes are two- to threefold increased in response to stimulus that activate glia, like forskolin or dibutyryl c-AMP.

Another important step in CNS steroidogenesis is the conversion of aromatizable androgens into estrogens. This nonreversible reaction is mediated by aromatase cytochrome P-450 19 (P-450-$_{ARO}$, EC 1.14.14), an enzyme located in the endoplasmic reticulum and first identified in brain during development, but today recognized in several CNS areas of adult vertebrates including humans, regardless of sex and normal or pathological condition.[46] Aromatase is the product of the *CYP 19* gene, which in humans has a coding region spanning nine exons (II-X). Upstream are several alternative 5'-untranslated first exons (Is) resulting from the use of different promoters that are tissue specific.[47] The aromatase protein encoded in each of these tissues is identical,[48] but the response elements of each promoter differ, and therefore regulation of aromatase transcription is not the same in all tissues.[47]

There is a large body of literature documenting the multiple regulators of aromatase gene in adipose tissue, bone, gonads, and placenta,[47,48] but little is known about the mechanisms that govern aromatase transcription in the nervous system. Regulators of aromatase expression in peripheral organs include testosterone, estradiol, orphan receptor ligands, cytokines, growth factors, such as insulin-like growth factor–I (IGF-I) and certain hormones, such as FSH.[47–49] In the CNS, the enzyme is regulated by neurotransmitters that act though PKC or PKG.[50] Testosterone has been described as an enhancer of aromatase synthesis in certain brain areas.[51] However, the actual activator is not testosterone itself, but its metabolite estradiol, acting in an estrogen receptor–dependent process.[52] Furthermore, posttranslational modifications of aromatase account for fast changes in enzymatic activity, such as those observed in hypothalamic preoptic area homogenates.[52] Among the candidates for posttranslation regulation of aromatase are the kinase PKC and one or several Ca^{2+}/calmodulin kinases.[52]

AROMATASE EXPRESSION BY GLIA

Aromatase expression in mammalian CNS is restricted, under normal conditions, to certain neuronal populations. These are mainly located in hypothalamus and limbic system. However, aromatase-expressing neurons are also present in the cerebral cortex.[53] In contrast with mammals, aromatase is expressed in radial glia in the brain of teleost fishes under normal conditions.[54] Furthermore, aromatase has been detected in astrocytes isolated from the cerebral cortex of neonatal rats.[42,55] In agreement with these *in vitro* results, we have observed a constitutive aromatase expression in hippocampal astrocytes cultured from postnatal rats. The immunostaining clearly delimitates the endoplasmic reticulum of GFAP-positive cells. Confocal microscopy shows that aromatase staining is present in GFAP unstained regions of the cytoplasm (FIG. 1). Interestingly, aromatase expression in hippocampal astrocytes is enhanced by different stress conditions, such as after serum deprivation or addition of glutamate to the cultures (FIG. 2). This result agrees with recent findings showing a robust expression of both mRNA[56] and protein[57] in reactive astrocytes in the brain of birds and mammals after brain injury *in vivo*. Aromatase-expressing reactive astrocytes are observed in all injured brain areas, including the cortex, corpus callosum, striatum, hippocampus, thalamus, and hypothalamus,[57] indicating that astrocytes from most brain areas have the potential for expressing aromatase, and therefore to produce estradiol, in response to injury.

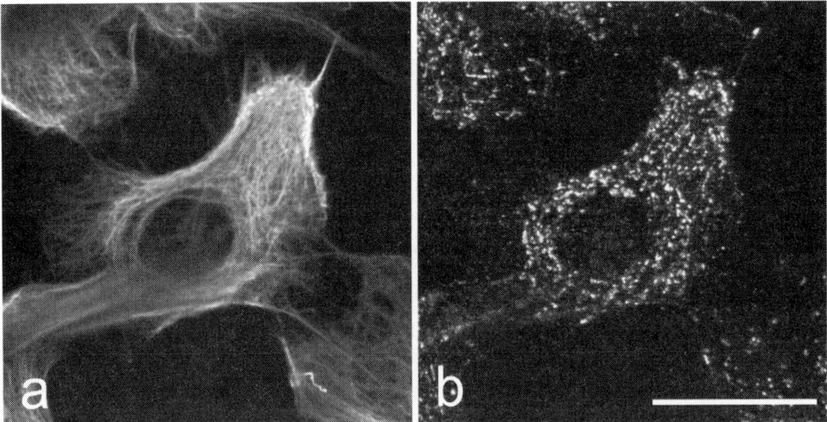

FIGURE 1. Confocal image of rat hippocampal astrocytes in culture immunostained against GFAP (**a**) and aromatase (**b**). Scale bar = 30 μm.

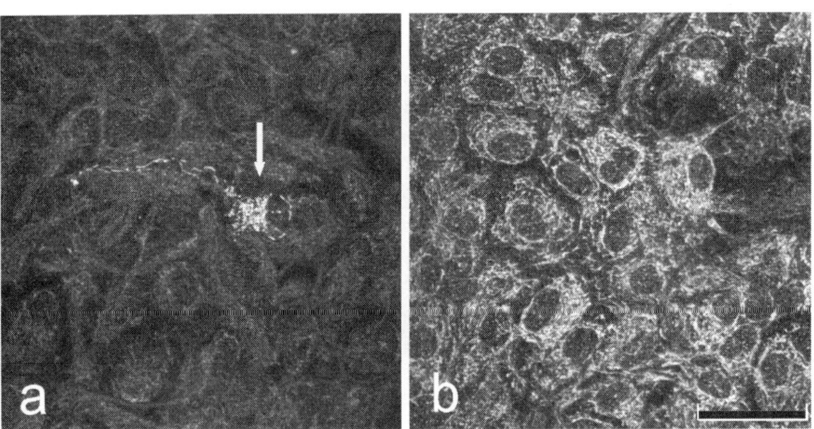

FIGURE 2. Aromatase immunoreactivity in rat hippocampal astrocytes. Under control conditions (**a**), constitutive aromatase expression is low except in a few cells (*arrow*). After serum deprivation (**b**), aromatase immunostaining is greatly enhanced. Scale bar = 50 μm.

AROMATASE IS NEUROPROTECTIVE

Considering the neuroprotective properties of estradiol,[9] it seems reasonable to infer that the expression of aromatase in astrocytes after brain injury may play some role in neuroprotection. To test this hypothesis, we infused the specific aromatase inhibitor fadrozole in the lateral cerebral ventricle of male rats. The effect of inactivating brain aromatase on the response to neurotoxic stimuli was assessed using kainic acid, a well-characterized neurotoxin for hippocampal neurons in the rat. Kainic acid was administered at a dose that does not affect hippocampal neurons in intact male rats but results in a significant neuronal loss in the hippocampus of castrated rats. Treatment with kainic acid did not affect the number of hippocampal neurons in animals infused in the lateral cerebral ventricle with vehicle. However, kainic acid resulted in a significant neuronal loss in the hippocampus of the animals that were infused in the cerebral ventricle with the aromatase inhibitor.[58] This finding indicates that local cerebral aromatase activity is involved in neuroprotection. Therefore, the induction of aromatase in astroglia after brain injury and the local formation of estradiol by these cells may represent a response of the injured neural tissue to limit the neurodegenerative damage.

The neuroprotective effect of aromatase has been confirmed using aromatase knockout mice. These animals show an enhanced hippocampal neurodegeneration in response to neurotoxins compared to wild-type mice.[58] Furthermore, neuroprotective effects of aromatase have been observed in other brain areas, such as the olivocerebellar system.[59] The inferior olivary nucleus is the source of climbing fibers, the most potent excitatory input to cerebellar Purkinje cells. Rat inferior olivary neurons are highly sensitive to the toxicity of 3-acetylpirydine (3AP), an antimetabolite of nicotinamide. The destruction of the inferior olive with 3AP results in loss of climbing fiber input to cerebellar Purkinje neurons,[60] and this deafferentation leads to ataxia.[61] Inferior olivary neurons express both aromatase[59] and estrogen receptors[62] and estradiol protects inferior olivary neurons from 3AP toxicity.[59] In contrast, the administration of the aromatase inhibitor fadrozole to male rats results in an increased neuronal death of inferior olivary neurons after 3AP treatment.[59] The enhanced neuronal death observed in the inferior olivary nuclei and hippocampus of rats treated with fadrozole and 3AP or kainic acid, respectively, was counterbalanced by the administration of estradiol.[58,59] This indicates that the toxic effect of fadrozole is caused by the inhibition of aromatase and not to another unknown effect of the drug. Therefore, we may conclude that neuroprotective effects of aromatase are mediated by the formation of estradiol.

THERAPEUTIC IMPLICATIONS

Neural tissue shows several physiopathological responses in adaptation to neurodegenerative conditions, such as the activation of glial cells—astrocytes and microglia—around neurodegenerative foci. Activated or reactive astrocytes are the source of neuroprotective molecules that decrease neuronal damage. The data reviewed here indicate that estradiol is one of such neuroprotective factors produced by reactive astrocytes. Therefore, it may be useful to exploit the endogenous capacity of astrocytes to express aromatase and synthesize estradiol to develop specific neuroprotective pharmacological tools for the therapy or prevention of neurodegenerative diseases. Because the human aromatase gene has several promoters that are regulated by different transcription factors and signaling pathways, it is theoretically possible to specifically enhance estradiol production by reactive astrocytes at the sites of brain injury.

ACKNOWLEDGMENTS

This study has been supported by grants from the Commission of the European Communities, specific RTD program "Quality of Life and Management of Living Resources," QLK6-CT-2000-00179 and from Ministerio de Ciencia y Tecnología, Spain, SAF 2002-00652.

REFERENCES

1. SIMERLY, R.B. 2002. Wired for reproduction: organization and development of sexually dimorphic circuits in the mammalian forebrain. Annu. Rev. Neurosci. **25:** 507–536.
2. WANG, L. *et al.* 2003. Estrogen receptor (ER)beta knockout mice reveal a role for ERbeta in migration of cortical neurons in the developing brain. Proc. Natl. Acad. Sci. USA **100:** 703–708.
3. RUPPRECHT, R. & F. HOLSBOER. 1999. Neuroactive steroids: mechanisms of action and neuropsychopharmacological perspectives. Trends Neurosci. **22:** 410–416.
4. MCEWEN, B. *et al.* 2001. Tracking the estrogen receptor in neurons: implications for estrogen-induced synapse formation. Proc. Natl. Acad. Sci. USA **98:** 7093–7100.
5. MCEWEN, B. 2002. Estrogen actions throughout the brain. Recent Prog. Horm. Res. **57:** 357–384.
6. RUDICK, C.N. & C.S. WOOLLEY. 2003. Selective estrogen receptor modulators regulate phasic activation of hippocampal CA1 pyramidal cells by estrogen. Endocrinology **144:** 179–187.
7. KARISHMA, K.K. & J. HERBERT. 2002. Dehydroepiandrosterone (DHEA) stimulates neurogenesis in the hippocampus of the rat, promotes survival of newly formed neurons and prevents corticosterone-induced suppression. Eur. J. Neurosci. **16:** 445–453.
8. SHINGO, T. *et al.* 2003. Pregnancy-stimulated neurogenesis in the adult female forebrain mediated by prolactin. Science **299:** 117–120.
9. GARCIA-SEGURA, L.M., I. AZCOITIA & L.L. DONCARLOS. 2001. Neuroprotection by estradiol. Prog. Neurobiol. **63:** 29–60.
10. SAWADA, H. & S. SHIMOHAMA. 2000. Neuroprotective effects of estradiol in mesencephalic dopaminergic neurons. Neurosci. Biobehav. Rev. **24:** 143–147.
11. STEIN, D.G. 2001. Brain damage, sex hormones and recovery: a new role for progesterone and estrogen? Trends Neurosci. **24:** 386–391.
12. COMPTON, J., T. VAN AMELSVOORT & D. MURPHY. 2002. Mood, cognition and Alzheimer's disease. Best. Pract. Res. Clin. Obstet. Gynaecol. **16:** 357–370.
13. FILLIT, H.M. 2002. The role of hormone replacement therapy in the prevention of Alzheimer disease. Arch. Intern. Med. **162:** 1934–1942.
14. KOLSCH, H. & M.L. RAO. 2002. Neuroprotective effects of estradiol-17beta: implications for psychiatric disorders. Arch. Women Ment. Health. **5:** 105–110.
15. LU, A. *et al.* 2002. 17-beta-estradiol induces heat shock proteins in brain arteries and potentiates ischemic heat shock protein induction in glia and neurons. J. Cereb. Blood Flow Metab. **22:** 183–195.
16. OKUN, M.S., W.M. MCDONALD & M.R. DELONG. 2002. Refractory nonmotor symptoms in male patients with Parkinson disease due to testosterone deficiency: a common unrecognized comorbidity. Arch. Neurol. **59:** 807–811.
17. RAPKIN, A.J. *et al.* 2002. The clinical nature and formal diagnosis of premenstrual, postpartum, and perimenopausal affective disorders. Curr. Psychiatry Rep. **4:** 419–428.
18. JONES, K.J. *et al.* 2000. Gonadal steroid enhancement of facial nerve regeneration: role of heat shock protein 70. J. Neurocytol. **29:** 341–349.
19. AZCOITIA, I. *et al.* 2003. Progesterone and its derivatives dihydroprogesterone and tetrahydroprogesterone reduce myelin fiber morphological abnormalities and myelin fiber loss in the sciatic nerve of aged rats. Neurobiol. Aging **24:** 853–860.

20. GARCIA-SEGURA, L.M., I. TORRES-ALEMAN & F. NAFTOLIN. 1989. Astrocytic shape and glial fibrillary acidic protein immunoreactivity are modified by estradiol in primary rat hypothalamic cultures. Brain Res. Dev. Brain Res. **47:** 298–302.
21. DEL CERRO, S., J. GARCIA-ESTRADA & L.M. GARCIA-SEGURA. 1995. Neuroactive steroids regulate astroglia morphology in hippocampal cultures from adult rats. Glia **14:** 65–71.
22. AMATEAU, S.K. & M.M. MCCARTHY. 2002. Sexual differentiation of astrocyte morphology in the developing rat preoptic area. J. Neuroendocrinol. **14:** 904–910.
23. LUQUIN, S., F. NAFTOLIN & L.M. GARCIA-SEGURA. 1993. Natural fluctuation and gonadal hormone regulation of astrocyte immunoreactivity in dentate gyrus. J. Neurobiol. **24:** 913–924.
24. JUNG-TESTAS, I. *et al.* 1992. Demonstration of steroid hormone receptors and steroid action in primary cultures of rat glial cells. J. Steroid Biochem. Mol. Biol. **41:** 621–631.
25. MAGNAGHI, V. *et al.* 2001. Neuroactive steroids and peripheral myelin proteins. Brain Res. Brain Res. Rev. **37:** 360–371.
26. BRUCE-KELLER, A.J. *et al.* 2000. Antiinflammatory effects of estrogen on microglial activation. Endocrinology **141:** 3646–3656.
27. JUNG-TESTAS, I. & E.E. BAULIEU. 1998. Steroid hormone receptors and steroid action in rat glial cells of the central and peripheral nervous system. J. Steroid Biochem. Mol. Biol. **65:** 243–251.
28. HOSLI, E. *et al.* 2001. Colocalization of androgen, estrogen and cholinergic receptors on cultured astrocytes of rat central nervous system. Int. J. Dev. Neurosci. **19:** 11–19.
29. VEGETO, E. *et al.* 2001. Estrogen prevents the lipopolysaccharide-induced inflammatory response in microglia. J. Neurosci. **21:** 1809–1818.
30. JORDAN, C.L., R.H. PRICE, JR. & R.J. HANDA. 2002. Androgen receptor messenger RNA and protein in adult rat sciatic nerve: implications for site of androgen action. J. Neurosci. Res. **69:** 509–518.
31. GUDINO-CABRERA, G. & M. NIETO-SAMPEDRO. 1999. Estrogen receptor immunoreactivity in Schwann-like brain macroglia. J. Neurobiol. **40:** 458–470.
32. AZCOITIA, I., A. SIERRA & L.M. GARCIA-SEGURA. 1999. Localization of estrogen receptor beta-immunoreactivity in astrocytes of the adult rat brain. Glia **26:** 260—-267.
33. MILNER, T.A. *et al.* 2001. Ultrastructural evidence that hippocampal alpha estrogen receptors are located at extranuclear sites. J. Comp. Neurol. **429:** 355–371.
34. FINLEY, S.K. & M.F. KRITZER. 1999. Immunoreactivity for intracellular androgen receptors in identified subpopulations of neurons, astrocytes and oligodendrocytes in primate prefrontal cortex. J. Neurobiol. **40:** 446–457.
35. GARCIA-OVEJERO, D. *et al.* 2002. Glial expression of estrogen and androgen receptors after rat brain injury. J. Comp. Neurol. **450:** 256–271.
36. PUY, L. *et al.* 1995. Immunocytochemical detection of androgen receptor in human temporal cortex characterization and application of polyclonal androgen receptor antibodies in frozen and paraffin-embedded tissues. J. Steroid Biochem. Mol. Biol. **55:** 197–209.
37. DUENAS, M. *et al.* 1994. Gonadal hormone regulation of insulin-like growth factor-I-like immunoreactivity in hypothalamic astroglia of developing and adult rats. Neuroendocrinology **59:** 528–538.
38. SOLUM, D.T. & R.J. HANDA. 2002. Estrogen regulates the development of brain-derived neurotrophic factor mRNA and protein in the rat hippocampus. J. Neurosci. **22:** 2650–2659.
39. FLORES, C. *et al.* 1999. Ovariectomy of adult rats leads to increased expression of astrocytic basic fibroblast growth factor in the ventral tegmental area and in dopaminergic projection regions of the entorhinal and prefrontal cortex. J. Neurosci. **19:** 8665–8673.
40. MCCARTHY, J.B. *et al.* 2002. TrkA immunoreactive astrocytes in dendritic fields of the hippocampal formation across estrous. Glia **38:** 36–44.
41. IVANOVA, T., M. KAROLCZAK & C. BEYER. 2001. Estrogen stimulates the mitogen-activated protein kinase pathway in midbrain astroglia. Brain Res. **889:** 264–269.

42. Zwain, I.H. & S.S. Yen. 1999. Neurosteroidogenesis in astrocytes, oligodendrocytes, and neurons of cerebral cortex of rat brain. Endocrinology **140:** 3843–3852.
43. Mellon, S.H. & L.D. Griffin. 2002. Neurosteroids: biochemistry and clinical significance. Trends Endocrinol. Metab. **13:** 35–43.
44. Schumacher, M. *et al.* 2000. Steroid synthesis and metabolism in the nervous system: trophic and protective effects. J. Neurocytol. **29:** 307–326.
45. King, S.R. *et al.* 2002. An essential component in steroid synthesis, the steroidogenic acute regulatory protein, is expressed in discrete regions of the brain. J. Neurosci. **22:** 10613–10620.
46. Stoffel-Wagner, B. 2001. Neurosteroid metabolism in the human brain. Eur. J. Endocrinol. **145:** 669–679.
47. Simpson, E.R. *et al.* 2002. Aromatase—a brief overview. Annu. Rev. Physiol. **64:** 93–127.
48. Kamat, A. *et al.* 2002. Mechanisms in tissue-specific regulation of estrogen biosynthesis in humans. Trends Endocrinol. Metab. **13:** 122–128.
49. Silva, J.M. & C.A. Price. 2002. Insulin and IGF-I are necessary for FSH-induced cytochrome P450 aromatase but not cytochrome P450 side-chain cleavage gene expression in oestrogenic bovine granulosa cells in vitro. J. Endocrinol. **174:** 499–507.
50. Abe-Dohmae, S., Y. Takagy & N. Harada. 1996. Neurotransmitter-mediated regulation of brain aromatase: protein kinase C- and G-dependent induction. J. Neurochem. **67:** 2087–2095.
51. Abdelgadir, S.E. *et al.* 1994. Androgens regulate aromatase cytochrome P450 messenger ribonucleic acid in rat brain. Endocrinology **135:** 395–401.
52. Balthazart, J., M. Baillien & G.F. Ball. 2001. Phosphorylation processes mediate rapid changes of brain aromatase activity. J. Steroid Biochem. Mol. Biol. **79:** 261–277.
53. MacLusky, N.J., F. Naftolin & P.S. Goldman-Rakic. 1986. Estrogen formation and binding in the cerebral cortex of the developing rhesus monkey. Proc. Natl. Acad. Sci. USA **83:** 513–516.
54. Forlano, P.M., *et al.* 2001. Anatomical distribution and cellular basis for high levels of aromatase activity in the brain of teleost fish: aromatase enzyme and mRNA expression identify glia as source. J. Neurosci. **21:** 8943–8955.
55. Zwain, I.H., S.S. Yen & C.Y. Cheng. 1997. Astrocytes cultured in vitro produce estradiol-17beta and express aromatase cytochrome P-450 (P-450 AROM) mRNA. Biochim. Biophys. Acta **1334:** 338–348.
56. Peterson, R.S., C.J. Saldanha & B.A. Schlinger. 2001. Rapid upregulation of aromatase mRNA and protein following neural injury in the zebra finch (*Taeniopygia guttata*). J. Neuroendocrinol. **13:** 317–323.
57. Garcia-Segura, L.M. *et al.* 1999. Aromatase expression by astrocytes after brain injury: implications for local estrogen formation in brain repair. Neuroscience **89:** 567 578.
58. Azcoitia, I. *et al.* 2001. Brain aromatase is neuroprotective. J. Neurobiol. **47:** 318–329.
59. Sierra, A., I. Azcoitia & L.M. Garcia-Segura. 2003. Endogenous estrogen formation is neuroprotective in a model of cerebellar ataxia. Endocrine **21:** 43–51.
60. Baetens, D., L.M. Garcia-Segura & A. Perrelet. 1982. Effects of climbing fiber destruction on large dendrite spines of Purkinje cells. Exp. Brain Res. **48:** 256–262.
61. Fernandez, A.M. *et al.* 1999. Neuroprotective actions of peripherally administered insulin-like growth factor I in the injured olivo-cerebellar pathway. Eur. J. Neurosci. **11:** 2019–2030.
62. Shughrue, P.J., M.V. Lane & I. Merchenthaler. 1997. Comparative distribution of estrogen receptor-alpha and -beta mRNA in the rat central nervous system. J. Comp. Neurol. **388:** 507–525.

Neurotrophic Factors and Estradiol Interact To Control Axogenic Growth in Hypothalamic Neurons

H.F. CARRER, M.J. CAMBIASSO, V. BRITO, AND S. GOROSITO

Instituto de Investigación Médica M. y M. Ferreyra, INIMEC-CONICET, Casilla de Correo 389, 5000 Córdoba, Argentina

ABSTRACT: Previous work from our laboratory has shown that in cultures of hypothalamic neurons obtained from male fetuses at embryonic day 16, the axogenic response to estrogen (E2) is contingent on coculture with target glia or target glia-conditioned media (CM). Neither the estrogen receptor blockers tamoxifen nor ICI 182,780 prevented the axogenic effects of the hormone. Estradiol made membrane-impermeable by conjugation to a protein of high molecular weight (E2-BSA) preserved its axogenic capacity, suggesting the possibility of a membrane effect responsible for the action of E2. Western blot analysis of extracts from homogenates of cultured neurons grown with E2 and CM from target glia had more TrkB than cultures with CM alone or E2 alone. To further investigate the interaction between E2 and the neurotrophin receptors, we used a specific antisense oligonucleotide (AS) to prevent the estradiol-induced increase of TrkB. The effect of E2 was suppressed in cultures in which TrkB was down-regulated by the AS, showing decreased axonal elongation when compared with neurons treated with E2 without AS or with sense TrkB. In cultures grown with AS, the axonal length of E2-treated cultures was not different from cultures without E2. Evidence suggesting cross-talk between E2 and neurotrophic factor(s) prompted investigation of signaling along the MAPK cascade. Immuno blotting of E2-treated cultures showed increased levels of phosphorylated ERK1 and ERK2. UO126 but not LY294002 blocked E2-induced axonal elongation, suggesting that the MAPKs are involved in this response.

KEYWORDS: sexual differentiation; hypothalamus; TrkB; MAPK; ERK1/2; PI3

Work from several laboratories has brought to the fore evidence indicating the interaction of estrogen and neurotrophic factors in the development of neurites and differentiation of neurons (for review see Toran Allerand *et al.*[1] and Chowen *et al.*[2]). Work from the laboratory of Toran Allerand initially demonstrated coexpression of estrogen receptor mRNA with the mRNAs for neurotrophins and their receptors, differential and reciprocal up-regulation of estrogen, and NGF receptor mRNA and protein expression by estrogen in adult female rat sensory neurons, PC12 cells, and cerebral cortical cultures. They also found evidence for putative estrogen response

Address for correspondence: Hugo F. Carrer, Instituto Ferreyra, Casilla de Correo 389, 5000 Córdoba, Argentina. Voice: 54-351-4681465, ext. 109, fax: 54-351-4695163.
hfcarrer@immf.uncor.edu

Ann. N.Y. Acad. Sci. 1007: 306–316 (2003).
doi: 10.1196/annals.1286.029

elements (EREs) in the NGF, TrkA, p75, and BDNF genes and further showed that estrogen and neurotrophin receptor coexpression may result in convergence or cross-coupling of their signaling pathways. E2 could increase the amount of trophic factors released to the medium by glial cells, the number and/or sensitivity of receptors, or a combination of these mechanisms. The capacity of glial cells from a variety of brain regions to produce the appropriate growth factors has been documented.[3]

Previous work from our laboratory has shown that the axogenic effect of estradiol on male-derived hypothalamic neurons is dependent on the presence of soluble factor(s) produced by target glia,[4] and this effect was found to correlate with an increase in receptors for the neurotrophic factor IGF-I and TrkB but not TrkA and TrkC.[5] In sexually segregated cultures of dissociated neurons taken from ventromedial hypothalamus of rat fetuses at gestation day 16 (GD16), only neurons from males respond with increased axonal growth to the addition of 17β-estradiol to the culture medium.[4] Moreover, this response is contingent on coculture with heterotopic glia (mostly astrocytes) from a target region (amygdala) harvested from same-sex fetuses, whereas, in the presence of homotopic glia or in cultures without glia, E2 had no effect. It was concluded that at GD16 the axogenic effect of E2 depends on interaction between neurons and glia from a target region and that neurons from fetal male donors appear to mature earlier than neurons from females, a differentiated response that appears to take place before differential exposure to gonadal secretions.

The fact that in our experiments both E2 and coculture with target glia were necessary for the axogenic response to appear argues in favor of a triple interaction between E2, neurons equipped with the necessary receptors, and the appropriate glia releasing to the medium some factor(s) which produces the observed effect in all or most neurons present in the culture. Alternatively, the simpler explanation that most or all neurons responded to E2 because they are equipped with ER also must be considered.

THE AXOGENIC EFFECT OF ESTRADIOL REQUIRES GLIA-DERIVED SOLUBLE FACTORS

With this evidence in mind, the interaction between glia and neurons was investigated further by us in a study designed to establish whether the E2-dependent capability of target astroglia to support axonal growth depends either on cell surface interactions between neurons and glia or on differences in soluble factors released by glia. With this purpose, we studied the effects of target and nontarget glia-conditioned media (CM) on the E2-induced growth of neuronal processes of hypothalamic neurons obtained from sexually segregated fetal donors. Glia cells, mainly astrocytes, were cultured without addition of E2, to isolate the effects of the hormone on neurons themselves.

The growth and differentiation of hypothalamic neurons was differentially affected by E2 and the astroglia-CMs depending on the genetic sex of the neurons, confirming the results observed in cocultures with glia.[4] Hypothalamic neurons from males were particularly sensitive to the presence of astroglia-CM, because media conditioned by target (ventral mesencephalon) and nontarget (striatum or cerebral cortex) glia modified the number of primary neurites and the growth of axons, whereas, in female cells, only target-derived CM affected axonal growth. The lack of an E2 effect on female-derived neurons was not caused by a generalized deficit in growth capacity in these cultures, as demonstrated by the fact that NGF and target-derived CM did induce additional axon growth.

The evidence obtained support the hypothesis that the developmental actions of estrogen on neurite growth and differentiation can result from modulatory interactions with endogenous growth factors, rather than directly from estrogenic action alone. In fact, the most obvious explanation of our results is that the axogenic effect of E2 depends on the participation of a soluble factor released by glia to the culture medium.

Apart from the sexual differences in response to E2 made evident in our sexually segregated cultures, it is important to keep in mind that gonadal steroid hormones have dynamic effects on neuritogenesis that are regionally specific. Whereas in hypothalamic and hippocampal neurons an axogenic effect has been observed,[6,7] in neurons from the amygdala the effect was exerted on dendritic arborization.[8] On the other hand, in the arcuate nucleus E2 causes a *decrease* of axosomatic synapses,[9,10] whereas cerebellar cells fail to respond to variations in gonadal hormone levels.[11] In males astroglia-CM from areas that cannot be regarded as target for hypothalamic neurons (cortex or striatum) had an *inhibitory* effect on axon growth that was not demonstrated in female-derived neurons. Our results and those from other laboratories[12] underline the highly dynamic and mutually interactive nature of neuron–glia relations. These interactions are age dependent and region specific, so that generalizations about their influence and outcome should be made with caution, particularly if during experimental procedures separation of neurons and glia may have modified the growth of certain surviving cell lineages or cell subtypes.

THE AXOGENIC EFFECT PERSISTS IN THE PRESENCE OF ESTROGEN RECEPTOR BLOCKERS

It is not yet known whether the ER that mediates the neurotrophin–estrogen interaction controlling neuritogenic effects in the brain is ERα, ERβ, or other as yet unidentified receptor. This question also was investigated in our model using specific nuclear ER blockers.[13] Although the presence of ERα mRNA was demonstrated in the donor tissues as well as in the neurons cultured with or without E2, neither the Type III steroidal receptor blocker tamoxifen nor Type I antiestrogen ICI 182,780, a nonsteroidal receptor antagonist, prevented the axogenic effects of the hormone. Tamoxifen as well as ICI 182,780 were added at a concentration 10-fold greater (1×10^{-6} M) than estradiol, a dose relationship that effectively blocks classic receptor-mediated estrogenic effects.[14] ICI in particular has been shown to block ERα and ERβ,[15] but despite this capacity it did not interfere with the effects observed by us. The efficacy of these and other ER antagonists has been characterized on the basis of their ability to prevent the transcriptional activation of genes containing an estrogen response element (ERE). Therefore, it is possible that this "nongenomic" effect of estradiol escaped the blockade by acting upstream of any potential interaction with ERE[16] or cross-coupling with neuritotrophic signaling cascades such as MAPK or PKA[17,18] in the cytoplasm.

The insertion of the receptor protein in the cell membrane could equally explain the inability of tamoxifen and ICI 182,780 to block the effect of estradiol, a possibility we investigated using a membrane-impermeable E2-albumin construct (E2-BSA). Estradiol conjugated to a protein of high molecular weight preserved its axogenic capacity, suggesting the possibility of a membrane effect responsible for the action of E2.

The mechanisms of estrogen receptor signaling can be mediated by at least four pathways.[19] Two of these mechanisms require estrogen receptor binding within the cell and therefore are not likely to be responsible for the neuritogenic effects we observed. A third mechanism posits the activation of intracellular kinase pathways leading to phosphorylation and activation of ER at ERE-containing promoters in a ligand-independent manner. This pathway is used by growth factors and may possibly explain the promiscuous interaction between E2 and neurotrophins and their receptors: in theory, E2 could activate the neurotrophin receptors and/or the neurotrophins could activate the ER and indeed several instances of this type of effect have been documented (see Cenni and Picard.[20]). This does not appear to be the case in our model, because tamoxifen and ICI 182,780 did not block the axogenic effect, and, moreover, in male neurons from GD16 *both* E2 and CM were necessary. In this instance, the simultaneous activation of the estrogenic and trophic signaling pathways through membrane-bound specific receptors parsimoniously explains the results. This interpretation coincides with the fourth mechanism, characterized as nongenomic or membrane signaling,[19] which requires the activation of a membrane associated binding site, in the form of a different, albeit unknown, type of ER linked to an intracellular signaling pathway.

Direct membrane effects of E2 have been observed repeatedly, but the identity of the receptor responsible for this effect remains elusive. Although the presence of ERα anchored to the membrane of cultured hippocampal neurons has been demonstrated,[21] the existence of a hitherto unidentified isoform of ER has gained ground.[22] Singh *et al.*[17] postulate that a membrane-bound ER may be part of a multimeric complex including also hsp90 and B-Raf. Evidence has been obtained that both cytosolic and membrane-bound ERα as well as ERβ originate from a single transcript,[23] suggesting that a posttranslational modification of the amino acid sequence allows the insertion in the cell membrane.[24] More recently, the laboratory of Toran Allerand addressed with surprising results the question of the identity of the receptor mediating these effects: neither ERα nor ERβ mediated activation of the MAP kinase cascade. The existence of a putative, novel, estradiol-sensitive receptor, designated ER-X placed within plasma membrane caveolae was proposed[25] and recently confirmed.[26] It is also important to recall the work of Moats and Ramirez [27] showing that E2-BSA is bound to clathrin-coated pits and the isolation of a membrane-bound protein identified as glyceraldehyde-3-phosphate dehydrogenase (GAPDH), which binds estrogen and varies with the estrous cycle and hormonal manipulations.[28] This membrane-dependent mechanism would explain how cells could respond to E2 without the participation of cytosolic ERs. Altogether, these findings supply a mechanism explaining the effects of E2-BSA in our experiments.

ESTROGEN INCREASES THE EXPRESSION OF NEUROTROPHIN RECEPTORS

The results described above suggested a dynamic interaction between some neurotrophic factor(s) present in the astroglia-CM and neurons cultured in the presence of E2. This interaction may be instrumented through the regulation of the respective receptors, thus modulating the effect of the specific ligands. This possibility was investigated by semiquantitative analysis by SDS-PAGE of the trophic factor receptors tyrosine kinase type A (TrkA), type B (TrkB), type C (TrkC), and insulin-like growth factor receptor (IGF)–I, in extracts from homogenates of cultured hypothalamic neurons. Western blot analysis showed that in cultures of male-derived neurons grown with E2 and CM from target glia, the amounts of TrkB had increased notably. Densitometric quantification showed that these cultures had more TrkB than cultures with CM alone or E2 alone. On the contrary, in cultures of female-derived neurons, the presence of CM alone induced maximal levels of TrkB, which were not further increased by E2. Levels of TrkC were not modified by any experimental condition in male- or female-derived cultures and Trk A was not found in the homogenates.

Electrophoretic analysis of these extracts showed that they also contained a protein migrating in SDS-PAGE at 97 kDa, characteristic for the IGF-I receptor. This band reacted with the polyclonal antibody against the β subunit of this receptor. The IGF-I R_β was found only in cultures of male-derived neurons grown with both CM and E2, but not in controls without E2 or without astroglia-CM or female-derived neurons in all conditions. The close correlation between an increase in receptors for the neurotrophic factor IGF-I and TrkB but not TrkA and TrkC[5] supported the conclusion that E2 and the trophic factors released by astrocytes may be acting simultaneously and concurrently to induce axonal growth. The finding that in neurons from males at GD16 neither astroglia-CM, nor estradiol alone are able to promote the neuritogenic response, supports this possibility.

To further investigate the interaction between E2 and the neurotrophin receptors, we used a specific antisense oligonucleotide (AS) that affects neuritic growth in a dose-dependent manner (FIG. 1). A dose (5 mM) that did not affect growth in control conditions could block the increase in axonal length and TrkB expression produced by E2. In cultures grown with AS the axonal length of E2-treated cultures was not different from cultures without E2. In cells grown with sense TrkB, neurite length as well as number of minor processes were not different from cells grown with vehicle, and the axogenic effect of estradiol was preserved. In light of these results, it is reasonable to assume that the effects observed in cultures treated with AS can be attributed to inhibited synthesis of TrkB protein, rather than to nonspecific effects of the added nucleotide.

The simplest interpretation of our results would be that the TrkB antisense prevented the axogenic response to estradiol because the increased TrkB levels normally observed in neurons treated with estradiol is a necessary requirement for the accelerated axon growth. This explanation agrees with our previous results[5] indicating that estradiol and trophic factors released by astrocytes from a target region may act concurrently to induce axon elongation. In fact, it has been shown that estrogen and nerve growth factor may regulate receptor and/or ligand availability through reciprocal regulation at the level of gene transcription (for review, see Toran Allerand *et al.*,[1] Kato *et al.*,[29] and Garcia Segura *et al.*[30]). This convergence could explain why for the axogenic effect to occur the concurrent action of both estrogen and soluble trophic factor(s) from target astroglia is necessary. It has been shown that the inhibition of the synthesis of the growth factor IGF-I and its receptor prevented the effect of estrogen on the number and arborization of arcuate nucleus neurons.[31,32] Moreover, both an estrogen receptor antagonist and an IGF-I receptor antagonist blocked the estrogen-induced synaptic decrease in the arcuate nucleus.[33]

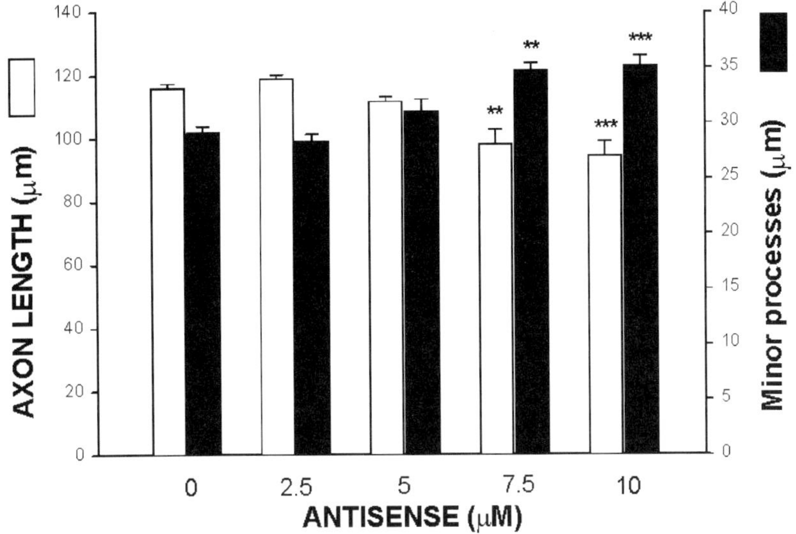

FIGURE 1. Effect of different doses of antisense oligonucleotide against TrkB mRNA on axon and minor process length (left and right axes, respectively) of male fetal hypothalamic neurons grown for 48 h *in vitro*. Data represent mean ± SEM.; $N = 4$ different cultures for each dose of antisense; 60 neurons were measured for each culture and dose. Axon length: overall ANOVA $F(4,10) = 11.97$, $P < 0.001$; minor processes length: overall ANOVA $F(4, 10) = 16.75$, $P < 0.001$. Post hoc test indicated $^{**}P \leq 0.01$ and $^{***}P \leq 0.001$ versus control cultures without antisense.

SIGNALING CASCADES ARE MODULATED BY ESTROGEN

Even if E2 can activate a signaling cascade independent of any classic genomic regulation, changes in protein transcription at some level are indispensable to explain the hormonal effects. Among the signal cascades studied so far in neural cells, estrogen has been shown to stimulate the formation of cAMP,[34] the phosphorylation of the cAMP response element binding protein CREB,[35] the formation of IP3,[36] the transient increase of intracellular Ca^{2+} levels,[37] and to activate the MAP kinase signaling pathway in a neuroblastoma cell line[38] and in cerebral cortical explants.[17] Also in organotypic slice cultures of the developing mouse cerebral cortex, cells that respond to estradiol treatment by phosphorylation of ERK1 and ERK2 have been identified. The requirement for Hsp90 in estrogen-induced activation of ERK1 and ERK2 by MEK2 was demonstrated, providing an insight into the mechanisms by which estradiol may influence cytoplasmic and nuclear events in responsive neurons via the MAP kinase cascade.[39]

The putative participation of the MAP kinase cascade was investigated in our model evaluating activation of ERK1/2. After 48 h in culture with E2 and astroglia-CM, a 3-h washout period was performed. The cultures were pulsed with estradiol 10 nM for 30 and 60 min or with BDNF 50 ng/mL for 60 min and harvested for Western blot analysis of ERK phosphorylation. An increase of phosphorylated ERK1/2

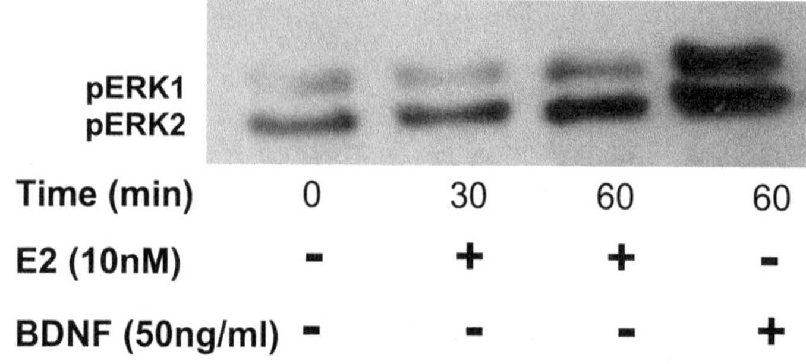

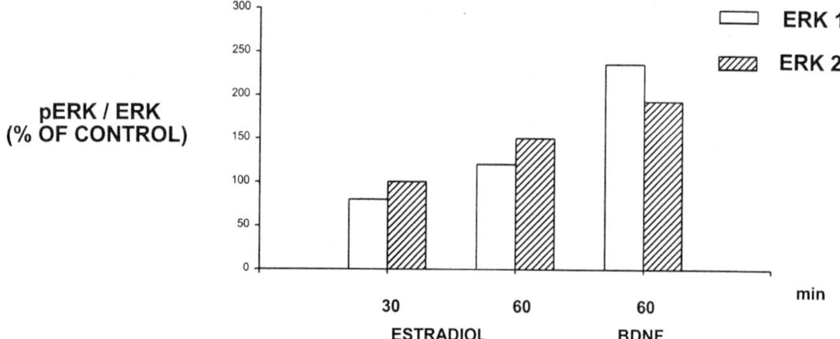

FIGURE 2. Effect of estradiol and BDNF on phosphorylation of ERK1/2. Dissociated hypothalamic neurons taken from GD 16 male fetuses were grown in astroglia-conditioned medium and estradiol 10 nM for 48 h. After 3-h washout, cultures were pulsed for the indicated times with E2 or BDNF and harvested for Western blotting. (*top*) Example of immunoblot showing an increase of phosphorylated ERK1/2 in cultures treated with E2 for 1 h. (*bottom*) Ratio of readings for pERK/ERK bands in arbitrary densitometric units expressed as percent of control (time 0). Each ratio was calculated for bands measured in the same membranes.

was observed in cultures treated with E2 for 1 h. As expected, BDNF also increased phosphorylated ERK1/2 (FIG. 2). This question was further investigated in our model by growing neurons with target astroglia-CM and E2 in the presence of LY294002 (a specific inhibitor of PI 3-kinase) or UO126, which inhibits MEK1 and MEK2. Only UO126 effectively blocked E2-induced axonal elongation (FIGS. 3 and 4), thus confirming the participation of ERK1/2. Additional experiments are necessary to establish (1) if activated ERK produces changes at transcriptional levels or direct phosphorylation of cytosolic proteins like tubuline; (2) if ERK phosphorylation depends on activation of membrane and/or nuclear ER; and (3) the identity of this ER (α, β, or X). Evidently, more experiments are necessary to define the precise mechanisms and complete the model of E2-neurotrophic factor interaction explaining axon elongation of hypothalamic neurons in males.

The consequence of a change in genetic activity could be a direct increase of the cytosqueletal proteins involved in neurite growth and/or the production of receptors

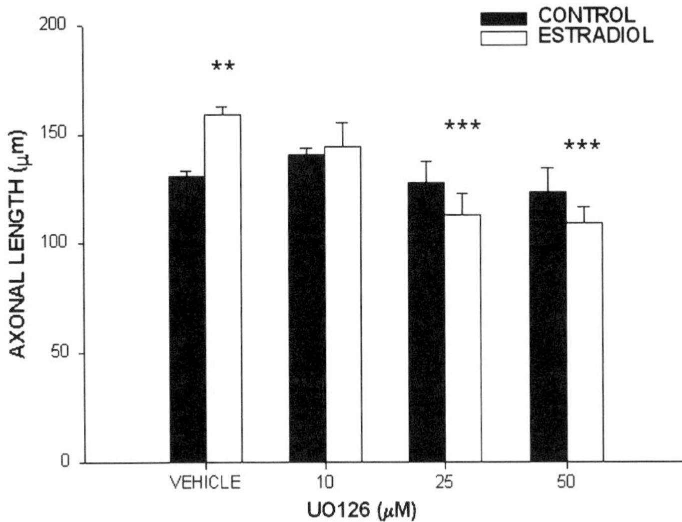

FIGURE 3. Effect of MEK1/2 inhibition by UO126 on the axogenic effect of estradiol. Dissociated hypothalamic neurons taken from GD 16 male fetuses were grown in astroglia-conditioned medium without (Control) or with estradiol 10 nM for 24 h. After 3-h washout, cultures were treated with 10, 25, or 50 mM UO126 for 1h, and then estradiol was added back for an additional 24 h. Data represent mean ± SEM; $N = 3–5$ different cultures for each condition; 60 neurons were measured for each culture and condition. Two-way ANOVA showed significant hormone X inhibitor interaction $F(3, 24) = 3.66$, $P = 0.02$. Post hoc test indicated $^{**}P \leq 0.01$ versus control and $^{***}P \leq 0.001$ versus estradiol-treated cultures without UO126.

for neurotrophic factors or their specific ligands. It is also possible that the increase of specific receptors be one step further removed from the hormone's action, if trophic factors act in an autocrine fashion to up-regulate the levels of their respective receptors, as discussed above.

CONCLUSIONS

Estrogen availability to the brain cells at particular times and places affects the growth, differentiation, and selective survival of neurons and glia ordaining the sex-specific synaptic connections and their functional profile. This complex process requires the participation of specific receptors for estrogen as well as for neurotrophic factors, some of them from glial origin. Apart from the genomic effects resulting from the translocation of the liganded nuclear estrogen receptor, there are second messenger effects mediated through a membrane-associated ER. This pathway would follow the MAPK signaling cascade (ERK1/2) to activate genes controlling synthesis of neurotrophin receptors and other growth-associated proteins. This signaling cascade may be one of the putative sites of cross talk between the estrogen and neurotrophic signals resulting in additive, potentiating, or interdependently

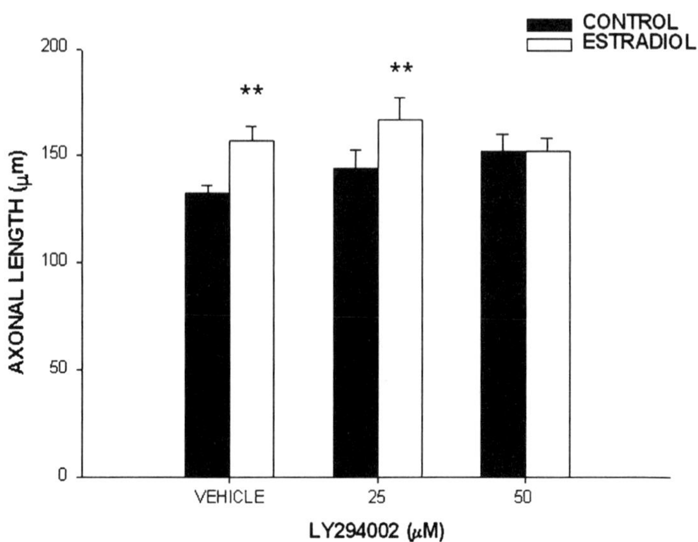

FIGURE 4. Effect of PI 3 kinase inhibition by LY294002 on the axogenic effect of estradiol. Dissociated hypothalamic neurons taken from GD 16 male fetuses were grown in astroglia-conditioned medium without (Control) or with estradiol 10 nM. After 3-h washout, cultures were treated with 25 or 50 μM LY294002 for 1 h and then estradiol was added back for an additional 24 h. Data represent mean ± SEM.; $N = 3–5$ different cultures for each condition; 60 neurons were measured for each culture and condition. Two-way ANOVA showed significant hormone X inhibitor interaction F (2, 16) = 6.96, $P = 0.006$. Post hoc test indicated $^{**}P \leq 0.01$ versus control.

complementary effects on growth and differentiation. In view of the multiple and varied alternatives succinctly described above, it seems superfluous to state that the precise mechanisms involved from E2 activation of receptors to neurite growth are still not definitely established.

ACKNOWLEDGMENTS

Work from the authors' laboratory was supported by grants from Agencia Córdoba Ciencia, Agencia Nacional de Promoción Científica y Tecnológica, Consejo Nacional de Investigaciones Científicas y Técnicas (CONICET) of Argentina, and the European Commission. H.F.C. and M.J.C. are career members of CONICET.

REFERENCES

1. Toran Allerand, C.D., M. Singh & G. Setalo. 1999. Novel mechanisms of estrogen action in the brain: new players in an old story. Front. Neuroendocrinol. **20:** 97–121.
2. Chowen, J.A., I. Azcoitia, G.P. Cardona Gomez & L.M. Garcia Segura. 2000. Sex steroids and the brain: lessons from animal studies. J. Pediatr. Endocrinol. Metab. **13:** 1045–1066.

3. LABOURDETTE, G. & M. SENSENBRENNER. 1995. Growth factors and their receptors in the central nervous system. *In* Neuroglia. H. Kettenmann & B.R. Ransom, Eds.: 441–459. Oxford University Press. New York.
4. CAMBIASSO, M.J., H. DIAZ, A. CACERES & H.F. CARRER. 1995. Neuritogenic effect of estradiol on rat ventromedial hypothalamic neurons co-cultured with homotopic or heterotopic glia. J. Neurosci. Res. **42:** 700–709.
5. CAMBIASSO, M.J., J.A. COLOMBO & H.F. CARRER. 2000. Differential effect of oestradiol and astroglia-conditioned media on the growth of hypothalamic neurons from male and female rat brains. Eur. J. Neurosci. **12:** 2291–2298.
6. BLANCO, G., H. DIAZ, H.F. CARRER & L. BEAUGE. 1990. Differentiation of rat hippocampal neurons induced by estrogen in vitro—effects on neuritogenesis and Na,K-ATPase activity. J. Neurosci. Res. **27:** 47–54.
7. DIAZ, H., A. LORENZO, H.F. CARRER & A. CACERES. 1992. Time lapse study of neurite growth in hypothalamic dissociated neurons in culture—sex differences and estrogen effects. J. Neurosci. Res. **33:** 266–281.
8. LORENZO, A., H. DIAZ, H.F. CARRER & A. CACERES. 1992. Amygdala neurons in vitro—neurite growth and effects of estradiol. J. Neurosci. Res. **33:** 418–435.
9. PÁRDUCZ, A., J. PEREZ & L.M. GARCIA SEGURA. 1993. Estradiol induces plasticity of gabaergic synapses in the hypothalamus. Neuroscience **53:** 395–401.
10. NAFTOLIN, F., L.M. GARCIA SEGURA, D. KEEFE, *et al.* 1990. Estrogen effects on the synaptology and neural membranes of the rat hypothalamic arcuate nucleus. Biol. Reprod. **42:** 21–28.
11. LUQUIN, S., F. NAFTOLIN & L.M. GARCIA SEGURA. 1993. Natural fluctuation and gonadal hormone regulation of astrocyte immunoreactivity in dentate gyrus. J. Neurobiol. **24:** 913–924.
12. GARCIA-SEGURA, L.M., M. DUEÑAS, S. BUSIGUINA, *et al.* 1995. Gonadal hormone regulation of neuronal-glial interactions in the developing neuroendocrine hypothalamus. J. Steroid Biochem. Mol. Biol. **53:** 293–298.
13. CAMBIASSO, M.J. & H.F. CARRER. 2001. Nongenomic mechanism mediates estradiol stimulation of axon growth in male rat hypothalamic neurons in vitro. J. Neurosci. Res. **66:** 475–481.
14. MURPHY, D.D. & M. SEGAL. 1996. Regulation of dendritic spine density in cultured rat hippocampal neurons by steroid hormones. J. Neurosci. **16:** 4059–4068.
15. KUIPER, G.G., B. CARLSSON, K. GRANDIEN, *et al.* 1997. Comparison of the ligand binding specificity and transcript tissue distribution of estrogen receptors alpha and beta. Endocrinology **138:** 863–870.
16. SUKOVICH, D.A., R. MUKHERJEE & P.A. BENFIELD. 1994. A novel, cell-type-specific mechanism for estrogen receptor-mediated gene activation in the absence of an estrogen-responsive element. Mol. Cell Biol. **14:** 7134–7143.
17. SINGH, M., G. SETALO, X.P. GUAN, *et al.* 1999. Estrogen-induced activation of mitogen-activated protein kinase in cerebral cortical explants: convergence of estrogen and neurotrophin signaling pathways. J. Neurosci. **19:** 1179–1188.
18. BEYER, C. & M. KAROLCZAK. 2000. Estrogenic stimulation of neurite growth in midbrain dopaminergic neurons depends on cAMP/protein kinase A signaling. J. Neurosci. Res. **59:** 107–116.
19. HALL, J.M., J.F. COUSE & K.S. KORACH. 2001. The multifaceted mechanisms of estradiol and estrogen receptor signaling. J. Biol. Chem. **276:** 36869–36872.
20. CENNI, B. & D. PICARD. 1999. Ligand-independent activation of steroid receptors: new roles for old players. Trends Endocrinol. Metab. **10:** 41–46.
21. CLARKE, C.H., A.M. NORFLEET, M.S.F. CLARKE, *et al.* 2000. Perimembrane localization of the estrogen receptor alpha protein in neuronal processes of cultured hippocampal neurons. Neuroendocrinology **71:** 34–42.
22. SHUGHRUE, P.J., G.R. ASKEW, T.L. DELLOVADE & I. MERCHENTHALER. 2002. Estrogen-binding sites and their functional capacity in estrogen receptor double knockout mouse brain. Endocrinology **143:** 1643–1650.
23. RAZANDI, M., A. PEDRAM, G.L. GREENE & E.R. LEVIN. 1999. Cell membrane and nuclear estrogen receptors (ERs) originate from a single transcript: studies of ER alpha and ER beta expressed in Chinese hamster ovary cells. Mol. Endocrinol. **13:** 307–319.

24. LEVIN, E.R. 1999. Cellular functions of the plasma membrane estrogen receptor. Trends Endocrinol. Metab. **10:** 374–377.
25. TORAN ALLERAND, C.D. 2000. Novel sites and mechanisms of oestrogen action in the brain. Novartis Found. Symp. **230:** 56–69.
26. TORAN ALLERAND, C.D., X. GUAN, N.J. MACLUSKY, *et al.* 2002. ER-X: a novel, plasma membrane-associated, putative estrogen receptor that is regulated during development and after ischemic brain injury. J. Neurosci. **22:** 8391–8401.
27. MOATS, R.K. & V.D. RAMIREZ. 2000. Electron microscopic visualization of membrane-mediated uptake and translocation of estrogen-BSA: colloidal gold by Hep G2 cells. J. Endocrinol. **166:** 631–647.
28. RAMIREZ, V.D., J.L. KIPP & I. JOE. 2001. Estradiol, in the CNS, targets several physiologically relevant membrane-associated proteins. Brain Res. Brain Res. Rev. **37:** 141–152.
29. KATO, S., Y. MASUHIRO, M. WATANABE, *et al.* 2000. Molecular mechanism of a cross-talk between oestrogen and growth factor signalling pathways. Genes Cells **5:** 593–601.
30. GARCIA SEGURA, L.M., F. NAFTOLIN, J.B. HUTCHISON, *et al.* 1999. Role of astroglia in estrogen regulation of synaptic plasticity and brain repair. J. Neurobiol. **40:** 574–584.
31. CHOWEN, J.A., I. TORRES ALEMÁN & L.M. GARCÍA SEGURA. 1992. Trophic effects of estradiol on fetal rat hypothalamic neurons. Neuroendocrinology **56:** 895–901.
32. DUEÑAS, M., I. TORRES ALEMAN, F. NAFTOLIN & L.M. GARCIA SEGURA. 1996. Interaction of insulin-like growth factor-I and estradiol signaling pathways on hypothalamic neuronal differentiation. Neuroscience **74:** 531–539.
33. CARDONA GOMEZ, G.P., J.L. TREJO, A.M. FERNANDEZ & L.M. GARCIA SEGURA. 2000. Estrogen receptors and insulin-like growth factor-I receptors mediate estrogen-dependent synaptic plasticity. Neuroreport **11:** 1735–1738.
34. GU, Q. & R.L. MOSS. 1996. 17 Beta-estradiol potentiates kainate-induced currents via activation of the cAMP cascade. J. Neurosci. **16:** 3620–3629.
35. ZHOU, Y., J.J. WATTERS & D.M. DORSA. 1996. Estrogen rapidly induces the phosphorylation of the cAMP response element binding protein in rat brain. Endocrinology **137:** 2163–2166.
36. FAVIT, A., L. FIORE, F. NICOLETTI & P.L. CANONICO. 1991. Estrogen modulates stimulation of inositol phospholipid hydrolysis by norepinephrine in rat brain slices. Brain Res. **555:** 65–69.
37. BEYER, C. & H. RAAB. 1998. Nongenomic effects of oestrogen: embryonic mouse midbrain neurones respond with a rapid release of calcium from intracellular stores. Eur. J. Neurosci. **10:** 255–262.
38. WATTERS, J.J., J.S. CAMPBELL, M.J. CUNNINGHAM, *et al.* 1997. Rapid membrane effects of steroids in neuroblastoma cells: effects of estrogen on mitogen activated protein kinase signalling cascade and c-fos immediate early gene transcription. Endocrinology **138:** 4030–4033.
39. SETALO, G., M. SINGH, X.P. GUAN & C.D. TORAN ALLERAND. 2002. Estradiol-induced phosphorylation of ERK1/2 in explants of the mouse cerebral cortex: the roles of heat shock protein 90 (Hsp90) and MEK2. J. Neurobiol. **50:** 1–12.

Steroid Effects on Glial Cells

Detrimental or Protective for Spinal Cord Function?

ALEJANDRO F. DE NICOLA,[a] FLORENCIA LABOMBARDA,[a] SUSANA L. GONZALEZ,[a] MARIA CLAUDIA GONZALEZ DENISELLE,[a] RACHIDA GUENNOUN,[b] AND MICHAEL SCHUMACHER[b]

[a]*Laboratory of Neuroendocrine Biochemistry, Instituto de Biologia y Medicina Experimental, and Department of Biochemistry, Faculty of Medicine, University of Buenos Aires, Buenos Aires, Argentina*

[b]*INSERM U488, Hôpital de Bicêtre, 94276 Bicêtre, France*

ABSTRACT: Repair of damage and recovery of function are fundamental endeavors for recuperation of patients and experimental animals with spinal cord injury. Steroid hormones, such as progesterone (PROG), show regenerative and myelinating properties following injury of the peripheral and central nervous system. In this work, we studied PROG effects on glial cells of the normal and transected (TRX) spinal cord, to complement previous studies in motoneurons. Both neurons and glial cells expressed the classical PROG receptor (PR), suggesting that genomic mechanisms participated in PROG action. In TRX rats, PROG treatment stimulated the number of NADPH-diaphorase (nitric oxide synthase) active astrocytes, whereas the number of astrocytes expressing the glial fibrillary acidic protein (GFAP) was stimulated in control but not in TRX rats. PROG also stimulated the immunocytochemical staining for myelin-basic protein (MBP) and the number of oligodendrocyte precursor cells expressing the chondroitin sulfate proteoglycan NG2 in TRX rats. In terms of beneficial or detrimental consequences, these PROG effects may be supportive of neuronal recuperation, as shown for several neuronal functional parameters that were normalized by PROG treatment of spinal cord injured animals. Thus, PROG effects on glial cells go in parallel with morphological and biochemical evidence of survival of damaged motoneurons.

KEYWORDS: progesterone; spinal cord injury; astrocytes; oligodendrocytes; myelin basic protein; glial fibrillary acidic protein; nitric oxide synthase; NG2 cells; neuroprotection

INTRODUCTION

Traumatic spinal cord injury constitutes a devastating event that often results in complete loss of motor function. All cell types populating the spinal cord are profoundly affected following injury.[1] Neurons, especially ventral horn motoneurons,

Address for correspondence: Alejandro F. De Nicola, Instituto de Biologia y Medicina Experimental, Obligado 2490, 1428 Buenos Aires, Argentina. Voice: + 54-11-4783-2869; fax: +54-11-4786-2564.
denicola@dna.uba.ar

**Ann. N.Y. Acad. Sci. 1007: 317–328 (2003). © 2003 New York Academy of Sciences.
doi: 10.1196/annals.1286.030**

show early degeneration and chromatolysis, with death occurring by necrosis or apoptosis, depending on the severity of the lesion. Astroglial cells become strongly activated, with increased expression of the intermediate filament, glial fibrillary acidic protein (GFAP). Activated astrocytes bring protection to damaged neurons by producing trophic factors; they also increase the uptake of toxic levels of glutamate and potassium and release lactate that becomes a glucose precursor in neurons. Astrogliosis, however, may also impose a barrier to axonal regeneration. Oligodendrocytes, the myelinating cells of the central nervous system (CNS), show changes typical of apoptosis, and axons are markedly demyelinated. The resulting myelin debris becomes a source of myelin-associated inhibitors of axonal regeneration.[2] Lastly, resting microglia become activated, increasing their mobility, secretion of cytokines, and mounting an inflammatory response.[1]

Repair of damage and recovery of function are fundamental endeavors for recuperation of patients or experimental animals with spinal cord injury. Strategies employed to fill these objectives include transplant of peripheral nerves, olfactory ensheathing cells, stem cells, Schwann cells, and enhancement of axonal growth using fibronectin conduits.[3] Pharmacological treatments include delivery of neurotrophic factors, antioxidant compounds, antiglutamatergic drugs, and steroids.[3,4]

Steroid hormones show promising therapeutic perspectives during the acute phase of spinal cord injury because of their protective effects on damaged neurons.[4–7] Glucocorticoids are highly effective for recovery in patients with spinal cord trauma, and in rats in contusion and transection models.[4] However, gonadal steroids, including progesterone (PROG), also provide neuroprotection in spinal cord injury and lesions of brain-stem motor nuclei.

Thus, PROG prevents neuronal loss following contusion, ischemia, and edema of the brain, and preserves neurons after cuts to the hypoglossal and facial motor nuclei.[7] In the spinal cord, treatment of rats with PROG increases motoneuron survival after axotomy or injury, protects cultured neurons against glutamate toxicity, and normalizes defective functional parameters of injured neurons.[8,9] In rats with complete spinal cord transection (TRX), deafferentiation reduces the levels of choline acetyltransferase (ChAT) and $\alpha 3$ subunit mRNA of the Na,K-ATPase, while moderately up-regulating the mRNA of the growth-associated protein GAP-43.[10] *In vivo* PROG treatment during 72 h restores levels of the sodium pump mRNA and ChAT to normal, whereas levels of GAP-43 mRNA are further enhanced.[10] These responses are interpreted as protective and regenerative of damaged tissue.

PROG also stimulates myelination. In Schwann cells (the myelinating glial of the peripheral nervous system), PROG and its reduced metabolites activate genes encoding the myelin proteins Po and PMP22 and induce the expression of Krox 20, a transcription factor related to myelinogenesis.[11,12] In the regenerating sciatic nerve of male mice, endogenously formed PROG promotes the formation of new myelin sheaths after a cryolesion.[13] In cultures of oligodendrocytes, the myelin-producing glia of the CNS, PROG increases the expression of the myelin basic protein (MBP).[13] Finally, PROG also regulates GFAP-labeled astrocytes in the CNS after a penetrating brain injury. In this study, proliferation of GFAP-immunoreactive astrocytes in the vicinity of the wound is decreased in steroid-treated rats.[14]

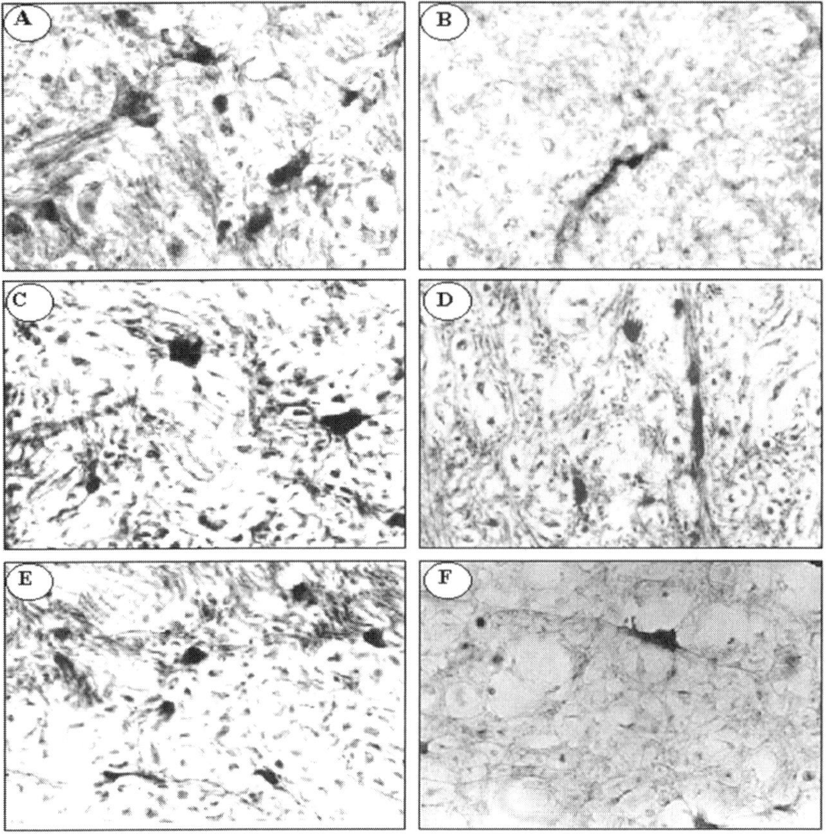

FIGURE 1. PR immunoreactive glial cells in the spinal cord gray matter **(A, C, E)** and white matter **(B, D, F)**. **A, B:** ovariectomized (OVX) rat; **C, D:** OVX rat treated with estradiol; **E, F:** untreated male rat. Magnification: 1000×. (Modified from Labombarda *et al.*[15])

PROG RECEPTORS IN THE SPINAL CORD

Both spinal cord motoneurons and glial cells expressed PROG receptors (PR).[15] Immunocytochemistry, using the KC 146 monoclonal antibody recognizing the B-form of PR, demonstrated that not only neurons from ventral horn and lamina IX, but also those from glial cells in gray and white matter (FIG. 1) and ependymal cells were PR-positive. Evidence of estrogen inducibility of PR in ovariectomized rats (FIG. 1; A, B vs. C, D) or of gender differences in neuronal PR immunostaining intensity were not obtained in the spinal cord (A, B vs. E, F). In pituitary and uterus from estrogenized female rats, which showed the expected estrogen dependency, PR showed a strict nuclear localization; whereas in neurons and glial cells of the spinal cord, PR localized in cytoplasm and/or nucleus as well as in some cell processes. Although the type of glial cells expressing PR was not identified, expression of PR in astrocytes and oligodendrocytes was suggested in this work.[15]

In a second study, two binding molecules for PROG in the control and in the injured spinal cord were investigated: the classical PR and a recently discovered PROG membrane-binding site called 25-Dx.[16] For both molecules, RT-PCR was employed to determine the relative mRNA levels, whereas cellular receptor localization was investigated by immunocytochemistry. We observed that spinal cord PR mRNA was estrogen insensitive, as it occurred in some brain areas, and amounted to a third of that measured in the estradiol-stimulated uterus of female ovariectomized rats. In male rats with complete spinal cord TRX, levels of PR mRNA significantly decreased, while mRNA of the novel membrane receptor for progesterone 25-DX were unchanged with respect to those of control animals. When spinal cord–injured animals received PROG treatment during 75 h, the PR mRNA levels were similar to those of nontreated animals, while the 25-DX mRNA levels significantly increased. As in the first study, immunostaining of PR showed intracellular localization in neurons and glial cells, whereas 25-DX immunoreactivity localized to the plasma membrane of dorsal horn and central canal neurons. Since the two binding systems for PROG differed in their response to lesion, hormone treatment, and regional localization, their function may also differ under normal and pathological conditions. However, because only PR was detected in glial cells, genomic mechanisms may play some role on PROG effects in astrocytes and oligodendrocytes. Nevertheless, the fact that PR mRNA declined after spinal cord TRX suggested that alternative mechanisms were also taking place in the injured tissue.

EXPERIMENTAL SPINAL CORD INJURY AND HORMONE TREATMENT

Sprague-Dawley male rats (250–300 g) were deeply anesthetized, and spinal cord TRX was carried out at thoracic level T10, using the sharp edge of a 25-G needle.[10,15] Sham-operated rats were not transected. For PROG treatment, four injections of 4 mg/kg PROG dissolved in vegetable oil was given at 1 h (i.p.), 24 h, 48 h, and 72 h (s.c.) post-lesion. This PROG dose prevented neuronal degeneration and loss after brain injury.[8] Animals were used for the different experiments 75 h after sham surgery or TRX, and 3 h after receiving the last injection.

EFFECTS OF PROG ON ASTROCYTES

Two proteins were analyzed in astrocytes from rats with spinal cord TRX, namely, the GFAP and the NADPH-diaphorase. As already mentioned, GFAP constitutes a useful marker of astroglial activation after injury. NADPH-diaphorase, an accepted histochemical marker for nitric oxide synthase (NOS), has a restricted distribution in normal neurons, but is found in resting astrocytes. In contrast to astrocytes, oligodendrocytes are devoid of nitric oxide synthase. It is known that injury, ischemia, and cytokines stimulate astroglial NOS.[17] Therefore, the objectives of this study were first to assess the response of NOS after hormone treatment, while considering the duel roles of NO, not only in cytotoxicity but also in the enhancement of cell function.[18] And, second, to elucidate the response of GFAP, in view of its importance for astrocyte function and its postulated role in myelin repair and deposition.[19]

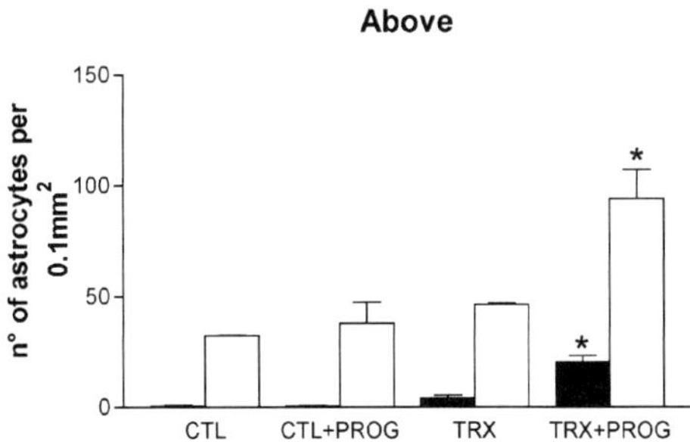

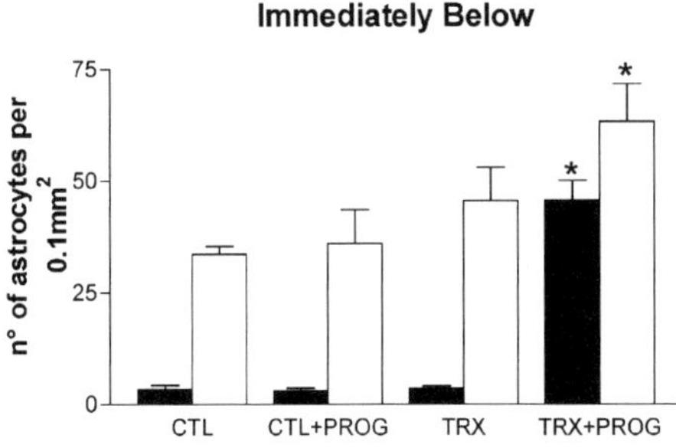

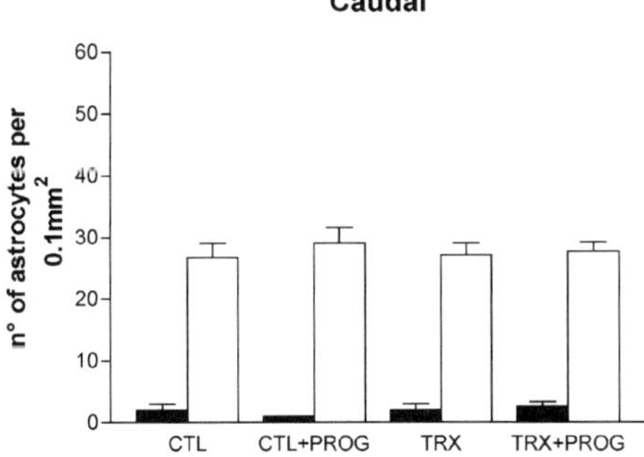

FIGURE 2. Progesterone (PROG) effects on the number of NADPH-diaphorase positive astroctes of normal and transected spinal cords. Data correspond to the number of cells per 0.1 mm^2 in the white matter (lateral funiculus, *white bars*) and gray matter (Lamina IX, *dark bars*). Group labeling: CTL, control sham-operated rats; CTL + PROG, controls receiving PROG; TRX, spinal cord transection; TRX + PROG, transection plus PROG. Cells were counted above (T5 level, *upper graph*), immediately below (L1 level, *middle graph*) or caudal (L3 level, *lower graph*) to the lesion placed at T10. The results represented the mean ± SEM of $n = 4$ animals per group. Statistical significance was carried out by ANOVA and post-hoc tests. For white and gray matter astrocytes located above and immediately below the lesion: * TRX + P4: $P < 0.05$ vs. all other groups. (From Labombarda *et al.*[17] Reprinted with permission from Elsevier.)

NADPH-diaphorase activity was determined in cryostat sections of spinal cord regions taken above (T5 level), immediately below (L1 level), and caudal to the lesion (L3 level). Equivalent regions were dissected from the spinal cord of sham-operated rats. Data of NADPH-diaphorase histochemistry in control, control + PROG, TRX and TRX + PROG groups are shown (FIG. 2). In controls, PROG had no effect on the total number of NADPH-diaphorase positive astrocytes on all levels of the spinal cord analyzed. In animals with TRX that did not receive hormone, the number of NADPH-diaphorase active astrocytes remained similar to the controls and controls plus PROG. However, in the TRX group PROG increased the total number of NADPH-diaphorase active cells in white and gray matter above and immediately below, but not caudal to the lesion ($P < 0.05$ or less, FIG. 2). We also observed that large-sized NADPH-diaphorase positive astrocytes, measuring >55 mm^2 in the gray matter and >70 mm^2 in the white matter, were more frequent in the TRX + PROG group than in the other groups, both above and immediately below the lesion (FIG. 3).

With regard to GFAP response: In controls, PROG produced a strong up-regulation of the total number of GFAP-expressing astrocytes in gray and white matter at all levels of the spinal cord (control + PROG: $P < 0.05$ or less vs. control group (FIG. 4). Spinal cord TRX, per se, was also a powerful stimulus for GFAP expression in gray and white mater distributed above, immediately below and caudal to the lesion (TRX $P < 0.05$ or less vs. sham-operated controls). After TRX, PROG treatment did not modify the already high GFAP immunoreactivity. The exception to this finding was a TRX + PROG effect in the gray matter astrocytes, caudal to the lesion ($P < 0.05$ vs. TRX alone). We also observed that large stellate GFAP-positive astrocytes predominated in white matter (>70 μm^2) and gray matter (>55 μm^2) in control + PROG, TRX and TRX + PROG groups, over the sham-operated control animals. Thus, while spinal cord lesion due to complete TRX was a powerful stimulus for GFAP expression, PROG effects on this protein required quiescent astrocytes, as shown in control rats.

It seems important to speculate about the possible role of PROG on these two astrocyte proteins: first, because PROG effects on NADPH-diaphorase were only obtained in astrocytes from lesioned spinal cord, it is likely that the response of the enzyme to PROG was potentiated by environmental factors released during injury, which then conditioned the sensitivity to PROG in reactive astrocytes; and, second, because these factors affected proximal astrocytes (i.e., above and immediately below the lesion site), they may be acting locally without diffusion to the caudal region of the spinal cord.

NADPH-diaphorase staining, however, did not indicate which enzyme isoform was the target of PROG effects. Astrocytes can express all known NOS isoforms. Preliminary experiments demonstrated abundant nNOS-positive astrocytes in the spinal cord from rats with TRX receiving PROG. In these experiments, astrocytes remained iNOS negative, whereas LPS-stimulated peritoneal macrophages strongly reacted with the iNOS antibody (unpublished data). Increased NO generation may be neurotoxic or cytoprotective, with literature reports supporting both alternatives. Thus, stimulated astrocytes may be neurotoxic via a NO-mediated mechanism, and NO is involved in spinal cord cavitation. In contrast, other authors considered that NOS expression by neurons is associated with axonal sprouting and growth in the spinal cord, and increased NO may be beneficial to neuronal function after a region has been damaged.[18]

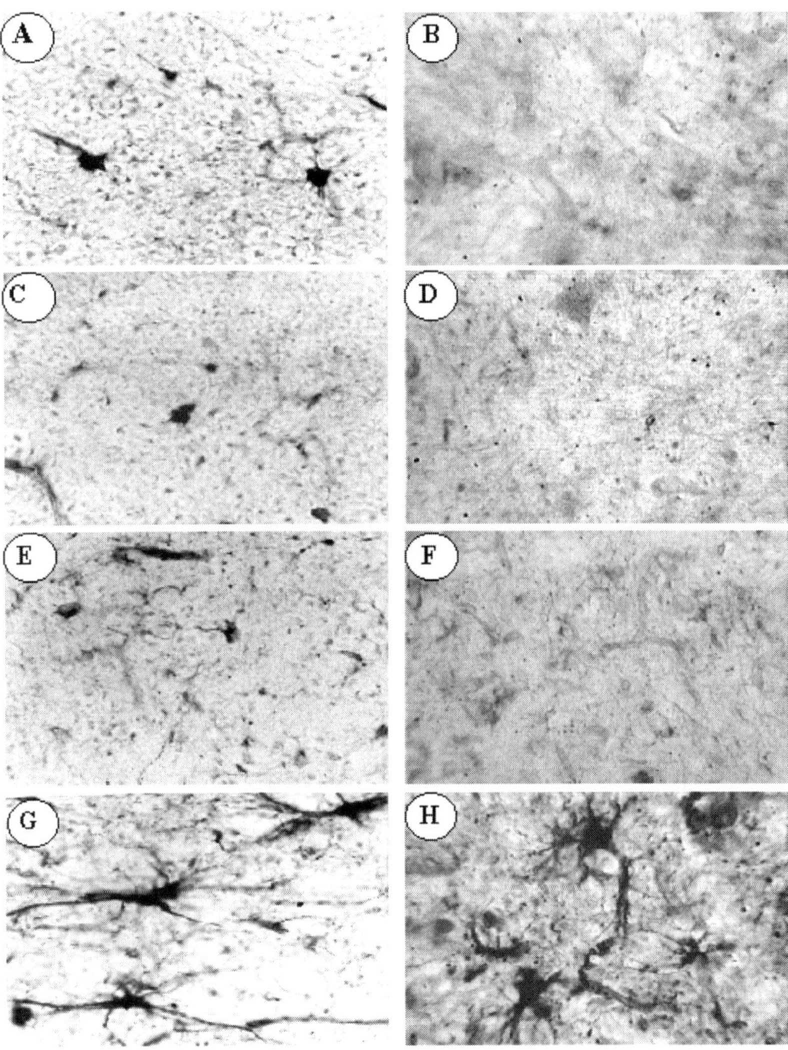

FIGURE 3. Representative NADPH-diaphorase staining of astrocytes from the white matter **(A, C, E, G)** and gray matter **(B, D, F, H)** localized below the lesion at T10 or a similar region taken from sham-operated rats. Group labeling as in the legend to FIGURE 2. The photomicrographs represent CTL **(A, B)**, CTL + PROG **(C, D)**, TRX **(E, F)** and TRX + PROG **(G, H)** groups. Staining of large, stellate astrocytic forms predominated in **G** and **H**. Magnification: 1000×, no counterstaining. (From Labombarda *et al.*[17] Repinted with permission from Elsevier).

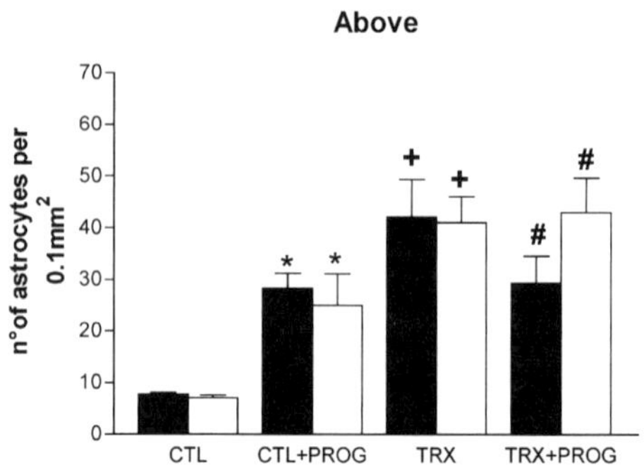

Immediately Below

n° of astrocytes per 0.1mm^2

100

75

50

25

0

CTL CTL+PROG TRX TRX+PROG

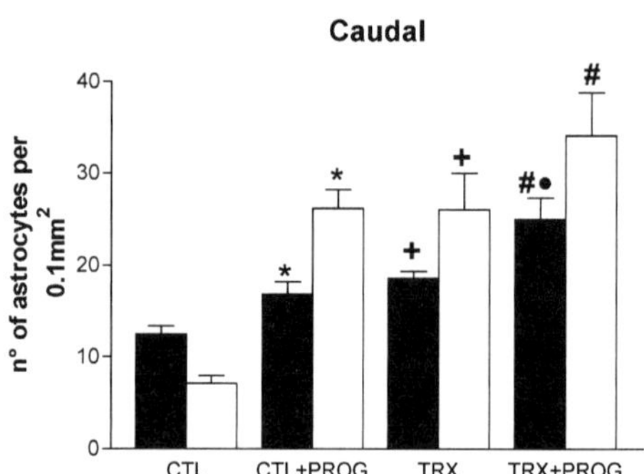

FIGURE 4. Progesterone (PROG) effects on the total number of immunoreactive GFAP astrocytes of normal and transected spinal cords. Data corresponded to astrocyte number per 0.1 mm^2 in the white matter (*white bars*) and gray matter (*dark bars*). Group labeling is the same as in the legend to FIGURE 2. Significance: For white and gray matter astrocytes located above, immediately below, and caudal to the lesion: *CTL + PROG: $P < 0.05$ vs. CTL; $^+$TRX and $^\#$TRX + PROG: $P < 0.05$ vs. CTL. However, TRX vs. TRX + PROG: NS. For gray matter astrocytes of the caudal region: ● TRX + PROG: $P < 0.05$ vs. all other groups. (From Labombarda *et al.*[17] Reprinted with permission from Elsevier).

Effects of PROG on GFAP protein expression, instead, differed from those on NADPH-diaphorase activity. Thus, PROG increased the number and area of GFAP-expressing astrocytes resident in the gray and white matter at all levels of the spinal cord from sham-operated rats. However, except for the gray matter in the caudal region, it was ineffective in rats with TRX. This finding suggests that up-regulation of GFAP by PROG involved resting astrocytes distributed throughout the spinal cord. Furthermore, GFAP-positive astrocytes from PROG-treated animals, as well as those from rats with TRX, presented long processes and a stellated morphology. Regarding the mechanism for PROG up-regulation of GFAP, the reported elevation of the GFAP mRNA by PROG and 5-dihydroprogesterone[20] suggests a regulatory effect at the level of gene expression.

One other report considered PROG effects on GFAP-immunolabeled reactive astrocytes after CNS injury. After a penetrating brain injury, decreased proliferation of GFAP-immunoreactive astrocytes in the vicinity of the wound is obtained in PROG-treated rats,[14] in contrast to our data in the spinal cord. However, brain and spinal cord astrocytes may respond differently to injury, because pronounced astrocyte heterogeneity exists in the CNS. Besides, after spinal cord lesion, the GFAP gene may be unresponsive to hormonal treatment, suggesting that local injury takes precedence over hormone-mediated responses at the GFAP gene.

The induction of a reactive response in quiescent astrocytes by PROG may have functional consequences. Although traditionally astrocytosis is considered a negative factor for neuronal trophism and regeneration, recent data support that reactive astrocytes may help neuronal regeneration and stop neuronal death by secretion of growth factors, substrate-bound neurite promoting factors, removal of neurotoxins and glutamate, and provision of glucose precursors to neurons.[21] GFAP-expressing astrocytes may be also necessary for myelination and normal white matter architecture.[19] If true for the spinal cord, PROG might help myelin synthesis in the control spinal cord.

PROG EFFECTS ON MYELIN BASIC PROTEIN AND OLIGODENDROCYTE PRECURSOR CELLS

Previous reports on PROG induction of myelin genes in Schwann cells and cultured oligodendrocytes suggest that PROG might also increase myelinogenesis in the spinal cord. To this end, we studied (1) the effects of spinal cord TRX and PROG treatment on the expression of MBP, a component of CNS myelin, and (2) the number of oligodendrocyte precursors using an antibody recognizing the surface oligodendrocyte precursor cells (NG2) proteoglycan. Spinal cord injury constitutes a powerful stimulus for proliferation of NG2 oligodendrocyte precursors.[22] In addition, a role of PROG on the olidodendrocyte cell lineage has been already postulated.[23]

Therefore, employing an antibody reacting against MBP, we determined the immunoreaction-staining intensity of the corticospinal tract (CST), the dorsal ascending funiculus (DAT), and the ventral funiculus (VF). These areas of white matter were selected considering that after spinal cord TRX, CST fibers represented axons undergoing axonal degeneration, whereas those in DAT represented the response of proximal axons. VF staining was the response of ventral roots originating in motoneurons. After TRX, MBP-staining intensity in CST immediately below the lesion site was reduced by half of the control, sham-operated animals (controls 0.069 ± 6.5×10^{-3}; TRX 0.042 ± 3.8×10^{-3}, $P < 0.05$), whereas in TRX rats receiving PROG it reverted to near control levels (TRX + PROG 0.08 ± 5.5×10^{-3}, $P < 0.05$ vs. TRX). A similar response was found for DAT (controls 0108 ± 0.015; TRX 0.067 ± 8.7×10^{-3}, $P < 0.05$; TRX + PROG 0.13 ± 9.11×10^{-3}, $P < 0.05$ vs. TRX). In contrast, staining intensity in VF remained unchanged, indicating some region specificity in response to steroid treatment.

In order to explain the enhanced MBP immunostaining of TRX rats receiving PROG, we envisaged two mechanisms: first a direct participation of PROG in myelination, as shown in the PNS and cultured oligodendrocytes;[1–13] and, second, the PROG stimulation of oligodendrocyte development, and differentiation. The latter hypothesis was tested by measuring the number of premyelinating oligodendrocyte precursor cells using an antibody recognizing the NG2 proteoglycan. The number of NG2 cells/200 mm^2 area was determined immediately below the lesion (thoracic level) and caudal to TRX (L4 region). In agreement with McTigue *et al.*,[22] the TRX powerfully stimulated NG2 cell number, as these cells were practically absent in control rats receiving vehicle or PROG treatment. PROG treatment of TRX rats significantly increased NG2 number immediately below the lesion (TRX 41.5 ± 5.4; TRX + PROG 62.5 ± 1.5, $P < 0.05$) and also distant to it. Therefore, the powerful effect of PROG on NG2-expression may ultimately contribute to myelin production. Although NG2 cells are MBP negative, they are able to migrate, proliferate, and differentiate into mature oligodendrocytes.[23] This combined action of PROG on MBP immunostaining and NG2 cells in rats with TRX suggests that the steroid contributed to remyelination of the damaged spinal cord.

CONCLUSION

Our data demonstrated that in rats with TRX, PROG induced an up-regulation of glial cell parameters, including astrocyte NADPH-diaphorase, oligodendrocyte MBP staining, and the number of NG2 cells. These PROG effects on glial cells may be supportive of neuronal recuperation. As previously shown, deafferented motoneurons from spinal cord–lesioned animals present several biochemical abnormalities involving the acetylcholine-synthesizing enzyme, the sodium pump mRNA, BDNF mRNA, and the GAP 43 mRNA. These parameters are reverted to normal after PROG treatment is given to TRX animals, with the exception of GAP 43 mRNA, which is further enhanced. As further evidence for PROG neuroprotection, we recently observed that chromatolysis, originating in motoneurons of rats with TRX, was considerably prevented when the animals received an intensive PROG treatment. Thus, PROG effects on glial cells go in parallel with morphological and biochemical evidence of survival of damaged motoneurons. This process favors the view that PROG-supported spinal cord function is by a dual action on neurons and glial cells.

ACKNOWLEDGMENTS

This research was supported by a collaborative program between the governments of France and Argentina (ECOS/ SECYT # A98SO1), the University of Buenos Aires (M048), CONICET (PIP 02007), FONCYT (BID 802 OC AR PICT 2000 05-08663), and Fundacion Antorchas.

REFERENCES

1. BEATTIE, M.S., A.A. FAROOQUI & J.E. BRESNAHAN. 2000. Review of current evidence for apoptosis after spinal cord injury. J. Neurotrauma **17:** 915–923.
2. FOURNIER, A.E. & S.M. STRIITTMATTRER. 2001. Repulsive factors and axon regeneration in the CNS. Curr. Opin. Neurobiol. **11:** 89–94.
3. PRIESTLEY, J.V., M.S. RAMER, V.R. KING, *et al.* 2002. Stimulating regeneration in the damaged spinal cord. J. Physiol. (Paris) **96:** 123–133.
4. HALL, E.D. 2001. Pharmacological treatment of acute spinal cord injury: how do we build on past success? J. Spinal Cord Med. **24:** 142–146.
5. DE NICOLA, A.F. 1993. Steroid hormones and neuronal regeneration. Adv. Neurol. **59:** 199–206.
6. HALL, E. 1993. Neuroprotective actions of glucocorticoid and non-glucocorticoid steroids in acute neuronal injury. Cell. Mol. Neurobiol. **13:** 415–432.
7. JONES, K.J., S.M. DRENGLER & M. OBLINGER. 1997. Gonadal steroid regulation of growth-associated protein mRNA expression in axotomized hamster facial motor neurons. Neurochem. Res. **22:** 1367–1374.
8. STEIN, D.G. & Z.L. FULOP. 1998. Progesterone and recovery after traumatic brain injury: an overview. Neuroscientist **4:** 435–442.
9. ROOF, R. & E. HALL. 2000. Gender differences in acute CNS trauma and stroke: neuroprotective effects and progesterone. J. Neurotrauma **17:** 367–388.
10. LABOMBARDA, F., S. GONZALEZ, M.C. GONZALEZ DENISELLE, *et al.* 2002. Cellular basis for progesterone neuroprotection in the injured spinal cord. J. Neurotrauma **19:** 343–355.
11. DESARNAUD, F., A.N. DO THI, A.M. BROWN, *et al.* 1998. Progesterone stimulates the activity of the promoters of peripheral myelin protein-22 and protein zero genes in Schwann cells. J. Neurochem. **71:** 1765–1768.
12. MELCANGI, R.C., V. MAGNAGHI & L. MARTINI. 2000. Aging in peripheral nerves: regulation of myelin protein genes by steroid hormones. Prog. Neurobiol. **60:** 291–308.
13. SCHUMACHER, M., I. AKWA, R. GUENNOUN, *et al.* 2000. Steroid synthesis and metabolism in the nervous system: trophic and protective effects. J. Neurocytol. **29:** 307–326.
14. GARCIA-ESTRADA, J., J.A. DEL RIO, S. LUQUIN, *et al.* 1993. Gonadal hormones down-regulate reactive gliosis and astrocyte proliferation after a penetrating brain injury. Brain Res. **628:** 271–278.
15. LABOMBARDA, F., R. GUENNOUN, S. GONZALEZ, *et al.* 2000. Immunocytochemical evidence for a progesterone receptor in neurons and glial cells of the rat spinal cord. Neurosci. Lett. **288:** 29–32.
16. KREBS, C.J., E.D. JARVIS, J. CHAN, *et al.* 2000. A membrane-associated progesterone-binding protein, 25-Dx, is regulated by progesterone in brain regions involved in female reproductive behaviors. Proc. Natl. Acad. Sci. USA **97:** 12816–12821.
17. LABOMBARDA, F., S. GONZALEZ, P. ROIG, *et al.* 2000. Modulation of NADPH-diaphorase and glial fibrillary acidic protein by progesterone in astrocytes from normal and injured rat spinal cord. J. Steroid Biochem. Mol. Biol. **73:** 159–169.
18. STOJKOVIC, T., C. COLIN, F. LE SAUX & C. JACKE. 1998. Specific pattern of nitric oxide synthase expression in glial cells after hippocampal injury. Glia **22:** 329–327.
19. LIEDTKE, W., W. EDELMAN, P.L. BIERI, *et. al.* 1996. GFAP is necessary for the integrity of CNS white matter architecture and long-term maintenance of myelination. Neuron **17:** 607–615.
20. MELCANGI, R.C., M.A. RIVA, F. FUMAGALLI, *et al.* 1996. Effect of progesterone, testosterone and their 5 alpha-reduced metabolites on GFAP gene expression in type 1 astrocytes. Brain Res. **711:** 10–15.
21. MULLER, H.W., H.P. MATTHIESE, C. SCHMALENBACH & W.O. SCHROEDER. 1991. Glial support of CNS neuronal survival, neurite growth and regeneration. Rest. Neurol. Neurosci. **2:** 229–232.

22. McTigue, D.M., P. Wei & B.T. Stokes. 2001. Proliferation of NG2-positive cells and altered oligodendrocyte numbers in the contused spinal cord. J. Neurosci. **21:** 3392–3400.
23. Gago, N., Y. Akwa, N. Sananes, R. Guennoun, *et al.* 2001. Progesterone and the oligodendroglial lineage: Stage-dependent biosynthesis and metabolism. Glia **36:** 295–308.

Sex Steroid Regulation of Microglial Cell Activation

Relevance to Multiple Sclerosis

PAUL D. DREW, JANET A. CHAVIS, AND RENU BHATT

Department of Anatomy and Neurobiology, University of Arkansas for Medical Sciences, Little Rock, Arkansas 72205, USA

ABSTRACT: Multiple sclerosis (MS) occurs more commonly in females than males. However, the mechanisms resulting in gender differences in MS are unknown. Several studies have suggested that sex steroids influence the development and severity of MS. For example, pregnancy influences MS symptoms, with remission in the third trimester of gestation, followed by exacerbation in the postpartum period. In addition, oral contraceptives containing female sex steroids have been associated with a lower risk of developing MS and decreased disability. Experimental autoimmune encephalomyelitis (EAE) is an autoimmune disorder initiated by T cells reactive against central nervous system (CNS) antigens. EAE is characterized by inflammation and demyelination of the CNS, and by remittent paralysis—features consistent with MS. Recent studies have suggested that female sex steroids may modulate EAE, at least in part, through effects on T cells. For example, sex steroids shift T cells toward a Th2 phenotype *in vitro*, and cytokines produced by Th2 cells generally suppress EAE. Activated microglia also are believed to contribute to MS pathology; perhaps due in part to production of nitric oxide (NO) and TNF-α, molecules which can be toxic to CNS cells, including oligodendrocytes. We are currently investigating the role of sex steroids in modulating microglial cell function in relation to MS. It is hoped that elucidation of the mechanisms by which sex steroids modulate CNS inflammation will lead to future therapies in the treatment of MS.

KEYWORDS: microglia; nitric oxide; TNF-α; estrogen; progesterone

INTRODUCTION

In the United States, it is estimated that 250,000–350,000 people have physician-diagnosed multiple sclerosis (MS).[1] The cause of MS is unknown. However, because MS is characterized by perivascular mononuclear-cell inflammatory infiltrates and demyelination, features also characteristic of experimental autoimmune encephalomyelitis (EAE), an autoimmune process is thought to be involved in its pathogenesis.[2] Epidemiological studies, as well as studies examining identical twins, suggest

Address for correspondence: Paul D. Drew, Ph.D., University of Arkansas for Medical Sciences, Department of Anatomy and Neurobiology, Slot 510, Shorey Bldg., Rm. 922, 4301 W. Markham St., Little Rock, AR 72205. Voice: 501-296-1265; fax: 501-686-6382.
drewpauld@uams.edu

Ann. N.Y. Acad. Sci. 1007: 329–334 (2003).
doi: 10.1196/annals.1286.031

that both genetics and environment, particularly viral infection, may play a role in the pathogenesis of MS.[2] Multiple drugs have been approved for use in the treatment of MS, but because these agents are not a cure for the disease, the need remains for the development of better treatment strategies in MS.

MS occurs more frequently in females than males.[3] This is consistent with many other autoimmune diseases including rheumatoid arthritis, systemic lupus erythematosus, and Hashimoto's thyroiditis, in which women are also disproportionately affected.[4,5] Gender disparity in these autoimmune diseases could result from factors including (1) sex steroid hormones, (2) sex-linked genetic inheritance, and (3) sexual dimorphic immune responses.[6]

However, the precise mechanisms resulting in gender disparity in autoimmune diseases have not been elucidated. Several studies have suggested that sex steroids influence the development and severity of MS. For example, pregnancy influences MS symptoms, with remission in the third trimester of gestation, followed by exacerbation in the postpartum period.[7] In addition, oral contraceptives containing female sex steroids have been associated with a lower risk of developing MS and decreased disability.[8]

EFFECTS OF SEX STEROIDS ON T CELLS

Studies using an animal model of MS have suggested that female sex steroids may modulate EAE, at least in part, through their effects on T cells. For example, investigators have demonstrated that not only are female SJL mice more susceptible than are males to EAE, but also that T cells from female mice produce more severe disease when adoptively transferred into recipients.[9,10] In addition, estrogens[11–13] and testosterone[9] have been demonstrated to repress EAE. Furthermore, EAE is repressed during late pregnancy, which is characterized by elevated serum levels of estrogens and progesterone.[14,15] Sex steroids also shift T cells toward a Th2 phenotype *in vitro*,[9,16,17] and cytokines produced by Th2 cells generally suppress EAE.[18] Collectively, these studies suggest that sex steroids modulate EAE, in part through their effects on T-cell phenotype.

EFFECTS OF SEX STEROIDS ON MICROGLIA

In addition to autoreactive T cells, activated microglia participate in pathology associated with MS.[19,20] However, the effect of sex steroids upon activation of microglia has not been thoroughly investigated. Microglia are resident CNS cells that function in host defense. These cells may serve as antigen-presenting cells and can be phagocytic. Upon CNS injury or inflammation, microglia become activated, resulting in increased proliferation and altered morphology. Activated microglia exhibit increased MHC class II expression and produce a variety of molecules including NO and cytokines, including TNF-α.[19]

NO is a gaseous molecule produced by a series of three enzymes, termed nitric oxide synthases (NOS), that perform a wide variety of cellular functions: endothelial NOS (eNOS) and neuronal NOS (nNOS) occur constitutively, are Ca^{2+} dependent, and mediate vasodilation and neurosignaling, respectively. Inducible NOS (iNOS) was first demonstrated in monocytes, but is now known to be expressed in a variety of cells including microglia. iNOS is a Ca^{2+} and calmodulin-independent enzyme, which is induced by a variety of inflammatory cytokines and bacterial products including lipopolysaccharide (LPS).[21] TNF-α is also produced by cells of monocyte origin, including microglia, in response to inflammatory stimuli.[19]

Although molecules including NO and TNF-α are toxic to pathogens, these agents can also be toxic to CNS cells including myelin-producing oligodendrocytes,[19] which are compromised in the course of MS.[22] These molecules also may be toxic to neurons, and thus may contribute to the axonal degeneration that is characteristic of MS.[23] It should be noted that NO and TNF-α have alternatively been reported to protect CNS cells.[24,25] Inhibition of NO and TNF-α synthesis blocks development of EAE.[26–29] Thus, agents that inhibit NO and TNF-α synthesis may be effective in the treatment of MS.

Previously, we demonstrated that sex steroids, including β-estradiol, estriol, and progesterone, inhibit lipopolysachharide (LPS) induction of NO production in primary rat microglia and in the mouse N9 microglial cell line.[30] These hormones acted by inhibiting the production of iNOS, which catalyzes the synthesis of NO. Estriol likely inhibits iNOS gene expression because the hormone blocks LPS induction of iNOS RNA levels.

The proinflammatory cytokines IFN-γ and TNF-α are believed to be important modulators of MS. We demonstrated that estrogens and progesterone also inhibit NO production by microglial cells activated in response to these cytokines. Activated microglia elicit TNF-α in addition to NO, and we further demonstrated that estrogens and progesterone repress TNF-α production by these cells. Finally, estriol and progesterone, at concentrations consistent with late pregnancy, inhibited NO and TNF-α production by activated microglia, suggesting that hormone inhibition of microglial cell activation may contribute to the decreased severity of MS symptoms commonly associated with pregnancy.[30]

Studies by Vegeto *et al.* have demonstrated that microglia express both ER-α and ER-β receptors.[31] These studies further demonstrated that estrogen inhibition of microglial cell activation is blocked by estrogen receptor agonists. This supports a model in which estrogen modulates microglial activation via classical intracellular estrogen receptors.

Studies by Bruce-Keller *et al.* support the concept that estrogens inhibit microglial cell activation via classical estrogen receptors and further demonstrate that these estrogen-mediated effects on microglial cell activation involve stimulation of MAP kinase signal transduction pathways.[32,33]

We recently obtained evidence suggesting that female sex steroids inhibit LPS induction of IL-12 by N9 microglial cells (Drew *et al.*, unpublished data). IL-12 is critical in the differentiation of T cells toward a Th1 phenotype, and Th1 cells are believed to contribute to the pathology associated with MS.[34] These *in vito* studies suggest that sex steroids may inhibit the differentiation of encephalitogenic Th1 cells, and thus may be therapeutic in the treatment of MS. In addition, we have data that indicate that estrogens and progesterone are capable of protecting CG4 oligodendrocyte cells from hydrogen-peroxide mediated toxicity (Drew *et al.*, unpublished data).

We are currently analyzing the effects of sex steroids directly on primary oligodendrocyte viability, as well as the effects of these hormones on oligodendrocyte vi-

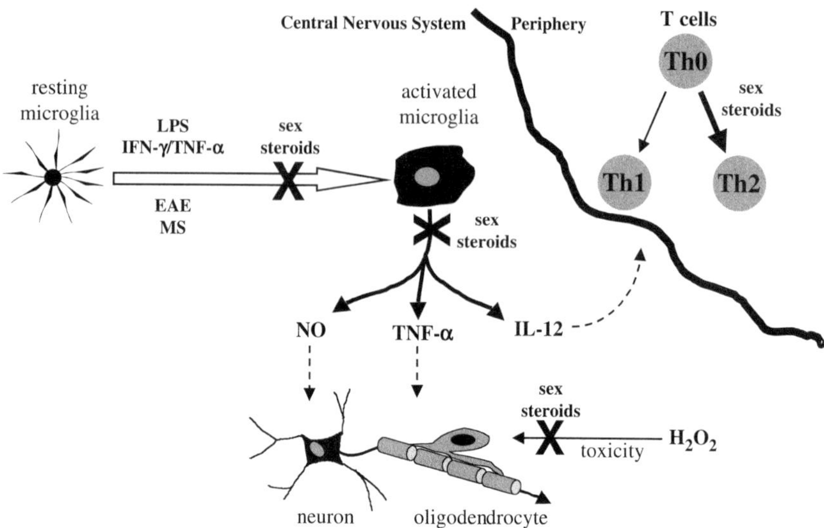

FIGURE 1. Sex steroid modulation of MS: potential mechanisms. Sex steroids are believed to alter T-cell differentiation that results in a skewing toward a Th2 phenotype, which is believed to protect against EAE/MS. Sex steroids also block the activation of microglial cells, which results in repression of NO and TNF-α expression. This likely protects oligodendrocytes and neurons from the toxic effects of NO and TNF-α. Sex steroids may also inhibit IL-12 production by microglia. Because IL-12 plays a critical role in Th1 differentiation, sex steroids may induce skewing toward a protective Th2 phenotype. Sex steroids may also directly protect oligodendrocytes from toxic agents including hydrogen peroxide.

ability, indirectly through effects on NO and TNF-α production by microglia. Furthermore, our studies indicate that female sex steroids inhibit production of MHC II, iNOS, and TNF-α by primary human microglia (Drew *et al.*, unpublished data). These studies support the notion that our previous studies with rodent microglia are relevant to human disease processes. The effects of sex steroids on microglial cell function are summarized in FIGURE 1. Collectively, these studies support the concept that sex steroids may be therapeutic in the treatment of MS. In fact, recent clinical studies suggest that the pregnancy hormone estriol is effective in the treatment of MS.[35]

ACKNOWLEDGMENTS

This work was supported by grants from the National Multiple Sclerosis Society (RG 3198A1) and the National Institutes of Health (NS 042860).

REFERENCES

1. ANDERSON, D.W., J.H. ELLENBERG, C.M. LEVENTHAL, *et al.* 1992. Revised estimate of the prevalence of multiple sclerosis in the United States. Ann. Neurol. **31:** 333–336.

2. MARTIN, R., H.F. MCFARLAND & D.E. MCFARLIN. 1992. Immunological aspects of demyelinating diseases. Annu. Rev. Immunol. **10:** 151–187.
3. DUQUETTE, P. & M. GIRARD. 1993. Hormonal factors in susceptibility to multiple sclerosis. Curr. Opin. Neurol. Neurosurg. **6:** 195–201.
4. BEESON, P.B. 1994. Age and sex associations of 40 autoimmune diseases. Am. J. Med. **96:** 457–462.
5. JACOBSON, D.L., S.J. GRANGE, N.R. ROSE, *et al.* 1997. Epidemiology, and estimated population burden of selected autoimmune diseases in the United States. Clin. Immunol. Immunopathol. **84:** 223–243.
6. WHITACRE, C.C., S.C. REINGOLD, P.A. O'LOONEY, *et al.* 1999. A gender gap in autoimmunity. Science **283:** 1277–1278.
7. CONFAVREUX, C., M. HUTCHINSON, M.M. HOURS, *et al.* 1998. Rate of pregnancy-relapse in multiple sclerosis: pregnancy in multiple sclerosis group. N. Engl. J. Med. **339:** 285–291.
8. VILLARD-MACINTOSH, L. & M.P. VESSEY. 1993. Oral contraception and reproductive factors in multiple sclerosis incidence. Contraception **47:** 161–168.
9. DALAL, M., S. KIM & R.R. VOSKUHL. 1997. Testosterone therapy ameliorates experimental autoimmune encephalomyelitis and induces a T helper 2 bias in the antigen-specific T lymphocyte response. J. Immunol. **159:** 3–6.
10. DING, M., J.L. WONG, N.E. ROGERS, *et al.* 1997. Gender differences of inducible nitric oxide production in SJL/J mice with experimental autoimmune encephalomyelitis. J. Neuroimmunol. **77:** 99106.
11. ARNASON, B.G. & D.P. RICHMAN. 1969. Effect of oral contraceptives on experimental demyelinating disease. Arch. Neurol. **21:** 103–108.
12. JANSSON, L., T. OLSSON & R. HOLMDAHL. 1994. Estrogen induces a potent suppression of experimental autoimmune encephalomyelitis and collagen induced arthritis in mice. J. Neuroimmunol. **53:** 203–207.
13. KIM, S., S.M. LIVA, M.A. DALAL, *et al.* 1999. Estriol ameliorates autoimmune demyelinating disease: implications for multiple sclerosis. Neurology **52:** 1230–1238.
14. VOSKUHL, R.R. & K. PALASZYNSKI. 2001. Sex hormones in experimental autoimmune encephalomyelitis: implications for multiple sclerosis. Prog. Clin. Neurosci. **7:** 258–270.
15. LANGER-GOULD, A., H. GARREN, A. SLANSKY, *et al.* 2002. Late pregnancy suppresses relapses in experimental autoimmune encephalomyelitis: evidence for a suppressive pregnancy-related serum factor. J. Immunol. **169:** 1084–1091.
16. CORREALE, J., M. ROJANY & L.P. WEINER. 1998. Steroid hormone regulation of cytokine secretion by proteolipid protein-specific CD4$^+$ T cell clones isolated from multiple sclerosis patients and normal control subjects. J. Immunol. **161:** 3365–3374.
17. GILMORE, W., L.P. WEINER & J. CORREALE. 1997. Effect of estradiol on cytokine secretion by proteolipid protein-specific T cell clones isolated from multiple sclerosis patients and normal control subjects. J. Immunol. **158:** 446–451.
18. OLSSON, T. 1995. Critical influences of the cytokine orchestration on the outcome of myelin antigen-specific T-cell autoimmunity in experimental autoimmune encephalomyelitis and multiple sclerosis. Immunol. Rev. **144:** 245–268.
19. BENVENISTE, E.N. 1997. Role of macrophages/microglia in multiple sclerosis and experimental allergic encephalomyelitis. J. Mol. Med. **75:** 165–173.
20. SRIRAM, S. & M. RODRIGUEZ. 1997. Indictment of microglia as the villain in multiple sclerosis. Neurology **48:** 464–470.
21. MACMIKING, J., Q. XIE & C. NATHAN. 1997. Nitric oxide and macrophage function. Annu. Rev. Immunol. **15:** 323–350.
22. RAINE, C.S. 1997. The Norton Lecture: a review of the oligodendrocyte in the multiple sclerosis lesion. J. Neuroimmunol. **77:** 135–152.
23. TRAPP, B.D., J. PETERSON, R.M. RANSOHOFF, *et al.* 1998. Axonal transection in the lesions of multiple sclerosis. N. Engl. J. Med. **338:** 278–285.
24. MATTSON, M.P., S.W. BARGER, K. KURUKAWA, *et al.* 1997. Cellular signaling roles of TGF beta, TNF alpha, and beta APP in brain injury responses and Alzheimer's disease. Brain Res. Brain Res. Rev. **23:** 47–61.

25. MUNOZ-FERNANDEZ, M.A. & M. FRESNO. 1998. The role of tumor necrosis factor, interleukin 6, interferon-gamma, and inducible nitric oxide synthase in the development and pathology of the nervous system. Prog. Neurobiol. **56:** 307–340.
26. RUDDLE, N.H., C.M. BERGMAN, K.M. MCGRATH, *et al.* 1990. An antibody to lymphotoxin and tumor necrosis factor prevents transfer of experimental allergic encephalomyelitis. J. Exp. Med. **172:** 1193–1200.
27. SELMAJ, K., C.S. RAINE & A.H. CROSS. 1991. Anti-tumor necrosis factor therapy abrogates autoimmune demyelination. Ann. Neurol. **30:** 694–700.
28. ZHOU, W., R.G. TILTON, J.A. CORBETT, *et al.* 1996. Experimental allergic encephalomyelitis in the rat is inhibited by aminoguanidine, an inhibitor of nitric oxide synthase. J. Neuroimmunol. **64:** 123–133.
29. DING, M., M. ZHANG, J.L. WONG, *et al.* 1998. Antisense knockdown of inducible nitric oxide synthase inhibits induction of experimental autoimmune encephalomyelitis in SJL/J mice. J. Immunol. **160:** 2560–2564.
30. DREW, P.D. & J.A. CHAVIS. 2000. Female sex steroids: Effects upon microglial cell activation. J. Neuroimmunol. **111:** 77–85.
31. VEGETO, E., C. BONINCONTRO, G. POLLIO, *et al.* 2001. Estrogen prevents the lipopolysaccharide-induced inflammatory response in microglia. J. Neurosci. **21:** 1809–1818.
32. BRUCE-KELLER, A.J., J.L. KEELING, J.N. KELLER, *et al.* 2000. Antiinflammatory effects of estrogen on microglial activation. Endocrinology **141:** 3646–3656.
33. BRUCE-KELLER, A.J., S.W. BARGER, N.I. MOSS, *et al.* 2001. Pro-inflammatory and prooxidant properties of the HIV protein Tat in a microglial cell line: attenuation by 17 beta-estradiol. J. Neurochem. **78:** 1315–1324.
34. ADORINI, L. 1999. Interleukin-12, a key cytokine in Th1-mediated autoimmune diseases. Cell. Mol. Life Sci. **55:** 1610–1625.
35. SICOTTE, N.L., S.M. LIVA, R. KLUTCH, *et al.* 2002. Treatment of multiple sclerosis with the pregnancy hormone estriol. Ann. Neurol. **52:** 421–428.

Neurogenesis in the Subependymal Layer of the Adult Rat

A Role for Neuroactive Derivatives of Progesterone

CLAUDIO GIACHINO,[a] MARIARITA GALBIATI,[b] ALDO FASOLO,[a] PAOLO PERETTO,[a] AND ROBERTO MELCANGI[b]

[a]*Department of Animal and Human Biology, University of Turin, Via Accademia Albertina 13, 10123 Turin, Italy*

[b]*Department of Endocrinology and Center of Excellence on Neurodegenerative Diseases, University of Milan, Via Balzaretti 9, 20133 Milan, Italy*

ABSTRACT: The subependymal layer (SEL) of the adult mammalian brain provides a continuous supply of newborn cells that migrate to the olfactory bulb (OB) where they differentiate into interneurons. These newly generated cells migrate tangentially to the OB within a dense meshwork of astrocytic cells, organized to form tangentially oriented channels (glial tubes). The central nervous system is able to synthesize a variety of steroids. Among these, we analyzed the effects of progesterone (P) and its neuroactive metabolites dihydroprogesterone (DHP) and tetrahydroprogesterone (THP), administered by intraventricular injection, on the SEL of the adult rat. We found that THP and DHP, but not their precursor P, modify glial tubes organization and decrease immunoreactivity for glial associated proteins in SEL astrocytes. Moreover P metabolites reduce the proliferative activity within the SEL.

KEYWORDS: neuroactive steroids; progesterone metabolites; subependymal layer; glial tubes; adult neurogenesis; neurogenetic niche

INTRODUCTION

The subependymal layer (SEL) of the adult mammalian forebrain retains the capacity to generate new neurons virtually throughout life.[1] Newly generated cells deriving from the SEL migrate towards the olfactory bulb where they differentiate into interneurons.[1] There is a peculiar glial organization within the SEL of adult rodents, consisting of long astrocytic channels (glial tubes) enwrapping chains of tangential migrating cells.[2,3] Glial tubes separate the chains of proliferating/migrating cells from the surrounding mature tissue and may play a crucial role creating a permissive environment (niche) for adult neurogenesis.[4–6]

Address for correspondence: Claudio Giachino, Department of Animal and Human Biology, University of Turin, Via Accademia Albertina 13, 10123 Turin, Italy. Voice: +39 011 670 4683; fax: + 39 011 670 4692.

claudio.giachino@unito.it

Ann. N.Y. Acad. Sci. 1007: 335–339 (2003). © 2003 New York Academy of Sciences. doi: 10.1196/annals.1286.032

Hormones can modulate adult neurogenesis in the SEL-OB system during behaviorally relevant processes, such as estrous induction and pregnancy.[7,8] Although it has been suggested that estrogens can be responsible for the increased proliferation observed in the SEL of prairie voles during estrous induction, intraventricular injections of estradiol performed on adult mice do not change cell proliferation within this system.[7,8] These data indicate that hormones and mechanisms implicated in SEL neurogenesis are poorly investigated. In particular, the regulative role of neurosteroids and neuroactive steroids on adult SEL neurogenesis has not been addressed. These classes of steroid hormones can be synthesized directly in the central nervous system.[9] For example, progesterone (P) may be metabolized within the brain into dihydroprogesterone (DHP) and subsequently into tetrahydroprogesterone (THP).[9] Although the distribution of classical steroid receptors within the SEL has not been investigated, recent studies indicate that in the neonatal rat, SEL migrating neuroblasts express functional $GABA_A$ receptor,[10] which represents a membrane receptor for THP.[9] Moreover, astrocytes, which form the glial tubes and play a crucial role in SEL neurogenesis,[1,11] express both progesterone receptor (PR) and $GABA_A$ receptor.[12] We have analyzed whether P and its neuroactive metabolites DHP and THP may influence *in vivo* the SEL of the adult male rat. We have injected P, DHP, or THP into the lateral ventricle and analyzed after 2 days the SEL by immunohistochemistry. Anti-GFAP and anti-vimentin antibodies were used to label the glial tubes. The immunoreactivity for bone morphogenetic protein 7 (BMP7), a molecule associated with the glial tubes,[6] was also analyzed. Moreover, the proliferating neuroblasts were identified by means of anti-PSA-NCAM antibody by using intraventricular injections of the exogenous marker of proliferation 5-bromo-2′-deoxyuridine (BrdU) detected immunohistochemically.

RESULTS AND DISCUSSION

By using anti-GFAP antibody to recognize the SEL glial compartment, we found that treatments with THP and, to a lesser extent, DHP (but not P) lead to a reduction of GFAP immunoreactivity, specifically within the SEL region (Fig. 1A and B). Modifications of the typical structural organization of the glial tubes are particularly evident at the level of the SEL-rostral extension in THP-treated rats (Fig. 1). Comparison between injected and controlateral hemispheres of THP and DHP treated rats shows that GFAP immunoreactivity is reduced within the SEL, mainly in the injected hemisphere (data not shown). In agreement with the data *in vivo*, our previous results demonstrated that DHP and THP down-regulate GFAP gene expression in cultures of protoplasmic astrocytes.[13] It is important to highlight that while DHP is able to bind to the progesterone receptor (PR) in the same manner as P, THP represents a potent ligand of the $GABA_A$ receptor.[9] Since astrocytes express both classical (i.e., PR) and nonclassical (i.e., $GABA_A$ receptor) steroid receptors,[12] the effects exerted by DHP and THP *in vivo* might be ascribed to interaction with either PR or $GABA_A$ receptor, or to a mixed action. To identify the SEL glial compartment, we also used an antibody directed against vimentin, an intermediate filament protein, which is abundantly expressed by immature glial cells and retained by glial tubes astrocytes.[3,4] Anti-vimentin analysis demonstrated the presence of labeled astrocytic processes along the xtent of the SEL, in both the control and the treated animals.

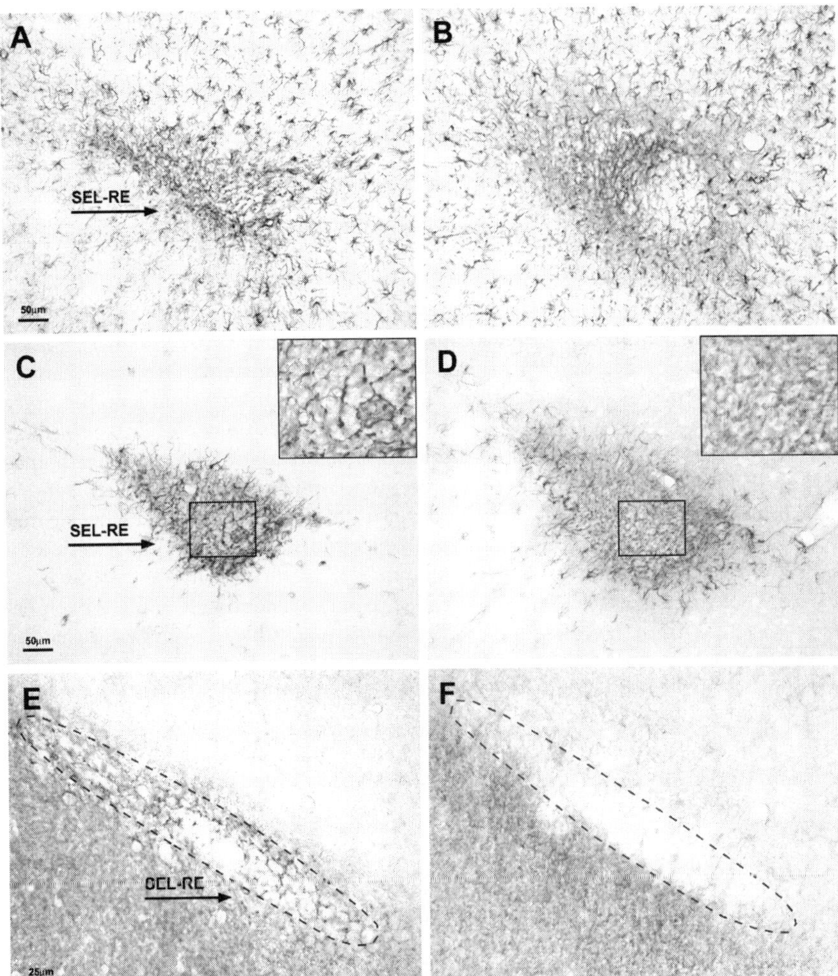

FIGURE 1. Immunostaining for GFAP **(A, B)**, vimentin **(C, D)**, and BMP7 **(E, F)** in coronal sections cut at the level of the SEL-rostral extension (SEL-RE) of the control **(A, C, E)** and THP treated **(B, D, F)** rats. Note the structural disorganization of the glial tubes and the reduction of the immunoreactivity for glial-associated proteins in treated rats.

Nevertheless, a reduction of the immunoreactivity was observed after THP treatment (FIG. 1C and D). This suggests that P metabolites induce the down-regulation of glial-specific proteins in this region, without a disappearance of astrocytic glial cells after treatment.

We also analyzed the immunoreactivity for bone morphogenetic protein 7 (BMP7), a molecule expressed within the SEL and probably secreted by glial tubes.[6] It is noteworthy that BMP proteins are expressed in regions of the adult nervous system characterized by neural plasticity and these molecules are among the fundamental components of the SEL neurogenetic niche.[5,6,11] Our data indicate that the immunoreactivity for BMP7 is reduced after THP treatment, specifically within the SEL region (FIG. 1E,F). These results further suggest modifications of the SEL glial compartment after THP treatment.

Also of importance, in addition to the effects exerted by neuroactive metabolites of P on the glial tubes, THP and DHP reduced BrdU immunostaining within the entire extent of the SEL (data not shown) two days after BrdU injection. Cell counts confirmed that the number of BrdU-labeled proliferating cells within the SEL of the olfactory bulb was reduced by about fivefold in THP- and DHP-treated animals, compared to those of the control and to the P-treated rats ($P < 0.05$). Conversely, the immunoreactivity for PSA-NCAM, a molecule associated in the SEL with proliferating/migrating neuroblasts,[4] was not modified by treatments.[14]

In spite of several studies showing that some classes of steroid hormones can act on adult hippocampal neurogenesis by modulating cell proliferation,[15] no literature shows a direct action of P and its neuroactive derivatives on neuroblasts proliferation. However, a recent work demonstrating that neuronal progenitors of the neonatal rat SEL express functional $GABA_A$ receptors[10] might suggest that THP acts on SEL proliferation by activating this neurotransmitter receptor. If we hypothesize that THP is responsible for the effect on neuroblasts proliferation, the effect exerted by DHP might be explained with conversion into THP by the action of the 3α-hydroxysteroid dehydrogenase enzyme. On the other hand, considering the putative importance of astrocytic glial cells of this system, it is also possible to hypothesize that the effects exerted by neuroactive steroids on glial tubes might indirectly account for the reduced cell proliferation observed within the SEL after THP and DHP treatments.

Altogether, the present results indicate that neuroactive derivatives of P (i.e., DHP and THP) exert direct effects on both neuroblasts and astrocytes of the SEL, reducing cell proliferation and expression of glial associated proteins. This suggests that the steroidal environment of the brain, besides modulating adult hippocampal neurogenesis, may also play a role in SEL neurogenesis. Future experiments will be requested to explain the kind of receptor involved in such effects.

ACKNOWLEDGMENTS

This work was supported by grants from MURST, Compagnia di San Paolo, and by the Commission of the European Communities, specific RTD program "Quality of Life and Management of Living Resources," QLK6-CT-2000-00179.

REFERENCES

1. ALVAREZ-BUYLLA, A. & J.M. GARCIA-VERDUGO. 2002. Neurogenesis in adult subventricular zone. J. Neurosci. **22:** 629–634.
2. LOIS, C., J.M. GARCIA-VERDUGO & A. ALVAREZ-BUYLLA. 1996. Chain migration of neuronal precursors. Science **271:** 978–981.
3. PERETTO, P. *et al.* 1997. Glial tubes in the rostral migratory stream of the adult rat. Brain Res. Bull. **42:** 9–21.
4. PERETTO, P. *et al.* 1999. The subependymal layer in rodents: a site of structural plasticity and cell migration in the adult mammalian brain. Brain Res. Bull. **49:** 221–243.

5. LIM, D.A. *et al.* 2000. Noggin antagonizes BMP signaling to create a niche for adult neurogenesis. Neuron **28:** 713–726.
6. PERETTO, P. *et al.* 2002. BMP mRNA and protein expression in the developing mouse olfactory system. J. Comp. Neurol. **451:** 267–278.
7. SHINGO, T. *et al.* 2003. Pregnancy-stimulated neurogenesis in the adult female forebrain mediated by prolactin. Science **299:** 117–120.
8. SMITH, M.T. *et al.* 2001. Increased number of BrdU-labeled neurons in the rostral migratory stream of the estrous prairie vole. Horm. Behav. **39:** 11–21.
9. MELCANGI, R.C. *et al.* 2001. Formation and effects of neuroactive steroids in the central and peripheral nervous system. Int. Rev. Neurobiol. **46:** 145–176.
10. STEWART, R.R. *et al.* 2002. Neural progenitor cells of the neonatal rat anterior subventricular zone express functional GABA(A) receptors. J. Neurobiol. **50:** 305–322.
11. DOETSCH, F. *et al.* 1999. Subventricular zone astrocytes are neural stem cells in the adult mammalian brain. Cell **97:** 703–716.
12. MELCANGI, R.C. *et al.* 2001. Glial cells: a target for steroid hormones. Prog. Brain Res. **132:** 31–40.
13. MELCANGI, R.C. *et al.* 1996. Effect of progesterone, testosterone and their 5 alpha-reduced metabolites on GFAP gene expression in type 1 astrocytes. Brain Res. **711:** 10–15.
14. GIACHINO, C. *et al.* Effects of progesterone derivatives, dihydroprogesterone and tetrahydroprogesterone, on the subependymal layer of the adult rat. J. Neurobiol. In press.
15. FUCHS, E. & E. GOULD. 2000. In vivo neurogenesis in the adult brain: regulation and functional implications. Eur. J. Neurosci. **12:** 2211–2214.

Steroid Hormone Signaling between Schwann Cells and Neurons Regulates the Rate of Myelin Synthesis

PAUL M. RODRIGUEZ-WAITKUS,[a] ANDREW J. LaFOLLETTE,[b] BENJAMIN K. NG,[a] THANT S. ZHU,[a] H. EDWARD CONRAD,[a] AND MICHAEL GLASER[a,b]

[a]*Department of Biochemistry and* [b]*Neuroscience Program, University of Illinois, Urbana, Illinois 61801, USA*

Abstract: Fluorescence digital imaging microscopy was used to develop a method that allows the continuous monitoring and quantitative measurement of a single myelin internode throughout its development. Using this technique, steroid hormones such as progesterone and dexamethasone were shown to reduce the time required for the initiation and to regulate the rate of myelin synthesis. Progesterone was capable of increasing the rate of myelin synthesis in Schwann cell/neuronal co-cultures in a dose-dependent manner. RT-PCR and *in situ* hydridization studies revealed that the mRNAs for P450scc and 3β-hydroxysteroid dehydrogenase, the enzymes involved in progesterone biosynthesis, were induced at the onset of myelin synthesis. The progesterone receptor protein translocated into the nucleus of the neurons during myelin synthesis, suggesting that progesterone could also be affecting neuronal gene expression. Changes in gene expression caused by progesterone are being examined to identify additional factors that may control myelin formation.

Keywords: steroids; Schwann cell/neuronal co-cultures; myelin

INTRODUCTION

The myelin sheath is a specialized membrane in the nervous system that facilitates the transmission of nerve impulses in a fast and efficient manner. Steroids hormones can be synthesized *de novo* in the nervous system,[1,2] and the possible regulation of myelin synthesis by these molecules has been the focus of recent research. Progesterone, in particular, is synthesized by Schwann cells in the peripheral nervous system,[1,3] and it is capable of regulating the rate of myelin synthesis.[4]. There is extensive signaling and cross talk between the myelin-forming cell and the neuron to control the various stages of myelin formation, e.g., cell proliferation, migration, and differentiation. Steroid hormones andgrowth factors are potential regulators of these events. The goal of the research discussed in this article is to

Address for correspondence: Michael Glaser, Department of Biochemistry, University of Illinois, 600 S. Mathews Ave. Urbana, IL 61801. Fax: 217-244-5858.
m-glaser@uiuc.edu

**Ann. N.Y. Acad. Sci. 1007: 340–348 (2003). © 2003 New York Academy of Sciences.
doi: 10.1196/annals.1286.033**

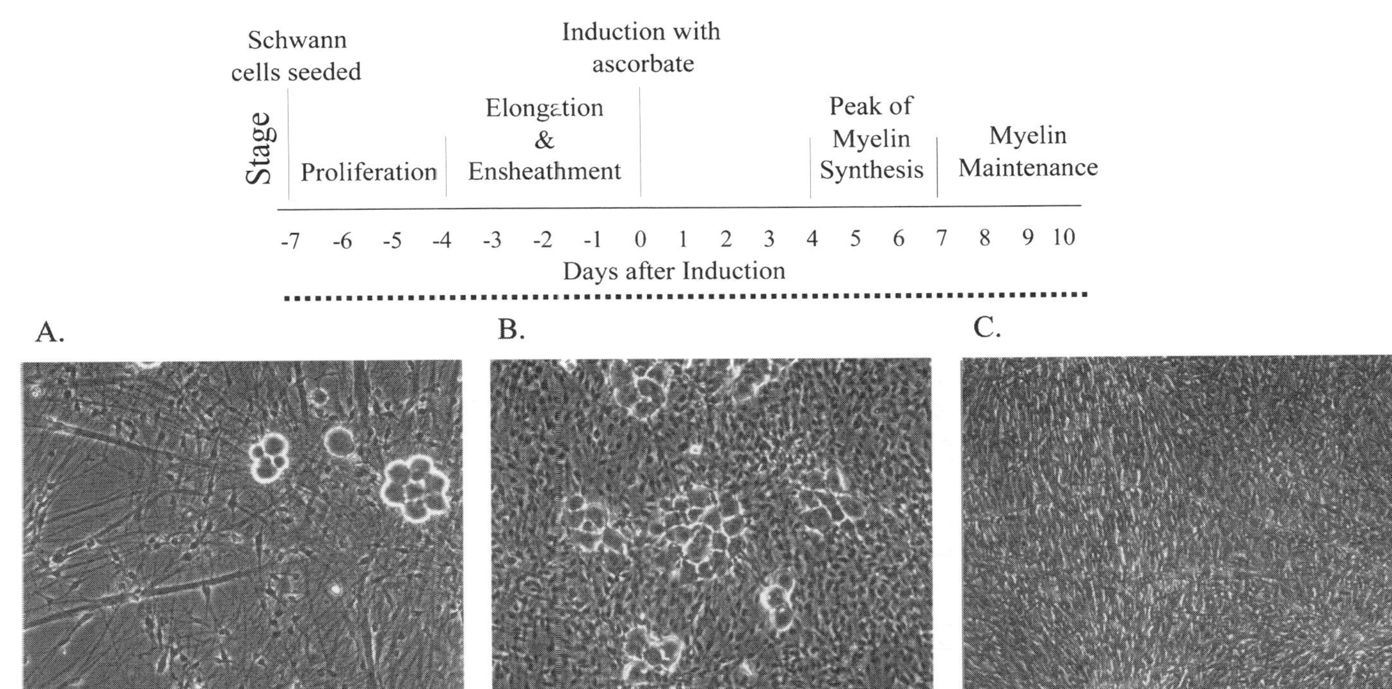

FIGURE 1. Establishment of Schwann cell/neuronal co-cultures. Purified Schwann cells were seeded onto the DRG neurons (**A**). Once the Schwann cells had proliferated and reached concluency (**B**), the cells were induced to synthesize myelin by the addition of ascorbic acid. Days 4 to7 after induction represent the peak of myelin synthesis (**C**).

understand the cell–cell signal transduction pathways involved in regulating the initiation and rate of myelin synthesis, with emphasis on the effects of steroid hormones in Schwann cell/neuronal co-cultures.

Schwann Cell/Neuronal Co-Cultures

Schwann cell/neuronal co-cultures represent a unique system to study the different developmental stages leading to myelin synthesis. The signaling processes and changes in gene expression that occur at the initiation of myelin synthesis can be studied using this system. A key feature in using co-cultures is that myelin synthesis can be made to occur synchronously,[5] and the changes in gene expression can be determined at different times during the myelination process.

Purified neuronal and Schwann cell cultures were prepared using methods basically described by Eldridge *et al.*[6] Briefly, neuronal cultures were established from dorsal root ganglia (DRG) neurons obtained from 15-day-gestation rat embryos. Schwann cells were isolated from the sciatic nerve of 2-day-old rat pups.[7] The purified Schwann cells were used to seed the neuronal cells and establish co-cultures. After seeding, the Schwann cells proliferated and ensheathed the axons in the culture. The time for this to occur was variable from culture to culture. However, after this process has occurred, further differentiation did not occur until ascorbate was added. Myelin synthesis was induced by the addition of ascorbate, added fresh to the culture media every third day. The cells proceeded to synthesize myelin in a synchronous and reproducible manner with a peak rate of myelin synthesis occurring 4 to 7 days later. Thus, the expression of different factors can be monitored through the different steps in myelin synthesis. Co-cultures can be examined during (a) the period when Schwann cells are proliferating, (b) the period when proliferation has stopped and the Schwann cells fully occupy and ensheath the axons, (c) the premyelinating period after ascorbate has been added, (d) The period of active myelin synthesis, and (e) the period of maintenance of the myelin sheath (FIG. 1).

Rate of Myelin Synthesis

Previous studies on myelin synthesis have provided limited information concerning the dynamics of the process, including the initiation, the rate of synthesis, and the extent of myelination. In order to follow the effects of different growth factors and hormones on myelin synthesis at specific stages in the myelination process, a novel method was developed that allows the continuous monitoring and quantitative measurement of myelin formation at a single internode.[5]

Using the fluorescent ceramide analogues, *N*-[5-(5,7-dimethyl BODIPY)-1 pentanoyl]D-erythrosphingosine (C5-DMB-ceramide), *N*-[4-(4,4-difluoro-5-(2-thi-enyl BODIPY) phenoxy acetyl sphingosine (C4-DFB ceramide), and a fluorescently-labeled free fatty acid(C5-DMB-hexadecanoic acid) (Molecular Probes, Inc., Eugene, OR), Schwann cell/neuronal co-cultures were observed to metabolize the fluorescent lipid precursors and incorporate them into the myelin sheath.[4,5] Using digital imaging fluorescence microscopy, the relative amount of fluorescent lipid precursors were measured quantitatively as they were incorporated into newly synthesized myelin. The rate of myelin synthesis was calculated from the changes in fluorescent intensity as a function of time. FIGURE 2A shows a fully myelinated

A.

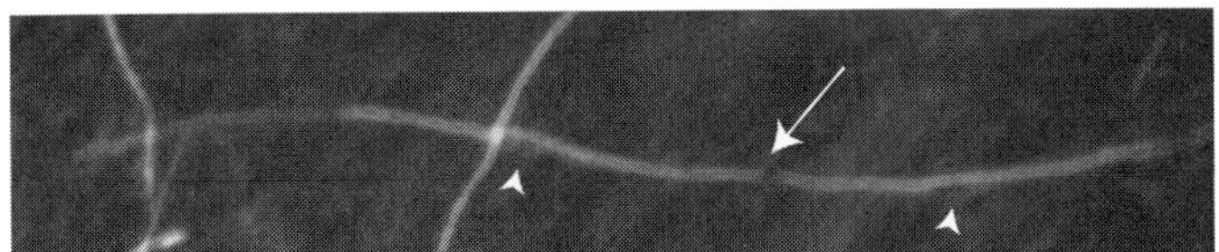

B.

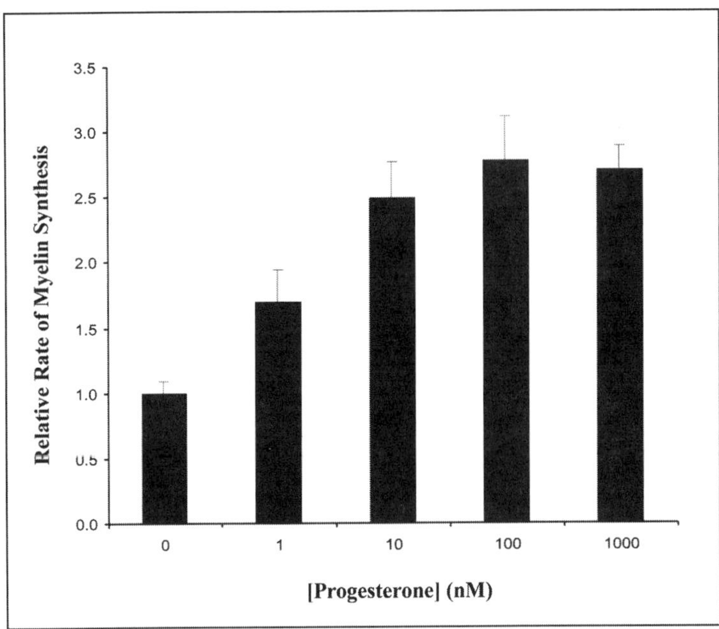

FIGURE 2. Fluorescent lipid incorporation to measure the rate of myelin synthesis. (**A**) Shows a fluorescence micrograph of internodes after incorporation of the fluorescently labeled free fatty acid during myelin synthesis. *Arrowheads* point to two myelinating Schwann cell bodies on the same axons. *Arrow* points to the node of Ranvier between these two internodes. (**B**) Progesterone increased the rate of myelin synthesis in a dose-dependent manner. Different concentrations of progesterone were added to Schwann cell/neuronal co-cultures from the day of induction to 4 days after induction. Fluorescent lipid incorporation into newly synthesized myelin was measured for cells cultured under these conditions. The rate of myelin synthesis increased as the concentration of progesterone increased. A three-fold increase in the rate of myelin synthesis relative to the control (no progesterone added) was observed using 100 nM progesterone.

internode at day 7 after induction that had incorporated fluorescently labeled free fatty acids. Previous studies in our laboratory showed that progesterone and dexamethasone accelerated the time of initiation by 24 h and enhanced the peak rate of myelin synthesis in Schwann cell/neuronal co-cultures.[4] RU-486, a competitive antagonist of progesterone and glucocorticoids, inhibited the initiation and formation of myelin. These results indicated that endogenously synthesized steroid hormones were important for proper myelin synthesis.

Exogenous progesterone increased the rate of myelin synthesis in the co-cultures in a dose-dependent manner. Starting at the day of induction, co-cultures were treated with four different concentrations of progesterone: 1 nM, 10 nM, 100 nM, and 1 μM. On the fourth day, the rate of fluorescent lipid incorporation into newly synthesized myelin was measured using the procedure outlined above. FIGURE 2B shows that increasing concentrations of progesterone produced increased rates of myelin synthesis when compared to control co-cultures that were not treated with exogenous progesterone. A nearly threefold increase in the rate of myelin synthesis was observed at a concentration of 100 nM progesterone. At concentrations above 100 nM, no further increase in the rate of myelin synthesis occurred. Because endogenously produced progesterone was present in the co-cultures, the effect of progesterone on the rate of myelin synthesis was much greater than threefold.

Cytochrome P450scc, 3β-Hydroxysteroid Dehydrogenase and the Progesterone Receptor Expression in Schwann Cell/Neuronal Co-Cultures

The presence of enzymes responsible for progesterone biosynthesis, particularly cytochrome P450scc (converts cholesterol to pregnenolone) and 3β-hydroxysteroid dehydrogenase (3β-HSD) (converts pregnenolone to progesterone), has been localized to different regions of the nervous system. The expression of these enzymes in Schwann cells and the effects of steroid hormones on myelin synthesis suggested the potential of steroids as signaling molecules between glia and neurons. Determining the spatial and temporal expression of these enzymes and the progesterone receptor during Schwann cell/neuronal co-culture development could elucidate signaling mechanisms and determine the paracrine and/or autocrine pathways in which these factors are involved.

RT-PCR experiments revealed that the transcripts for P450scc, 3β-HSD and the progesterone receptor were expressed in Schwann cell/neuronal co-cultures. Cytochrome P450scc was found to be induced by 17-fold, 3β-HSD was induced by 30-fold, while the progesterone receptor expression increased by 10-fold between 3–5 days after induction.[4] In order to localize the expression of these enzymes, *in situ* hybridization studies were performed. In premyelinating (2–3 days after induction) co-cultures, cytochrome P450scc, and 3β-HSD transcripts were detected at very low amounts, while in actively myelinating co-cultures (4–7 days after induction) mRNA of both enzymes was induced in Schwann cells.[8] The majority of the Schwann cells that stained more intensely for P450scc and 3β-HSD were elongated and actively forming myelin.

Immunocytochemistry was performed to determine the localization of the progesterone receptor in Schwann cell/neuronal co-cultures. The progesterone receptor staining was positive in dorsal root ganglia neurons, and the receptor was localized in the nucleus during myelin synthesis. There was minor staining in the

Schwann cells compared with the neurons. These results suggest a translocation of the progesterone receptor into the nucleus of the neurons during myelin synthesis. Futhermore, the translocation of PR into the nucleus signifies that progesterone was being synthesized during this time.

Differential Display PCR Analysis

The fact that Schwann cells primarily expressed the enzymes responsible for progesterone synthesis and that the progesterone receptor was primarily localized in the nucleus of the neurons during myelin synthesis suggested that this steroid could be affecting neuronal gene expression. mRNA Differential Display PCR (DDPCR) was employed in an attempt to identify novel neuronal genes induced by progesterone during myelin synthesis.[4] DDPCR allows the identification of differentially expressed genes and requires very low amounts of RNA compared to other methods like microarrays.[9]

DRG neurons were cultured in media lacking any steroid hormones. These neurons were treated with or without 100 nM of progesterone for 24 h, and the RNA was

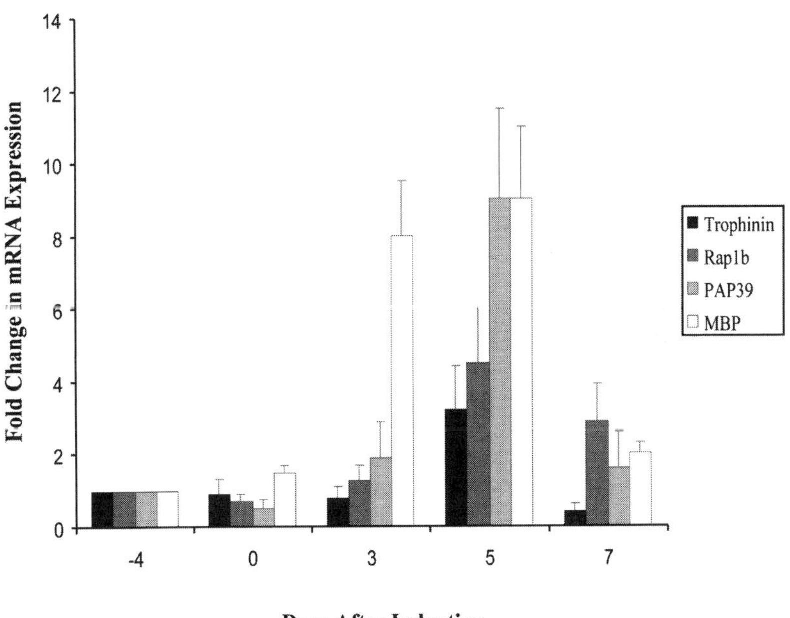

FIGURE 3. Differential display PCR was employed to identify genes induced by progesterone in neurons. The induction of mRNA expression of these genes during the different stages of co-culture development was measured relative to co-cultures 4 days before induction. Rap1b, PAP-39, and trophinin mRNA expression increased during myelin synthesis. Rap1b and PAP-39 were found to be induced by 5-fold and 9-fold, respectively, while trophinin increased by 3-fold during myelin synthesis. Myelin basic protein (MBP) was used as a control to show when myelin was being synthesized.

extracted and used for DDPCR analysis. PCR products were run in duplicate to minimize the frequency of false positives. Several new genes have been identified and are being characterized. These include rap1b, a small GTPase protein; a gene similar to mouse trophinin, a cell adhesion molecule; and PRPP-associated protein-39 kDa (PAP-39), a protein regulator of PRPP synthase activity. Expression of these genes increased in Schwann cell/neuronal co-cultures during myelin synthesis (FIG. 3) and can be decreased by addition of RU-486.[8] Rap1b was found to be induced by fivefold, PAP-39 was induced by ninefold, while trophinin increased by threefold during myelin synthesis. Addition of progesterone to neurons cultured alone showed an increase in the expression of these genes, while other steroids like dexamethasone did not induce the genes. The role of these genes in neurons presumably involves preparing the axons for myelination and subsequent electrical activity. Rap1b could be involved in vesicle and axonal transport and could also be rearranging the neuronal cytoskeleton for myelination. PAP-39 could be regulating PRPP synthase activity and metabolism of nucleotides and neurotransmitters such as ATP. Trophinin, a homophilic cell adhesion molecule found to be involved during the implantation process was recently discovered in mouse.[13] This protein was found to be expressed at high levels in the brain compared to other tissues and hormonally regulated in the uterus by estrogen instead of progesterone.[14] RT-PCR experiments performed in our laboratory showed that both Schwann cells and neurons expressed trophinin. This molecule could play a role in Schwann cell/neuronal interactions.

Other gene candidates have been identified by DDPCR. Among these are MSS4, a GDP-releasing factor and Rab regulatory factor; a brain tropomyosin, L31 ribosomal protein; a voltage-dependent anion channel (VDAC), and a deafness/dystonia peptide-2 (DDP-2). Identification of these progesterone inducible genes could provide new insights in the signaling cascades that progesterone may trigger and the cellular changes that occur during myelin synthesis.

CONCLUSION

Recent literature supports the idea that progesterone is a regulator of the rate of myelin synthesis, but the mechanism of action remains unclear. Some possible scenarios include the following: (1) Progesterone could be increase the expression of myelin proteins via its classical steroid receptor expressed in Schwann cells, and thereby enhance myelin synthesis.[3,10] The presence of the progesterone receptor in Schwann cells has been previously demonstrated.[11] (2) It could enhance myelin genes through signaling cascades stimulated by progesterone metabolites interacting with GABA receptors.[12] (3) Progesterone could induce neuronal genes that prepare the neurons for myelin synthesis.[8] Progesterone could also stimulate secretion of neuronal factors to signal Schwann cells to initiate myelin synthesis. A combination of these three mechanisms may be occurring.

Our data using Schwann cell/neuronal co-cultures suggests that Schwann cells express both cytochrome P450 side chain cleavage and 3β-hydroxysteroid dehydrogenase, which are the enzymes involved in progesterone biosynthesis. These two enzymes are upregulated in Schwann cells during myelin synthesis. The progesterone receptor is induced and translocates into the nucleus of DRG neurons. Thus, progesterone acts in a paracrine fashion to induce neuronal genes that may help neurons

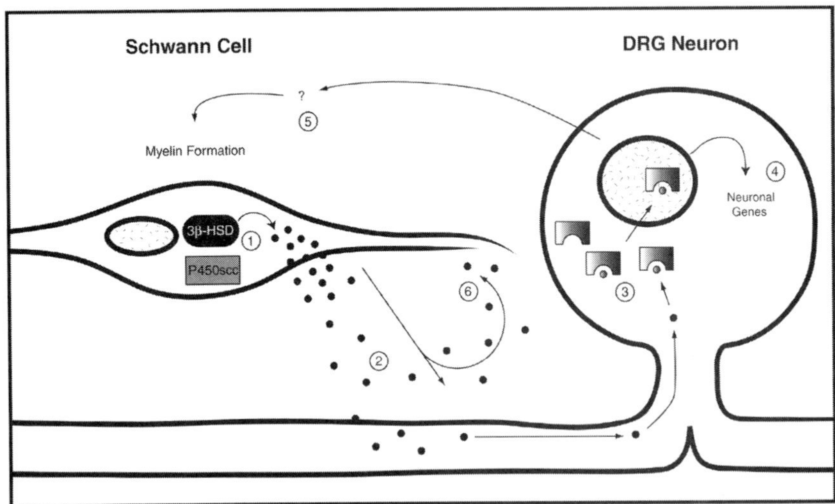

FIGURE 4. Model for the progesterone mechanism of action during myelin synthesis. Schwann cells express both cytochrome P450 side chain cleavage and 3β-hydroxysteroid dehydrogenase (1), which are the enzymes involved in progesterone biosynthesis. These two enzymes are upregulated in Schwann cells during myelin synthesis. The progesterone synthesized by Schwann cells (2) binds the progesterone receptor that is expressed in DRG neurons (3). Progesterone acts to induce neuronal genes in a paracrine fashion. (4) These gene products subsequently help neurons prepare for the myelinating stage and could signal Schwann cells (5) to start myelin formation. (6) Progesterone can also act in an autocrine fashion directly on Schwann cells.

prepare for myelination (FIG. 4). In addition, progesterone can also act directly on Schwann cells to upregulate genes in myelin synthesis.[3,10,12]

Neuronal signals are necessary for Schwann cells to form myelin, and progesterone is part of the cross talk that prepares neurons for myelination. Recently in our laboratory, it has been shown that a platelet-derived growth factor (PDGF) isoform may contribute to these neuronal-signaling events. The long form PDGF-A chain (LF-PDGF-A) isoform has been identified through RT-PCR, *in situ* hybridization, and immunocytochemical analyses in co-cultures.[15] Expression of LF-PDGF-A and their corresponding receptors seem to be upregulated during myelin synthesis.[15] It has also been shown that PR translocation in neurons during myelin synthesis was reduced dramatically when LF-PDGF-A action was abolished. These experiments have provided evidence that growth factors, in synergy with steroids hormones, contribute to a series of events which ultimately regulate myelin synthesis.

ACKNOWLEDGMENTS

This work was supported in part by the Multiple Sclerosis Society (Grant PP0918) and the American Heart Association (Midwest Affiliate) (Grant 0255980Z).

REFERENCES

1. KOENIG, H.L. *et al.* 1995. Progesterone synthesis and myelin formation by Schwann cells. Science **268:**1500–1503.
2. MELLON, S.H. & L.D. GRIFFIN. 2002. Neurosteroids: biochemistry and clinical significance. Trends Endocrinol. Metab. **13:** 35–43.
3. BAULIEU, E. & M. SCHUMACHER. 2000. Progesterone as a neuroactive neurosteroid, with special reference to the effect of progesterone on myelination. Steroids **65:** 605–612.
4. CHAN, J.R. *et al.* 1998. Glucocorticoids and progestins signal the initiation and enhance the rate of myelin formation. Proc. Natl. Acad. Sci. USA **95:** 10459–10464.
5. BILDERBACK, T. *et al.* 1997. Measurement of the rate of myelination using a fluorescent analogue of ceramide. J. Neurosci. Res. **49:** 497–507.
6. ELDRIDGE, C.F. *et al.* 1987. Differentiation of axon-related Schwann cells in vitro. I. Ascorbic acid regulates basal lamina formation and myelin formation. J. Cell Biol. **105:** 1023–1034.
7. BROCKES, J.P., K.L. FIELDS & M.C. RAFF. 1979. Studies on cultured rat Schwann cells. I. Establishment of purified populations from cultures of peripheral nerve. Brain Res. **165:** 105–118.
8. CHAN, J.R. *et al.* 2000. Progesterone synthesized by Schwann cells during myelin formation regulates neuronal gene expression. Mol. Biol. Cell **11:** 2283–2295.
9. LIANG, P. & A.B. PARDEE. 1992 Differential display of eukaryotic messenger RNA by means of the polymerase chain reaction. Science **257:** 967–971.
10. JUNG-TESTAS, I. *et al.* 1996. The neurosteroid progesterone increases the expression of myelin proteins (MBP and CNPase) in rat oligodendrocytes in primary culture. Cell. Mol. Neurobiol. **16:** 439–443.
11. JUNG-TESTAS, I. *et al.* 1996. Demonstration of progesterone receptors in rat Schwann cells. J. Steroid Biochem. Mol. Biol. **58:** 77–82.
12. MELCANGI, R.C. *et al.* 1999. Progesterone derivatives are able to influence peripheral myelin protein 22 and P0 gene expression: possible mechanisms of action. J. Neurosci. Res. **15:** 349–357.
13. FUKUDA, M.N. *et al.* 1995. Trophinin and tastin, a novel cell adhesion molecule complex with potential involvement in embryo implantation. Genes Dev. **9:** 1199–1210.
14. SUZUKI, N. *et al.* 2000. Trophinin expression in the mouse uterus coincides with implantation and is hormonally regulated but not induced by implanting blastocysts. Endocrinology **141:** 4247–4254.
15. NG, B.K. *et al.* 2003. The expression of an alternatively spliced variant of PDGF A-chain modulates *in vitro* myelin synthesis. In preparation.

Ndrg2, a Novel Gene Regulated by Adrenal Steroids and Antidepressants, Is Highly Expressed in Astrocytes

NANCY R. NICHOLS

Department of Physiology, Monash University, Victoria 3800, Australia

ABSTRACT: Previously, we cloned a gene from rat hippocampus that now shows homology to Ndrg2, a member of the N-myc downregulated gene (NDRG) family with putative roles in neural differentiation, synapse formation, and axon survival. Following adrenalectomy, hippocampal Ndrg2 mRNA increased in response to glucocorticoids. Ndrg2 mRNA was also upregulated by corticosterone in cerebral cortex and heart. Since Ndrg2 mRNA increased in response to glucocorticoid treatment of cultured astrocytes, we examined its cellular localization in adult brain by *in situ* hybridization. Ndrg2 mRNA is a prevalent message that is widely expressed throughout the brain, but is more abundant in gray matter than in white matter. Predominant mRNA expression was found in neurogenic regions of the adult brain. Furthermore, Ndrg2 mRNA in these regions was localized to GFAP-positive astrocytes or radial glia. In one of these regions, the subgranular zone of the dentate gyrus, Ndrg2 expression was decreased after adrenalectomy, and was restored to sham-operated levels by corticosterone, indicating that it is under positive regulation by glucocorticoids *in vivo.* Recently, another group reported that Ndr2/Ndrg2 transcripts in rat frontal cortex were decreased by chronic antidepressant treatment. Because antidepressants may alleviate symptoms of depression by reversing the effects of glucocorticoids, these data suggest that further study of Ndrg2 regulation and function in glia could contribute to understanding the pathogenesis and treatment of depression.

KEYWORDS: depression; glia; glial fibrillary acidic protein; neurogenesis; N-myc downstream-regulated gene 2

INTRODUCTION

Glucocorticoids have diverse actions in the central nervous system (CNS), including regulation of development, plasticity, homeostasis, and behavior. Two types of corticosteroid receptors mediate the actions of glucocorticoids in the brain: high-affinity mineralocorticoid receptors (MR) and lower-affinity glucocorticoid receptors (GR). Both receptors are located in the principal cell types of the CNS and are most abundant in the hippocampus.[1–3] Cellular responses to glucocorticoids result from transcriptional effects when steroid-receptor complexes translocate to the

Address for correspondence: Nancy R. Nichols, Department of Physiology, Building 13F, Monash University, Victoria 3800, Australia. Voice: +61-3-9905-2516; fax: +61-3-9905-2547. nancy.nichols@med.monash.edu.au

Ann. N.Y. Acad. Sci. 1007: 349–356 (2003). © 2003 New York Academy of Sciences. doi: 10.1196/annals.1286.034

TABLE 1. Cloning of Ndrg2 and GFAP from rat hippocampus as differential responses to corticosterone[a]

Clones	CR62	CR43,46,59,69
Response to corticosterone[b]	Increase	Decrease
Intact/ADX (-fold)[c]	2.5	0.4
Sequence identity	Ndrg2	GFAP

[a]Except for sequence identity of Ndrg2, these data were previously described.[3,4]

[b]Rats were adrenalectomized (ADX) and injected subcutaneously with 40 mg/kg corticosterone in oil or oil vehicle for 3 days. PolyA-containing RNA was isolated from the hippocampus for construction and screening of a cDNA library. Direction of response was based on results of tertiary screening using DNA slot blots and RNA hybridization analysis.

[c]Rats were ADX for 7 days and fold-change was determined by RNA blot hybridization analysis using hippocampal total RNA.

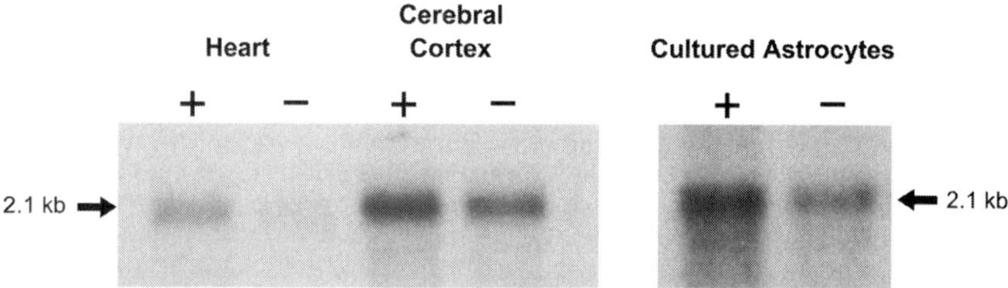

FIGURE 1. Ndrg2 mRNA is upregulated by glucocorticoids in heart, cerebral cortex, and cultured astrocytes. RNA blot hybridization analysis was performed as previously described.[10] Male Fischer 344 rats (2–3 months) were adrenalectomized and treated with 10 mg corticosterone/day for 3 days (+) or vehicle (−) for preparation of total RNA from cerebral cortex and polyA-containing RNA from the heart. Cultured astrocytes from neonatal forebrain were treated for 16 h with 1 μg/mL hydrocortisone (+) or vehicle (−) for preparation of total RNA. Total mRNA (4 μg) and polyA-containing RNA (0.1 μg) were run on denaturing gels, transferred to nylon, and hybridized with Ndrg2 ^{32}P-cRNA probes before being exposed to Kodak X-OMAT AR film for 4–5 days. Previous experiments using these samples indicated decreases or no change in other cloned mRNAs.[3,4,10] Size was determined by comparison with an RNA ladder and was within the size range reported for Ndrg2 mRNA (2.1–2.4 kb). Magnitude of change was determined by computerized videodensitometry and ranged from 2-fold for cerebral cortex to ~10-fold for the heart.

nucleus and bind response elements in target genes. To identify responses to glucocorticoids in target cells of the brain, we previously cloned mRNAs from the rat hippocampus that were increased or decreased in response to corticosterone, the endogenous glucocorticoid of the rat. Eight different mRNAs were isolated, including glial fibrillary acidic protein (GFAP), glutamine synthetase, glycerol phosphate dehydrogenase, transforming growth factor-β1, and four unknown sequences.[3,4]

Earlier we showed that GFAP, a marker of astrocytes, is under negative regulation by corticosterone (TABLE 1). Furthermore, GFAP dramatically increased in the subgranular zone of the dentate gyrus after adrenalectomy. This effect was dependent on the presence of dying granule neurons that was a response to removal of trophic adrenal steroids.[5] Based on these data, we proposed that GFAP downregulation is an adaptive effect of glucocorticoids that which returns astrocytes to a normal state after their reactivity in response to insults and neurodegeneration.[3,6] From the same hippocampal cDNA library, we cloned an unknown gene (CR62) as an increase in response to corticosterone (TABLE 1). FIGURE 1 shows that it recognized a 2.1-kb mRNA that increased in response to glucocorticoid treatment in the heart (ventricle), cerebral cortex, and cultured astrocytes. More recently, we identified the gene encoded by this mRNA and showed that it is a novel glial response to glucocorticoids.

Identification of Ndrg2 cDNA and Hybrid-Selected In Vitro *Translation Products*

CR62 was isolated as a 2-kb clone from a rat hippocampal cDNA library. Partial sequencing of the ends revealed a 3′-polyA tail but no homology with known genes in nucleic acid sequence databases. In 1996, however, two matches were found in GenBank with unidentified expressed sequence tags (ESTs) from human and mouse brain libraries. However, in 2000 when we had sequenced ~1.5 kb of CR62 cDNA by automated sequencing methods, a BLAST search showed homology with mouse Ndr2/Ndrg2.[7] Ndrg2 is a member of a new gene family, the N-myc downstream-regulated gene (NDRG) family. More recent searches showed identity to rat Ndrg2 from frontal cortex[8] and kidney.[9]

Characterization of the rat NDRG2 protein was performed using the cDNA for hybrid of the mRNA from total RNA isolated from rat brain followed by *in vitro* translation and resolution on two-dimensional gels as described previously.[10] A 42 kDa, pI 5.4 polypeptide was selected along with eight additional isoforms ranging from 43- to 46-kDa and pI from 5.3–5.1. The members of the NDRG family are highly conserved, diverging at their N- and C-terminals. The sizes of the NDRG2 polypeptides are similar to those described for other members of the family. In addition, alternate transcripts and isoforms exist for members of this gene family, including Ndrg2.[8,9] It is unknown whether the different brain NDRG2 polypeptides result from alternately spliced mRNAs or from *in vitro* posttranslational modifications.

NDRG Family: Expression, Regulation, and Possible Functions

Four NDRG proteins belong to a new family of differentiation-related genes. The functions of NDRG1-4 proteins are of major interest because of their expression in the developing and adult nervous system and their suggested roles in neural differentiation, synapse formation, and axonal survival. Their expression is also increased in adult tissues, suggesting a role in maintenance of the differentiated state. The first member of this family, NDRG1, was discovered based on its upregulation in N-myc knockout mice.[11] These studies showed that NDRG1 expression increased during embryonic development at the time when N-myc expression decreased and cells began to differentiate. Although members of the NDRG family are similar in their amino acid sequences, they differ in tissue distribution, and only NDRG1 is regulated by N-myc and cellular stress.[7] TABLE 2 compares some of the major findings on Ndrg2 and Ndrg1 expression. In contrast to the upregulation of Ndrg2 mRNA by glucocorticoids, Ndrg1 is highly homologous (>95% similarity) to TDD5, an androgen

TABLE 2. Chromosomal location, disease association, and expression characteristics of Ndrg2 and Ndrg1 expression[7,9,13,14]

Characteristics	Ndrg2	Ndrg1
Chromosomal location	14q11.1-.2	8q24.3
Disease association	None identified	Peripheral neuropathy, HMSNL[a] in Roma Gypsies
N-myc repression	No	Yes
Tissue expression	Brain, spinal cord, skeletal muscle, heart > kidney and liver	Ubiquitously expressed
Cell expression	Astrocytes and classical aldosterone target epithelia	Schwann cells and many other cell types

[a]HMSNL (Hereditary Motor and Sensory Neuropathy-Lom) mutation results in premature termination codon.

target gene that is repressed by testosterone and dihydrotestosterone.[12] These data suggest that NDRG proteins may serve similar functions in different tissues where they are regulated by different factors.

Recently, functional genomics was used to determine that a mutation in NDRG1 was the cause of an autosomal recessive peripheral neuropathy predominantly found in the Roma Gypsy community in Europe (TABLE 2).[13] A single mutation occurs in Gypsies of different identities and histories of migration, which predates their divergence when small nomadic bands left India about 1000 AD. Because NDRG1 is highly expressed in Schwann cells, the mutation may result in impaired Schwann cell differentiation and axon–glial interactions, disrupting signaling important for axon survival in the peripheral nervous system.[14]

Sequence alignments indicate that NDRG2 and NDRG4 belong to a separate subfamily and both of these genes are highly expressed in adult human and rat brain and heart.[15] NDRG4/Bdm1 is expressed in neurons of the brain and spinal cord and is more abundant in adult than in fetal brain.[16] Different isoforms of NDRG4 are expressed at different times during development, and they possibly have unique roles to play in cellular differentiation and neurite outgrowth.[15] In contrast to predominant expression of Ndrg4 mRNA in the postnatal brain at the time of synapse formation and programmed cell death,[16] Ndrg2 mRNA is initially expressed in the embryonic ventricular zone throughout the CNS, which suggests a role in formation of the brain and spinal cord.[7] FIGURE 1 shows that Ndrg2 mRNA is increased in response to glucocorticoids in the adult rat heart (ventricles), cerebral cortex, and cultured astrocytes. In contrast, Boulkroun *et al.* isolated Ndrg2 as a gene that was upregulated in response to aldosterone in kidney and other aldosterone target epithelia specialized for sodium reabsorption, but not in the heart.[9] They also showed that Ndrg2 mRNA was an early, transcription-dependent mineralocorticoid-specific response to aldosterone *in vitro* in a collecting duct cell line, but it did not respond to the GR agonist, dexamethasone. The human Ndrg2 promoter contains a glucocorticoid response element (GRE) half-site upstream from the 5′-untranslated region.[9] Preliminary data (not shown) indicate that regulation of Ndrg2 is not mineralocorticoid-specific in the hippocampus because a GR-specific agonist has a similar effect to corticosterone. Together these data point to differential regulation of Ndrg2 expression by adrenal steroids in different target tissues.

Ndrg2: a Role in Depression?

Recent studies also indicate a role for Ndrg2 in regulation of structural changes in the adult brain. In a preliminary study, Takahashi *et al.* reported that two slice variants of Ndrg2 in rat frontal cortex were downregulated by chronic use of antidepressants or electroconvulsive shock treatment, another effective therapy for depression.[8] High levels of glucocorticoids accompany many cases of depression and can damage the brain resulting in loss of neuronal connections, reduced neurogenesis, and mental deficits. Antidepressants may alleviate symptoms of depression by reversing the effects of glucocorticoids.[17] Our data show that Ndrg2 mRNA is upregulated by glucocorticoids, in the opposite direction to that of antidepressants. Furthermore, glucocorticoids decrease neurogenesis in the adult dentate gyrus and antidepressants increase neurogenesis after several weeks, a time frame that corresponds to the length of treatment required for their effectiveness in reducing symptoms of depression.[18–20] Therefore, regulation of Ndrg2 may be a molecular correlate of morphological and functional changes in the hippocampus (and possibly other brain regions) that are related to depression.

Glial Expression of Ndrg2 mRNA in Neurogenic Zones of Adult Brain

Since glucocorticoids increased Ndrg2 mRNA in cultured astrocytes, we examined its cellular localization and regulation in adult brain by *in situ* hybridization (FIG. 2). Ndrg2 mRNA is highly expressed throughout the brain hemisections in a pattern similar to GFAP mRNA, except it is more prevalent in gray matter than in white matter. GFAP mRNA is dramatically increased in the subgranular zone of the dentate gyrus in response to adrenalectomy-induced apoptosis.[5] In contrast to GFAP, Ndrg2 mRNA does not show large-magnitude changes to glucocorticoid manipulation. However, darkfield and brightfield microscopy of grain clusters (not shown) confirmed expression of this mRNA in two neurogenic zones, including the subgranular zone of the dentate gyrus and the subventricular zone of the lateral ventricle, in comparison with sense controls that did not detect grains above background. Ndrg2 expression was quantified in the subgranular zone of the dentate gyrus by computer-assisted grain counting after emulsion autoradiography. Percent cellular area covered by grains was determined for 20 cells on each side of the dentate gyrus per rat and analyzed by analysis of variance with Tukey post-hoc test at the 0.05 level of significance. In this neurogenic region, Ndrg2 mRNA decreased by 3 days after adrenalectomy and was restored to sham-operated levels by corticosterone replacement (mean ± standard deviation, $n = 5$–6; Sham = 6.62 ± 1.14; ADX = 4.93 ± 0.86; ADX + CORT = 7.18 ± 0.80; $P < 0.05$, ADX versus Sham and ADX + CORT groups). The demonstration that Ndrg2 expression in the subgranular zone of the dentate gyrus is under positive regulation by glucocorticoids suggests that it could be involved in inhibition of neurogenesis or in cell differentiation.

The subgranular zone of the dentate gyrus is also an area enriched in GFAP-expressing astrocytes and radial glia. Therefore, we combined GFAP immunohis-

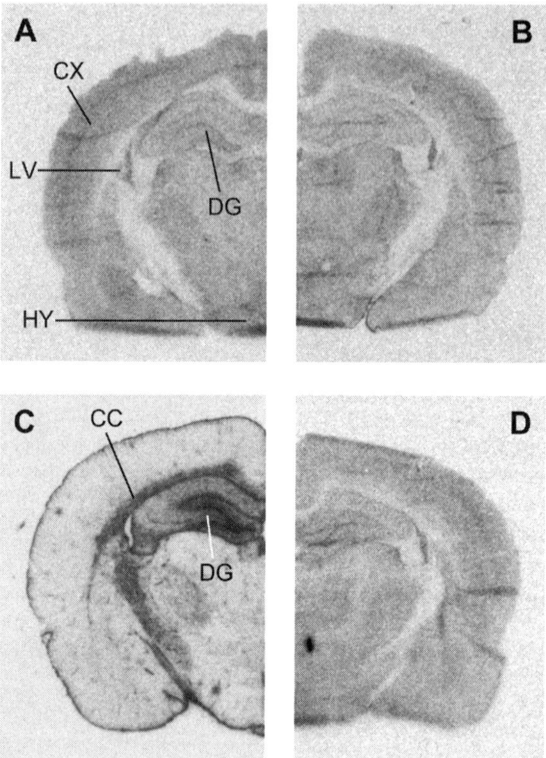

FIGURE 2. Ndrg2 mRNA is highly expressed throughout the adult rat brain, including neurogenic regions. Male Fischer 344 rats (2–3 months) were sham-operated (Sham) or adrenalectomized (ADX) for 3 days with or without corticosterone (CORT) replacement (200 μg/mL) in drinking water (0.9% NaCl). *In situ* hybridization was performed on brain sections that were hybridized with radiolabeled cRNA probes as previously described[5] and exposed to Kodak Biomax MR film for 6–16 h. (**A**) Ndrg2 Sham, (**B**) Ndrg2 ADX, (**C**) GFAP ADX, and (**D**) Ndrg2 ADX + CORT. *Abbreviations*: CX, cerebral cortex; LV, lateral ventricle; DG, dentate gyrus; HY, hypothalamus; CC, corpus callosum.

tochemistry with Ndrg2 *in situ* hybridization to determine whether mRNA expression was localized to astrocytes or radial glia in the neurogenic regions. We found high expression of Ndrg2 in GFAP-positive cell bodies in a laminar pattern along both zones, but not over dentate granule neurons, and also in the neuropil adjacent to the lateral ventricle and in some but not all GFAP-positive processes in both locations. The expression of Ndrg2 mRNA is consistent with an astrocytic pattern of expression. Astrocytes are involved in the origin of new neurons in the adult hippocampus in two ways: (1) they can induce neurogenesis from neural stem cells[21] and (2) dividing astrocytes in the subgranular zone are precursors for new neurons.[22] It will be important to determine the function of Ndrg2 in astrocytes in relation to gliogenesis and neurogenesis. However, we have not yet examined other markers to determine whether Ndrg2 is also expressed in radial glia or other cell types in neurogenic regions of the adult brain.

CONCLUSIONS

Similar to its strong expression in the embryonic ventricular zone, Ndrg2 is predominately expressed in two neurogenic regions in the adult brain. Glucocorticoid upregulation of Ndrg2 mRNA in a neurogenic region suggests that it could be involved in inhibitory effects of corticosterone on neurogenesis or in maintenance of the differentiated state. We have shown that Ndrg2 is a novel glial gene that may be useful in studying glial-cell abnormalities in major psychiatric disorders[23,24] and in investigating the role of reactive astrocytes in regulating axonal growth and CNS regeneration.[25] The expression of Ndrg2 in astrocytes or radial glia and downregulation by antidepressants implicate glia as a potential target for these therapeutic drugs in the brain.[23] Since antidepressants may alleviate symptoms of depression by reversing the effects of glucocorticoids, Ndrg2 expression may be a molecular correlate of morphological and functional changes in the hippocampus that are related to depression. Studying the differential regulation of Ndrg2 and neurogenesis by antidepressants and glucocorticoids in animal models may contribute to understanding their interaction in depression.

ACKNOWLEDGMENTS

This work was supported in part by grants from the Department of Veterans' Affairs, Australia and a Monash Small Grant. The author thanks students Christopher Choy, Angelina Mercuri, Lisa Pullen, Catherine Upton, and Nicole Bye for technical assistance and Michelle Mulholland for help with image processing; Jean deVellis, University of California, Los Angeles for treated astrocyte cultures; and Heinz Osterburg for assistance with hybrid selection/*in vitro* translation experiments in Caleb Finch's laboratory at the University of Southern California, Los Angeles.

REFERENCES

1. Bohn, M.C., E. Howard, U. Vielkind, *et al.* 1991. Glial cells express both mineralocorticoid and glucocorticoid receptors. J. Steroid Biochem. Mol. Biol. **40:** 105–111.
2. Tanaka, J., H. Fujita, S. Matsuda, *et al.* 1997. Glucocorticoid and mineralocorticoid receptors in microglial cells: the two receptors mediate differential effects of corticosteroids. Glia **20:** 23–37.
3. Nichols, N.R. & C.E. Finch. 1994. Gene products of corticosteroid action in hippocampus. Ann. N.Y. Acad. Sci. **746:** 145–154.
4. Nichols, N.R., J.N. Masters & C.E. Finch. 1994. Cloning of steroid-responsive mRNAs by differential hybridization. Methods Neurosci. **22:** 296–313.
5. Bye, N. & N.R. Nichols. 1998. Adrenalectomy-induced apoptosis and glial responsiveness during aging. Neuroreport **9:** 1179–1184.
6. Nichols, N.R. 1999. Glial responses to steroids as markers of brain aging. J. Neurobiol. **40:** 585–601.
7. Okuda, T. & H. Kondoh. 1999. Identification of new genes, *Ndr2* and *Ndr3*, which are related to *Ndr1/RTP/Drg1* but show distinct tissue specificity and response to N-myc. Biochem. Biophys. Res. Commun. **266:** 208–215.

8. TAKAHASHI, K., M. YAMADA, M. HIRANO, *et al.* 2001. Expression of two novel splice variants for putative rat *NDR2* gene after chronic treatment with antidepressant and ECT [abstract]. 31st Annual Meeting of the Society for Neuroscience: 218.17.
9. BOULKROUN, S., M. FAY, M.-C. ZENNARO, *et al.* 2002. Characterization of rat *NDRG2* (N-Myc Downstream Regulated Gene 2), a novel early mineralocorticoid-specific induced gene. J. Biol. Chem. **277:** 31506–31515.
10. NICHOLS, N.R., H.H. OSTERBURG, J.N. MASTERS, *et al.* 1990. Messenger RNA for glial fibrillary acidic protein is decreased in rat brain following acute and chronic corticosterone treatment. Mol. Brain Res. **7:** 1–7.
11. SHIMONO, A., T. OKUDA & H. KONDOH. 1999. N-myc-dependent repression of Ndr1, a gene identified by direct subtraction of whole mouse embryo cDNAs between wild type and N-myc mutant. Mech. Dev. **83:** 39–52.
12. LIN, T-M. & C. CHANG. 1997. Cloning and characterization of TDD5, an androgen target gene that is differentially repressed by testosterone and dihydrotestosterone. Proc. Natl. Acad. Sci. USA **94:** 4988–4993.
13. KALAYDIJEVA, L., J. HALLMAYER, D. CHANDLER, *et al.* 1996. Gene mapping in Gypsies identifies a novel demyelinating neuropathy on chromosome 8q24. Nature Genet. **14:** 214–217.
14. KALAYDJIEVA, L., D. GRESHAM, R. GOODING, *et al.* 2000. N-myc downstream-regulated gene 1 is mutated in hereditary motor and sensory neuropathy-Lom. Am. J. Hum. Genet. **67:** 47–58.
15. QU, X., Y. ZHAI, H. WEI, *et al.* 2002. Characterisation and expression of three novel differentiation-related genes belonging to the human NDRG gene family. Mol. Cell. Biochem. **229:** 35–44.
16. YAMAUCHI, Y., S. HONGO, T. OHASHI, *et al.* 1999. Molecular cloning and characterization of a novel developmentally regulated gene, Bdm1, showing predominant expression in postnatal rat brain. Mol. Brain Res. **68:** 149–158.
17. CZEH, B., T. MICHAELIS, T. WATANABE, *et al.* 2001. Stress-induced changes in cerebral metabolites, hippocampal volume, and cell proliferation are prevented by antidepressant treatment with tianeptine. Proc. Natl. Acad. Sci. USA **98:** 12796–12801.
18. GOULD, E. 1999. Serotonin and hippocampal neurogenesis. Neuropsychopharmacology **21:** 46S–51S.
19. JACOBS, B.L., H. VAN PRAAG & F.H. GAGE. 2000. Adult brain neurogenesis and psychiatry: a novel theory of depression. Mol. Psychiatry **5:** 262–269.
20. DUMAN, R.S., J. MALBERG & S. NAKAGAWA. 2001. Regulation of adult neurogenesis by psychotropic drugs and stress. J. Pharmacol. Exp. Ther. **299:** 401–407.
21. SONG, H., C.F. STEVENS & F.H. GAGE. 2002. Astroglia induce neurogenesis from adult neural stem cells. Nature **417:** 39–44.
22. SERI, B., J.M. GARCIA-VERDUGO, B.S. MCEWEN, *et al.* 2001. Astrocytes give rise to new neurons in the adult mammalian hippocampus. J. Neurosci. **21:** 7153–7160.
23. COTTER, D.R., C.M. PARIANTE & I.P. EVERALL. 2001. Glial cell abnormalities in major psychiatric disorders: the evidence and implications. Brain Res. Bull. **55:** 585–595.
24. ONGUR, D., W.C. DREVETS & J.L. PRICE. 1998. Glial reduction in the subgenual prefrontal cortex in mood disorders. Proc. Natl. Acad. Sci. USA **95:** 13290–13295.
25. RIDET, J.L., S.K. MALHOTRA, A. PRIVAT, *et al.* 1997. Reactive astrocytes: cellular and molecular clues to biological function. Trends Neurosci. **20:** 570–577.

11β-Hydroxysteroid Dehydrogenases in the Brain

Two Enzymes Two Roles

MEGAN C. HOLMES, JOYCE L.W. YAU, YURI KOTELEVTSEV,[a]
JOHN J. MULLINS,[b] AND JONATHAN R. SECKL

Molecular Endocrinology, Molecular Medicine Centre, [a]Biomedical Sciences and [b]Molecular Physiology, College of Medicine and Veterinary Sciences, University of Edinburgh, Edinburgh, United Kingdom

ABSTRACT: Glucocorticoids affect a wide range of processes in the brain, altering neurotransmission, electrophysiological activity, metabolism, cell division, and death. These actions are mediated by corticosteroid receptors (glucocorticoid and mineralocorticoid) that modify transcriptional activity of target genes. The amount of steroid available to activate these receptors is not only dependent on the circulating levels but also on pre-receptor metabolism of glucocorticoids occurring intracellularly. This metabolism is carried out by the enzymes 11β-hydroxysteroid dehydrogenases (11β-HSDs). There are two distinct isozymes, the products of distantly related genes. 11β-HSD type 2 inactivates glucocorticoids to its inert 11-keto derivative, while 11β-HSD type 1 elevates intracellular glucocorticoid levels by regenerating active glucocorticoids from circulating 11-dehydrocorticosterone or cortisone. This review highlights the important and very different roles the two enzymes play in the brain, outlining recent results obtained from studying mice with a targeted gene deletion in the 11β-HSD1 or 11β-HSD2 genes.

KEYWORDS: glucocorticoids; 11β-hydroxysteroid dehydrogenases; HPA axis; cerebellum; programming

INTRODUCTION

Glucocorticoids have a plethora of effects that influence many systems of the body, including the brain. Most neural pathways are modified by glucocorticoids, because target genes include neurotransmitter synthesis enzymes, receptors as well as enzymes involved in calcium activation and ion channels (e.g., K^+ channels). High levels of glucocorticoids are deleterious to the homeostasis of the body at all stages of life, causing abnormalities in development through to potentiation of cognitive deficiencies seen in aging. Normally, glucocorticoid levels are strictly controlled by a negative feedback action of glucocorticoids on the hypothalamo-

Address for correspondence: Dr. Megan C. Holmes, Molecular Endocrinology, Molecular Medicine Centre, Western General Hospital, Edinburgh EH4 2XU, UK. Voice: 44-131-651-1033; fax: 44-131-651-1085.
Megan.Holmes@ed.ac.uk

**Ann. N.Y. Acad. Sci. 1007: 357–366 (2003). © 2003 New York Academy of Sciences.
doi: 10.1196/annals.1286.035**

pituitary-adrenal (HPA) axis; impairments in this regulation modify lifetime levels of glucocorticoids' generating maladaptive effects in the brain.

11β-HYDROXYSTEROID DEHYDROGENASES

11β-Hydroxysteroid dehydrogenases (11β-HSDs) are enzymes that metabolize glucocorticoids and hence regulate the intracellular levels of steroid available to activate corticosteroid receptors. There are two isozymes, 11β-HSD type 1 and type 2, which in most tissues and conditions drive the enzyme reaction in opposite directions. 11β-HSD2 inactivates glucocorticoids (corticosterone in the rat or mouse, cortisol in humans) by removing a proton from the hydroxyl group at C11 and thus generating a ketone (producing 11-dehydrocorticosterone [11-DHC] or cortisone). The 11-keto steroids do not bind to or activate corticosteroid receptors. 11β-HSD2 acts *solely* as a dehydrogenase (unidirectional) with physiological corticosteroids, uses nicotinamide adenine dinucleotide (NAD) as a co-factor, has a low Km for corticosterone, and is highly expressed in classical aldosterone-selective target tissues (distal nephron, colon, sweat glands).[1] 11β-HSD1, however, is bidirectional *in vitro* but generally acts as a reductase, regenerating corticosterone from the inactive 11-keto derivative *in vivo* or in intact cells. It uses NAD phosphate (NADP) as co-factor and acts as a lower-affinity, high-capacity enzyme with a general distribution of many metabolically active tissues in the body, notably in liver, adipose tissue, bone, the gonads (in some species), and the brain.[2,3]

Until recently, research into the roles of these two enzymes have been severely hampered by the lack of specific inhibitors. The most effective inhibitors are glycyrrhetinic acid and its derivatives (such as carbenoxolone), which exhibit nonselective inhibition of both enzymes.[4,5] Therefore, the approach of this laboratory was to investigate the consequence of removing each enzyme independently in mice by targeted gene deletion.

THE METABOLIC PHENOTYPE OF 11β-HSD1 KNOCKOUT MICE

Mice homozygous for targeted disruption of the 11β-HSD1 gene had no detectable 11β-HSD1 mRNA and also no 11-reductase activity as demonstrated by the failure to convert 11-DHC to corticosterone.[6] The knockout mice thrived, were fertile, and did not exhibit any overt phenotypical abnormalities. However, upon closer examination, it was determined that glucocorticoid-induced responses were attenuated in the 11β-HSD1 knockout (–/–) mice, consistent with the hypothesis that 11β-HSD1 activity contributes significantly to the active intracellular glucocorticoid pool. For example, the 11β-HSD1 null mice generate reduced induction of phosphoenolpyruvate carboxykinase (PEPCK) and glucose-6-phosphatase (key glucocorticoid-inducible gluconeogenic and glycolytic enzymes) following a fast, compared to wild-type controls. Furthermore, after 4 weeks fat feeding or following an acute stressor, the 11β-HSD1 knockout mice had lower levels of fasting (overnight) plasma glucose.[6] More detailed analysis of these mice suggest that 11β-HSD1 deficiency produces a "cardioprotective" lipid profile due, at least in part, to increased beta oxidation in the liver, hepatic insulin sensitization, and reduced fibrinogen synthesis.[7]

11β-HSD1 expression is switched on fairly late in gestation,[8] and loss of expression does not lead to manifestation of a gross developmental phenotype; the mice appear healthy and robust. However, some caution should be observed for inhibiting the enzyme in pregnancy because on some murine genetic backgrounds pups appear to be born significantly heavier, and their growth during the early neonatal period is greater than wild-type mice (Holmes, unpublished observation). Moreover, 11β-HSD1 null mice have subtle but significant perinatal developmental changes in their lungs, compatible with modest immaturity of the surfactant system.[9] Any consequences of these early effects remain to be elucidated.

11β-HSD1 AND HPA AXIS REGULATION

11β-HSD1 is also highly expressed in many regions of the brain, including the hippocampus, cerebellum, and neocortex. What is its role there? It has been postulated that 11β-HSD1 may play a role in modulating glucocorticoid effects on mood, learning, and memory. Significantly, areas of 11β-HSD1 expression include central sites of negative feedback of glucocorticoids, which autoregulate HPA activity and hence corticosterone levels in a tight feedback loop.

What is the effect of removal of 11β-HSD1 on the HPA axis? 11β-HSD1(–/–) mice have hypertrophied adrenals and elevated basal ACTH and corticosterone levels at the nadir of the rhythm.[6,10] The increased ACTH level is apparently sufficient to underpin the adrenal hypertrophy. Moreover, *in vitro*, 11β-HSD1(–/–) adrenal glands are hyperesponsive to ACTH. These effects are compatible with the decreased half-life of active glucocorticoids in this mutant due to lack of regeneration in the liver and other sites. Furthermore, CRF mRNA levels in the paraventricular nucleus (PVN) of the hypothalamus are unaltered, suggesting the net effect (of increased corticosterone, decreased half-life, and decreased regeneration occurring centrally) of 11β-HSD1(–/–) is to maintain normal central drive. Other factors that regulate glucocorticoid action such as corticosteroid binding globulin (CBG) and glucocorticoid receptors (GR) are also not affected by loss of 11β-HSD1 activity.[10]

When the HPA axis is activated by restraint stress, the peak corticosterone response is exaggerated in 11β-HSD1 null mice, but peak ACTH levels are unaltered.[10] These data suggest that the corticosterone hypersecretion is mainly due to the hypersensitive adrenal. However, the turn-off phase of the ACTH response, which correlates with glucocorticoid negative-feedback efficiency, is delayed. It was also observed that administration of a dose of cortisol, 2 h prior to restraint stress, causes a greater inhibition of a subsequent corticosterone response to restraint stress in wild-type mice compared to 11β-HSD1(–/–) mice, providing further evidence for attenuated negative feedback in the null mice. It therefore appears that although elevated levels of corticosterone are circulating, there is an impaired glucocorticoid signal at feedback sites, due to the loss of 11ß-HSD1 activity.[10] This is consistent with the finding that the brain accumulates significantly less ^{3}H-corticosterone after a 7-day infusion in knockout mice compared to wild-type, suggesting 11b-HSD1 activity is required for normal intracellular glucocorticoid levels in the brain.[11]

Stress itself has been shown to regulate 11β-HSD1 expression in a time- and tissue-dependent manner. While shorter-term stressors or glucocorticoid treatment of 2–10 days induces a rise in hippocampal 11β-HSD1 expression,[12] more chronic (one month) psychosocial stress causes a decrease in expression.[13] This suggests the rise in 11β-HSD1 activity in response to the acute stress is a compensatory action to increase the negative feedback signal to switch off the HPA axis, whereas the protective response against chronic stress is to ameliorate the metabolic effects of glucocorticoid excess.

The circadian periodicity of plasma corticosterone is also modified in 11β-HSD1-null mice. The evening elevation in corticosterone is shifted much earlier, producing an extended period of hypersecretion. 11β-HSD1 activity is not thought to be regulated in a circadian pattern, because 11β-HSD1 mRNA expression is unaltered at 8 A.M. versus 8 P.M.[10] It therefore is possible that 11β-HSD1 may modify central glucocorticoid signaling on circadian pathways. The mechanisms and loci of these interesting effects remain to be determined.

11β-HSD1 AND BRAIN AGING

Glucocorticoids are considered a major risk factor in aging processes, potentiating age-related cognitive impairments.[14] Although the hippocampus requires glucocorticoids for neuronal function and survival, it is also particularly vulnerable to the adverse effects of chronic glucocorticoid excess, which produces atrophy of dendrites, neuronal and cognitive dysfunction, and even, in some strains of rats, neuronal loss. In primary cultures of hippocampal cells, 11β-HSD1 is the sole isozyme expressed, and it again acts as a reductase, converting inert into active glucocorticoids. This results in a potentiation of kainic acid-induced neurotoxicity in hippocampal cells in primary culture by the usually inert 11-DHC, unless the 11β-HSD1 activity is inhibited by carbenoxolone.[15] Similar data have also been reported *in vivo*. In a subgroup of aged rodents, an association is found between cognitive decline with a chronic elevation of plasma corticosterone levels and a loss of circadian periodicity. If glucocorticoids are maintained at low levels, by adrenalectomizing the rats and replacing with a constant low-dose release of corticosterone, they are less susceptible to age-related cognitive impairment.[16,17] Old (24-month) wild-type mice, as aged rats, show glucocorticoid-associated impairments in hippocampus-dependent learning and memory tasks in the water maze. Young 11β-HSD1(–/–) mice, despite elevated plasma corticosterone levels, perform as young wild types. Strikingly, aged 11β-HSD1 null mice also learn as well as young mice and avoid the cognitive decline seen in the majority of aged wild-type animals.[11] This cognitive protection associates with reduced intrahippocampal corticosterone levels, in the face of elevated plasma levels, indicating the potency of intracellular metabolism by 11β-HSDs in determining effective glucocorticoid action upon target receptors.

Interestingly, 11β-HSD1 mRNA levels decrease within the hippocampus in aged rats, which inversely correlate with their increase in plasma corticosterone levels.[18] We hypothesize that reduction in 11β-HSD1 activity would impair glucocorticoid feedback and hence may underpin HPA axis hyperactivity with aging. However, these effects will be balanced by the lower intracellular glucocorticoid levels (with less regenerated active glucocorticoid) protecting the vulnerable hippocampus.

In general, reduction of 11β-HSD1 activity results in beneficial consequences to the animal. Although there are elevated circulating corticosterone levels and impaired HPA regulation, the lower intracellular corticosterone levels in brain (and other tissues) result in a neuroprotective profile. Very recently, a new class of selective 11β-HSD1 inhibitors have been found to reduce blood glucose levels in hyperglycemic mice.[19,20] It will be interesting to see whether they access the central nervous system (CNS) and can also produce the beneficial cognitive effects seen in the study of 11β-HSD1(–/–) mice.

THE ROLE OF 11β-HSD2

The most important role of 11β-HSD2 in the periphery is to protect the intrinsically nonselective mineralocorticoid receptors (MR) of the kidney from being illicitly activated by corticosterone instead of their primary *in vivo* ligand, aldosterone.[21] Without this pre-receptor metabolism MR are activated by corticosterone producing the syndrome of apparent mineralocorticoid excess (SAME). This is seen in patients with reduced activity of 11β-HSD2 due to mutations in the 11β-HSD2 gene.[22] Mice homozygous for targeted disruption of the 11β-HSD2 gene faithfully reproduce the phenotype, showing polyuria, hypertension, sodium retention, potassium loss, and distal nephron pathology, as well as overt mineralocorticoid activity of corticosterone not seen in wild-type mice.

11β-HSD2 IN THE BRAIN

In the brain of the rat, 11β-HSD2 is expressed in a few, discrete nuclei mostly regulating central control of salt/water balance and blood pressure (e.g., SCO, subcommissural organ; NTS, nucleus tractus solitarius; amygdala).[23,24] In the mouse, there is an even more limited expression because no expression is observed in the SCO (Robson and Holmes, unpublished observation), consistent with the different salt regulation in the mouse, which is less mineralocorticoid dependent, compared to the rat.[25] The central regulation of blood pressure and salt balance is mediated by aldosterone actions and not reproduced by corticosterone, indicating aldosterone-selective MR in these specific actions. Thus, 11β-HSD2 in the adult brain is thought to protect MR from activation by corticosterone.[26,27] When carbenoxolone was infused into the lateral ventricles of intact rats, at a dose that had no effect when given peripherally, it caused an increase in blood pressure within 3 days, demonstrating the importance of central 11β-HSD2 in regulating blood pressure.[27]

High levels of glucocorticoids have deleterious actions in development, inhibiting cell proliferation and differentiation. The brain is an important target for these effects. 11β-HSD2 acts as a major barrier to glucocorticoids reaching the fetus and the neonate. It is highly expressed in the placenta, inactivating corticosterone prior to reaching the fetus. Perhaps as a further layer of defense, 11β-HSD2 is expressed in the developing brain. Central expression is observed from midgestation in a wide range of central sites, but the expression is switched off as each nucleus develops.[8,28] At birth, the main areas of expression are in the thalamus and cerebellum, which are areas still developing postnatally, but by postnatal day 21 11β-HSD2 expression in the CNS is confined to those few areas seen in the adult.

GLUCOCORTICOID EFFECTS ON CEREBELLAR POSTNATAL DEVELOPMENT

Several previous studies in the rat have shown that postnatal treatment with glucocorticoids (hydrocortisone, dexamethasone, corticosterone) results in a delayed and malformed development of the cerebellum. The cerebellum is still proliferating postnatally, and a considerable amount of cell migration and differentiation as well as cerebellar secondary folding is taking place between P1–28. Neonatal adrenalectomy prolongs mitosis and delays disappearance of the external granule layer (EGL), a secondary germinal zone present on the surface of the developing cerebellum. Exogenously administered glucocorticoids accelerate the disappearance of the EGL due to premature cessation of granule cell division and an inhibition of cell proliferation, which results in a decrease in cell numbers within the internal granule layer (IGL) and abnormalities in the secondary folding of the lobes (most marked in lobes VIII and IX of the cerebellar cortex).[29,30] Since the EGL has particularly high expression of 11β-HSD2, does loss of this GC protective enzyme mimic the effects of exogenously elevated glucocorticoids? The mice used for these studies have the 11β-HSD2 gene deletion bred onto an inbred strain (C57BL/6) to facilitate investigation of the phenotype, and these mice exhibit much milder symptoms of SAME compared to those reported in the MF1 strain. In preliminary studies we find that cerebellar growth is significantly impaired in 11βHSD2(–/–) mice, consistent with a neuroprotective role for 11β-HSD2 in postnatal cerebellar development.

PRENATAL GLUCOCORTICOID PROGRAMMING AND THE ROLE OF 11β-HSD2

The early-life effects of glucocorticoids in the rodent have been studied in some detail in the rat, though effects in the mouse are less well documented. Other species have also been studied such as the guinea-pig and sheep, and correlations have been made with human data.[31–33] In the rat, exogenous administration of corticosterone or the synthetic glucocorticoid, dexamethasone, during pregnancy can have life-long effects on the offspring, making them more susceptible to pathology in adult life. These effects are called glucocorticoid "programming," and the brain is a prime site of action. Prenatal dexamethasone, a poor 11β-HSD2 substrate that therefore crosses the placenta intact, results in offspring with increased HPA axis activity demonstrated by elevated basal corticosterone levels. This is thought to be the consequence of altered expression of corticosteroid receptors at sites of glucocorticoid feedback such as the PVN, hippocampus, and/or amygdala.[34] The precise pattern of GR/MR changes is dependent on the window of time of the glucocorticoid exposure. Furthermore, as adults these prenatal dexamethasone-exposed rats develop behavioral abnormalities consistent with a more anxious phenotype. Similar data have been obtained in rats that have been exposed to prenatal stress (a consequence of which will be elevation of endogenous glucocorticoids),[35] as well as offspring of pregnant rats treated with carbenoxolone, which inhibits placental 11βHSD2 activity to elevate glucocorticoid exposure to the fetus.[36]

The next question is, are the 11β-HSD2(–/–) mice behaving as a glucocorticoid programmed animal? Before addressing this question, we must outline some of the

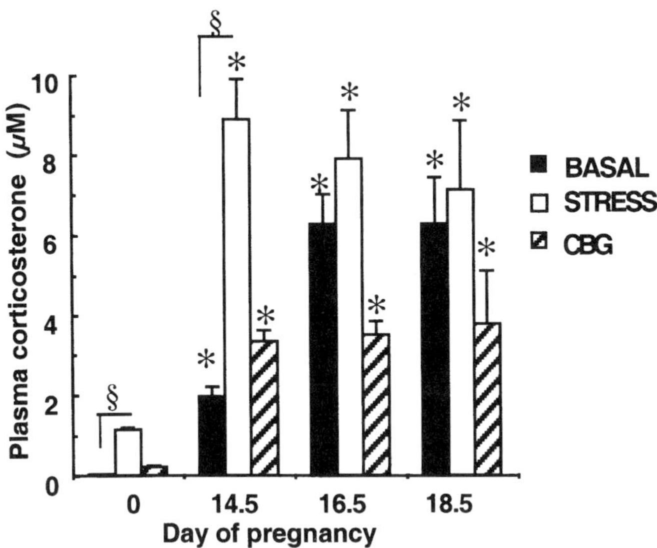

FIGURE 1. Plasma corticosterone and CBG levels in pregnant mouse dams at different stages of pregnancy. Both basal and stress induced plasma corticosterone levels are greatly increased in pregnancy, which are compensated only in part by an increase in plasma CBG levels. Samples were taken prior to (basal; *black columns*) and after (stress; *open columns*) 10-min restraint stress. Values are means ± SEM, $n = 5$. $^{*}P < 0.01$ compared to respective nonpregnant control (0); $^{\S}P < 0.01$ compared to basal.

key differences in glucocorticoid regulation and secretion during pregnancy of the rat versus the mouse that could potentially modify maternal environment and programming. The pregnant rat maintains an environment of low levels of glucocorticoids by becoming less responsive to stress.[37] Consequently, the placental barrier of 11β-HSD2 is less likely to be breached to affect fetal development. However, in the mouse, basal levels of plasma corticosterone rise dramatically throughout pregnancy to reach a plateau by day 16 when they are approximately 50–100 times higher than nonpregnant levels (FIG. 1). Induction of CBG occurs in an attempt to buffer this astronomical rise in plasma corticosterone, but although CBG levels increase over 10-fold, full buffering of corticosterone is not accomplished. Not surprisingly, restraint stress could not induce further increases in corticosterone, so paradoxically they appear to be stress hyporesponsive. However, throughout pregnancy a circadian rhythm of plasma corticosterone is preserved, and only peak levels of corticosterone penetrate the 11β-HSD2 barrier,[38] providing essential glucocorticoids for normal developmental processes such as maturation of the lung.

In the rat, central programming by glucocorticoids alters HPA activity and behavior such that the rats appear more anxious. At present we have insufficient evidence for programming of the HPA axis in the 11β-HSD2(–/–) mouse. Basal and peak stress corticosterone responses appear normal; more detailed experiments, however, are necessary to determine whether there is altered "switch-off" characteristics comparable to that seen in prenatally stressed animals. Furthermore, the 11β-HSD2(–/–) mice have significantly smaller adrenals (C.J. Kenyon and M.C. Holmes, unpublished observation) compared to wild-type mice, which may be due to the SAME phenotype but which may mask any hyperactivity of the HPA axis induced by glucocorticoid programming. Alternatively, the mouse may be more resistant to glucocorticoid programming of the HPA axis than the rat, perhaps reflecting the difference in maternal glucocorticoid environment. However, preliminary experiments suggest that the 11β-HSD2(–/–) mice have a programmed phenotype of elevated anxiety, consistent with phenotype of prenatal glucocorticoid exposure (Holmes, unpublished observations). In conclusion, the 11β-HSD2(–/–) mice exhibit developmental abnormalities and an adult phenotype, reflecting the deleterious consequences of elevated glucocorticoid exposure during the vulnerable stages of brain development.

SUMMARY

11β-HSD knockout mice have been invaluable in dissecting the roles of both isozymes in many systems, but particularly in the brain. The lack of tissue-specific glucocorticoid regeneration in the 11β-HSD1(–/–) mice attenuates glucocorticoid effects within the brain producing a deficit in the tight regulation of the HPA axis and a consequent rise in plasma corticosterone concentrations. However, the loss of the enzyme in central regions results in low intracellular corticosterone levels, even with the increase in plasma levels, generating an attenuation of glucocorticoid-induced cognitive decline with age. In general, a more advantageous phenotype is observed with low 11β-HSD1 activity; the converse, however, is seen in 11β-HSD2 knockout mice. 11β-HSD2 inactivation of glucocorticoids is crucial in two ways: it protects (1) MR from promiscuous activation by corticosterone and (2) GR from activation at critical times during development where glucocorticoids will cause long-lasting deleterious effects. Loss of this enzyme results in SAME, with the consequent hypertension and salt/water imbalance and also produces profound developmental defects. To further elucidate the roles of each enzyme in central regions, it would be useful to study transgenic mice with tissue-specific and temporal regulation of enzyme expression.

REFERENCES

1. Brown, R.W., K.E. Chapman, Y. Kotelevtsev, *et al.* 1996. Cloning and production of antisera to human placental 11β-hydroxysteroid dehydrogenase type 2. Biochem. J. **313:** 1007–1017.
2. Moisan, M.-P., J.R. Seckl & C.R.W. Edwards. 1990. 11β-hydroxysteroid dehydrogenase bioactivity and messenger RNA expression in rat forebrain: localization in hypothalamus, hippocampus and cortex. Endocrinology **127:** 1450–1455.
3. Seckl, J.R. & B.R. Walker. 2001. Minireview: 11 beta-hydroxysteroid dehydrogenase type 1—a tissue-specific amplifier of glucocorticoid action. Endocrinology **142:** 1371–1376.
4. Teelucksingh, S., R. Benediktsson, R.S. Lindsay, *et al.* 1991. Liquorice. Lancet **337:** 1549.
5. Monder, C. 1991. Corticosteroids, kidneys, sweet roots and dirty drugs. Mol. Cell. Endocrinol. **78:** C95–C98.

6. KOTELEVTSEV, Y., M.C. HOLMES, A. BURCHELL, *et al.* 1997. 11beta-hydroxysteroid dehydrogenase type 1 knockout mice show attenuated glucocorticoid-inducible responses and resist hyperglycemia on obesity or stress. Proc. Natl. Acad. Sci. USA **94:** 14924–14929.
7. MORTON, N.M., M.C. HOLMES, C. FIEVET, *et al.* 2001. Improved lipid and lipoprotein profile, hepatic insulin sensitivity, and glucose tolerance in 11 beta-hydroxysteroid dehydrogenase type 1 null mice. J. Biol. Chem. **276:** 41293–41300.
8. DIAZ, R., R.W. BROWN & J.R. SECKL. 1998. Distinct ontogeny of glucocorticoid and mineralocorticoid receptor and 11β-hydroxysteroid dehydrogenase types I and II mRNAs in the fetal rat brain suggest a complex control of glucocorticoid actions. J. Neurosci. **18:** 2570–2580.
9. HUNDERTMARK, S., A. DILL, A. EBERT, *et al.* 2002. Foetal lung maturation in 11 beta-hydroxysteroid dehydrogenase type 1 knockout mice. Horm. Metab. Res. **34:** 545–549.
10. HARRIS, H.J., Y. KOTELEVTSEV, J.J. MULLINS, *et al.* 2001. Intracellular regeneration of glucocorticoids by 11beta-hydroxysteroid dehydrogenase (11beta-HSD)-1 plays a key role in regulation of the hypothalamic-pituitary-adrenal axis: analysis of 11beta-HSD-1-deficient mice. Endocrinology **142:** 114–120.
11. YAU, J.L.W., J. NOBLE, C.J. KENYON, *et al.* 2001. Lack of tissue glucocorticoid reactivation in 11 beta-hydroxysteroid dehydrogenase type 1 knockout mice ameliorates age-related learning impairments. Proc. Natl. Acad. Sci. USA **98:** 4716–4721.
12. JAMIESON, P.M., E. FUCHS, G. FLUGGE, *et al.* 1997. Attenuation of hippocampal 11beta-hydroxysteroid dehydrogenase type 1 by chronic psychosocial stress in the tree shrew. Stress **2:** 123–132.
13. SECKL, J.R. 1997. 11beta-hydroxysteroid dehydrogenase in the brain: a novel regulator of glucocorticoid action? Front. Neuroendocrinol. **18:** 49–99.
14. SAPOLSKY, R.M., L.C. KREY & B.S. MCEWEN. 1986. The neuroendocrinology of stress and ageing. The glucocorticoid cascade hypothesis. Endocr. Rev. **7:** 284–301.
15. RAJAN, V., C.R.W. EDWARDS & J.R. SECKL. 1996. 11β-hydroxysteroid dehydrogenase in cultured hippocampal cells reactivates inert 11-dehydrocorticosterone, potentiating neurotoxicity. J. Neurosci. **16:** 65–70.
16. LANDFIELD, P.W., R.K. BASKIN & T.A. PITLER. 1981. Brain aging correlates: retardation by hormonal-pharmacological treatments. Science **214:** 581–584.
17. LANDFIELD, P.W., J.C. WAYMIRE & G. LYNCH. 1978. Hippocampal aging and adrenocorticoids: quantitative correlations. Science **202:** 1098–1102.
18. YAU, J.L.W. & J.R. SECKL. 2001. 11 Beta–hydroxysteroid dehydrogenase type I in the brain; thickening the glucocorticoid soup. Mol. Psychiatr. **6:** 611–614.
19. BARF, T., J. VALLGARDA, R. EMOND, *et al.* 2002. Arylsulfonamidothiazoles as a new class of potential antidiabetic drugs. Discovery of potent and selective inhibitors of the 11 beta-hydroxysteroid dehydrogenase type 1. J. Med. Chem. **45:** 3813–3815.
20. ALBERTS, P., L. ENGBLOM, N. EDLING, *et al.* 2002. Selective inhibition of 11 beta-hydroxysteroid dehydrogenase type 1 decreases blood glucose concentrations in hyperglycaemic mice. Diabetologia **45:** 1528–1532.
21. EDWARDS, C.R.W., P.M. STEWART, D. BURT, *et al.* 1988. Localisation of 11β-hydroxysteroid dehydrogenase-tissue specific protector of the mineralocorticoid receptor. Lancet **ii:** 986–989.
22. WHITE, P.C., T. MUNE & A.K. AGARWAL. 1997. 11 Beta-hydroxysteroid dehydrogenase and the syndrome of apparent mineralocorticoid excess. Endocr. Rev. **18:** 135–156.
23. ROBSON, A.C., C.M. LECKIE, J.R. SECKL, *et al.* 1998. 11Beta-hydroxysteroid dehydrogenase type 2 in the postnatal and adult rat brain. Mol. Brain Res. **61:** 1–10.
24. ROLAND, B.L., K.X.Z. LI & J.W. FUNDER. 1995. Hybridization histochemical localization of 11β-hydroxysteroid dehydrogenase type 2 in rat brain. Endocrinology **136:** 4697–4700.
25. ROWLAND, N.E. & M.J. FREGLY. 1988. Sodium appetite: species and strain differences and role of renin-angiotensin-aldostyerone system. Appetite **11:** 143–178.
26. GOMEZ-SANCHEZ, E.P. 1986. Intracerebroventricular infusion of aldosterone induces hypertension in rats. Endocrinology **118:** 819–823.
27. GOMEZ-SANCHEZ, E.P. & C.E. GOMEZ-SANCHEZ. 1992. Central hypertensinogenic effects of glycyrrhizic acid and carbenoxolone. Am. J. Physiol. **263:** E1125–E1130.

28. BROWN, R.W., R. DIAZ, A.C. ROBSON, *et al.* 1996. The ontogeny of 11β-hydroxysteroid dehydrogenase type 2 and mineralocorticoid receptor gene expression reveal intricate control of glucocorticoid action in development. Endocrinology **137:** 794–797.
29. BOHN, M.C. 1980. Granule cell genesis in the hippocampus of rats treated neonatally with hydrocortisone. Neuroscience **5:** 2003–2012.
30. BOHN, M.C. & J.M. LAUDER. 1978. The effects of neonatal hydrocortisone on rat cerebellar development: an autoradiographic and light microscopic study. Dev. Neurosci. **1:** 250–266.
31. MATTHEWS, S.G. 2002. Early programming of the hypothalamo-pituitary-adrenal axis. Trends Endocrinol. Metab. **13:** 373–380.
32. WELBERG, L.A.M. & J.R. SECKL. 2001. Prenatal stress, glucocorticoids and the programming of the brain. J. Neuroendocrinol. **13:** 113–128.
33. WEINSTOCK, M. 2001. Alterations induced by gestational stress in brain morphology and behaviour of the offspring. Prog. Neurobiol. **65:** 427–451.
34. WELBERG, L.A.M., J.R. SECKL & M.C. HOLMES. 2001. Prenatal glucocorticoid programming of brain corticosteroid receptors and corticotrophin-releasing hormone: Possible implications for behaviour. Neuroscience **104:** 71–79.
35. MACCARI, S., P.V. PIAZZA, M. KABBAJ, *et al.* 1995. Adoption reverses the long-term impairment in glucocorticoid feedback induced by prenatal stress. J. Neurosci. **15:** 110–116.
36. WELBERG, L.A., J.R. SECKL & M.C. HOLMES. 2000. Inhibition of 11beta-hydroxysteroid dehydrogenase, the foeto-placental barrier to maternal glucocorticoids, permanently programs amygdala GR mRNA expression and anxiety-like behaviour in the offspring. Eur. J. Neurosci. **12:** 1047–1054.
37. JOHNSTONE, H.A., A. WIGGER, A.J. DOUGLAS, *et al.* 2000. Attenuation of hypothalamic-pituitary-adrenal axis stress responses in late pregnancy: changes in feedforward and feedback mechanisms. J. Neuroendocrinol. **12:** 811–822.
38. VENIHAKI, M., A. CARRIGAN, P. DIKKES, *et al.* 2000. Circadian rise in maternal glucocorticoid prevents pulmonary dysplasia in fetal mice with adrenal insufficiency. Proc. Natl. Acad. Sci. USA **97:** 7336–7341.

Hippocampal and Hypothalamic Function after Chronic Stress

M. JOËLS, J.M. VERKUYL, AND E. VAN RIEL

Swammerdam Institute for Life Sciences, Section Neurobiology, University of Amsterdam, 1098 SM Amsterdam, the Netherlands

ABSTRACT: **Hyperactivity of the hypothalamo-pituitary-adrenal (HPA) axis is often observed in association with and even prior to the onset of major depression. It is presently unclear (1) which molecular and cellular processes contribute to hyperactivity of parvocellular hypothalamic neurons (key regulators of the HPA system) and (2) how HPA axis hyperactivity can lead to attenuation of central serotonergic transmission, a crucial factor in the onset of clinical symptoms. In an attempt to address these issues in an experimental model we used rats exposed to chronic unpredictable stressors, a paradigm causing prolonged HPA-axis hyperactivity. In the first study spontaneous and evoked GABA-mediated input to parvocellular neurons in the paraventricular hypothalamic nucleus was recorded with the whole cell patch-clamp technique. The frequency, but not other properties, of spontaneous GABA-mediated inhibitory postsynaptic currents was reduced after chronic stress, resulting in a reduced amplitude of the evoked GABA current. This potentially would disinhibit parvocellular neurons, provided that other inputs are unchanged. In the second study, responses of CA1 hippocampal neurons to serotonin were recorded with microelectrodes. It appeared that the membrane hyperpolarization caused by activation of serotonin-1A receptors is attenuated in tissue from chronically stressed rats. However, no apparent changes in expression of the serotonin-1A or corticosteroid receptors were observed. This supports the notion that chronic stress eventually results in attenuation of serotonergic responsiveness by a mechanism not involving transcriptional regulation of the receptor. Follow-up studies will need to examine whether treatment with corticosteroid receptor antagonists can normalize the attenuated transmission after chronic stress.**

KEYWORDS: **corticosterone; electrophysiology; GABA; serotonin; depression**

INTRODUCTION

The paraventricular nucleus of the hypothalamus (PVN) plays a key role in the activity of the hypothalamo-pituitary-adrenal (HPA) system. Upon stressful stimuli, corticotropin-releasing hormone (CRH) is released from terminals of parvocellular PVN neurons into the median eminence, reaching the anterior pituitary via portal

Address for correspondence: M. Joëls, Swammerdam Institute for Life Sciences, Section Neurobiology, University of Amsterdam, Kruislaan 320, 1098 SM Amsterdam, the Netherlands. Voice: 0031-20-5257626; fax: 0031-20-5257709.
joels@science.uva.nl

Ann. N.Y. Acad. Sci. 1007: 367–378 (2003).
doi: 10.1196/annals.1286.036

vessels. Subsequently released adrenocorticotropin hormone induces secretion of cortisol (in humans; corticosterone in most rodents) from the adrenal cortex, which feeds back negatively onto the anterior pituitary and parvocellular PVN neurons. Corticosteroid hormones also reach higher brain areas like the hippocampus, where they bind to intracellular receptors.[1] Two types of receptors are distinguished by distinct binding properties: the mineralocorticoid receptor (MR), which displays high affinity for the endogenous hormones, cortisol (or corticosterone) and aldosterone; and the glucocorticoid receptor (GR), exhibiting a nearly ten-fold-lower affinity for cortisol but effectively binding synthetic glucocorticoids like dexamethasone.[2,3] Owing to its high affinity, the MR is already substantially activated when corticosteroid levels are low, for example, under rest at the trough of the circadian release pattern. By contrast, GRs only become fully occupied when corticosteroid levels are high such as occurs after exposure to stress. The two receptor types show different distribution patterns within the brain.[3] MRs are, for instance, highly expressed in limbic areas, including the hippocampal subregions and some of the amygdala nuclei. GRs are very abundant in the PVN—the main site of feedback after a stress-induced rise in corticosteroid level—but are also enriched in the hippocampal CA1 region and dentate gyrus. Principal neurons in the CA1 area contain MRs as well as GRs and the influence of corticosteroid hormones on CA1 cell function therefore depends on the relative occupation of these two receptor types. The two corticosteroid receptor types both act as transcriptional regulators, either by binding as homodimers to response elements in gene promoter sequences or by interacting as monomers with other transcription factors, a process not requiring binding of the corticosteroid receptor itself to the DNA.[4,5]

Dysregulation of the HPA-axis occurs in association with many diseases. *Hypo*activity is observed, for instance, in patients suffering from posttraumatic stress disorder or fibromyalgia.[6,7] *Hyper*activity of the HPA axis is seen in association with, for example, Alzheimer's disease and major depression.[8–10] Hyperactivity is usually characterized by elevated basal circulating levels of corticosteroid hormones and less efficient feedback action at the level of the pituitary and PVN. Although HPA-axis hyperactivity does not occur in all patients with major depression, aberrations can be seen in a considerable subgroup when tested with the combined dexamethasone-CRH challenge test.[10] Several factors indicate that dysregulation of the HPA axis may even be causal to the precipitation of clinical symptoms in depression. Thus, hyperactivity of the HPA axis is partly normalized when patients are treated with antidepressants; the degree of normalization correlates negatively with relapse probability.[10] Moreover, high-risk probands of patients with major depression display significantly raised HPA-axis activity prior to the manifestation of the disease.[10,11]

At present, it is not quite clear how the HPA system can become gradually unhinged and why repetition of otherwise harmless stressors can result in persistent hyperactivity of the axis, in particular of CRH-producing cells in the PVN. One of the many theories proposed is that chronic stress exposure upregulates the co-secretagogue vasopressin, which is less susceptible to negative feedback via GRs.[12] This apparent GR resistance may be amplified by small variations in the GR gene—polymorphisms, which occur surprisingly often[13]—or by differential expression of co-activators or co-repressors.[14] Another possibility is that neuronal inputs to the PVN gradually and persistently change after prolonged exposure to stress, eventually disinhibiting the CRH-producing cells. These cells receive (among others) inputs mediated by noradrenaline, glutamate, and GABA, of which the latter input is prominent[15] and in part relays projections from higher limbic areas.[16]In the next section we will describe the role of corticosterone on GABAergic input to parvocellular neurons in the PVN and present preliminary data about changes in GABAergic transmission in the PVN after chronic stress.

A second issue that needs to be resolved is how hyperactivity of the HPA axis affects higher brain regions such that the elevated corticosteroid levels eventually facilitate the precipitation of clinical symptoms. In the case of major depression, two features of higher brain regions are of particular interest. First, the responsiveness to serotonin (5-hydroxytryptamine, 5-HT): this is supposedly attenuated in depressed patients in view of the effectiveness of current antidepressants which increase the availability of 5-HT in brain.[17] Second, the structural integrity and amino acid neurotransmission: recent MRI studies in patients have demonstrated a reversible decrease in hippocampal volume in association with major depression.[18] It has been assumed that excitatory amino acids may play an important role in such morphological changes. In this chapter we will briefly review how HPA axis hyperactivity gradually changes responses to serotonin and excitatory amino acids in the hippocampus.

PARVOCELLULAR NEURONS IN THE PVN

Parvocellular neurons in the PVN receive a strong GABAergic input, in part conveying information directly from other hypothalamic nuclei, but also relaying inputs from higher brain regions like the cingulate cortex and hippocampus.[16] The GABAergic input is particularly strong, as evidenced by the fact that about 50% of the hypothalamic synapses are GABAergic and nearly all CRH parvocellular neurons express GABA receptors.[19,20] Earlier studies suggested that the GABAergic input and the humoral input to CRH-producing PVN neurons do not act independently. Thus, injection of the $GABA_A$ receptor antagonist bicuculline close to the PVN caused an increase of CRH, AVP, and c-FOS expression in the parvocellular subregion of the PVN, and increased circulating corticosterone levels.[15] Conversely, removal of the humoral feedback by adrenalectomy (ADX) led to increased benzodiazepine binding as measured in whole hypothalamus preparations of the rat. This effect was reversed by corticosteroid substitution.[21] These observations instigated a recent study examining the effect of ADX on spontaneous $GABA_A$ receptor–mediated responses of parvocellular PVN neurons.[22]

Parvocellular neurons in a rat transversal brain slice containing the PVN were identified based on the location and shape of their cell body. Spontaneous GABAergic input to these neurons was recorded with the whole cell patch-clamp method, in the presence of tetrodotoxin (miniature inhibitory postsynaptic currents, mIPSCs). It was found that thus-identified parvocellular neurons differed in many respects from magnocellular neurons: The former compared to the latter had on average a lower membrane capacitance, and a lower frequency and amplitude of the mIPSCs. In the absence of endogenous corticosteroid hormones, the mIPSC frequency was significantly enhanced in parvocellular but not magnocellular PVN neurons. The absence of corticosteroids did not affect the amplitude nor the decay of the mIPSCs (FIG. 1). Replacement of ADX animals with a moderately high dose of corticosterone was sufficient to restore the mIPSC properties to those of sham-operated control rats.

The amplitude and decay of mIPSCs reflect properties of GABA receptors on the postsynaptic membrane, whereas the frequency is determined presynaptically. The data therefore indicate that presynaptic aspects of the GABAergic innervation of the PVN are changed in the absence of corticosterone, either caused by an increased release probability or an increased number of GABAergic synapses. The latter was in-

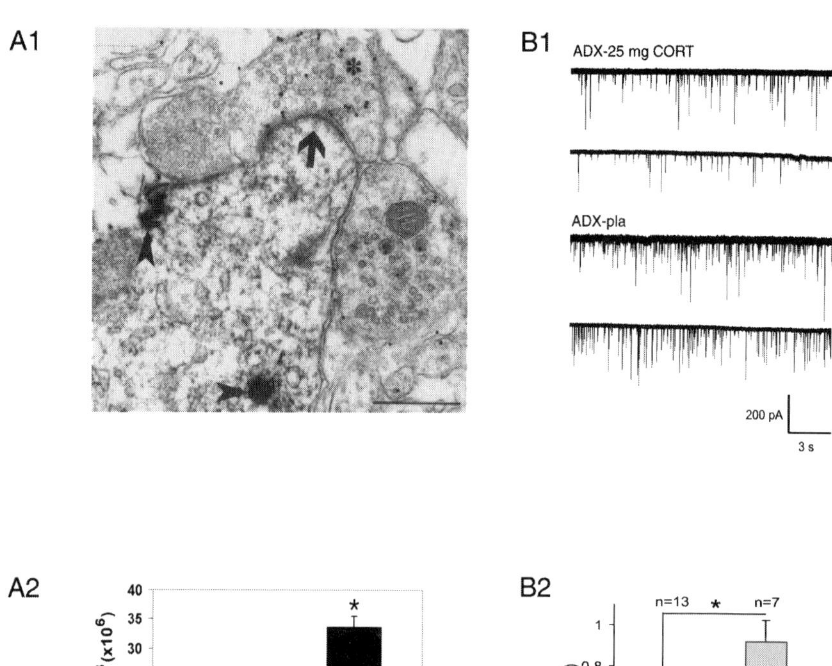

FIGURE 1. (**A1**) Electromicroscopic image of GABAergic synapses onto a CRH-producing parvocellular neuron in the PVN. (**A2**) The number of synapses is increased in the absence of corticosterone, compared to the control situation. (After Miklos and Kovacs.[23]) (**B1**) Typical traces from a parvocellular neuron in the PVN, showing miniature GABA-mediated inhibitory postnsynaptic currents (mIPSCs). (**B2**) In the absence of corticosterone, the frequency of the mIPSCs is enhanced compared to the situation where corticosterone is present. (After Verkuyl and Joëls.[22])

deed confirmed in an electronmicroscopic study showing an enhanced number of GABAergic synapses onto CRH-producing PVN cells after ADX (Ref. 23; see FIG. 1). The increased GABAergic innervation in the absence of corticosterone may serve to restrain local network activity, a function normally exerted by the humoral feedback signal.

Apparently, the spontaneous (local) GABAergic innervation of PVN parvocellular neurons is normally suppressed by moderately high levels of corticosterone, an effect that is overridden by the humoral suppression of CRH synthesis and release when corticosteroid levels are high. In a follow-up study we investigated how the GABAergic innervation is affected by persistent activation of hypothalamic GRs. To this end rats were exposed twice daily for 21 days to unpredictable stressors. This paradigm, which is accompanied by reduced body weight gain and adrenal hypertrophy,[24,25] was earlier found to reduce the expression of specific $GABA_A$ receptor subunits.[24] In accordance, preliminary data show that parvocellular PVN neurons recorded one day after the last stress exposure—when basal (trough) corticosterone levels are low—exhibited a reduced mIPSC frequency, in the absence of changes on either amplitude or kinetic properties. The reduced mIPSC frequency was accompanied by a reduction of the maximal GABA receptor–mediated current, evoked by synaptic stimulation. Double-pulse stimulation experiments revealed that the reduced mIPSC frequency is not due to a decreased release probability of GABA-containing vesicles, but probably to a decrease in the number of GABAergic synapses. Collectively, this suggests that after chronic stress, a diminished GABAergic tone of parvocellular PVN neurons occurs already at very low circulating corticosterone levels, potentially giving rise to elevated basal levels of corticosteroid hormones.

NEUROTRANSMISSION IN THE HIPPOCAMPUS

A prolonged period in which the HPA axis is hyperactive is expected to affect processes in the brain, resulting from the overexposure to corticosterone. This certainly holds for the hippocampal formation, an area involved in mood and memory formation and endowed with a high abundance of corticosteroid receptors. Studies examining the functional consequences of prolonged overexposure to corticosterone in the hippocampus so far have concentrated on the responsiveness to 5-HT in the CA1 hippocampal area and to excitatory amino acids in the dentate gyrus and CA3 region.

Serotonin

Earlier, acute shifts in circulating corticosterone level were found to affect responses of CA1 hippocampal pyramidal neurons to 5-HT.[26] After binding of 5-HT to the 5-HT1A receptor, a G protein is activated, resulting in opening of an inwardly rectifying potassium channel (GIRK).[27] Opening of this GIRK channel typically leads to a decrease of the membrane resistance and hyperpolarization of a CA1 pyramidal neuron (FIG. 2). When corticosterone levels are low, thus preferentially activating MRs, 5-HT1A receptor–mediated responses were found to be small.[26] After a brief rise in corticosterone level (e.g., evoked by an acute stress), the 5-HT response increases in magnitude through a process requiring DNA-binding of GR homodimers.[26,28–30] Corticosteroid modulation of 5-HT responses mediated via other

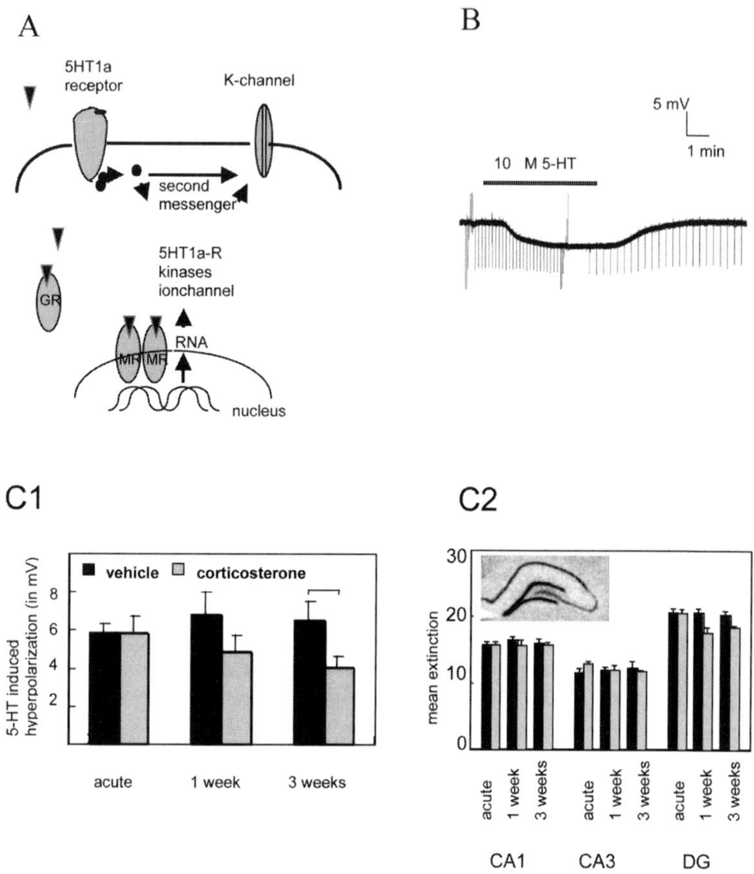

FIGURE 2. (**A**) Schematic representation of the 5-HT1A receptor signaling cascade. After binding of 5-HT to the 5-HT1A receptor, a G-protein is activated resulting in opening of an inwardly rectifying potassium channel (GIRK). Corticosterone enters the cell and binds to MR and/or GR. This complex translocates to the nucleus, where it interacts with the DNA. Responsive genes could include the 5-HT1A receptor but, for example, also kinases that modulate 5-HT1A receptor function through posttranslational modification. (**B**) Opening of the GIRK channel typically leads to a decrease of the membrane resistance and hyperpolarization of a CA1 pyramidal neuron. The trace depicts the course of the membrane potential in time. Negative deflections represent the voltage change due to a constant current pulse of 200-ms duration. The reduced voltage change during 5-HT application (bar on top) reflects a decrease in input resistance of the cell. (**C1**) A single exogenous administration of a high dose of corticosterone does not influence the 5-HT-induced membrane hyperpolarization, compared to injection with the vehicle. However, daily injections of corticosterone but not vehicle gradually attenuate the response to 5-HT. (**C2**) Expression of the 5-HT1A receptor mRNA in the CA1 hippocampal area does not change when animals receive high doses of corticosterone for 1 day or 1 or 3 weeks. (After Karten *et al.*[35])

receptors appears to be relatively limited.[26,31] The mechanism underlying the corticosteroid modulation of 5-HT1A receptor–mediated responses is still not quite resolved. Although transcriptional regulation of the 5-HT1A receptor has been reported, the time-frame and steroid receptor dependency of this molecular pathway do not support a role in the functional changes observed.[32] Similarly, corticosteroid-dependent modulation of G-protein subunits or the GIRK channel cannot explain the observed functional effects.[33,34] Possibly corticosteroids alter 5-HT1A receptors posttranslationally, changing the coupling between the receptor and the G protein.

Chronic elevation of corticosteroid levels, by injecting rats once daily with a high dose of corticosterone for 21 days was found to attenuate 5-HT1A receptor–mediated responses.[35] This appears to be a gradual process, since no differences with the vehicle-injected controls was observed after a single injection; after one week a tendency towards a decrease was observed, but significant attenuation was only seen after three weeks. A similar attenuation of 5-HT1A receptor–mediated responses was seen in adrenalectomized rats that were implanted with high-dose corticosterone pellets for two weeks.[36] The attenuated functional response occurred in the absence of downregulation of the 5-HT1A receptor mRNA expression, as demonstrated both with *in situ* hybridization and with a single-cell RNA survey of identified CA1 neurons.[35] The attenuated 5-HT responses after chronic exogenous corticosterone administration may have been caused by a resistance of GRs to increase 5-HT responses as normally seen. Alternatively, chronic corticosterone administration may impair the 5-HT1A receptor signaling cascade at some place. The latter is expected to attenuate 5-HT responses regardless of the degree of MR and/or GR activation.

Chronic corticosterone administration largely downregulates the HPA-axis activity. In a follow-up study, rats were studied under conditions that corticosterone levels were elevated overall due to HPA-axis hyperactivity. The same chronic unpredictable stress paradigm as described in the previous section was applied. It appeared that in this model, too, 5-HT1A receptor–mediated responses were attenuated, one day after a 21-day period of variable stress exposure, in the absence of changes in the 5-HT1A mRNA expression in the CA1 region.[37] Most of the cells in this study were recorded when the circulating corticosterone concentration was low, favoring the view that the 5-HT1A receptor signaling cascade becomes impaired after chronic overexposure to corticosterone. In agreement, additional GR activation *in vitro* resulted in an enhanced response to 5-HT, comparable to what is seen in control animals. This suggests that 5-HT responses are not impaired due to a general GR resistance.

Excitatory Amino Acids

From the same animals subjected to chronic unpredictable stress, responses of dentate granule cells to perforant path stimulation were recorded. The perforant path projection is mediated by glutamate. In dentate cells from all animals, responses mediated via AMPA receptors were distinguished from those via NMDA receptors, based on inactivation and kinetic properties and using pharmacological tools.[25] Several hours after *in vitro* activation of GRs in control animals, AMPA and NMDA receptor–mediated responses were comparable to those seen in tissue obtained from rats with low corticosterone levels (under rest, at the circadian trough), that is, in which mostly MRs but not GRs were occupied. By contrast, in chronically stressed rats, *in vitro* GR activation resulted in markedly enhanced AMPA receptor–mediated responses, while NMDA–mediated responses were not significantly affected.

Interestingly, different results were obtained in CA3 pyramidal neurons after a prolonged period of restraint stress.[38] These neurons are known to undergo considerable atrophy of their apical dendrites after a prolonged period of stress, as demonstrated in rats and monkeys as well as tree shrews.[39–41] It has been proposed that excitatory amino acid projections cause the dendritic atrophy, since treatment with NMDA-receptor blockers prevents atrophy.[42,43] In accordance, prolonged exposure to restraint stress was found to enhance the NMDA– but not AMPA receptor–mediated responses to commissural fiber stimulation.[38] This effect was prevented by the antidepressant tianeptine, suggesting that NMDA receptor–caused atrophy may play a role in depression. It should be noted, though, that tianeptine itself (in non-stressed controls) already altered transmission. Apparently, excitatory amino acid–mediated transmission in at least two hippocampal areas is enhanced after prolonged exposure to stress, supposedly rendering cells more susceptible to degenerative processes. The mechanism, though, may be region-specific and the outcome may also depend on the properties of the neurons involved, the local circuitry, intrinsic factors and other inputs.

CONCLUDING REMARKS

Corticosteroid hormones clearly affect hippocampal function under physiological conditions, for example, after acute stress exposure.[44] However, pathological situations associated with hyperactivity of the HPA axis resulting in a more persistent overexposure of the brain to corticosteroids also profoundly alter neurotransmission in the hippocampus as well as other areas such as the PVN. So far, the effects seen in animal models with HPA-axis hyperactivity are not a mere extrapolation of effects seen after acute stress exposure: Potentiation as well as attenuation has been observed.

Hyperactivity of the HPA axis occurs in association with many pathological conditions, including major depression. Why stressful situations in susceptible individuals eventually dysregulate HPA function is presently still an enigma. We here addressed one possibility, that is, that the neuronal inhibitory control over CRH producing neurons in the PVN exerted by GABA gradually lessens. Both *in situ* hybridization[24] and functional investigations indeed support a diminished GABA-ergic innervation of parvocellular neurons in the PVN after a period of chronic stress. However, this story is far from complete. First, CRH-producing cells make up only part of the parvocellular neurons in the PVN. Our functional studies did not allow distinction between CRH- and non-CRH-producing parvocellular neurons, so that it is not proven that the decreased GABAergic tone involves CRH-producing cells. Second, our study only examined neurons one day after the final stressor. From this single timepoint it is impossible to conclude that the GABAergic tone of parvocellular neurons is gradually impaired by chronic stress. Also, the mechanism leading to decreased GABAergic innervation can not be deciphered from the present study. Most importantly, CRH-producing neurons receive many inputs, in addition to the GABAergic pathway, which collectively determine the excitability of the neurons. Although it was recently concluded that the GABAergic as opposed to the glutamatergic pathway plays a crucial role in control of the HPA axis,[15] the effect of chronic stress in the PVN can only be fully appreciated when all major inputs are examined. At present, we can only tentatively conclude that the diminished GABAergic innervation seen in chronically stressed rats may lead to a gradual disinhibition of parvocellular PVN cells, particularly with basal corticosterone concentrations, provided that other inputs to these cells are not largely altered. Disinhibition of CRH-producing cells would then result in HPA axis hyperactivity. Consequently, the brain (but also other organs) will be daily overexposed to corticosteroids.

The functional consequences of such overexposure were examined in the hippocampus. It is these consequencs that might explain the increased likelihood for the precipitation of clinical symptoms in susceptible individuals. Interestingly, responsiveness to 5-HT was largely attenuated after chronic stress. This seems to be due to an impaired 5-HT1A receptor signaling cascade rather than resistance to GR-mediated effects. Since chronic stress and exogenous corticosterone administration affected the 5-HT system similarly, it is tempting to conclude that the elevation of corticosterone levels rather than of other HPA-axis factors plays a crucial role. When corticosteroid levels are high, the attenuation of 5-HT responsiveness is indeed a gradual process that takes weeks to fully develop. Whether this can explain the risk factor imposed by chronic stress in susceptible subjects to precipitate major depression, of course, remains to be seen. Our studies focused specifically on postsynaptic 5-HT1A receptor–mediated responses. However, it is well documented that glucocorticoids affect 5-HT responsiveness in other areas,[45] but also 5-HT synthesis and turnover. Furthermore, the central 5-HT system in turn adds to the control of the HPA-axis activity (for review, see Refs. 46 and 47), which makes it difficult to decide on the sequence of events.

Not only the 5-HT mediated transmission in the hippocampus is affected by chronic stress: Recent studies also show that excitatory amino acid–mediated input is also profoundly altered after stress. In general, postsynaptic responses to glutamate were increased, although the receptor involved showed regional differences. It is presently unclear whether these enhanced glutamatergic responses develop gradually. Similarly, the underlying mechanism is totally unknown. It needs to be tested in more detail[48,49] whether GR activation in chronically stressed animals enhances glutamatergic transmission through transcriptional regulation of NMDA and/or AMPA receptors. It has been assumed that enhanced glutamatergic transmission may underlie dendritic atrophy of at least CA3 neurons. This causal relationship, however, still awaits firm proof.

One issue not addressed in the studies about functional changes after chronic stress is the reversibility of events. On the basis of observations in humans it is expected that the disinhibition of PVN cells and attenuated 5-HT responses in the hippocampus will be persistent, although some normalization over time and particularly after treatment with antidepressants may occur. Future studies will need to address this important aspect. Also, the mechanism by which adaptations in the central neurotransmitter systems occur over time is still unresolved. In the case of 5-HT, post-translational modification rather than transcriptional regulation of the 5-HT1A receptor seems to be involved, but how the former is accomplished is still open for investigation.

It remains to be seen whether central neurotransmitter systems in humans deviate in a comparable manner from their normal function as here reviewed for animal models after chronic stress. If so, timely treatment with compounds normalizing HPA-axis activity or balancing central effects of corticosteroids might be able to prevent such deviations. Evidence so far supports that treatment with such compounds may indeed be beneficial in a subgroup of individuals with major depression.[50]

ACKNOWLEDGMENTS

The contribution by I.M. Miklos and K. Kovacs to FIGURE 1 is gratefully acknowledged.

REFERENCES

1. McEWEN, B.S., E.R. DE KLOET & W. ROSTENE. 1986. Adrenal steroid receptors and actions in the nervous system. Physiol. Rev. **66:** 1121–1188.
2. REUL, J.M. & E.R. DE KLOET. 1985. Two receptor systems for corticosterone in rat brain: microdistribution and differential occupation. Endocrinology **117:** 2505–2511.
3. DE KLOET, E.R. 1991. Brain corticosteroid receptor balance and homeostatic control. Front. Neuroendocrinol. **12:** 95–164.
4. BEATO, M. & A. SANCHEZ-PACHECO. 1996. Interaction of steroid hormone receptors with the transcription initiation complex. Endocr. Rev. **17:** 587–609.
5. McEWAN, I.J., A.P. WRIGHT & J.A. GUSTAFSSON. 1997. Mechanism of gene expression by the glucocorticoid receptor: role of protein-protein interactions. Bioessays **19:** 153–160.
6. YEHUDA, R. 2001. Biology of posttraumatic stress disorder. J. Clin. Psychiatry **62:** 41–46.
7. GRIEP, E.N., J.W. BOERSMA, E.G. LENTJES, *et al.* Function of the hypothalamic-pituitary-adrenal axis in patients with fibromyalgia and low back pain. J. Rheumatol. **25:** 1374–1381.
8. AISEN, P.S. & G.M. PASINETTI. 1998. Glucocorticoids in Alzheimer's disease: the story so far. Drugs Aging **12:** 1–6.
9. GOLD, P.W. & G.P. CHROUSOS. 2002. Organization of the stress system and its dysregulation in melancholic and atypical depression: high vs low CRH/NE states. Mol. Psychiatry **7:** 254–275.
10. HOLSBOER, F. & N. BARDEN. 1996. Antidepressants and hypothalamic-pituitary-adrenocortical regulation. Endocr. Rev. **17:** 187–205.
11. MODELL, S., M. ISING, F. HOLSBOER, *et al.* 2002. The Munich Vulnerability Study on Affective Disorders: stability of polysomnographic findings over time. Biol. Psychiatry **52:** 430–437.
12. DE KLOET, E.R., E. VREUGDENHIL, M. OITZL, *et al.* 1998. Brain corticosteroid receptor balance in health and disease. Endocr. Rev. **19:** 269–301.
13. IKEDA, Y., T. SUEHIRO, S. TSUZURA, *et al.* 2001. A polymorphism in the promoter region of the glucocorticoid receptor gene is associated with its transcriptional activity. Endocr. J. **48:** 723–726.
14. MEIJER, O.C. 2002. Coregulator proteins and corticosteroid action in the brain. J. Neuroendocrinol. **14:** 499–505.
15. COLE, R.L. & P.E. SAWCHENKO. 2002. Neurotransmitter regulation of cellular activation and neuropeptide gene expression in the paraventricular nucleus of the hypothalamus. J. Neurosci. **22:** 959–969.
16. HERMAN, J.P. & W.E. CULLINAN. 1997. Neurocircuitry of stress: central control of the hypothalamo-pituitary- adrenocortical axis. Trends Neurosci. **20:** 78–84.
17. CRYAN, J.F. & B.E. LEONARD. 2000. 5-HT1A and beyond: the role of serotonin and its receptors in depression and the antidepressant response. Hum. Psychopharmacol. **15:** 113–135.

18. SAPOLSKY, R.M. 2000. Glucocorticoids and hippocampal atrophy in neuropsychiatric disorders. Arch. Gen. Psychiatry **57:** 925–935.
19. DECAVEL, C. & A.N. VAN DEN POL. 1990. GABA: a dominant neurotransmitter in the hypothalamus. J. Comp. Neurol. **302**: 1019–1037.
20. CULLINAN, W.E. 2000. GABA(A) receptor subunit expression within hypophysiotropic CRH neurons: a dual hybridization histochemical study. J. Comp. Neurol. **419:** 344–351.
21. GOEDERS, N.E., E.B. DE SOUZA, *et al.* 1986. Benzodiazepine receptor GABA ratios: regional differences in rat brain and modulation by adrenalectomy. Eur. J. Pharmacol. **129:** 363–366.
22. VERKUYL, J.M. & M. JOËLS. 2003. Effect of adrenalectomy on minature inhibitory postsynaptic currents in the paraventricular nucleus of the hypothalamus. J. Neurophysiol. **89:** 237–245.
23. MIKLOS, I.H. & K.J. KOVACS. 2002. GABAergic innervation of corticotropin-releasing hormone (CRH)-secreting parvocellular neurons and its plasticity as demonstrated by quantitative immunoelectron microscopy. Neuroscience **113:** 581–592.
24. CULLINAN, W.E. & T.J. WOLFE. 2000. Chronic stress regulates levels of mRNA transcripts encoding beta subunits of the GABA(A) receptor in the rat stress axis. Brain Res. **887:** 118–124.
25. KARST, H. & M. JOËLS. 2003. Effect of chronic stress on synaptic currents in rat hippocampal dentate gyrus neurons. J. Neurophysiol. **89:** 625–633.
26. JOËLS, M., W. HESEN & E.R. DE KLOET. 1991. Mineralocorticoid hormones suppress serotonin-induced hyperpolarization of rat hippocampal CA1 neurons. J. Neurosci. **11:** 2288–2294.
27. ANDRADE, R., R.C. MALENKA & R.A. NICOLL. 1986. A G protein couples serotonin and GABAB receptors to the same channels in hippocampus. Science **234:** 1261–1265.
28. BECK, S.G., K.C. CHOI, T.J. LIST, *et al.* 1996. Corticosterone alters 5-HT_{1A} receptor-mediated hyperpolarization in area CA1 hippocampal pyramidal neurons. Neuropsychopharmacology **14:** 27–33.
29. HESEN, W. & M. JOËLS. 1996. Modulation of 5HT1A responsiveness in CA1 pyramidal neurons by in vivo activation of corticosteroid receptors. J. Neuroendocrinol. **8:** 433–438.
30. KARST, H., Y.J. KARTEN, H.M. REICHARDT, *et al.* 2000. Corticosteroid actions in hippocampus require DNA binding of glucocorticoid receptor homodimers. Nat. Neurosci. **3:** 977–978.
31. BIRNSTIEL, S. & S.G. BECK. 1995. Modulation of the 5-hydroxytryptamine4 receptor-mediated response by short-term and long-term administration of corticosterone in rat CA1 hippocampal pyramidal neurons. J. Pharmacol. Exp. Ther. **273:** 1132–1138.
32. MEIJER, O.C. & E.R. DE KLOET. 1998. Corticosterone and serotonergic neurotransmission in the hippocampus: functional implications of central corticosteroid receptor diversity. Crit. Rev. Neurobiol. **12:** 1–20.
33. OKUHARA, D.Y., S.G. BECK & N.A. MUMA. 1997. Corticosterone alters G protein alpha-subunit levels in the rat hippocampus. Brain Res. **745:** 144–151.
34. MUMA, N.A. & S.G. BECK. 1999. Corticosteroids alter G protein inwardly rectifying potassium channels protein levels in hippocampal subfields. Brain Res. **839:** 331–335.
35. KARTEN, Y.J.G., S.M. NAIR, L. VAN ESSEN, *et al.* 1999. Long-term corticosterone application decreases serotonin responses of CA1 neurons in the rat hippocampus. Proc. Natl. Acad. Sci. USA **96:** 13456–13461.
36. MUELLER, N.K. & S.G. BECK. 2000. Corticosteroids alter the 5-HT(1A) receptor-mediated response in CA1 hippocampal pyramidal cells. Neuropsychopharmacology **23:** 419–427.
37. VAN RIEL, E., O.C. MEIJER, P.J. STEENBERGEN & M. JOËLS. 2002. Chronic unpredictable stress causes attenuation of serotonin responses in cornu ammonis 1 pyramidal neurons. Neuroscience **120:** 649–658.
38. KOLE, M.H., L. SWAN & E. FUCHS. 2002. The antidepressant tianeptine persistently modulates glutamate receptor currents of the hippocampal CA3 commissural associational synapse in chronically stressed rats. Eur. J. Neurosci. **16:** 807–816.

39. Magarinos, A.M. & B.S. McEwen. 1995. Stress-induced atrophy of apical dendrites of hippocampal CA3c neurons: comparison of stressors. Neuroscience **69:** 83–88.
40. Sapolsky, R.M., H. Uno, C.S. Rebert, *et al.* 1990. Hippocampal damage associated with prolonged glucocorticoid exposure in primates. J. Neurosci. **10:** 2897–2902.
41. Magarinos, A.M., B.S. McEwen, G. Flugge *et al.* 1996. Chronic psychosocial stress causes apical dendritic atrophy of hippocampal CA3 pyramidal neurons in subordinate tree shrews. J. Neurosci. **16:** 3534–3540.
42. McEwen, B.S. 1999. Stress and hippocampal plasticity. Annu. Rev. Neurosci. **22:** 105–122.
43. Magarinos, A.M. & B.S. McEwen. 1995. Stress-induced atrophy of apical dendrites of hippocampal CA3c neurons: involvement of glucocorticoid secretion and excitatory amino acid receptors. Neuroscience **69:** 89–98.
44. Joëls, M. 1997. Steroid hormones and excitability in the mammalian brain. Front. Neuroendocrinol. **18:** 2–48.
45. Lanfumey, L., M.C. Pardon, N. Laaris, *et al.* 1999. 5-HT1A autoreceptor desensitization by chronic ultramild stress in mice. Neuroreport **10**: 3369–3374.
46. Dinan, T.G. 1996. Serotonin and the regulation of hypothalamic-pituitary-adrenal axis function. Life Sci. **58:** 1683–1694.
47. Lowry, C.A. 2002. Functional subsets of serotonergic neurones: implications for control of the hypothalamic-pituitary-adrenal axis. J. Neuroendocrinol. **14:** 911–923.
48. Watanabe, Y., N.G. Weiland & B.S. McEwen. 1995. Effect of adrenal steroid manipulations and repeated restraint stress on dynorphin mRNA levels and excitatory amino acid receptor binding in hippocampus. Brain Res. **680:** 217–225.
49. Schwendt, M. & D. Jezova. 2000. Gene expression of two receptor subunits in respose to repeated stress exposure in rat hippocampus. Cell. Mol. Neurobiol. **20:** 319–329.
50. Belanoff, J.K., A.J. Rothschild, F. Cassidy, *et al.* 2002. An open label trial of C-1073 (mifepristone) for psychotic major depression. Biol. Psychiatry **52:** 386–392.

Corticosteroid Receptor Transgenic Mice

Models for Depression?

ALEXANDRE URANI AND PETER GASS

Central Institute of Mental Health (CIMA), University of Heidelberg, D-68159 Mannheim, Germany

ABSTRACT: Dysregulations and dysfunctions of corticosteroids and their receptors have been implicated in the pathogenesis of stress-related disorders, in particular in depression. It is currently under debate, however, whether corticosteroid imbalances are a cause or rather a consequence of affective disorders. Corticosteroids exert their effects mainly by two receptors: glucocorticoid receptors (GRs) and mineralocorticoid receptors (MRs). We present here analyses made on several strains of mice with targeted mutations of corticosteroid receptors. The results help to understand how corticosteroid receptors regulate the hypothalamic-pituitary-adrenal (HPA) system. Furthermore, first behavioral analyses have indicated that corticosteroid receptor mutant mice show alterations in their emotional behavior. Certain mouse strains with specific alterations of GR or MR expression may represent genetic models of depression or at least have a predisposition to develop a depressive or a depression-resistant state upon exposure to stress. The corticosteroid receptor–regulated target genes to be identified in these models may code for proteins that could represent new drug-targets for the treatment of affective disorders.

KEYWORDS: depression; animal model; transgenic mice; mineralocorticoid receptor; glucocorticoid receptor

INTRODUCTION

Corticosteroids, Corticosteroid Receptors, and Depression

Affective disorders are influenced or even caused by genetic, developmental, and environmental events. All these factors become manifest at the biological level and lead to transient or persistent dysfunctional changes in several regions and/or systems of the brain. A key biological system disturbed in depressive illness is the hypothalamic-pituitary-adrenal (HPA) system.[1] Thus, many patients with a severe major depressive episode (MDE) have higher blood levels of cortisol than do healthy subjects, and a dysregulated circadian rhythm of cortisol secretion.[2–6] However, it must be noted that not all patients with major depression are hypercortisolemic when studied cross-sectionally.[7] Furthermore, hypercortisolism does not occur daily in depressed patients, and—if present—can return to normal even within the same day.[8]

Address for correspondence: Peter Gass, M.D., Central Institute of Mental Health, Mannheim J5, D-68159 Mannheim, Germany. Voice: ++49 621 1703 956; fax: ++49 621 1703 760. gass@as200.zi-mannheim.de

Ann. N.Y. Acad. Sci. 1007: 379–393 (2003). © 2003 New York Academy of Sciences. doi: 10.1196/annals.1286.037

Corticosteroids have been further implicated in the pathomechanisms of depression by the hypothesis that antidepressants may act through normalization of the HPA system.[9] Indeed, elevated cortisol levels observed in depressive patients usually return to normal under antidepressant treatment,[10] or once depression disappears.[11] So far, the pathomechanisms of the HPA system dysinhibition in depression have not been elucidated and could involve any level of regulation, from higher brain centers to the adrenals. However, increasing evidence has accumulated that a dysfunction of corticosteroid receptors may be implicated in the pathogenesis of depression.

Two hypotheses have been put forward: First, that high cortisol levels in depression may be caused by a deficient negative feedback on the hypothalamus due to diminished corticosteroid receptor expression or function. Alternatively, a primary upregulation of corticotropin-releasing hormone (CRH) could lead to a dysinhibition of the HPA system and a secondary corticosteroid receptor downregulation, which would also—by a vicious circle—cause excessive plasma cortisol levels. It has recently been shown in an open clinical study that a GR antagonist (RU486, mifepristone) is an effective treatment of psychotic major depression, the type of depression with the most severe abnormalities in HPA system activity.[12] This effect was obtained within a few days, in contrast to the few weeks conventional antidepressants need to become effective. Moreover, cortisol synthesis inhibitors such as ketoconazole have also shown benefits in the treatment of major depression.[13,14] Altogether these results indicate an important role for corticosteroid receptors in depression and make them a promising target for antidepressant treatment.[1]

Molecular and Functional Properties of Corticosteroid Receptors

Glucocorticoids exert their effects via two types of receptors: high-affinity receptors for cortisol called mineralocorticoid receptors (MRs), because of their ability to bind also mineralocorticoids (e.g., aldosterone), and low-affinity receptors called glucocorticoid receptors (GRs), which mainly bind cortisol. MRs are predominantly found in the limbic system, in particular in the hippocampus, whereas GRs are ubiquitously expressed throughout the central nervous system.[15] Functionally, MRs are thought to be involved in the physiological maintenance of the HPA system, while GRs are supposed to control the recovery from stress.[16,17] Corticosteroid receptors are intracellular proteins and function as transcription factors. Their ligands are lipophilic and can easily cross the cytoplasmic membrane. Inside the cell, activation of the receptors provokes their translocation to the nucleus, where they bind to specific sequences on the DNA (GREs, glucocorticoid response elements) and enhance or repress the transcription rate of their target genes.[18,19] GRs can also up- or downregulate gene transcription by direct interaction with other transcription factors such as CREB, AP-1, and Stat5.[20–22]

Activation of corticosteroid receptors in neurons can influence diverse cellular processes such as energy metabolism, signal transduction, and even structural plasticity. Functional consequences include the control of excitability in limbic brain regions, in particular in the hippocampus.[17,23–25] The corticosteroid receptor–mediated effects at the cellular level have consequences for processes in which the hippocampal formation plays an essential role, for example, in the neuroendocrine regulation of the HPA system, and also in behavior. Thus, corticosteroids influence perception and spontaneous behavior as well as learning and memory.[17]

ANIMAL MODELS OF DEPRESSION

A good animal model of human depression should fulfill the following criteria as best as possible: strong behavioral similarities (e.g., similar core symptoms), common etiology, similar pathophysiology, and common treatment. Such a model could then be used to elucidate molecular and biochemical mechanisms underlying the pathogenesis of depression. One of the core symptoms of severe depression in man and mice is anhedonia, that is, lack of interest in pleasurable activities. In mice, anhedonia can be measured by a loss of preference for sweet solutions over tap water.

Confusion should be avoided between a model and a test. A model can be defined as an organism or a particular state of an organism that reproduces aspects of the human pathology providing a certain degree of predictive validity. A test is an end-point behavioral or physiological measure designed to assess the effect of a pharmacological or environmental manipulation. In this respect, models of depression are different from the tests used to monitor the effects of antidepressants. "Behavioral despair" paradigms such as the Porsolt forced-swim test[26] and the tail suspension test[27] cannot be considered as models of depression, even though their efficiency to screen for antidepressant-like activity is widely accepted. Nevertheless, increased despair behavior in these tests can be regarded as part of a depressive syndrome.

Stress-Induced Models

Two paradigms induce anhedonia in mice: the chronic mild stress model and the learned helplessness paradigm. In the chronic mild stress model, animals are subjected for several weeks to a series of mild stressors (intermittent food and water deprivation, overnight illumination, cage tilt, noise, etc.[28,29]). This treatment induces a reduction of sucrose preference, decreased intracranial self-stimulation, altered sexual and aggressive behavior, loss of body weight, sleep disturbances, and overactivation of the HPA system. These symptoms are reversible upon administration of antidepressants.

In the learned helplessness paradigm, animals are exposed to inescapable electric footshocks, which induce a number of deficits similar to those observed after chronic stress: failure in avoidance learning, lower preference for sucrose solution, decreased appetite, loss of body weight, and overactivation of the HPA system. Again, these effects are reversed by the administration of antidepressants. Thus, the behavioral and somatic deficits observed in these two models mimic the human depressive syndrome.

Pharmacological Models

The most pharmacological models of depression are based on the monoaminergic hypothesis of depression, which conceptualizes the biological basis as a deficiency in one or several biogenic monoamines (serotonin, 5-HT; norepinephrine, NA; dopamine, DA). Antidepressant drugs are therefore classified according to their ability to improve monoaminergic transmission. Reserpine depletes the aminergic pools in the presynaptic nerve terminals, imitating the pathophysiology postulated for depressive patients. The reversal of some effects of reserpine administration (e.g., ptosis and hypothermia) is used to predict the antidepressant activity of drugs.[30,31] In animals treated with reserpine, a decrease in the preference for sucrose was also observed.[32] Antidepressant treatment, including lithium and electroconvulsive therapy (ECT), has been shown to reverse behavioral and biochemical deficits induced by reserpine.[33,34]

Based on the theory that depression can also result from excessive serotonergic neurotransmission, the 5-hydroxytryptophan model of depression has been developed. Indeed, administration of this serotonin precursor also produces depression-like symptoms in rodents, and this effect is attenuated by antidepressant treatment.[35]

Transgenic Models

A major drawback of the previous models is the difficulty to know whether the pathological changes observed are due to the animals' "depressive state" or rather reflect the manipulation by which this state was induced, for example, by stress or pharmacological treatment. An alternative animal model of affective disorders would be an endogenous, genetic model, independent of external factors, which mimics essential aspects of the human disorder and responds to standard regimens of therapy. Mouse mutants with altered HPA system activity are candidate strains for a murine depression-like syndrome, because HPA system imbalances are a key biological marker for a major depression in humans. In particular, alterations of corticosteroid receptors appear promising in modeling affective disorders. Different strains of mutant mice can be obtained by over- or underexpression of glucocorticoid receptors. Current techniques even allow a conditional gene disruption in specific brain regions, in the best case inducible at a specific timepoint.[36,37]

MICE WITH TARGETED MUTATIONS OF GR OR MR

Animal models of human diseases can be obtained by introduction of genes and/or disruption of genes through various techniques. Genetically modified animals also allow studying the role of a specific gene in the pathophysiology of a disease. Several mouse strains with specific alteration of genes implied in the HPA axis regulation have been obtained. Among them, we will focus on mice with modifications of GR and MR expression. The neuroendocrinological and behavioral phenotypes of these strains are subsequently described and also summarized in TABLE 1.

Transgenic Mice with Decreased GR Expression

A first mouse model with reduced GR expression was developed by transgenic expression of an antisense RNA sequence complementary to a fragment of the GR cDNA under the control of a human neurofilament promoter.[38] The exact mechanisms leading to an intracellular reduction of GR mRNA in these mice remains unclear. It was suggested that the antisense RNA forms hybrids with the endogenous mRNA, resulting in a specific decrease of the targeted mRNA and therefore a decrease—but not a complete suppression—of translation into the corresponding protein. The amount of GR reduction depends on the promoter activity of the antisense transgene and therefore varies from neuron to neuron.

TABLE 1. HPA system dysregulation and behavioral symptoms in mice with targeted mutations of GR and MR

	Baseline HPA System				Challenged HPA System			Behavior		
	Hypothalamic* CRH	Pituitary POMC/ ACTH	Plasma ACTH	Plasma CORT	Stress-ind* ACTH	Stress-ind* CORT	Dex/CRH-Test	Anxiety	Despair	Locomotion
Human depression	↑	n.d.	↑	↑	↓	↑	↑	↑	↑	
Tg mice with ↓ GR	↓	↔	↔	↔	↑	↓	↑	↓	↓	↔
GR knockout mice	↑	↑	n.d.	n.d.	n.d.	n.d.	n.d.	n.d.	n.d.	n.d.
GRNesCre mice	↑	↑	↓	↑	↓	↔	n.d.	↓	↓	↔
GRdim mice	↔	↑	↔	↑	n.d.	n.d.	n.d.			
Tg mice with ↑ GR	↓	↓	↑	↓	↑	↓	n.d.	↔	↔	↔
MR knockout mice	↑	↑	↓	↑	n.d.	n.d.	n.d.	↑	n.d.	n.d.

NOTE: Changes in human depression (↑ or ↓) were derived from comparisons with healthy control subjects. Changes in mutant mice were derived from comparisons with wild-type littermates. *CRH levels in patients were measured in the cerebrospinal fluid (after lumbar puncture), in mice by *in situ* hybridization or immunohistochemistry in the paraventricular hypothalamic nucleus. The HPA system in human depression and anxiety was challenged by CRH injection, not by stress. Locomotion as a behavioral parameter was not applicable to humans. Despair in the animals refers to a giving-up strategy in the Porsolt forced swim test (Tg = transgenic; n.d. = not done).

Under baseline conditions, these mice show reduced CRH expression in the hypothalamus and unaltered ACTH and corticosterone plasma levels in the morning as well as in the evening.[39–41] Under stress conditions, however, they reveal an upregulation of the HPA system[38,42] that is reversed by antidepressant treatment.[43,44] After a CRH challenge, transgenic mice reveal a hyperresponse in ACTH and a decreased response in corticosterone levels, just opposite as seen in depressive patients.[40] On the other hand, similarly to patients with major depression, mice with transgenic GR expression fail to respond to the dexamethasone suppression test.[40] Upon behavioral testing, transgenic mice display less anxiety in the elevated plus maze and also after exposure to an intense psychosocial stress.[43,45] This anxiolytic effect may be explained by the reduced CRH levels, because mice with impaired CHR receptor expression show a similar behavioral phenotype.[46–49] Transgenic mice also exhibit enhanced responses to novelty and increased conditioned approach responses, in contrast to what one would expect in depression.[50] In the Porsolt forced swim test, where immobility time reflects behavioral despair, transgenic mice show less floating, also suggesting a decreased depression-like behavior. Taken together, transgenic mice with reduced GR expression present only few of the neuroendocrine and behavioral features observed in depression. However, since many of the deficits observed in these mice are reversed by antidepressant treatment,[43] this strain may be a valuable tool for the discovery of new antidepressants.

GR Knockout Mice

Two distinct disruptions of the GR gene have been generated in mice by gene targeting. The first was achieved by insertion of a neomycin cassette into exon 2 of the GR gene, resulting in a hypomorphic allele (FIG. 1a).[51] In these mice, an mRNA splice variant persists which encodes an N-terminal truncated protein containing the DNA-binding domain and the ligand-binding domain.[19] On a C57BL6/129sv genetic background, 10% of the knockout mice survive until maturity. In these latter, a diminished but still present binding of dexamethasone could be measured, suggesting a residual expression of GR. In fact, this binding reflects aberrant expression of a truncated GR containing the GR ligand-binding domain. However, these mice present all the characteristics of insensitivity to glucocorticoids showing their inability to elicit transcription of a functional GR despite residual binding.[52] The second mutation results in deletion of a DNA segment that contains exon 3 of the GR gene (GR^{null}). This exon encodes the first zinc-finger of the DNA-binding domain. Its absence leads to a complete inactivation of the GR gene. Homozygosity of this mutation ($GR^{null/null}$) is incompatible with survival to adulthood in any genetic background tested. The $GR^{null/null}$ mice die a few minutes after birth from severe atelectasis of the lungs.

GR knockout mice show a reduced capacity to activate key gluconeogenic enzyme genes in the liver and impaired negative feedback in the HPA axis, resulting in markedly elevated plasma ACTH and corticosterone levels.[51,53] Homozygous knockout mice show enhanced transcription of both CRH in the hypothalamus and proopiomelanocortin (POMC) in the anterior lobe of the pituitary, as well as elevated corticosterone plasma levels.[54] These results confirm the role of the GR-mediated negative feedback in the HPA system via transcriptional repression. No behavioral testing on the surviving GR knockout mice has been published.

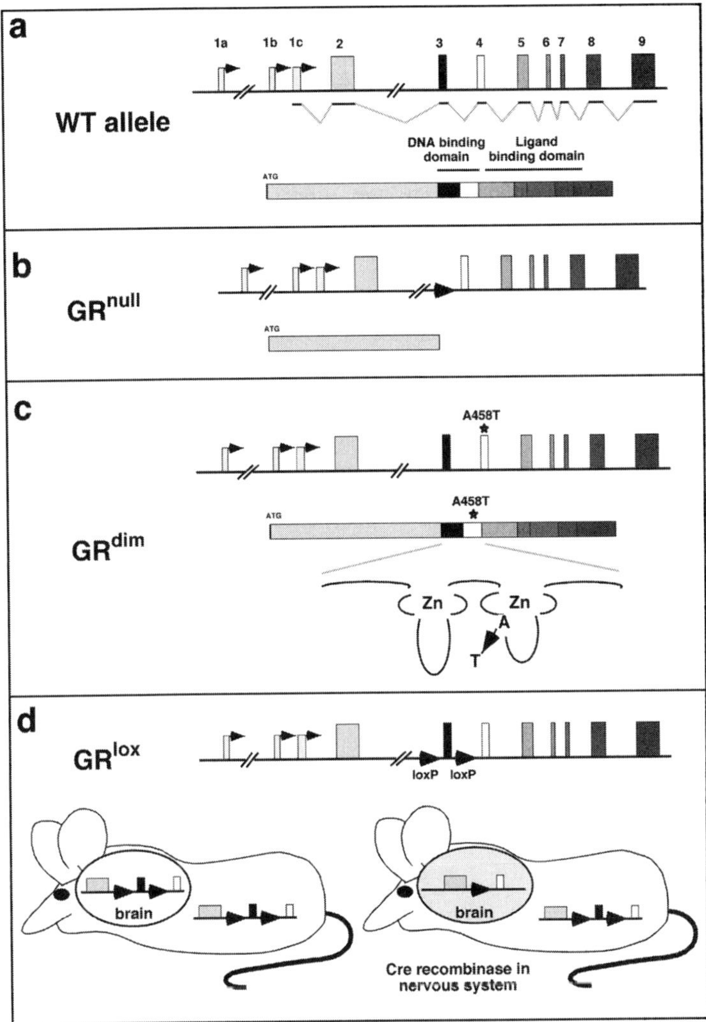

FIGURE 1. Schematic representation of different GR alleles used for homologous recombination in mice. (**a**) Organization of the wild-type (WT) GR gene. The *upper scheme* depicts the genomic structure of the GR gene with introns and numbered exons and the resulting mRNA. The *lower scheme* with the bars corresponding in grey to the respective exons represents the translated GR protein. The functional domains resulting from exon 3 and 4 (DNA-binding domain) and exon 5 to 9 (ligand-binding domain) are indicated. (**b**) The GR^{null} allele was obtained by deleting the third exon (and a subsequent frame shift) leading to a truncated GR protein without the important functional domains. (**c**) The GR^{dim} allele harbors a point mutation in exon 4 (alanine to threonine) that prevents the dimerization of the GR protein. This strategy selectively eliminates GR functions that require binding to GREs. (**d**) The GR^{lox} allele was generated by flanking exon 3 with loxP sites. This modification does not primarily impair expression and function of the GR gene but is sensitive to the (artificial) cellular expression of the enzyme Cre recombinase. When the Cre recombi-

Nervous System–Specific GR Knockout (GR^{NesCre}) Mice

Because a classical knockout of the GR causes perinatal lethality, a conditional disruption of this gene was generated using the Cre/loxP recombination system under the control of the rat nestin promoter.[55] This strategy resulted in viable mice (GR^{NesCre}) lacking GR in neurons and glial cells and allows the selective study of the role of GR in the nervous system (FIG. 1d).[55] The GR deficiency in the brain leads to a strong increase of CRH mRNA and protein in the hypothalamus. Thus, the GR-mediated negative feedback control at the level of the hypothalamus was confirmed for the first time by genetic tools. The HPA system shows a marked hyperactivity with strongly elevated ACTH levels in the pituitary, resulting in more than tenfold elevated plasma corticosterone levels.[55] However, levels of plasma ACTH were significantly reduced in GR^{NesCre} mice. This is most likely due to the intact (GR-mediated) suppression of ACTH secretion in the anterior pituitary, since this gland was not affected by the targeted GR disruption. The discordance between decreased circulating levels of ACTH and increased levels of corticosterone may be caused by an increased ACTH sensitivity of the adrenals or a direct stimulation of this gland (possibly by direct CRH effects and/or splanchnic innervation) that may develop under a chronic hyperactivation of the HPA system. Interestingly, a similar discrepancy in ACTH and cortisol plasma levels has been reported in patients with a major depressive episode.[56] Furthermore, the HPA system is still responsive to acute immobilization stress, resulting in increased levels of both circulating ACTH and corticosterone. Since elevated corticosterone levels can still act on peripheral tissues with preserved GR expression, GR^{NesCre} mice exhibit features reminiscent of Cushing's syndrome in humans.

In summary, the neuroendocrinological changes of the HPA system in GR^{NesCre} mice closely resemble those of patients with a major depression. Paradoxically, at the behavioral level, GR^{NesCre} mice display reduced anxiety. They spend more time in the anxiety-related lit compartment of the dark–light-box and in the open segments of the elevated O-maze.[55] In the forced swim test, GR^{NesCre} mice do not develop despair behavior, which is seen in control littermates upon repetitive swim stress exposure.[55] Thus, despite their depression-like hypercortisolism, GR^{NesCre} mice do not show, or are even resistant to develop, anxiety or depression. This paradoxical finding can be explained by the fact that the neurons of GR^{NesCre} mice lack GR, that is, the hypercortisolism cannot affect these neurons and cause relevant changes in behavior. Thus, despite their hypercortisolism, these mice most likely represent a genetically depression-resistant mouse strain. To prove this hypothesis, one has to subject these mice to a stress-induced depression model.

Mice with a DNA-Binding Defective GR (GR^{dim})

GR controls transcription by two major modes of action: (1) as dimer, binding to positive and negative GREs in the promoter of target genes; and (2) as monomer,

---

nase transgene is expressed in the same cell as GR^{lox}, the latter is turned into GR^{null} by deletion of exon 3 and a subsequent frame shift. When the Cre recombinase is expressed under the control of a promoter specific for the central nervous system, GR is deleted selectively in the brain and spinal cord, but is still normally expressed outside the nervous system. (Modified from Tronche *et al.*[19]).

modulating positively or negatively the activity of other transcription factors via protein–protein interactions.[57] The two modes of action can be dissected by introducing a point mutation (A458T) into the D-loop, that is, one of the dimerization domains of the GR (FIG. 1c).[58] This mutation was introduced in mice using a knock-in strategy replacing the endogenous GR gene.[59] The resulting GR^{dim} mice express GR molecules that cannot dimerize, but still act as monomers. Consequently, GR^{dim} mice are deficient in activating GRE-driven genes, but proficient in the modulation of other transcription factors, such as AP-1 and NF-κB.[59,60] In contrast to mice carrying disrupted alleles of GR, GR^{dim} mice are viable and can be used to study physiology and behavior in adulthood.[59]

Corticosterone levels in GR^{dim} mice are significantly higher than in wild-type animals. However, this mutation does not affect HPA axis feedback regulation at the level of hypothalamus, because CRH levels are similar to those of control animals. This result indicates that the control of CRH expression is independent of GR dimerization, despite a recently identified negative GRE in the CRH promoter.[61] ACTH immunostaining is increased in the anterior pituitary of GR^{dim} mice, but no difference is found in plasma levels. Since similar findings are also observed in GR^{NesCre} mice with intact GR function in the pituitary, the release of ACTH (in contrast to its synthesis) seems to be controlled by a dimerization-independent mechanism. POMC and prolactin mRNA are strongly upregulated in the anterior pituitary of GR^{dim} mice, suggesting a common mechanism of transcriptional regulation. For both genes functional nGREs requiring DNA-binding of GR have been described.[62, 63]

At the behavioral level, GR^{dim} mice display spatial memory deficits in the Morris watermaze. This impairment is not related to general cognitive deficits, since GR^{dim} mice reveal normal locomotion, exploration, and anxiety-related behavior.[64] Furthermore, GR^{dim} mice exhibit the same floating scores in the behavioral despair test as their wild-type littermates. Together with the findings reported for GR^{NesCre} mice, this may suggest that emotional behavior and learning are influenced by GRs via different molecular modes of action: learning and memory by GRE- or nGRE-dependent mechanisms, and anxiety-related behavior via protein–protein interactions of GRs. An electrophysiological correlate for the learning deficits in GR^{dim} mice could be altered calcium currents or a decreased serotonin responsiveness.[65]

Transgenic Mice with Increased GR Expression (YGR Mice)

GR overexpression in mice has been achieved by transgenic expression of two additional copies of the GR gene using a yeast artificial chromosome.[66] In these mice GR mRNA is overexpressed by 20 to 24%, and GR protein by 50%, thus demonstrating an autoregulation of the GR gene. YGR mice display a strong suppression of the HPA system with a more than two-fold reduction of CRH immunoreactivity, suggesting that overexpression of GR in the brain leads to increased repression of CRH production. In general, YGR mice show the opposite dysregulatory effects of the HPA system as GR^{NesCre} mice.[66] Preliminary behavioral tests with YGR mice show unaltered anxiety- and despair-related behavior (unpublished personal data). Similar to GR^{NesCre} mice, YGR mice should be subjected to a stress-induced depression model, since the increased stability of their HPA system may render them more stress-resistant on a behavioral level.

Conditional Overexpression of GR

Mice with a conditional overexpression of the GR have recently been generated under the forebrain-specific promoter calcium calmodulin dependent kinase II (CaMKII).[67] The HPA system of these mice does not seem to be affected, since plasma ACTH and corticosterone levels are not different from those of control animals. The only change observed is an increase of CRH mRNA expression in the rostral part of the central nucleus of the amygdala. These mice show normal locomotor activity, but increased anxiety-related behavior in the dark–light-box test. The authors claim that these animals may provide a useful model for increased anxiety-related behavior independent of circulating stress hormones. Further studies are necessary to assess the effect of this localized GR overexpression in a behavioral depression model.

MR Knockout Mice

MR knockout mice were generated by classical homologous recombination. Their phenotype is dominated by renal salt wasting, dehydration, and a failure to thrive, which is caused by the prominent role of MR for the expression and function of epithelial Na^+ channels in kidney and colon.[68] Untreated, they die between postnatal days 8 and 13, but can survive until adulthood when given external salt supply.[69,70] The rescued MR knockout mice show an upregulation of the whole HPA system, with elevated CRH levels in the PVN, higher amounts of POMC and ACTH in the anterior pituitary, and significantly elevated plasma corticosterone levels.[70] Since MR is not expressed in the HPA system itself, higher brain centers—for example, the hippocampus—are responsible for these effects. Inactivation of the MR produces a reduction of neurogenesis and of dentate granule cells, possibly due to the elevated corticosterone levels.[70] The postnatal exogenous salt supply has to be made by subcutaneous injection of physiological saline and involves daily handling of the animals during the complete early life period. This manipulation may have profound effects on both HPA system and behavior.[71] However, handling and exogenous salt supply most likely are not crucial factors for the HPA system overactivity in adult MR knockout mice, because this upregulation is already detected in MR knockout embryos at day E18.5. At this time point of development, the HPA system feedback regulation is well established, but salt and water homeostasis are maintained via the placental circulation.[54] Embryonic MR knockout animals, however, cannot serve as "handling controls" for behavioral testing. Preliminary experiments suggest increased anxious behavior in salt-rescued adult MR knockout mice. Due to the serious caveats mentioned, a thorough behavioral analysis needs to be performed in animals with a more elaborated (i.e., a brain- or hippocampus-specific) genetic disruption of the MR gene.

CONCLUSIONS

Targeting of corticosteroid receptor genes by homologous recombination in embryonic stem cells and by transgenic approaches has generated several strains of mutant mice with altered function of GR and MR. These mice allow the *in vivo* study of causal effects of the disrupted genes, and thus enable a correlation between GR or MR functioning and expression of target genes, endocrinology, and behavior. The endocrinological studies have yielded valuable insights into different feedback mechanisms of the HPA system controlled by MR and GR, respectively. Thus, the GR-mediated negative feedback control at the level of the hypothalamus was confirmed for the first time by genetic tools. The generation of dimerization-defective GR^{dim} mice allowed the distinction between negative transcriptional regulations of GR monomers at the level of the hypothalamus, and negative feedback of GR dimers at the level of the pituitary. In contrast, MR exerts its control on the HPA system selectively at higher brain centers such as the hippocampus.

Since dysfunction of the central stress hormone system is involved in the pathogenesis of anxiety and depression, mice with disrupted GRs or MRs could serve as models that mimic symptoms of these psychiatric disorders. Behavioral analyses of GR mutant mice revealed that emotional responses are controlled by GR monomers, since GR^{NesCre} but not GR^{dim} mice exhibited a significant decrease of anxious behavior in several tests. Therefore, mice with targeted mutations of the GR are candidate models for anxiety disorders, since all the genetically modified mice presented here (except GR^{dim}) exhibit alterations in anxiety-related behavior. However, the molecular mechanisms by which corticosteroid receptors influence anxiety behavior remain to be identified. With respect to modeling depression, the conclusions that can currently be drawn are less clear, because only a few of the strains presented here have been studied for the presence of depressive core symptoms such as anhedonia and despair. Among the genetically modified mice presented here, the most intensively studied strain at the behavioral level is the transgenic mouse with decreased GR expression. While this mouse strain failed to reproduce many of the neuroendocrinological and behavioral features of depression, the changes observed responded well to antidepressant treatment.[40,42,43,72] These data suggest that transgenic mice with reduced GR expression will prove useful to test the effect of antidepressant drugs, but cannot be considered as a proper animal model of depression.

So far, however, none of the mutants described here can be viewed as an animal model of a specific psychiatric disease defined by a common set of diagnostic criteria. Such criteria can be and have to be developed for mice. Genetic models for depression should demonstrate the presence of the core symptoms of anhedonia and despair. Further testing in a stress-induced model of depression should elaborate whether a specific mutation renders the GR- or MR-mutant mice more prone or more resistant to develop behavioral symptoms of depression. Such studies will be performed in the mouse strains reviewed in our laboratory in oncoming months.

Using promoters with neuroanatomically more restricted activity than the nestin promoter could lead to the identification of brain regions where GRs and MRs are involved in the symptomatology of affective disorders. Furthermore, molecular neurobiology will soon allow an inducible mutagenesis in adult mice. This will enable experiments, in which the behavior of an individual mouse can be studied before and after gene disruption. This progress may overcome some caveats against conventional gene-targeting techniques, concerning the influence of the genetic background of breeding animals and stem cells, the developmental compensation of mutations, etc.[23,73,74] Furthermore, the effect of antidepressant therapy could be assessed after defined onset of gene disruption without confounding variables such as developmental processes or stress-inducing measures. DNA microarray technology can be used for the identification of target genes regulated by GR and MR in brain areas responsible for specific depressive symptoms and responding to therapy. The identified corticosteroid receptor–regulated target genes may code for proteins that could turn out to represent new drug targets for the treatment of depression and anxiety.

ACKNOWLEDGMENTS

We would like to express our gratitude to Günther Schütz, whose laboratory generated most of the corticosteroid receptor mutant mice described and discussed in this paper. This work was supported by a grant from the Deutsche Forschungsgemeinschaft (427/4-2 to P.G.).

REFERENCES

1. HOLSBOER, F. 2000. The corticosteroid receptor hypothesis of depression. Neuropsychopharmacology **23:** 477–501.
2. GIBBONS, J.L. 1964. Cortisol secretion rate in depressive illness. Arch. Gen. Psychiatry **10:** 572–575.
3. DOLAN, R.J., S.P. CALLOWAY, *et al.* 1985. Life events, depression and hypothalamic-pituitary-adrenal axis function. Br. J. Psychiatry **147:** 429–433.
4. RUBIN, R.T., R.E. POLAND, *et al.* 1987. Neuroendocrine aspects of primary endogenous depression. I. Cortisol secretory dynamics in patients and matched controls. Arch. Gen. Psychiatry **44:** 328–336.
5. DEAKIN, J.F., I. PENNELL, *et al.* 1990. A neuroendocrine study of 5HT function in depression: evidence for biological mechanisms of endogenous and psychosocial causation. Psychopharmacology **101:** 85–92.
6. WONG, M.L., M.A. KLING, *et al.* 2000. Pronounced and sustained central hypernoradrenergic function in major depression with melancholic features: relation to hypercortisolism and corticotropin-releasing hormone. Proc. Natl. Acad. Sci. USA **97:** 325–330.
7. STRICKLAND, P.L., J.F. DEAKIN, *et al.* 2002. Bio-social origins of depression in the community. Interactions between social adversity, cortisol and serotonin neurotransmission. Br. J. Psychiatry **180:** 168–173.
8. GOLD, P.W., W.C. DREVETS, *et al.* 2002. New insights into the role of cortisol and the glucocorticoid receptor in severe depression. Biol. Psychiatry **52:** 381–385.
9. HOLSBOER, F. & N. BARDEN. 1996. Antidepressants and hypothalamic-pituitary-adrenocortical regulation. Endocr. Rev. **17:** 187–205.
10. BHAGWAGAR, Z., S. HAFIZI, *et al.* 2002. Acute citalopram administration produces correlated increases in plasma and salivary cortisol. Psychopharmacology **163:** 118–120.
11. STECKLER, T., F. HOLSBOER, *et al.* 1999. Glucocorticoids and depression. Baillieres Best Pract. Res. Clin. Endocrinol. Metab. **13:** 597–614.
12. BELANOFF, J.K., A.J. ROTHSCHILD, *et al.* 2002. An open label trial of C-1073 (mifepristone) for psychotic major depression. Biol. Psychiatry **52:** 386–392.
13. WOLKOWITZ, O.M., V.I. REUS, *et al.* 1993. Ketoconazole administration in hypercortisolemic depression. Am. J. Psychiatry **150:** 810–812.
14. WOLKOWITZ, O.M., V.I. REUS, *et al.* 1999. Antiglucocorticoid treatment of depression: double-blind ketoconazole. Biol. Psychiatry **45:** 1070–1074.
15. REUL, J.M. & E.R. DE KLOET. 1985. Two receptor systems for corticosterone in rat brain: microdistribution and differential occupation. Endocrinology **117:** 2505–2511.
16. DE KLOET, E.R. & J.M. REUL. 1987. Feedback action and tonic influence of corticosteroids on brain function: a concept arising from the heterogeneity of brain receptor systems. Psychoneuroendocrinology **12:** 83–105.
17. DE KLOET, E.R., E. VREUGDENHIL, *et al.* 1998. Brain corticosteroid receptor balance in health and disease. Endocr. Rev. **19:** 269–301.

18. JOELS, M. & E. VREUGDENHIL. 1998. Corticosteroids in the brain. Cellular and molecular actions. Mol. Neurobiol. **17:** 87–108.
19. TRONCHE, F., C. KELLENDONK, *et al.* 1998. Genetic dissection of glucocorticoid receptor function in mice. Curr. Opin. Genet. Dev. **8:** 532–538.
20. YANG-YEN, H.F., J.C. CHAMBARD, *et al.* 1990. Transcriptional interference between c-Jun and the glucocorticoid receptor: mutual inhibition of DNA binding due to direct protein-protein interaction. Cell **62:** 1205–1215.
21. IMAI, E., J.N. MINER, *et al.* 1993. Glucocorticoid receptor-cAMP response element-binding protein interaction and the response of the phosphoenolpyruvate carboxykinase gene to glucocorticoids. J. Biol. Chem. **268:** 5353–5356.
22. STOCKLIN, E., M. WISSLER, *et al.* 1996. Functional interactions between Stat5 and the glucocorticoid receptor. Nature **383:** 726–728.
23. JOELS, M. & E.R. DE KLOET. 1994. Mineralocorticoid and glucocorticoid receptors in the brain. Implications for ion permeability and transmitter systems. Prog. Neurobiol. **43:** 1–36.
24. DE KLOET, E. R., M.S. OITZL, *et al.* 1999. Stress and cognition: are corticosteroids good or bad guys? Trends Neurosci. **22:** 422–426.
25. JOELS, M. 2000. Modulatory actions of steroid hormones and neuropeptides on electrical activity in brain. Eur. J. Pharmacol. **405:** 207–216.
26. PORSOLT, R. D., M. LE PICHON, *et al.* 1977. Depression: a new animal model sensitive to antidepressant treatments. Nature **266:** 730–732.
27. STERU, L., R. CHERMAT, *et al.* 1985. The tail suspension test: a new method for screening antidepressants in mice. Psychopharmacology **85:** 367–370.
28. WILLNER, P. 1997. Validity, reliability and utility of the chronic mild stress model of depression: a 10-year review and evaluation. Psychopharmacology **134:** 319–329.
29. WILLNER, P., R. MUSCAT, *et al.* 1992. Chronic mild stress-induced anhedonia: a realistic animal model of depression. Neurosci. Biobehav. Rev. **16:** 525–534.
30. BOURIN, M. 1990. Is it possible to predict the activity of a new antidepressant in animals with simple psychopharmacological tests? Fundam. Clin. Pharmacol. **4:** 49–64.
31. ALMEIDA, R.N., D.S. NAVARRO, *et al.* 1998. Antidepressant effect of an ethanolic extract of the leaves of Cissampelos sympodialis in rats and mice. J. Ethnopharmacol. **63:** 247–252.
32. SKALISZ, L.L., V. BEIJAMINI, *et al.* 2002. Evaluation of the face validity of reserpine administration as an animal model of depression--Parkinson's disease association. Prog. Neuropsychopharmacol. Biol. Psychiatry **26:** 879–883.
33. REDROBE, J.P. & M. BOURIN. 1999. The effect of lithium administration in animal models of depression: a short review. Fundam. Clin. Pharmacol. **13:** 293–299.
34. VETULANI, J., L. ANTKIEWICZ-MICHALUK, *et al.* 1986. Effects of chronically administered antidepressants and electroconvulsive treatment on cerebral neurotransmitter receptors in rodents with 'model depression'. Ciba Found. Symp. **123:** 234–245.
35. NAGAYAMA, H., J.N. HINGTGEN, *et al.* 1980. Pre- and postsynaptic serotonergic manipulations in an animal model of depression. Pharmacol. Biochem. Behav. **13:** 575–579.
36. KELLENDONK, C., F. TRONCHE, *et al.* 1999. Mutagenesis of the glucocorticoid receptor in mice. J. Steroid Biochem. Mol. Biol. **69:** 253–259.
37. ROSSANT, J. & A. MCMAHON. 1999. "Cre"-ating mouse mutants-a meeting review on conditional mouse genetics. Genes Dev. **13:** 142–145.
38. PEPIN, M.C., F. POTHIER, *et al.* 1992. Impaired type II glucocorticoid-receptor function in mice bearing antisense RNA transgene. Nature **355:** 725–728.
39. KARANTH, S., A.C. LINTHORST, *et al.* 1997. Hypothalamic-pituitary-adrenocortical axis changes in a transgenic mouse with impaired glucocorticoid receptor function. Endocrinology **138:** 3476–3485.
40. BARDEN, N., I.S. STEC, *et al.* 1997. Endocrine profile and neuroendocrine challenge tests in transgenic mice expressing antisense RNA against the glucocorticoid receptor. Neuroendocrinology **66:** 212–220.
41. DIJKSTRA, I., F.J. TILDERS, *et al.* 1998. Reduced activity of hypothalamic corticotropin-releasing hormone neurons in transgenic mice with impaired glucocorticoid receptor function. J. Neurosci. **18:** 3909–3918.

42. PEPIN, M.C., F. POTHIER, *et al.* 1992. Antidepressant drug action in a transgenic mouse model of the endocrine changes seen in depression. Mol. Pharmacol. **42:** 991–995.
43. MONTKOWSKI, A., N. BARDEN, *et al.* 1995. Long-term antidepressant treatment reduces behavioural deficits in transgenic mice with impaired glucocorticoid receptor function. J. Neuroendocrinol. **7:** 841–845.
44. BARDEN, N. 1996. Modulation of glucocorticoid receptor gene expression by antidepressant drugs. Pharmacopsychiatry **29:** 12–22.
45. LINTHORST, A.C., C. FLACHSKAMM, *et al.* 2000. Glucocorticoid receptor impairment alters CNS responses to a psychological stressor: an in vivo microdialysis study in transgenic mice. Eur. J. Neurosci. **12:** 283–291.
46. HEINRICHS, S.C., J. LAPSANSKY, *et al.* 1997. Corticotropin-releasing factor CRF1, but not CRF2, receptors mediate anxiogenic-like behavior. Regul. Pept. **71:** 15–21.
47. TIMPL, P., R. SPANAGEL, *et al.* 1998. Impaired stress response and reduced anxiety in mice lacking a functional corticotropin-releasing hormone receptor 1. Nat. Genet. **19:** 162–166.
48. SMITH, G.W., J.M. AUBRY, *et al.* 1998. Corticotropin releasing factor receptor 1-deficient mice display decreased anxiety, impaired stress response, and aberrant neuroendocrine development. Neuron **20:** 1093–1102.
49. LIEBSCH, G., R. LANDGRAF, *et al.* 1999. Differential behavioural effects of chronic infusion of CRH 1 and CRH 2 receptor antisense oligonucleotides into the rat brain. J. Psychiatry Res. **33:** 153–163.
50. STECKLER, T. & F. HOLSBOER. 1999. Enhanced conditioned approach responses in transgenic mice with impaired glucocorticoid receptor function. Behav. Brain Res. **102:** 151–163.
51. COLE, T.J., J.A. BLENDY, *et al.* 1995. Targeted disruption of the glucocorticoid receptor gene blocks adrenergic chromaffin cell development and severely retards lung maturation. Genes Dev. **9:** 1608–1621.
52. COLE, T.J., K. MYLES, *et al.* 2001. GRKO mice express an aberrant dexamethasone-binding glucocorticoid receptor, but are profoundly glucocorticoid resistant. Mol. Cell. Endocrinol. **173:** 193–202.
53. CHRISTOFFELS, V. M., T. GRANGE, *et al.* 1998. Glucocorticoid receptor, C/EBP, HNF3, and protein kinase A coordinately activate the glucocorticoid response unit of the carbamoylphosphate synthetase I gene. Mol. Cell. Biol. **18:** 6305–6315.
54. REICHARDT, H.M. & G. SCHUTZ. 1996. Feedback control of glucocorticoid production is established during fetal development. Mol. Med. **2:** 735–744.
55. TRONCHE, F., C. KELLENDONK, *et al.* 1999. Disruption of the glucocorticoid receptor gene in the nervous system results in reduced anxiety. Nat. Genet. **23:** 99–103.
56. GOLD, P.W., F.K. GOODWIN, *et al.* 1988. Clinical and biochemical manifestations of depression. Relation to the neurobiology of stress (1). N. Engl. J. Med. **319:** 348–353.
57. REICHARDT, H.M. & G. SCHUTZ. 1998. Glucocorticoid signalling: multiple variations of a common theme. Mol. Cell. Endocrinol. **146:** 1–6.
58. HECK, S., M. KULLMANN, *et al.* 1994. A distinct modulating domain in glucocorticoid receptor monomers in the repression of activity of the transcription factor AP-1. EMBO J. **13:** 4087–4095.
59. REICHARDT, H.M., K.H. KAESTNER, *et al.* 1998. DNA binding of the glucocorticoid receptor is not essential for survival. Cell **93:** 531–541.
60. TUCKERMANN, J.P., H.M. REICHARDT, *et al.* 1999. The DNA binding-independent function of the glucocorticoid receptor mediates repression of AP-1-dependent genes in skin. J. Cell. Biol. **147:** 1365–1370.
61. MALKOSKI, S.P. & R.I. DORIN. 1999. Composite glucocorticoid regulation at a functionally defined negative glucocorticoid response element of the human corticotropin-releasing hormone gene. Mol. Endocrinol. **13:** 1629–1644.
62. DROUIN, J., Y.L. SUN, *et al.* 1993. Novel glucocorticoid receptor complex with DNA element of the hormone-repressed POMC gene. EMBO J. **12:** 145–156.
63. SAKAI, D.D., S. HELMS, *et al.* 1988. Hormone-mediated repression: a negative glucocorticoid response element from the bovine prolactin gene. Genes Dev. **2:** 1144–1154.

64. OITZL, M.S., H.M. REICHARDT, *et al.* 2001. Point mutation in the mouse glucocorticoid receptor preventing DNA binding impairs spatial memory. Proc. Natl. Acad. Sci. USA **98:** 12790–12795.
65. KARST, H., Y.J. KARTEN, *et al.* 2000. Corticosteroid actions in hippocampus require DNA binding of glucocorticoid receptor homodimers. Nat. Neurosci. **3:** 977–978.
66. REICHARDT, H.M., T. UMLAND, *et al.* 2000. Mice with an increased glucocorticoid receptor gene dosage show enhanced resistance to stress and endotoxic shock. Mol. Cell. Biol. **20:** 9009–9017.
67. WEI, Q., G.L. SCHAFER, *et al.* 2001. Tissue-specific overexpression of the glucocorticoid receptor in the brain. Soc. Neurosci. Abstr. **27**.
68. BERGER, S., M. BLEICH, *et al.* 1998. Mineralocorticoid receptor knockout mice: pathophysiology of Na+ metabolism. Proc. Natl. Acad. Sci. USA **95:** 9424–9429.
69. BLEICH, M., R. WARTH, *et al.* 1999. Rescue of the mineralocorticoid receptor knockout mouse. Pflugers Arch. **438:** 245–254.
70. GASS, P., O. KRETZ, *et al.* 2000. Genetic disruption of mineralocorticoid receptor leads to impaired neurogenesis and granule cell degeneration in the hippocampus of adult mice. EMBO Rep. **1:** 447–451.
71. ANISMAN, H., M.D. ZAHARIA, *et al.* 1998. Do early-life events permanently alter behavioral and hormonal responses to stressors? Int. J. Dev. Neurosci. **16:** 149–164.
72. BARDEN, N., J.M. REUL, *et al.* 1995. Do antidepressants stabilize mood through actions on the hypothalamic-pituitary-adrenocortical system? Trends Neurosci. **18:** 6–11.
73. GERLAI, R. 1996. Gene-targeting studies of mammalian behavior: is it the mutation or the background genotype? Trends Neurosci. **19:** 177–181.
74. GERLAI, R. 2000. Targeting genes and proteins in the analysis of learning and memory: caveats and future directions. Rev. Neurosci. **11:** 15–26.

High-Quality Antidepressant Discovery by Understanding Stress Hormone Physiology

FLORIAN HOLSBOER

Max Planck Institute of Psychiatry, D-80804 Munich, Germany

ABSTRACT: Compensating the consequences of impaired corticosteroid receptor signaling is a novel strategy to discover better antidepressants. The prevailing drugs gradually improve stress hormone regulation along with ameliorating psychopathology. The current understanding of how neuropeptides, such as corticotropin-releasing hormone (CRH) and vasopressin (AVP), drive cortisol secretion via corticotrophin has paved the way for CRH- and AVP-receptor antagonists. As alternative strategies, the blockade of corticosteroid receptors or inhibition of cortisol synthesis has emerged. All these strategies are not yet fully clinically developed, but preliminary data from basic and clinical research strongly underscore that such strategies may lead to innovative treatment modalities.

KEYWORDS: antidepressants; corticotropin-releasing hormone; vasopressin

INTRODUCTION

Several facts emerged that call for a paradigmatic shift in antidepressant drug discovery. (1) Depression will soon become the second leading cause for illness-related disability, trailing only cardiovascular disease. The impact of depression on general morbidity is further amplified, because mood disorders are one of the major risk factors for cardiovascular disease. (2) The list of top 10 medicines worldwide based on revenues in the year 2000 contained three antidepressants (Zoloft®, Prozac®, Paxil®). (3) Currently available antidepressants are based on a serendipitous observation in the 1950s, that is, that norepinephrine- and/or serotonin-reuptake inhibitory drugs are efficacious. Since then, all new antidepressants were developed analogous to this pharmacological principle. A common disadvantage of all these drugs is (1) that it takes too long until they work; (2) that they have too many adverse effects; and (3) that only 70–80% of the patients treated are cured. Also, although the scientific fundament on which currently available antidepressants are built is poor, there is growing evidence that the long-known stress hormone dysregulation seen among psychiatric patients is a causative mechanism leading to stress-related psychopathology.

Address for correspondence: Professor Florian Holsboer, M.D., Ph.D., Max Planck Institute of Psychiatry, Kraepelinstrasse 10, D-80804 Munich, Germany. Voice: 49-89-30-622-220; fax: 49-89-30-622-483.

holsboer@mpipsykl.mpg.de

**Ann. N.Y. Acad. Sci. 1007: 394–404 (2003). © 2003 New York Academy of Sciences.
doi: 10.1196/annals.1286.038**

The pharmaceutical industry has translated the impact of depression on illness-related disability and top revenues in medications into development and aggressive marketing of "more-of-the-same" products. At the same time, pharmaceutical industry and biotech companies embark on the opportunities of systematic, unbiased approaches. These include the search for targets using microarray technology that allows assessment of gene activity under experimentally defined conditions and subsequent identification of drugable targets. Once identified, high throughput screening, which makes possible the testing of every chemical available to see if something interesting happens to the targets, is initiated. The observed effects are further studied functionally in animal models before decisions are made whether or not a clinical development program is to be initiated. Although in principle this approach is very attractive and promises departure from the "usual suspects" approach, an entirely unfocused approach has provided huge, hard to digest, diverse databases. In this article, I delineate how the attrition rate that is currently plaguing high-quality drug discovery may be reduced by preferring precedented targets focusing on existing knowledge of stress hormone physiology.

CORTICOSTEROID RECEPTOR HYPOTHESIS OF DEPRESSION

The observed changes of hypothalamic-pituitary-adrenocortical (HPA) regulation are not specific for the diagnosis of depression or any other past, current, or (most likely) future diagnostic attribution according to manuals released by the World Health Organization or other authorities. Likewise, antidepressants are not specific treatments for any kind of current diagnosis. In contrast, their indication cuts across all syndromes characterized by depressed mood or various forms of anxiety. In all these clinical conditions, perturbed HPA activity either at baseline or in the context of function tests can be found with high frequency.

These changes were long considered as reflections of the stressful experience of affective illness. Several discoveries have challenged this interpretation and also have changed the previous view. The first study monitoring patients during the course of diverse antidepressant treatments revealed that initially abnormal dexamethasone suppression test results (i.e., inappropriately mute suppression of plasma cortisol concentrations by a low dose of the synthetic glucocorticoid dexamethasone [DEX] which acts mainly at the pituitary to suppress ACTH [the main peripheral stimulant for cortisol]) almost always normalizes before clinical remission of depression.[1] Furthermore, once a remitted patient shows high post–dexamethasone plasma cortisol levels, the patient has a much higher risk for relapse. This time grid suggests that HPA normalization is pertinent for recovery while a patient who continues to have or starts again developing HPA abnormality has some ongoing pathology in central neural circuits that leads to psychopathology through a mechanism that opposes antidepressant action.[2] At the same time, Vale's group isolated and characterized the hypothalamic factor that was suggested to be the key neuropeptide centrally governing the hormonal response to stress.[3] This factor, corticotropin-releasing hormone (CRH) was extensively used in animal studies, and it was suggested that CRH not only accounts for stress hormone release but also coordinates a large variety of behavioral adaptations (see Fig. 1).

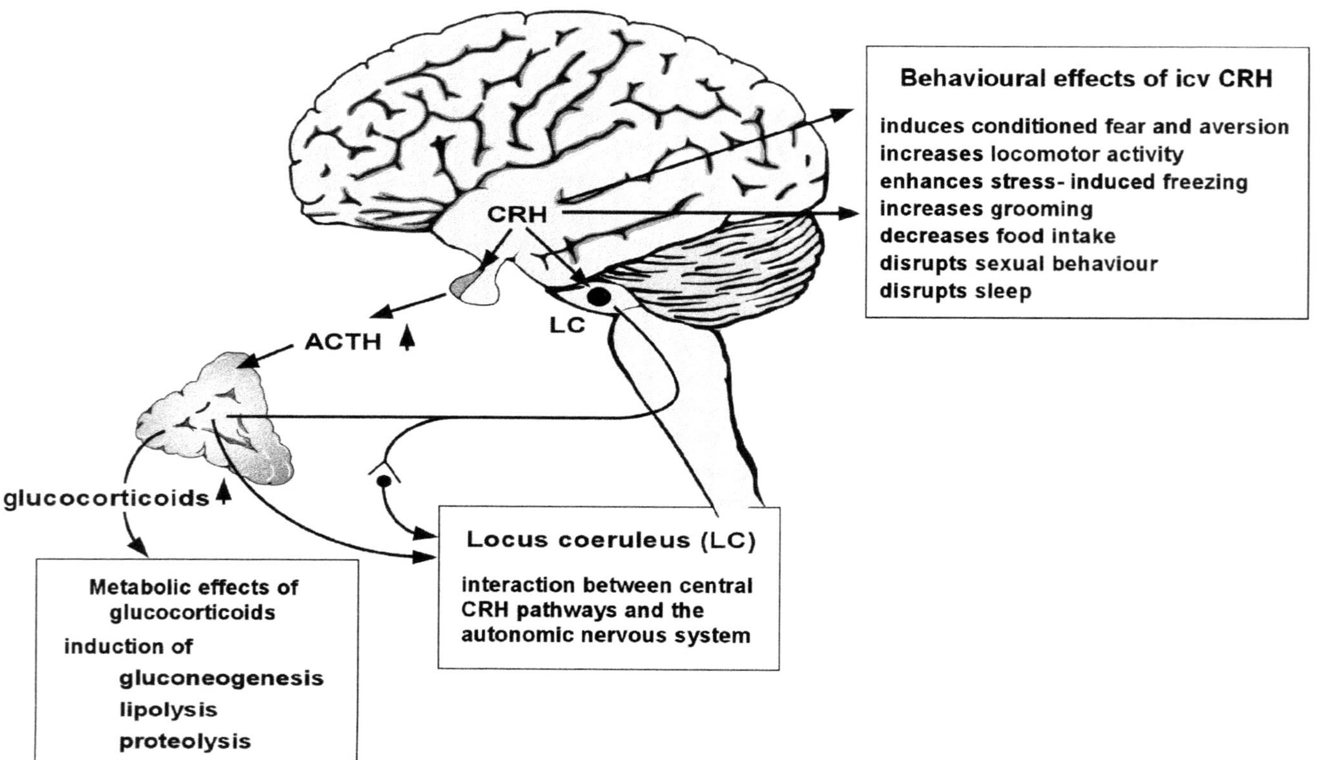

FIGURE 1. Increased levels of corticotropin-releasing hormone induce depresion-like symptoms in animals.

Also the first reports of CRH-induced hormone responses in depressives suggested a causal role for CRH in stress-related psychopathology. This conclusion was substantiated by human studies showing elevated CRH levels in cerebrospinal fluid (CSF) and reduced CRH binding in prefrontal cortex, the latter indicating CRH receptor desensitization by CRH excess. Finally, an increased number of CRH-producing neurons was found in the hypothalami of depressives. From there, nerve fibers project to many circuits in the brain that are implicated in pathophysiology of depression.[4] Of course, CRH does not act alone, and more recently vasopressin (AVP) has been characterized as another neuropeptide being a strong candidate in the development of stress-related disorders. Both neuropeptides, CRH and AVP, have in common that they are regulated by corticosteroid receptors. These receptors are located in the cytosol of nerve cells and kept by other proteins (mostly so-called chaperones) in a three-dimensional configuration, which allows high-affinity binding of cortisol (and other corticosteroids). There are two different corticosteroid receptors in the brain, glucocorticoid receptors (GRs, mainly binding cortisol in humans or corticosterone in rodents) and mineralocorticosteroid receptors (MRs, located mainly in the hippocampus and binding corticosteroids with 10-fold higher affinity, i.e., they are almost always occupied). Once activated by steroid hormones, these receptors dimerize forming homodimers (GR-GR, MR-MR) or heterodimers (GR-MR). These act as transcription factors and bind at specific DNA structures (glucocorticoid response elements [GREs]) which induces activation or repression of gene transcription. Alternatively, activated receptors can interact with other transcription factors and thus can indirectly modulate gene activity.[5]

The corticosteroid receptor hypothesis submits that corticosteroid receptor signaling is impaired in depression.[2] Specifically, if increased CRH and AVP are accounting for a high number of signs and symptoms prevalent in depression, it can be hypothesized that the corticosteroid receptor signaling which represses CRH and AVP gene expression is defunct. A function test was developed, to validate this hypothesis clinically, that probes corticosteroid receptor signaling with high sensitivity. This test combines the suppression of HPA activity by DEX with a CRH-induced ACTH activation and proved to pick up minor HPA changes with high sensitivity. A study by Modell *et al.*[6] used increasing doses of DEX among depressives and controls and showed that the (DEX) dose (ACTH, cortisol)–response curve in the DEX/CRH test was shifted among depressives toward lower dexamethasone sensitivity. Such a change is unlikely reflecting an inherited GR or MR gene defect but rather points to quantitative effects of coregulators, for example, the aforementioned chaperones. This view is supported by the occurrence of major HPA defects only in temporal proximity of affective episodes, but occurrence of GR or MR polymorphisms can not yet be fully excluded. Along this line, note that a sequence in the promoter of CRH was found that confers signals that are conveyed through antidepressants.[7] At this DNA sequence, called CRE (cyclic AMP response element), a transcription factor binds that is called CREB (CRE-binding protein) which activates CRH transcription. To do this, CREB needs to be phosphorylated by a kinase (PKA) which is a key element of a signaling pathway activated by antidepressants. The latter enhance biogenic amine concentrations at specific cell membrane receptors by inhibiting presynaptic reuptake transporters. After endured activation of these aminergic cell membrane receptors, a desensitization develops ultimately leading to decreased CREB phosphorylation and subsequently to decreased CRH gene expression.[8] This process needs time and may, at least in part, explain the long time to onset of clinical antidepressive effects. Note also that corticosteroids interact with G-protein–coupled receptor–cAMP-PKA pathways. For example, corticosteroids can abolish CREB phosphorylation in CRH neurons.[9] Against this background, it seems justified to investigate the HPA system thoroughly in humans and in appropriate animal models to discover novel targets.

CORTICOTROPIN-RELEASING HORMONE

The aforementioned biological actions of CRH are mediated via two types of G-protein–coupled receptors, CRHR1 and CRHR2, which contain seven transmembrane domains and share considerable sequence homology with one another. CRHR1 and CRHR2 have different expression patterns, and accordingly these receptors play distinct, though overlapping roles both in HPA-axis regulation and in stress-related behavioral effects.[10]

Several lines of evidence point to a key role of CRHR1 in mediating the CRH-elicited effects in depression and anxiety. Infusions of CRH into the rat brain produces anxiety-related behavior in a way similar to what transgenic overexpressing CRH in mouse mutants does.[11] Central administration of CRHR1 antisense probes restrains CRH-evoked and social defeat–evoked anxiety-like behaviors. In contrast, CRHR2 antisense does not produce an anxiolytic effect but does increase immobility in a forced swim test.[12] Because CRHR2 is activated not only by CRH but also by another neuropeptide, called urocortin (Ucn), it seems that a Ucn/CRHR2 system that plays a role in stress-coping behaviors also exists in the brain. Indeed, recently two selective ligands for CRHR2 were discovered (Ucn II, or stresscopin-related peptide, and Ucn III, or stresscopin). The role of CRHR2 is less clear than that of CRHR1, but it appears that CRHR2 has a dual mode of action: in the acute (early) phase CRHR2 is activated mostly through CRH and stresscopin, increasing emotionality (anxiety), whereas in the recovery phase it is also activated, presumably in the amygdala, basal nucleus of the stria terminalis and lateral septum, but now this contributes to reducing emotionality.[13]

One approach to study the effects of a receptor on complex systems such as behavior is to use mouse mutants in which the respective receptor has been deleted by genetic engineering. Mice, in which the CRHR1 gene had been inactivated, showed decreased anxiety-like behavior. The behavioral effect of this gene defect is not limited to anxiety but is also seen in other stress-related conditions such as withdrawal and abuse of alcohol.[14,15] Three lines of CRHR2-deficient mice were studied, but this did not provide a clear answer to the question of whether blockade of CRHR2 would ameliorate anxiety in stressful situations. In two lines of CRHR2 knockout mice increased anxiety-like behavior was found,[16,17] but in the third line no changes were found.[18] In addition, some sex differences in the phenotype were observed. Mouse mutants where both, CRHR1 and CRHR2, were knocked out showed a phenotype that was dominated by the absence of CRHR1.[19] The fact that these mice were viable, as were mutants with a CRH knockout, demonstrates that mammals do not need a functional CRH/CRHR-signaling system to live, making this a preferred system for drug targeting. Because the CRHR1 knockout mice also lacked CRHR1 at the pituitary and elsewhere in the organism, the possibility had to be rejected that their behavioral phenotype was secondary to the endocrine changes elicited by a CRH-refractory corticotrophic system leading to a diminished hormonal stress response. Therefore, a conditional mouse mutant was generated in which the gene deletion was restricted to the hippocampus and the prefrontal cortex, sparing the HPA axis. These mice also showed decreased anxiety-like behavior, whereas their endocrine system remained largely intact.[20]

These clinical and basic studies led several drug companies to develop specific and selective nonpeptide receptor antagonists with good oral bioavailability and rapid penetration across the blood–brain barrier. The recent advances in biotechnology in combination with optimized behavioral pharmacology techniques have led to the identification of several structural series of compounds that antagonize the effects of CRH at CRHR1.

The only drug that has so far been clinically tested is NBI-30775 (also referred to as R121919). This compound was first tested in a rat line with high innate anxiety and proved to reduce anxiety-like behavior. Interestingly, among those rats selectively bred to produce a low-anxiety phenotype, NBI-30775 did not show any behavioral response which is in accord with the view that neuropeptide receptors are only targets in the presence of pathophysiological mechanisms. Indeed, neuropeptides are usually only hypersecreted under certain physiological demands, such as adaptation to a stressor. A more recent study accords with the view that CRHR1 antagonists suppress stress-elicited behavioral changes in rats. A first clinical study designed as a safety and tolerability study but also rigidly monitoring psychopathological changes supported that CRHR1 antagonists are worthy to be further explored as novel antidepressants.[21] Also, studies investigating the effects of NBI-30775 in animal models and humans with depression underscored the potential of such drugs in the treatment of stress-related sleep disorders.[22,23] Whereas Johnson & Johnson (the licensee of R121919) decided to discontinue the clinical development of this drug, almost all big pharmaceutical companies are searching for new candidates directed against CRHR1 signaling.

VASOPRESSIN

Based on neuroendocrine studies in human and animal models, it was postulated that increased AVP secretion accounts for several signs and symptoms seen in depression.[24] This suggestion was confirmed by Purba *et al.*,[25] who found vasopressin to be increased in paraventricular nucleus neurons of depressives, by Dinan *et al.* ,[26] who showed that in depression vasopressinergic responsitivity is enhanced, and by van Londen *et al.*,[27] who found elevated plasma AVP concentrations in the same patients. In contrast with CRH, where elevations in CSF were repeatedly shown, AVP was not found to be elevated in depression.[28] However, it must be recognized that CSF neuropeptide contents do not necessarily reflect hypothalamic secretory activity. In rats, it was observed that cognitive stressors elicit AVP in the supraoptic nucleus.[29] Elevated AVP was also found in the hypothalamus of rats with innate high anxiety and postulated to mediate the increased ACTH and cortisol response in the DEX/CRH test. When treated with an antidepressant, the AVP content in the hypothalamus decreases in these rats along with normalization of initially abnormal DEX/CRH test results.[30] There are two AVP receptors in the brain V1a and V1b (also termed V3) which have locations that clearly favor the view that they also contribute to the behavioral phenotype implicated in stress-related disorders.[31] For example, V1a is expressed in the cortex, suprachiasmatic nucleus, central and medial amygdala, and hypothalamus; V1b is neuroanatomically less well studied but also occurs in cortex and amygdala as well as in supraoptic nucleus. The main physiological role of AVP receptors outside the brain is enhancement of corticosterone secretion, and neuroendocrine studies using a V1b-transgenic mouse overexpressing V1b receptors in corticotrophs confirmed this.[32]

In the light of the above findings, it was postulated that AVP hypersecretion exists in depression and that blocking this mechanism may reduce affective symptoms. A study by Landgraf *et al.*[29] used antisense probes directed against AVPmRNA in the septum and found reductions of anxiety-like behavior in rats. In the same vein are studies by Liebsch *et al.*[33]who injected a mixed V1a/V1b receptor antagonist in the rat septum and also found anxiolytic-like effects. These observations prompted the search for nonpeptide receptor antagonists[34] and recently Griebel *et al.*[35] were able to show that a synthetic V1b receptor antagonist also produces anxiolytic- and antidepressant-like effects and suggested that such drugs are worthy to be considered as novel candidates for antidepressant drug development.

GLUCOCORTICOID AND MINERALOCORTICOID RECEPTORS

Corticosteroid receptors constitute the relay between peripheral stress hormone secretion and modulation of behavioral processes in the brain. The hypersecretion of cortisol in depression as well as abnormal HPA function test results may well be secondary to impaired signaling due to inherited or acquired changes in the GR/MR pathways. In case of inherited HPA disturbance, either a polymorphism at the GR or at one or several genes coding for proteins that modulate pharmacological properties of GR (e.g., affinity) may be present.

Several polymorphisms in the glucocorticoid receptor gene had been discovered by Steven Lamberts's group in Rotterdam.[36] One of these polymorphisms consists of two linked point mutations separated by one base pair in codons 22 and 23 in exon 2 of the GR gene. The first mutation is silent, changing codon 22 from GAG to GAA, both coding for glutamic acid (E). The other mutation changes codon 23 from AGG to AAG resulting in an arginine (R) to lysine (K) amino acid exchange. Carriers of this ER22/23 EK allele were found to be less sensitive to the suppressive effect of low dose dexamethasone.[37] Because of the lower effect of cortisol on glucose metabolism, both glucose and insulin were lowered, resulting in a favorable metabolic health profile. Because patients with depression or individuals belonging to families with high genetic load for depression also have glucocorticoid receptor resistance, it would be worthwhile to study whether similar polymorphisms also exist in these patients. Although the most likely location for such a polymorphism would be a mutation in the ligand binding domain of GR,[38] it is yet not fully elucidated through which mechanism ER22/23EK confers glucocorticoid resistance. Alternatively, mutations in the promoter of genes coding for chaperones, for example, BAG-1 or FKBP51, resulting in overexpression of these proteins could lead to hypercortisolism.[39] It needs to be tested at the functional level whether gain or loss of functional activity of these chaperone molecules can be induced by drugs.

A more straightforward approach would be the partial blockade of corticosteroid receptors by low-dose antagonists. This strategy of decreasing cortisol bioavailability originally was advocated by B. E. P. Murphy, but only recently a substantial data base was published by Belanoff *et al.*[40] showing that mifepristone, a GR (and progesterone receptor) antagonist, rapidly ameliorates psychotic depression. The latter clinical condition is almost always associated with elevated cortisol secretion and according to a hypothesis by Piazza *et al.*,[41] this hypercortisolism may lead to increased dopaminergic activity. Notably, drugs that block central dopaminergic receptors are first-line treatments in psychotic states including psychotic depression.

A potential role of MR as a drug target is much less clear. Under conditions of stress, MR capacity increases by a mechanism implicating CRH action.[42] Also, antidepressants increase MR capacity in the rat hippocampus, pointing to a role of MR function in mediating the drug effect.[43] This is further underscored by a clinical study in which the antidepressant effect of amitriptyline was found to be decreased in case of coadministration of spironolactone, an MR antagonist.[44] Still another approach is the decrease of circulating cortisol by agents that block cortisol synthesis. One prominent agent is metyrapone which until recently had been studied only in very small open-label trials with mixed results. However, a study by Klaus Wiedemann's group showed that the effect of antidepressants can be significantly improved by coadministration of metyrapone.[45]

Although all these studies have potential merit for the clinician, it remains unclear by which mode of action antiglucocorticoid strategies may work. In case of GR or MR blockade, a myriad of different molecular events are set in motion, because of the pluripotent actions these ligand-activated nuclear receptors may induce. Similarly unclear are the effects of metyrapone, which results in a substantial increase of so-called neurosteroids. The latter are mainly binding at membrane-located $GABA_A$ receptors modulating their ion conductance which, in turn, translates into behavioral changes, for example, anxiolysis or sleep induction. Interestingly, antidepressants also can change neurosteroid concentrations in the CSF and plasma pointing to a function of these steroid derivatives.[46] There are some activities in pharmaceutical research to explore whether synthetic neurosteroids directed against certain specific $GABA_A$ receptor–mediated functions are possible drug candidates.

CONCLUSION

The currently available antidepressant drugs and anxiolytics have many disadvantages. Therefore, it is very likely that the rich knowledge based on stress hormone pharmacology that has been accumulated over the past decades will soon be exploited to find better drugs. Still, there is yet no CRHR1 antagonist that has proved to be efficacious in large double-blind controlled studies. Similarly, GR antagonists are yet not sufficiently well studied to allow firm predictions. The only exception is psychotic depression in which the data base available seems very promising. Even more in its infancy is the development of V1b antagonists in which only preliminary animal behavioral data exist.

I would not be surprised if the validation of all these "potential targets" that emerge from stress physiology would be validated only if human data from disease genetics are implemented. Maybe HPA-related drugs only work better than the currently available drugs in such cases in which a central HPA dysregulation exists (irrespective of whether this neuropathology is reflected by peripheral hypercortisolism or not). In any case, the more specific novel drugs get, the better they work among those where the specific neuropathology exists. On the other side, for those patients for whom mechanisms other than specific HPA-related neuropathology are causing the clinical condition, such drugs may not work at all. Therefore, the most important task for human stress hormone research will be precise phenotyping and genotyping of patients, allowing the clinician to choose the right drug at the right moment.

REFERENCES

1. Holsboer, F., R. Liebl & E. Hofschuster. 1982. Repeated dexamethasone suppression test during depressive illness. Normalization of test result compared with clinical improvement. J. Affect. Disord. **4:** 93–101.
2. Holsboer, F. 2000. The corticosteroid receptor hypothesis of depression. Neuropsychopharmacolgy **23:** 477–501.
3. Vale, W., J. Spiess, C. Rivier, *et al.* 1981. Characterization of a 41-residue ovine hypothalamic peptide that stimulates secretion of corticotropin and β-endorphin. Science **213:** 1394–1397.
4. Arborelius, L., M.J. Owens, P.M. Plotsky, *et al.* 1999. The role of corticotropin-releasing factor in depression and anxiety disorders. J. Endocrinol. **160:** 1–12.
5. Trapp, T. & F. Holsboer. 1996. Heterodimerization between mineralocorticoid and glucocorticoid receptor increases the functional diversity of corticosteroid action. Trends Pharmacol. Sci. **17:** 145–149.
6. Modell, S., A. Yassouridis, J. Huber, *et al.* 1997. Corticosteroid receptor function is decreased in depressed patients. Neuroendocrinology **65:** 216–222.
7. Spengler, D., R. Rupprecht, L. Phi Van, *et al.* 1992. Identification and characterization of a 3′,5′-cyclic adenosine monophosphate-response element in the human corticotropin-releasing hormone gene promoter. Mol. Endocrinol. **6:** 1931–1941.
8. Rossby, S.P., D.H. Manier, S. Liang, *et al.* 1999. Pharmacological actions of the antidepressant venlafaxine beyond aminergic receptors. Int. J. Neuropsychopharmacol. **2:** 1–8.
9. Legradi, G., D. Holzer, L.P. Kapcala, *et al.* 1997. Glucocorticoids inhibit stress-induced phosphorylation of CREB in corticotropin-releasing hormone neurons of the hypothalamic paraventricular nucleus. Neuroendocrinology **66:** 86–97.
10. Reul, J.M.H.M. & F. Holsboer. 2002. Corticotropin-releasing factor receptors 1 and 2 in anxiety. Curr. Opin. Pharmacol. **2:** 23–33.
11. Van Gaalen, M.M., M. Stenzel-Poore, F. Holsboer, *et al.* 2002. Effects of transgenic overproduction of CRH on anxiety-like behaviour. Eur. J. Neurosci. **15:** 2007–2015.
12. Liebsch, G., R. Landgraf, M. Engelmann, *et al.* 1999. Differential behavioural effects of chronic infusion of CRH_1 and CRH_2 receptor antisense oligodeoxynucleotides into the rat brain. J. Psychiatr. Res. **33:** 153–163.
13. Hsu, S.Y. & A.J.W. Hsueh. 2001. Human stresscopin-related peptide are selective ligands for the type 2 corticotropin-releasing hormone receptor. Nat. Med. **7:** 605–611.
14. Sillaber, I., G. Rammes, S. Zimmermann, *et al.* 2002. Enhanced and delayed stress-induced alcohol drinking in mice lacking functional CRH1 receptors. Science **296:** 931–933.
15. Timpl, P., R. Spanagel, I. Sillaber, *et al.* 1998. Impaired stress response and reduced anxiety in mice lacking a functional corticotropin-releasing hormone receptor 1. Nat. Genet. **19:** 162–166.
16. Bale, T.L., A. Contarino, G.W. Smith, *et al.* 2000. Mice deficient for corticotropin-releasing hormone receptor-2 display anxiety-like behaviour and are hypersensitive to stress. Nat. Genet. **24:** 410–414.

17. KISHIMOTO, T., J. RADULOVIC, M. RADULOVIC, *et al.* 2000. Deletion of Crh2 reveals an anxiolytic role for corticotropin-releasing hormone receptor-2. Nat. Genet. **24:** 415–419.
18. COSTE, S.C., R.A. KESTERSON, K.A. HELDWEIN, *et al.* 2000. Abnormal adaptations to stress and impaired cardiovascular function in mice lacking cortiotropin-releasing hormone receptor-2. Nat. Genet. **24:** 403–409.
19. PREIL, J., M.B. MÜLLER, A. GESING, *et al.* 2001. Regulation of the hypothalamic-pituitary-adrenocortical system in mice deficient for CRH receptors 1 and 2. Endocrinology **142:** 1–10.
20. MÜLLER, M.B., S. ZIMMERMANN, I. SILLABER, *et al.* 2003. Conditional inactivation of limbic corticotropin-releasing hormone receptor 1 reduces anxiety-related behavior. Nat. Neurosci. In press.
21. ZOBEL, A.W., T. NICKEL, H.E. KÜNZEL, *et al.* 2000. Effects of the high-affinity corticotropin-releasing hormone receptor 1 antagonist R121919 in major depression: the first 20 patients treated. J. Psychiatr. Res. **34:** 171–181.
22. LANCEL, M., P. MÜLLER-PREUSS, A. WIGGER, *et al.* 2002. The CRH-R1 antagonist R121919 attenuates stress-elicited sleep disturbances in rats, particularly in those with high innate anxiety. J. Psychiatr. Res. **36:** 197–208.
23. HELD, K., H. KÜNZEL, M. ISING, *et al.* 2002. Treatment with the CRH1-receptor-antagonist R121919 improves sleep-EEG in patients with depression. J. Psychiatr. Res. In press.
24. VON BARDELEBEN, U. & F. HOLSBOER. 1989. Cortisol response to a combined dexamethasone-hCRH challenge in patients with depression. J. Neuroendocrinol. **1:** 485–488.
25. PURBA, J.S., W.J.G. HOOGENDIJK, M.A. HOFMANN, *et al.* 1996. Increased number of vasopressin- and oxytocin-expressing neurons in the paraventricular nucleus of the hypothalamus in depression. Arch. Gen. Psychiatry **53:** 137–143.
26. DINAN, T.G., E. LAVELLE, L.V. SCOTT, *et al.* 1999. Desmopressin normalizes the blunted adrenocorticotropin response to corticotropin-releasing hormone in melancholic depression: evidence of enhanced vasopressinergic responsivity. J. Clin. Endocrinol. Metab. **84:** 2238–2240.
27. VAN LONDEN, L., J.G. GOEKOOP, G.M. VAN KEMPEN, *et al.* 1997. Plasma levels of arginine vasopressin elevated in patients with major depression. Neuropsychopharmacology **17:** 284–292.
28. HEUSER, I., G. BISSETTE, M. DETTLING, *et al.* 1998. Cerebrospinal fluid concentrations of corticotropin-releasing hormone, vasopressin, and somatostatin in depressed patients and healthy controls: response to amitriptyline treatment. Depress. Anxiety **8:** 71–79.
29. LANDGRAF, R., R. GERSTBERGER, A. MONTKOWSKI, *et al.* 1995. V1 vasopressin receptor antisense oligodeoxynucleotide into septum reduces vasopressin binding, social discrimination abilities, and anxiety-related behavior in rats. J. Neurosci. **15:** 4250–4258.
30. KECK, M.E., T. WELT, A. WIGGER, *et al.* 2001. The anxiolytic effect of the CRH_1 receptor antagonist R121919 depends on innate emotionality in rats. Eur. J. Neurosci. **13:** 373–380.
31. DE WIED, D., M. DIAMANT & M. FODOR. 1993. Central nervous system effects of the neurohypophyseal hormones and related peptides. Front. Neuroendocrinol. **14:** 251–302.
32. RENÉ, P., M. GRINO, C. VIOLLET, *et al.* 2002. Overexpression of the V3 vasopressin receptor in transgenic mice. Corticotropes leads to increased basal corticosterone. J. Neuroendocrinol. **14:** 737–744.
33. LIEBSCH, G., C.T. WOTJAK, R. LANDGRAF, *et al.* 1996. Septal vasopressin modulates anxiety-related behaviour in rats. Neurosci. Lett. **217:** 101–104.
34. MAYINGER, B. & J. HENSEN. 1999. Nonpeptide vasopressin antagonist: a new group of hormone blockers entering the scene. Exp. Clin. Endocrinol. Diabetes **107:** 157–165.
35. GRIEBEL, G., J. SIMIAND, C. SERRADEIL-LE GAL, *et al.* 2002. Anxiolytic- and antidepressant-like effects of the non-peptide vasopressin V_{1b} receptor antagonist, SSR149415, suggest an innovative approach for the treatment of stress-related disorders. Proc. Natl. Acad. Sci. USA **99:** 6370–6375.

36. KOPER, J.W., R.P. STOLK, P. DE LANGE, *et al.* 1997. Lack of association between five polymorphisms in the human glucocorticoid receptor gene and glucocorticoid resistance. Hum. Genet. **99:** 663–668.
37. VAN ROSSUM, E.F.C., J.W. KOPER, N.A.T.M. HUIZENGA, *et al.* 2002. A polymorphism in the glucocorticoid receptor gene, which decreases sensitivity to glucocorticoids in vivo, is associated with low insulin and cholesterol levels. Diabetes **51:** 3128–3134.
38. KINO, T. & G.P. CHROUSOS. 2001. Glucocorticoid and mineralocorticoid resistance/hypersensitivity syndromes. J. Endocrinol. **169:** 437–445.
39. SCHMIDT, U., G.M. WOCHNIK, M.C. ROSENHAGEN, *et al.* 2003. Essential role of the unusual DNA-binding motif of BAG-1 for inhibition of the glucocorticoid receptor. J. Biol. Chem. **278:** 4926–4931.
40. BELANOFF, J.K., A.J. ROTHSCHILD, F. CASSIDY, *et al.* 2002. An open label trial of C-1073 (mifepristone) for psychotic major depression. Biol. Psychiatry **52:** 386–392.
41. PIAZZA, P.V., F. ROUGÉ-PONT, V. DEROCHE, *et al.* 1996. Glucocorticoids have state-dependent stimulant effects on the mesencephalic dopaminergic transmission. Proc. Natl. Acad. Sci. USA **93:** 8716–8720.
42. GESING, A., A. BILANG-BLEUEL, S. DROSTE, *et al.* 2001. Psychological stress increases hippocampal mineralocorticoid receptor levels: involvement of corticotropin-releasing hormone. J. Neurosci. 4822–4829.
43. HOLSBOER, F. & N. BARDEN. 1996. Antidepressants and hypothalamic-pituitary-adrenocortical regulation. Endocr. Rev. **17:** 187–205.
44. HOLSBOER, F. 1999. The rationale for corticotropin-releasing hormone receptor (CRH-R) antagonists to treat depression and anxiety. J. Psychiatr. Res. **33:** 181–214.
45. JAHN, H., M. SCHICK, F. KIEFER, *et al.* 2002. Preliminary results of a prospective, double-blind, placebo controlled study of metyrapone as an adjunct in the treatment of major depression. Eur. Neuropsychopharmacol. **12** (Suppl.): 197.
46. RUPPRECHT, R. & F. HOLSBOER. 1999. Neuroactive steroids: mechanisms of action and neuropsychopharmacological perspectives. Trends Neurosci. **22:** 410–416.

Index of Contributors